Cardiopulmonary Resuscitation (CPR) 2005 Guidelines

Adult (>8yrs)	Child (1 to onset of puberty) & Infant (<1 yr)
Rescuer who is alone – alter sequence of rescue based on most likely cause • Sudden witnessed collapse – activate EMS, get and use AED as soon as possible, begin CPR • Hypoxic arrest (e.g., drowning) – provide 5 cycles (about 2 minutes) of CPR before alerting EMS and retrieving AED	Rescuer who is alone – alter sequence of rescue based on most likely cause • Sudden witnessed collapse – activate EMS, get and use AED as soon as possible, begin CPR • Hypoxic arrest (e.g., drowning) and unresponsive infants and children – provide 5 cycles (about 2 minutes) of CPR before alerting EMS
If spinal injury suspected, open airway with jaw thrust. Use head-tilt/chin-lift method to open airway if jaw thrust is not effective.	
Deliver 2 rescue breaths over 1 second each with just enough volume to produce chest rise.	
• Check for pulse • If no pulse within 10 seconds, begin CPR (30 compressions to 2 ventilations) at a rate of 100 compressions and 8-10 breaths per minute • Compressions should be 1½"-2" deep • Allow full recoil of chest after each compression (compression and recoil times should be equal) • Once advanced airway in place, do not stop compressions for ventilations	• Check for pulse • If no pulse within 10 seconds, begin CPR: *Child*: use heel of 1 or 2 hands at the nipple line *Infant*: use 2 fingers on breastbone just below the nipple line for 1-rescuer and 2 thumb-encircling hands technique for 2-rescuer • Immediately after giving rescue breaths (30 compressions and 2 breaths per cycle for 1-rescuer; 15 compressions and 1 breath for 2-rescuer) at a rate of 100 compressions and 12-20 breaths per minute • Compressions should be ½-⅓ the depth of the chest • Allow full recoil of chest after each compression (compression and recoil times should be equal) • Continue CPR for 2 minutes (5 cycles) • Once advanced airway in place, do not stop compressions for ventilations
Healthcare provider doing compressions should be relieved every 2 minutes to prevent fatigue	

ELSEVIER

evolve

:• *To access your Online Resources, visit:*

http://evolve.elsevier.com/Dictionary/

Evolve® provides online access to free resources designed specifically for you. Inside the site, you will find additional references not available in your printed dictionary, including…

- **Tabular Atlas of Human Anatomy**
  Describes position, connection, and function for hundreds of anatomical features.

- **Assessment Guides**
  Outlines the steps of complete and focused assessment of patients across the lifespan.

- **Health Promotion**
  Provides adult preventive care timelines for immunizations, general checkups, cancer screening, and more.

- **Infection Control**
  Offers information on immunization schedules, agents, and work restrictions for health care workers.

- **Common Drug Interactions**
  Describes common drug interactions by drug category, including the most significant effects.

- **Weblinks**
  Connects you with hundreds of thorough, reliable health care resources on the Internet.

MOSBY'S
DICTIONARY
OF MEDICINE, NURSING
& HEALTH PROFESSIONS

CONSULTANTS

Charlotte Andreasen, BS, PhD candidate
Research Assistant
University of Maryland, Baltimore
Department of Microbiology and
Immunology
Baltimore, Maryland

Aris J. Andrews, RN, MS
Assistant Professor
Creighton University
School of Nursing-Hastings Campus
Hastings, Nebraska

Carolyn Andrews, RN, MSN, ARNP-BC
Assistant Professor of Nursing,
Certified Registered Nurse
Practitioner
Troy University
School of Nursing
Troy, Alabama

Lori Ascher, BS, AAS, OTR, PTA

Patricia McCallig Bates, RN, BSN, CURN
Clinical Urology Staff Nurse
Kaiser Permanente
Portland, Oregon

Christina L. Baumer, RN, PhD, CNOR, CHES
Chair, Continuing Education Program
Director, Surgical Technology
Lancaster General College of Nursing
and Health Sciences
Lancaster, Pennsylvania

Colleen Becker, RN, MSN, CCRN
Patient Care Director
Barnes-Jewish Hospital
St. Louis, Missouri

Jane J. Benedict, RN, BSN, MSN
Associate Professor of Nursing
Pennsylvania College of Technology
Williamsport, Pennsylvania

Barbara Billek-Sawhney, PT, EdD
Associate Professor
Slippery Rock University
School of Physical Therapy
Slippery Rock, Pennsylvania

Jackie Birmingham, RN, BSN, MS, CMAC
Vice President, Professional Services
Curaspan, Inc./eDischarge
Newton, Massachusetts

Margie E. Brown, RNC, MS, ANP
Professor of Nursing
Long Beach City College
Department of Health and Science
Long Beach, California

Jeanie Burt, MSN, MA, RN
Assistant Professor
Harding University
College of Nursing
Searcy, Arkansas

Kathlyn Carlson, RN, MA, CPAN
Staff Nurse
Abbott-Northwestern Hospital
Post-Anesthesia Care Unit
Minneapolis, Minnesota

Paul W. Cascella, PhD
Associate Professor
Southern Connecticut State University
Department of Communication
Disorders
New Haven, Connecticut

Janice T. Chussil, MSN, DNC, ANP
Nurse Practitioner
Klein Dermatology and Associates
Portland, Oregon

Jeanenne F. Clark, RN, MSN, MPH
Patient Safety Specialist
Barnes-Jewish Hospital
Patient Safety and Quality
St. Louis, Missouri

Michael S. Clement, MD, FAAP
Clinical Lecturer
University of Arizona
Department of Family and Community
Medicine
Tucson, Arizona

Kathy Conley, BSN
Pediatric Nurse

Linda Copenhaver, MSN, RN
Associate Professor
Austin Community College
Associate Degree Nursing Program
Austin, Texas

Joyce E. Dains, PhD, JD, RN, FNP, BC, NP
Program Manager, Professional
Education for Prevention and
Early Detection
University of Texas
MD Anderson Cancer Center
Houston, Texas

Elaine S. Demeyer, RN, MSN, AOCN
President, CEO
Creative Cancer Concepts, Inc.
Faculty
Baylor University
Louise Herrington School of Nursing
Dallas, Texas

Deborah Oldenburg Erickson, MSN, RN
Assistant Professor
Bradley University
Department of Nursing
Peoria, Illinois

Mary G. Erslon, RN, MSN, CETN
Reimbursement Specialist
Mallinckrodt Inc.
Health Care Economics Department
St. Louis, Missouri

Susan S. Erue, RN, BSN, MSEd
Associate Professor
Iowa Wesleyan College
Division of Health and
Natural Sciences
Mount Pleasant, Iowa

John Fitzsimmons, MD
Assistant Professor of Anatomy
Michigan State University
Colleges of Medicine
Department of Radiology
East Lansing, Michigan

Donna G. Friedman, PhD
Professor of Chemistry
St. Louis Community College
at Florissant Valley
Chemistry Department
St. Louis, Missouri

John F. Fritz, MNRN
Formerly Director of Nursing
Education Informatics
Drexel University
College of Nursing and
Health Sciences
Philadelphia, Pennsylvania

Florencetta H. Gibson, BSN, MEd, MSN, PhD
Associate Professor-LMFT
University of Louisiana at Monroe
School of Nursing
Monroe, Louisiana

Mary B. Gilkey, APRN, BC, MSN
Director of Nursing
Virginia School of Technology
Virginia Beach, Virginia

Linda B. Haas, PhD, RN, CDE
Endocrinology Clinical Nurse
Specialist
VA Puget Sound Health Care System,
Seattle Division
Primary and Specialty Medical Care
Seattle, Washington

Dorothy G. Herron, PhD, RN, CS
Assistant Professor
University of Maryland
School of Nursing
Baltimore, Maryland

**Attila Hertelendy, MHSM,
CCEMT-P, NREMT-P**
Instructor
University of Mississippi Medical
Center
School of Health Related Professions
Jackson, Mississippi

Bonnie J. Hooper, RN, MSN
Adult Nurse Practitioner
Dermatology Associates of
San Diego County
Encinitas, California
La Jolla, California

Jené M. Hurlbut, RN, MSN, CFNP
Technical Instructor
University of New Mexico
Nursing Department
Gallup, New Mexico

Theresa G. Isom, BS, BSN, MS, RN
Nursing Coordinator
Tennessee Technology Center
at Memphis
Nursing Department
Memphis, Tennessee

Gail I. Jones, PhD, MT (ASCP), SC
Medical Technologist, Instructor
Texas Christian University
Biology Department
Fort Worth, Texas

JaCinda L. Jones, PharmD
Scientific Affairs Manager
Scios, Inc.
Jerseyville, Illinois

Tamara M. Kear, MSN, RN, CNN
Nursing Instructor
Gwynedd-Mercy College
School of Nursing
Gwynedd-Valley, Pennsylvania

Pamela D. Kortz, RN, BS, MS
Associate Professor of Nursing
Monroe Community College
Department of Nursing
Rochester, New York

**Judy LaBonte, MSN, APRN,
FNP, BC**
Assistant Professor
Baptist College of Health Sciences
Division of Nursing
Memphis, Tennessee

**Patricia A. Lamb, RN, MN, CNS,
CRNO**
President, Owner
Ophthalmic Nursing Care
of Arizona, Inc.
President
ASORN Grand Canyon
Phoenix, Arizona

Rae Langford, RN, EdD
Associate Professor
College of Nursing
Texas Woman's University
Houston, Texas

**Joyce E. Laurie, RN, MSN, APRN,
RN, CNS**
Laredo Medical Center
Laredo, Texas

David E. Lewis, PhD
Professor of Chemistry
University of Wisconsin-Eau Claire
Department of Chemistry
Eau Claire, Wisconsin

**Linda R. Littlejohns, RN, MSN,
CCRN, CNRN**
Vice President of Clinical
Development
Integra NeuroSciences Education
Institute
San Diego, California

Sharon Lytle, AAS, BSN, MSN
Professor
Nursing
Carl Sandburg College
Galesburg, IL

Lisa McClane, RNC, MSN, CWS
Administrator
Erlanger Health System
Women's and Infants' Services
Chattanooga, Tennessee

Mary S. Merchant, RN, MSN
Care Manager
Medical University of South Carolina
Division of Clinical Services
Charleston, South Carolina

Eva Moraa Mwancha, LPN
University of the District of Columbia
Nursing School
Washington DC

John J. Nagelhout, PhD, CRNA
Adjunct Professor
California State University, Fullerton
Fullerton, California
Director
Kaiser Permanente School
of Anesthesia
Pasadena, California

Elaine K. Neel, RN, BSN, MSN
Nursing Instructor
Graham Hospital
School of Nursing
Canton, Illinois

Patricia J. Nunn, RDH, MS
Professor and Chair
University of Oklahoma College
of Dentistry
Department of Dental Hygiene
Oklahoma City, Oklahoma

Jeffrey Papp, PhD, RT (R) (QM)
Professor, Physics and Diagnostic
Imaging
College of DuPage
Department of Health Sciences
Glen Ellyn, Illinois

Kevin T. Patton, PhD
Professor of Life Sciences
Saint Charles Community College
Saint Peters, Missouri
Adjunct Assistant Professor
of Physiology
Saint Louis University Medical School
Saint Louis, Missouri

Wendy M. Perry, RN, BSN, RNC
Registered Nurse
United States Army Nurse Corps
Elkridge, Maryland

Paul Philippe, RN, MS
New York State Board for Nursing
Adjunct Faculty
Long Island University
Brooklyn, New York

Leonard A. Piche, PhD, RD
Associate Professor
Nutrition Program
University of Western Ontario
Brescia College
London, Ontario

Roger Plaut, BS
Graduate Research Assistant
University of Maryland, Baltimore
Department of Microbiology
and Immunology
Baltimore, Maryland

Michele K. Plehn, BS, M (ASCP)
Lab Scientist, Medical Technologist
State of Maryland
Department of Health and Mental
  Hygiene
Baltimore, Maryland

Jean A. Proehl, RN, MN, CEN, CCRN
Emergency Clinical Nurse Specialist
Dartmouth-Hitchcock Medical Center
Lebanon, New Hampshire

Claudia Pucci, MD
Clinical Instructor in Psychiatry
Harvard Medical School
Beth Israel Deaconess Medical Center
Boston, Massachusetts
Dimock Community Health Center
Roxbury, Massachusetts

Diane P. Robinson, BSN, RN
Director of Nursing Services
Centre Medical and Surgical
  Associates
State College, Pennsylvania

Karen Robinson, RN, MN, MPM
Research Compliance Specialist
Allegheny General Hospital
Allegheny Singer Research
  Institutional Review Board
Pittsburgh, Pennsylvania

Debra Koss Rodriguez, RN, BSN
Staff Nurse
Inova Fairfax Hospital
Department of Labor and Delivery
Falls Church, Virginia

Natalia S. Rost, MD
Clinical Fellow in Neurology
Partners Healthcare System
Department of Neurology
Boston, Massachusetts

Kathy Sue Rowland, RN, BSEd
Registered Nurse
Barnes-Jewish Hospital
Surgical Services Education
St. Louis, Missouri

Susan C. Ruda, MS, APN, RN, ONC
Clinical Nurse Specialist
Parkview Musculoskeletal Institute
Palos Heights, Illinois

Darlene Schelper, RN, MSN, CEN, RN-C
Clinical Nurse Educator
Penn State Hershey Medical Center
Hershey, Pennsylvania

Jerry E. Seals, MD
Medical Doctor

A. Christy Seckman, RN, MSN
Associate Professor
Clarkson College
Nursing Department
Omaha, Nebraska

Sarah C. Smith, RN, MA, CRNO
Advanced Practical Nurse
University of Iowa
Department of Ophthalmology
Iowa City, Iowa

Adams O. Solola, PharmD
Staff Pharmacist
CVS Pharmacy
LaPlata, Maryland

Gary A. Thibodeau, PhD
Chancellor Emeritus and Professor
  Emeritus of Biology
University of Wisconsin—River Falls
River Falls, Wisconsin

Shannon Thomas, MS, MCG
Instructor
McLennan Community College
Health Sciences
Waco, Texas

Keith A. Wichinski, RN
Director of Clinical Services
National Nursing and Rehab
Corpus Christi, Texas

Juanita C. Widener, RN, BSN, MAEd
Nursing Instructor
Bainbridge College
Technical Studies Division
Bainbridge, Georgia

Mary E. Wilbur, RN, MSN
Care Manager
Medical University Hospital
Charleston, South Carolina

Susan F. Wilson, RN, PhD, FNP
Associate Professor
Texas Christian University
College of Health and
  Human Sciences
Harris School of Nursing
Fort Worth, Texas

Dennis W. Wolff, PhD
CEO
Medical Diagnoses Explained, Inc.
Omaha, Nebraska

Zoë Emma Violet Worthington, BS, PhD
Postdoctoral Fellow
University of Maryland, Baltimore,
  Medical School
Department of Microbiology
  and Immunology
Baltimore, Maryland

Nancy H. Wright, RN, BS, CNOR
Director of Surgical Techology
Virginia College
Birmingham, Alabama

Thomas J. Zwemer, DDS, MSD, ABO, FACD, FICD
Vice President for Academic Affairs
  Emeritus, Professor of Orthodontics
  Emeritus
Medical College of Georgia
Augusta, Georgia

A. ALPHABETIC ORDER

The entries are alphabetized in dictionary style, that is, letter by letter, disregarding spaces or hyphens between words:

analgesic	artificial lung
anal membrane	artificially acquired immunity
analog	artificial menopause

(Alphabetized in telephone-book style, that is, word by word, the order would be different: **anal membrane / analgesic / analog; artificial lung / artificial menopause / artificially acquired immunity.**)

The alphabetization is alphanumeric; that is, words and numbers form a single list, numbers being positioned as though they were spelled-out numerals: **Nilstat/90-90 traction/ninth nerve.** (An example of the few exceptions to this rule is the sequence **17-hydroxycorticosteroid / 11-hydroxyetiocholanolone / 5-hydroxyindoleacetic acid,** which can be found between the entries **hydroxochloroquine sulfate** and **hydroxyl,** not, as may be expected, **17-**... in letter "S," **11-**... in letter "E," and **5-**... in letter "F.")

Small subscript and superscript numbers are disregarded in alphabetizing: **No / N$_2$O / nobelium**

For the alphabetization of prefixes and suffixes, see F.

B. COMPOUND HEADWORDS

Compound headwords are given in their natural word order: **abdominal surgery,** not **surgery, abdominal; achondroplastic dwarf,** not **dwarf, achondroplastic.**

When appropriate, a reference is made elsewhere to the nonalphabetized element; the entry **dwarf,** for example, shows this indirect cross-reference: "... Kinds of dwarfs include **achondroplastic dwarf,** ..." (followed by additional terms ending in "dwarf").

There are few exceptions to this natural word order; nearly all of these concern formal classifications, for example: "**coping, defensive,** a nursing diagnosis accepted by the Eighth National Conference on the Classification of Nursing Diagnoses ..."

(NOTE: In this guide, the term "headword" is used to refer to any alphabetized and nonindented definiendum, be it a single-word term or a compound term.)

C. MULTIPLE DEFINITIONS

If a headword has more than one meaning, the meanings are numbered and are often accompanied by an indication of the field in which a sense applies: "**fraction, 1.** (in neurology) ... **2.** (in chemistry) ... **3.** (in bacteriology) ... **4.** (in histology) ... **5.** (in radiology) ..."

Smaller differences in meaning are occasionally separated by semicolons: "**enervation, 1.** the reduction or lack of nervous energy; weakness; lassitude, languor. **2.** removal of a complete nerve or of a section of nerve."

Words that are spelled alike but have entirely different meanings and origins are usually given as separate entries, with superscript numbers: "**aural**[1], pertaining to the ear or hearing ..." followed by "**aural**[2], pertaining to an aura."

For reference entries that appear in the form of numbered senses, see the example of **hyperalimentation** at E.

D. THE BOLDFACE ELEMENTS OF AN ENTRY

After the entry headword, which has large boldface type, the following elements may occur in boldface, in this order.

In boldface:

■ HEADWORD ABBREVIATIONS: **central nervous system (CNS)**

A corresponding abbreviation entry is listed: "**CNS,** abbreviation for **central nervous system.**" (For abbreviation entries, see F.)

Occasionally the order is reversed: "**DDT (dichlordiphenyltrichloroethane),**" with a corresponding reference entry: "**dichlordi-phenyltrichloroethane. See DDT.**" (For reference entries, see E below.)

■ PLURAL OR SINGULAR FORMS that are not obvious. The first form shown is the more common except when plurals are of more or less equal frequency: "**carcinoma,** *pl.* **carcinomas, carcinomata**"; "**cortex,** *pl.* **cortices**"; "**data,** *sing.* **datum**"

A reference entry is listed only when the terms are alphabetically separated; for example, there are several entries between **data** and "**datum. See data.**"

■ HIDDEN ENTRIES, that is, terms that can best be defined in the context of a more general entry. For example, the definition of the entry **equine encephalitis** continues as follows: "... **Eastern equine encephalitis (EEE)** is a severe form of the infection ... **western equine encephalitis (WEE),** which occurs ... **Venezuelan equine encephalitis (VEE),** which is common in ..."

The corresponding reference entries are "**eastern equine encephalitis. See equine encephalitis.**"; "**western equine encephalitis. See equine ...**"; and so forth. For further reference, from the abbreviations **EEE, WEE,** and **VEE,** see F.

■ INDIRECT CROSS-REFERENCES to other defined entries, shown as part of the definition and usually introduced by "Kinds of": "**dwarf,** ... Kinds of dwarfs include **achondroplastic dwarf, asexual dwarf,** ..., and **thanatophoric dwarf.**"

The entry referred to may or may not show a reciprocal reference, depending on the information value.

■ SYNONYMOUS TERMS, preceded by "Also called," "Also spelled," or, for verbs and adjectives, "Also": "**abducens nerve,** ... Also called **sixth nerve.**"

A corresponding reference entry is usually given: "**sixth nerve.** See **abducens nerve.**"

Occasionally the synonymous term is accompanied by a usage label: "**abdomen,** ... Also called *(informal)* **belly.**"

If a synonymous term applies to only one numbered sense, it precedes rather than follows the definition, to avoid ambiguity: "**algology, 1.** the branch of medicine that is concerned with the study of pain. **2.** also called **phycology,** the branch of science that is concerned with algae." (Whenever a synonymous term *follows* the last numbered sense, it applies to all senses of the entry.)

■ (DIRECT) CROSS-REFERENCES, preceded by "See also" or "Compare," referring to another defined entry for additional information: "**abdominal aorta,** ... See also **descending aorta.**"

The cross-reference may or may not be reciprocal.

Cross-references are also made to illustrations, to tables, to the color atlas, and to the appendixes.

For cross-references from an abbreviation entry (with "See"), see F.

■ PARTS OF SPEECH related to the entry headword, shown as run-on entries that do not require a separate definition: "**abalienation,** ... —**abalienate,** *v.,* **abalienated,** *adj.*"

E. REFERENCE ENTRIES

Reference entries are undefined entries referring to a defined entry. There, they usually correspond to the boldface terms for which reference entries are mentioned at D above.

However, many of the less frequently used synonymous terms are listed as a reference only; at the entry referred to, the reader's attention is not drawn to them with "Also called."

Some reference entries appear in the form of a numbered sense of a defined entry: "**hyperalimentation, 1.** overfeeding or the ... in excess of the demands of the appetite. **2.** See **total parenteral nutrition.**" The latter entry says "Also called **hyperalimentation.**"

If two or more alphabetically adjacent terms refer to the same entry or entries, they are styled as one reference entry: "**coxa adducta, coxa flexa. See coxa vara.**"

A reference entry that would be derived from a boldface term in an immediately adjacent entry is not listed again as a headword; it becomes a "hidden reference entry": **"acardius amorphus,** . . . Also called **acardius anceps."** But **acardius anceps** is not listed again as a reference entry because it would immediately *follow* the entry, the next entry being **acariasis.** Likewise: **"acoustic neuroma,** . . . Also called **acoustic neurilemmoma, acoustic neurinoma, acoustic neurofibroma."** But the three synonymous terms are not listed again as reference entries because they would immediately *precede* the entry, the entry ahead being **acoustic nerve.** Therefore:

> If a term is not listed at the expected place, the reader might find it among the boldface terms of the immediately preceding or the immediately following entry.

Selected British spellings are included where appropriate. These are included as reference entries which refer the reader to the American spelling containing the definition. After the definition, the British spelling is given as an alternate spelling. For example: **"haematology. See hematology."** The end of the definition for **hematology** says "Also spelled **haematology."** As with other reference entries, when the reference entry would immediately precede or follow the main entry, it is not included as a separate entry, such as **"hyperkalemia** . . . Also spelled **hyperkalaemia."**

F. OTHER KINDS OF ENTRIES

■ ABBREVIATION ENTRIES: Most abbreviation entries, including symbol entries, show the full form of the term in boldface: **"ABC, abbreviation for aspiration biopsy cytology." "H, symbol for the element hydrogen."** Implied reference is made to the entries **aspiration biopsy cytology** and **hydrogen** respectively.

Abbreviation entries for which there is no corresponding entry show the full form in italics: **"CBF, abbreviation for** *cerebral blood flow."* **"f, symbol for** *respiratory frequency."*

A combination of abbreviation entry and reference entry occurs when the abbreviation is that of a boldface or lightface term appearing under another headword. For example, the hidden entries at D (in addition to the reference entries shown there) are also referred to in the following manner: **"EEE, abbreviation for eastern equine encephalitis. See equine encephalitis."** An example with a lightface term: **"HLA-A, abbreviation for** *human leukocyte antigen A.* **See human leukocyte antigen."** The latter entry says ". . They are HLA-A, HLA-B, HLA-C . . ."

■ PREFIXES AND SUFFIXES: The large amount and the nature of prefix and suffix entries are an important feature of this dictionary. Through these entries the reader has additional access to the meanings of headwords and the words used in defining them. But such entries also give access to thousands of terms that are not included in this dictionary (and, to a large extent, are not found in any other reference work). For example, the entries **xylo-** and **-phage** (plus **-phagia, phago-,** and **-phagy**) may lead to the meaning of "xylophagous," namely, "wood-eating."

Prefix and suffix headwords consisting of variants are alphabetized by the first variant only. For example, **"epi-, ep-,** a prefix meaning 'on, upon' . . ." is followed by **epiblast** (notwithstanding **"ep-").** The other variant or variants are listed in their own alphabetical place as reference entries referring to the first variant: **"ep-. See epi-."**

■ ENTRIES WITH SPECIAL PARAGRAPHS: Among the entries on diseases, drugs, and procedures, at least 1100 feature special paragraphs, with headings such as:

observations, interventions, and *nursing considerations.* (for disease entries),

indications, contraindications, and *adverse effects.* (for drug entries),

method, nursing interventions, and *outcome criteria.* (for procedure entries).

G. FURTHER COMMENTS

■ EPONYMOUS TERMS THAT END IN "SYNDROME" OR "DISEASE" are given with an apostrophe (and "s" where appropriate) if they are based on the name of one person: **Adie's syndrome; Symmers' disease; Treacher Collins' syndrome** (the ophthalmologist Edward Treacher Collins). If they are based on the names of several people, they are without apostrophe: **Bernard-Soulier syndrome; Brill-Symmers disease.**

■ ABBREVIATIONS AND LABELS IN ITALIC TYPE: The abbreviations are *pl.* (plural), *npl.* (noun plural), *sing.* (singular); *n.* (noun), *adj.* (adjective), *v.* (verb). The recurring labels are *slang, informal, nontechnical, obsolete, archaic; chiefly British, Canada, U.S.*

■ DICTIONARY OF FIRST REFERENCE for general spelling preferences is *Webster's New Collegiate Dictionary;* thereafter: *Webster's Third New International Dictionary.*

H. PRONUNCIATION

■ SYSTEM: See the Pronunciation Key on p. xiv. The pronunciation system of this dictionary is basically a system that most readers know from their use of popular English dictionaries, especially the major college or desk dictionaries. All symbols for English sounds are ordinary letters of the alphabet with few adaptations, and with the exception of the schwa, /ə/ (the neutral vowel).

■ ACCENTS: Pronunciation, given between slants, is shown with primary and secondary accents, and a raised dot shows that two vowels or, occasionally, two consonants, between the slants are pronounced separately:

anoopsia /an′ō·op′sē·ə/
cecoileostomy /il′ē·os′tə mē/
methemoglobin /met′hēmə glō′bin, met·hē′mə glōbin/

Without the raised dot, the second /th/ in the last example would be pronounced as in "thin." (The pronunciation key lists the following paired consonant symbols as representing a single sound: /ch/, /ng/, /sh/, /th/, /ᵗh/, /zh/, and the foreign sounds /kh/ and /ᴋh/—if no raised dot intervenes.)

■ TRUNCATION: Pronunciation may be given in truncated form, especially for alternative or derived words:

defibrillate /difi′brilāt, difib′-/
bacteriophage /baktir′ē·ə fāj′, . . . —**bacteriophagy** /-of′ə jē/, *n.*

In the last example, the reader is asked to make the commonsense assumption that the primary accent of the headword becomes a secondary accent in the run-on term: /baktir′ē·of′ə jē/.

■ LOCATION: Pronunciation may be given for any boldface term and may occur anywhere in an entry:

aura /ôr′ə/, **1.** *pl.* **aurae** /ôr′ē/, a sensation . . . **2.** *pl.* **auras,** an emanation of light . . .
micrometer, 1. /mīkrom′ətər/, an instrument used for . . . **2.** /mī′krōmē′tər/, a unit of measurement . . .

Occasionally it is given for a lightface term:

b.i.d., (in prescriptions) abbreviation for *bis in die* /dē′ā/, a Latin phrase meaning . . .
boutonneuse fever. . . , an infectious disease . . . a tache noire /täshnô·är′/ or black spot . . .

■ LETTERWORD VERSUS ACRONYM: Letterwords are abbreviations that are pronounced by sounding the names of each letter, whereas acronyms are pronounced as words. If the pronunciation of an abbreviation is not given, the abbreviation is usually a letterword:

ABO blood groups [read /ā′bē′ō′/, not /ā′bō/]

If the pronunciation is an acronym, this is indicated by pronunciation:

AWOL /ā′wôl/

ANTERIOR VIEW OF SKULL

Frontal bone
Squama of frontal bone
Frontal eminence
Coronal suture
Glabella
Parietal bone
Superciliary ridge
Supraorbital foramen
Orbital plate of frontal bone
Supraorbital margin
Sphenoid (greater wing)
Zygomatic process of frontal bone
Superior orbital fissure
Temporal bone
Optic foramen
Nasal bone
Lacrimal bone
Zygomatic bone
Inferior orbital fissure
Infraorbital foramen
Nasal cavity
Maxilla
Middle and inferior nasal conchae
Ramus of mandible
Body of mandible
Mental foramen

FETAL SKULL

Parietal bone
Anterior fontanel
Frontal suture
Parietal eminence
Frontal bone
Frontal eminence
Posterior fontanel
Sphenoid fontanel
Occipital bone
Nasal bone
Lacrimal bone
Sphenoid
Maxilla
Mastoid fontanel
Zygomatic bone
Temporal bone (petrous portion)
Mandible
Temporal bone (squamous portion)
Tympanic ring
External auditory meatus

Coronal suture
Sagittal suture
Frontal bone
Superior temporal line
Parietal bone
Inferior temporal line
Superciliary ridge
Squamosal suture
Sphenoid (greater wing)
Supraorbital foramen
Temporal bone
Nasal bone
Occipital bone
Lacrimal bone
Lambdoidal suture
Infraorbital foramen
External occipital protuberance
Zygomatic bone
Maxilla
Mastoid process
External auditory meatus
Styloid process
RIGHT LATERAL VIEW OF SKULL
Zygomatic process of temporal bone
Mandible
Mental foramen

THORAX AND RIBS

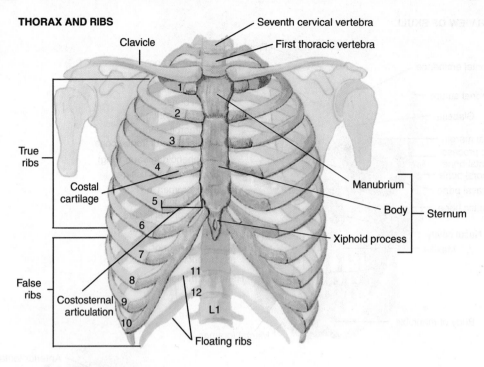

Seventh cervical vertebra

First thoracic vertebra

Clavicle

True ribs

Costal cartilage

Manubrium

Body

Xiphoid process

Sternum

False ribs

Costosternal articulation

1
2
3
4
5
6
7
8
9
10
11
12

L1

Floating ribs

PELVIS

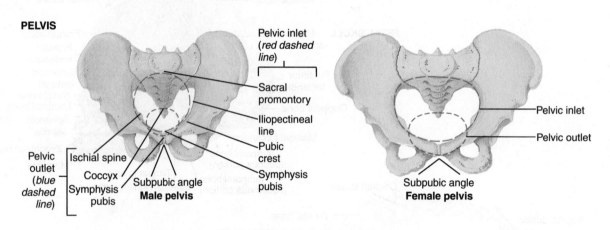

Pelvic inlet (*red dashed line*)

Sacral promontory

Iliopectineal line

Pubic crest

Symphysis pubis

Pelvic outlet (*blue dashed line*)

Ischial spine

Coccyx

Symphysis pubis

Subpubic angle

Male pelvis

Pelvic inlet

Pelvic outlet

Subpubic angle

Female pelvis

INDIVIDUAL VERTEBRA

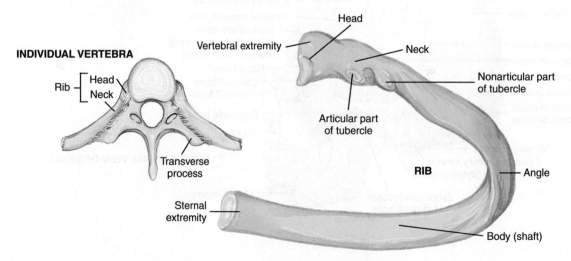

Rib

Head

Neck

Transverse process

Head

Vertebral extremity

Neck

Nonarticular part of tubercle

Articular part of tubercle

RIB

Angle

Sternal extremity

Body (shaft)

VERTEBRAL COLUMN

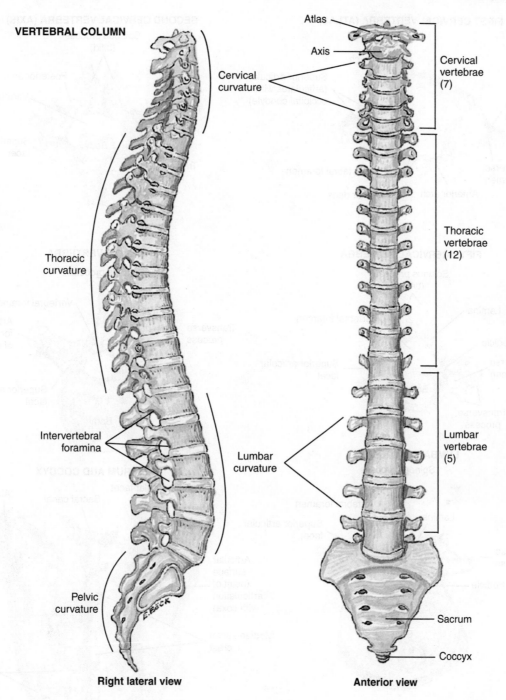

Atlas

Axis

Cervical curvature

Cervical vertebrae (7)

Thoracic curvature

Thoracic vertebrae (12)

Intervertebral foramina

Lumbar curvature

Lumbar vertebrae (5)

Pelvic curvature

Sacrum

Coccyx

E. Beck

Right lateral view

Anterior view

FIRST CERVICAL VERTEBRA (ATLAS)

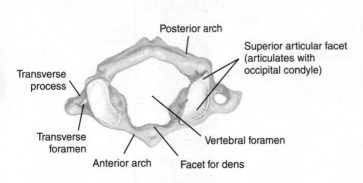

Posterior arch

Superior articular facet
(articulates with
occipital condyle)

Transverse
process

Transverse
foramen

Anterior arch

Vertebral foramen

Facet for dens

SECOND CERVICAL VERTEBRA (AXIS)

Spinous process
(bifid)

Posterior arch

Vertebral foramen

Transverse
process

Body

Superior articular
facet

Transverse
foramen

Dens

FIFTH CERVICAL VERTEBRA

Spinous process
(bifid)

Lamina

Vertebral foramen

Pedicle

Transverse
foramen

Body

Superior articular
facet

Transverse
process

THORACIC VERTEBRA

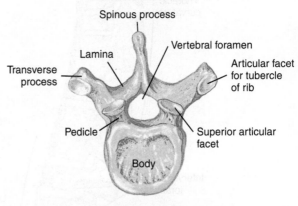

Spinous process

Lamina

Vertebral foramen

Transverse
process

Articular facet
for tubercle
of rib

Pedicle

Superior articular
facet

Body

LUMBAR VERTEBRA

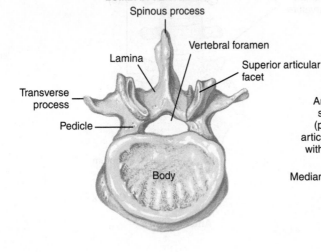

Spinous process

Lamina

Vertebral foramen

Superior articular
facet

Transverse
process

Pedicle

Body

SACRUM AND COCCYX

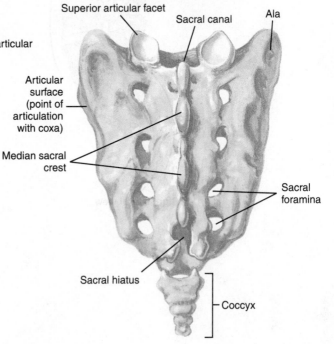

Superior articular facet

Sacral canal

Ala

Articular
surface
(point of
articulation
with coxa)

Median sacral
crest

Sacral
foramina

Sacral hiatus

Coccyx

MICROSCOPIC STRUCTURE OF BONE

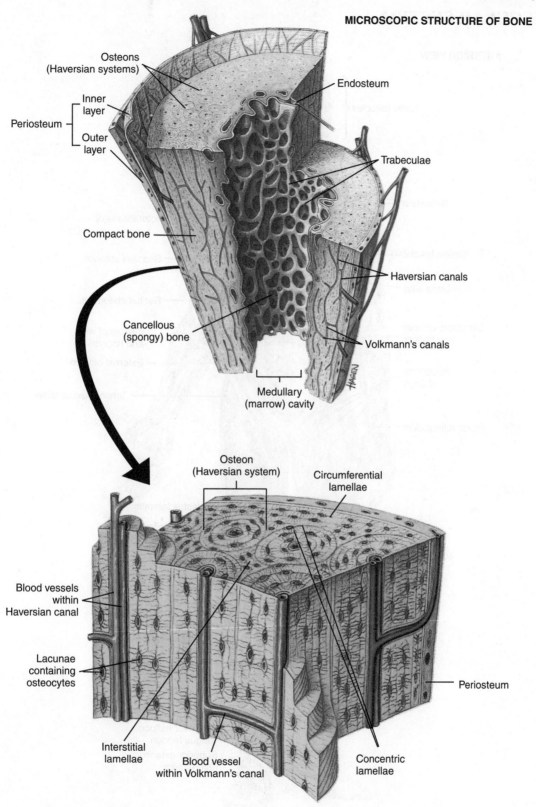

Osteons (Haversian systems)

Periosteum
- Inner layer
- Outer layer

Endosteum

Trabeculae

Compact bone

Haversian canals

Cancellous (spongy) bone

Volkmann's canals

Medullary (marrow) cavity

HAGEN

Osteon (Haversian system)

Circumferential lamellae

Blood vessels within Haversian canal

Lacunae containing osteocytes

Periosteum

Interstitial lamellae

Blood vessel within Volkmann's canal

Concentric lamellae

MUSCULAR SYSTEM

ANTERIOR VIEW

Cranial muscles

Facial muscles

Sternocleidomastoideus

Trapezius

Deltoideus

Pectoralis major

Biceps brachii

Serratus anterior

Linea alba

Rectus abdominis

Extensors of wrist and fingers

Flexors of wrist and fingers

Adductors of thigh

External oblique

Flexor retinaculum

Tensor fasciae latae

Sartorius

Vastus lateralis

Rectus femoris

Vastus medialis

Patella

Patellar tendon

Gastrocnemius

Tibialis anterior

Extensor digitorum longus

Peroneus longus

Peroneus brevis

Soleus

Extensor hallucis longus tendon

Superior extensor retinaculum

POSTERIOR VIEW

Sternocleidomastoideus

Splenius capitis

Seventh cervical vertebra

Trapezius

Deltoideus

Infraspinatus

Teres minor

Teres major

Portion of rhomboideus

Triceps

Latissimus dorsi

Extensors
of the wrist
and fingers

External oblique

Gluteus maximus

Semitendinosus

Adductor magnus

Biceps femoris

Gracilis
Iliotibial tract

Semimembranosus

Plantaris

Gastrocnemius

Gastrocnemius tendon
(Achilles tendon)

Peroneus longus

Soleus

Peroneus brevis

Superior peroneal retinaculum

**LATERAL AND ANTERIOR VIEWS OF
MUSCLES OF THE FACE AND ANTERIOR CRANIUM
AND SEVERAL MUSCLES OF MASTICATION**

Galea aponeurotica

Frontalis

Temporalis

Temporalis fascia

Auricularis superior

Auricularis anterior

Occipitalis

Auricularis posterior

Masseter

Sternocleidomastoideus

Trapezius

Orbicularis oculi

Corrugator

Procerus

Levator labii superioris alaeque nasi

Levator labii superioris

Zygomaticus minor

Levator anguli oris

Zygomaticus major

Orbicularis oris

Risorius (cut)

Mentalis

Depressor labii inferioris

Depressor anguli oris

Buccinator

Omohyoideus

Sternohyoideus

Galea aponeurotica
(frontal portion)

Medial palpebral ligament

Epicranius
(frontal belly)

Orbicularis oculi
(orbital portion)

Orbicularis oculi
(palpebral portion)

Levator labii superioris

Zygomaticus minor

Parotid gland

Zygomaticus (major)

Risorius

Levator anguli oris

Depressor anguli oris

Depressor labii inferioris

Procerus

Temporalis

Corrugator

Levator labii superioris alaeque nasi

Zygomaticus minor and major (cut)

Nasalis

Levator anguli oris (cut)

Masseter

Buccinator

Orbicularis oris

Mentalis

Platysma (part)

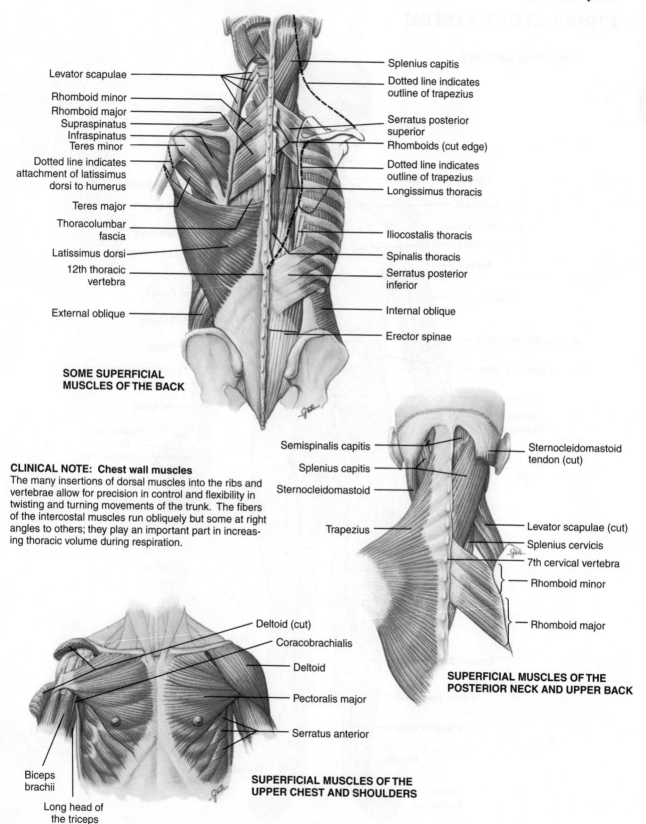

Levator scapulae

Rhomboid minor

Rhomboid major
Supraspinatus
Infraspinatus
Teres minor

Dotted line indicates
attachment of latissimus
dorsi to humerus

Teres major

Thoracolumbar
fascia

Latissimus dorsi

12th thoracic
vertebra

External oblique

Splenius capitis

Dotted line indicates
outline of trapezius

Serratus posterior
superior

Rhomboids (cut edge)

Dotted line indicates
outline of trapezius

Longissimus thoracis

Iliocostalis thoracis

Spinalis thoracis

Serratus posterior
inferior

Internal oblique

Erector spinae

**SOME SUPERFICIAL
MUSCLES OF THE BACK**

CLINICAL NOTE: Chest wall muscles
The many insertions of dorsal muscles into the ribs and
vertebrae allow for precision in control and flexibility in
twisting and turning movements of the trunk. The fibers
of the intercostal muscles run obliquely but some at right
angles to others; they play an important part in increasing thoracic volume during respiration.

Semispinalis capitis

Splenius capitis

Sternocleidomastoid

Trapezius

Sternocleidomastoid
tendon (cut)

Levator scapulae (cut)

Splenius cervicis

7th cervical vertebra

Rhomboid minor

Rhomboid major

**SUPERFICIAL MUSCLES OF THE
POSTERIOR NECK AND UPPER BACK**

Deltoid (cut)

Coracobrachialis

Deltoid

Pectoralis major

Serratus anterior

Biceps
brachii

Long head of
the triceps

**SUPERFICIAL MUSCLES OF THE
UPPER CHEST AND SHOULDERS**

CIRCULATORY SYSTEM

PRINCIPAL ARTERIES

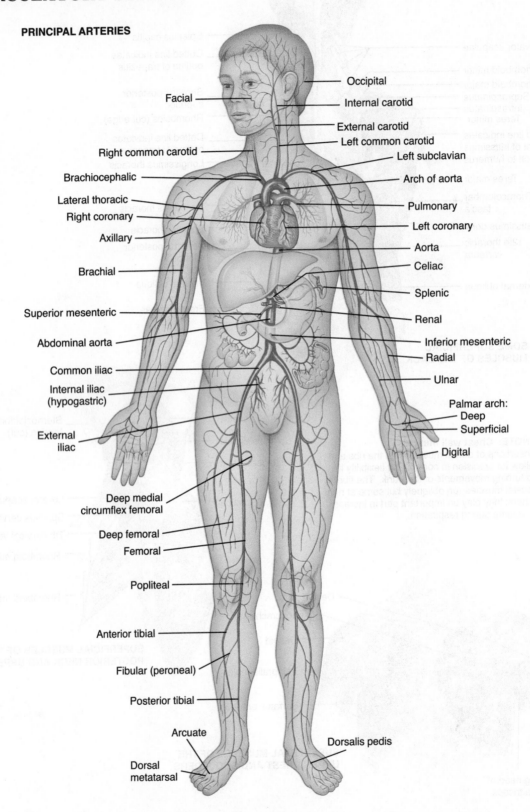

Occipital

Facial

Internal carotid

External carotid

Left common carotid

Right common carotid

Left subclavian

Brachiocephalic

Arch of aorta

Lateral thoracic

Pulmonary

Right coronary

Left coronary

Axillary

Aorta

Brachial

Celiac

Splenic

Superior mesenteric

Renal

Abdominal aorta

Inferior mesenteric

Radial

Common iliac

Ulnar

Internal iliac
(hypogastric)

Palmar arch:
Deep
Superficial

External
iliac

Digital

Deep medial
circumflex femoral

Deep femoral

Femoral

Popliteal

Anterior tibial

Fibular (peroneal)

Posterior tibial

Arcuate

Dorsalis pedis

Dorsal
metatarsal

PRINCIPAL VEINS

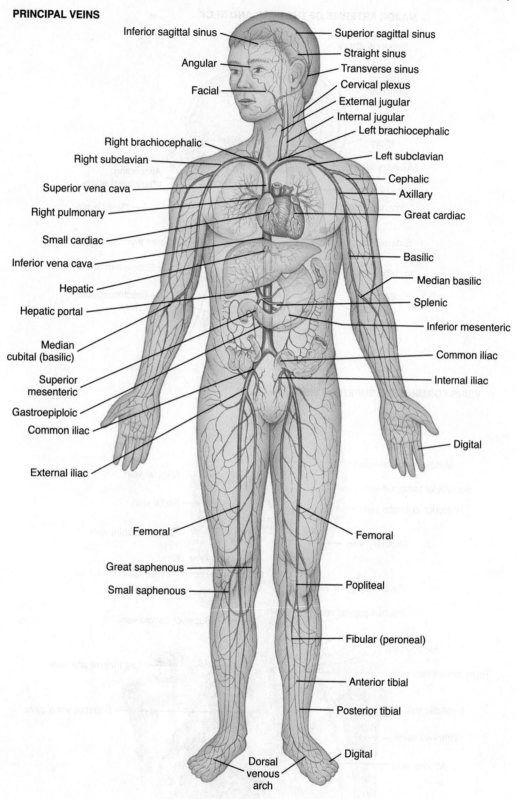

Inferior sagittal sinus
Superior sagittal sinus
Angular
Straight sinus
Facial
Transverse sinus
Cervical plexus
External jugular
Internal jugular
Left brachiocephalic
Right brachiocephalic
Left subclavian
Right subclavian
Cephalic
Superior vena cava
Axillary
Right pulmonary
Great cardiac
Small cardiac
Basilic
Inferior vena cava
Median basilic
Hepatic
Splenic
Hepatic portal
Inferior mesenteric
Median cubital (basilic)
Common iliac
Superior mesenteric
Internal iliac
Gastroepiploic
Common iliac
Digital
External iliac
Femoral
Femoral
Great saphenous
Small saphenous
Popliteal
Fibular (peroneal)
Anterior tibial
Posterior tibial
Digital
Dorsal venous arch

MAJOR ARTERIES OF THE HEAD AND NECK

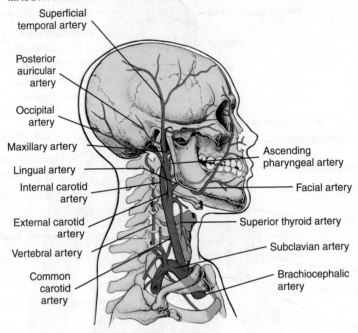

Superficial temporal artery

Posterior auricular artery

Occipital artery

Maxillary artery

Lingual artery

Internal carotid artery

External carotid artery

Vertebral artery

Common carotid artery

Ascending pharyngeal artery

Facial artery

Superior thyroid artery

Subclavian artery

Brachiocephalic artery

VEINS FORMING THE SUPERIOR VENA CAVA

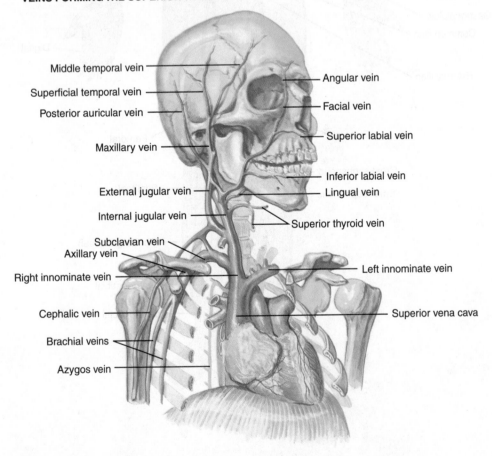

Middle temporal vein

Superficial temporal vein

Posterior auricular vein

Maxillary vein

External jugular vein

Internal jugular vein

Subclavian vein

Axillary vein

Right innominate vein

Cephalic vein

Brachial veins

Azygos vein

Angular vein

Facial vein

Superior labial vein

Inferior labial vein

Lingual vein

Superior thyroid vein

Left innominate vein

Superior vena cava

ANTERIOR VIEW OF THE HEART

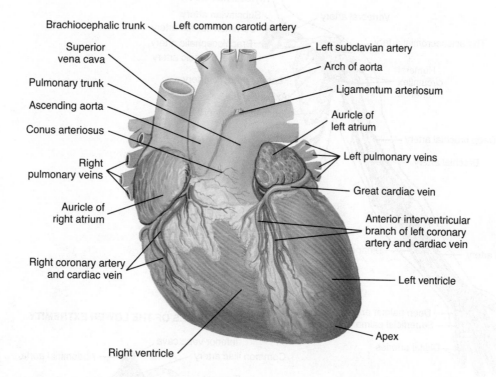

Brachiocephalic trunk

Left common carotid artery

Superior
vena cava

Left subclavian artery

Arch of aorta

Pulmonary trunk

Ligamentum arteriosum

Ascending aorta

Conus arteriosus

Auricle of
left atrium

Right
pulmonary veins

Left pulmonary veins

Auricle of
right atrium

Great cardiac vein

Anterior interventricular
branch of left coronary
artery and cardiac vein

Right coronary artery
and cardiac vein

Left ventricle

Apex

Right ventricle

POSTERIOR VIEW OF THE HEART

Left common carotid artery

Left subclavian artery

Brachiocephalic trunk

Aortic arch

Left pulmonary artery

Superior vena cava

Right pulmonary artery

Left pulmonary veins

Auricle of left atrium

Right pulmonary veins

Left atrium

Great cardiac vein

Right atrium

Inferior vena cava

Posterior artery
and vein of
left ventricle

Coronary sinus

Posterior interventricular
branch of right coronary
artery

Left ventricle

Middle cardiac vein

Apex

Right ventricle

Posterior interventricular sulcus

Circulatory system

MAJOR ARTERIES OF THE UPPER EXTREMITY

Vertebral artery
Thyrocervical trunk
Subclavian artery
Common carotid artery
Thoracicoacromial artery
Brachiocephalic artery
Internal thoracic artery
Humeral circumflex arteries
Lateral thoracic artery
Axillary artery
Subscapular artery

Deep brachial artery

Brachial artery

Radial artery — Ulnar artery

Deep palmar arch
Superficial palmar arch

Digital arteries

MAJOR ARTERIES OF THE LOWER EXTREMITY

Inferior vena cava
Common iliac artery
Abdominal aorta
Median sacral artery
External iliac artery
Internal iliac (hypogastric) artery
Superior gluteal artery
Lateral sacral artery
Internal pudendal artery
Inferior gluteal artery
Obturator artery

Deep femoral artery
Femoral artery

Descending branch of lateral circumflex artery
Genicular arteries

Popliteal artery

Fibular (peroneal) artery
Anterior tibial artery
Posterior tibial artery

Dorsalis pedis artery
Lateral plantar arch
Medial plantar artery
Plantar arch
Digital arteries

MAJOR VEINS OF THE UPPER EXTREMITY

Internal jugular vein

Subclavian vein

Brachiocephalic vein

Axillary vein

Cephalic vein

Brachial veins

Basilic vein

Median cubital (basilic) vein

Ulnar vein

Radial vein

MAJOR VEINS OF THE LOWER EXTREMITY

Common iliac vein

Inferior vena cava

Internal iliac vein

Internal iliac vein

Femoral vein

Great saphenous vein

Popliteal vein

Small saphenous vein

Fibular (peroneal) vein

Anterior tibial vein

Posterior tibial vein

Great saphenous vein

Dorsal veins of the foot

Dorsal venous arch

Digital vein

ENDOCRINE SYSTEM

GLANDS OF THE ENDOCRINE SYSTEM

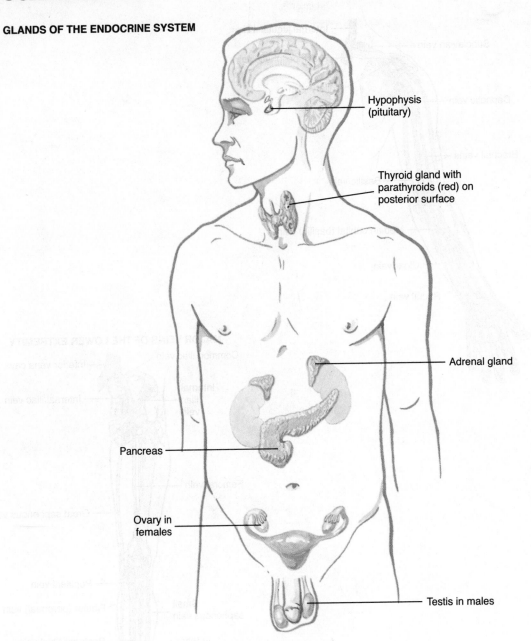

Hypophysis (pituitary)

Thyroid gland with parathyroids (red) on posterior surface

Adrenal gland

Pancreas

Ovary in females

Testis in males

LOCATION OF THE PITUITARY AND PINEAL GLANDS

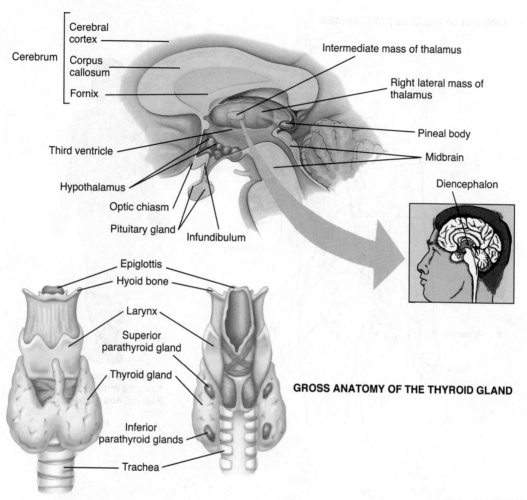

Cerebrum
- Cerebral cortex
- Corpus callosum
- Fornix

Intermediate mass of thalamus

Right lateral mass of thalamus

Pineal body

Midbrain

Diencephalon

Third ventricle

Hypothalamus

Optic chiasm

Pituitary gland

Infundibulum

Epiglottis

Hyoid bone

Larynx

Superior parathyroid gland

Thyroid gland

Inferior parathyroid glands

Trachea

GROSS ANATOMY OF THE THYROID GLAND

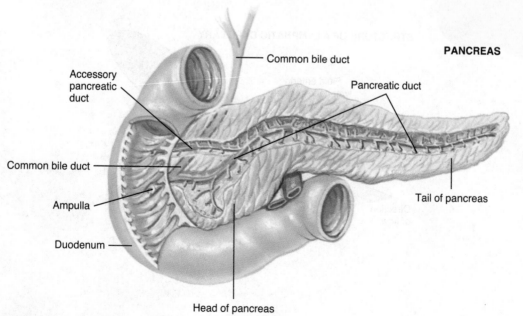

PANCREAS

Common bile duct

Accessory pancreatic duct

Pancreatic duct

Common bile duct

Ampulla

Tail of pancreas

Duodenum

Head of pancreas

LYMPHATIC SYSTEM

ORGANS OF THE LYMPHATIC SYSTEM

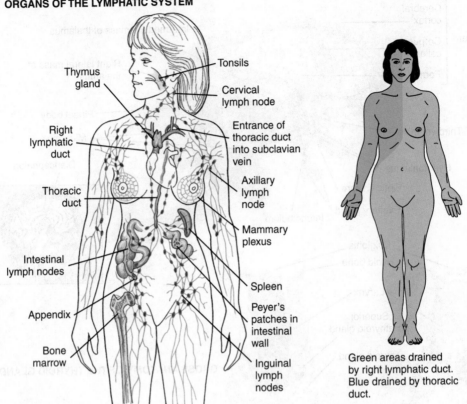

Thymus gland

Right lymphatic duct

Thoracic duct

Intestinal lymph nodes

Appendix

Bone marrow

Tonsils

Cervical lymph node

Entrance of thoracic duct into subclavian vein

Axillary lymph node

Mammary plexus

Spleen

Peyer's patches in intestinal wall

Inguinal lymph nodes

Green areas drained by right lymphatic duct. Blue drained by thoracic duct.

STRUCTURE OF A LYMPHATIC CAPILLARY

Fluid entering lymphatic capillary

Valve closed

Valve open

Overlapping endothelial cells

Direction of flow

STRUCTURE OF THE SPLEEN

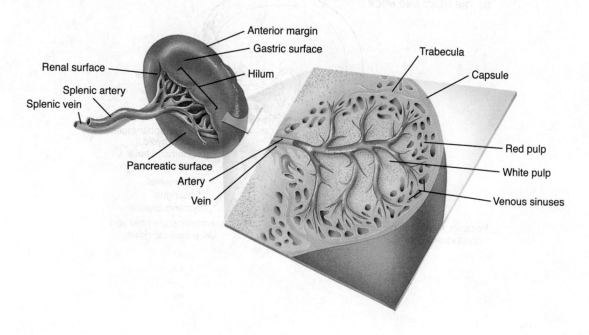

Anterior margin
Gastric surface
Renal surface
Hilum
Splenic artery
Splenic vein
Pancreatic surface
Artery
Vein

Trabecula
Capsule
Red pulp
White pulp
Venous sinuses

LOCATION AND GROSS ANATOMY OF THE THYMUS

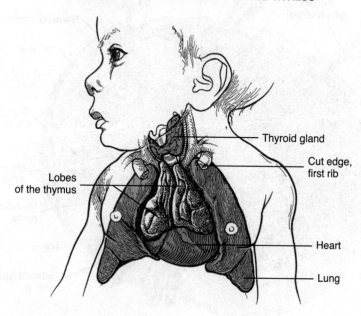

Thyroid gland
Cut edge,
first rib
Lobes
of the thymus
Heart
Lung

LYMPHATIC DRAINAGE SYSTEM OF THE HEAD AND NECK

Preauricular

Suboccipital

Mastoid (postauricular)

Parotid

Retropharyngeal

Suprahyoid

Submandibular (submaxillary)

Posterior cervical spinal nerve chain

Submental

Sublingual

Thyrolinguofacial

Posterior superficial cervical chain (transverse cervical artery chain)

Internal jugular chain

Anterior superficial and deep cervical chain

SCHEMATIC SECTION OF A LYMPH NODE

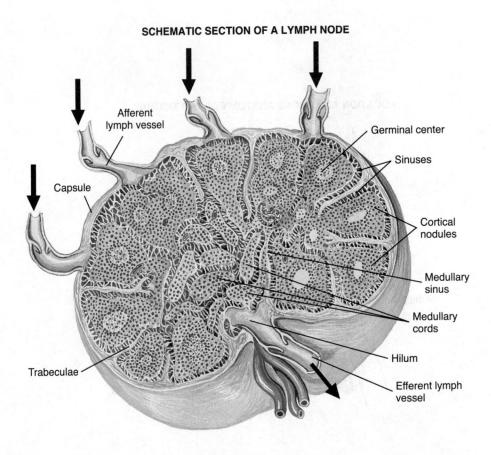

Afferent lymph vessel

Germinal center

Sinuses

Capsule

Cortical nodules

Medullary sinus

Medullary cords

Hilum

Trabeculae

Efferent lymph vessel

NERVOUS SYSTEM

SIMPLIFIED VIEW OF THE NERVOUS SYSTEM

Cerebrum

Cerebellum

Brachial plexus

Musculocutaneous nerve

Spinal cord

Intercostal nerves

Cauda equina

Femoral nerve

Ischial nerve

Femoral cutaneous nerve

Saphenous nerve

Tibial nerve

Peroneal nerve

Digital nerves

GROSS ANATOMY OF THE SPINAL CORD

Cervical vertebrae
C1
C2
C3
C4
C5
C6
C7

Brachial plexus

Thoracic vertebrae
T1
T2
T3
T4
T5
T6
T7
T8
T9
T10
T11
T12

Lumbar vertebrae
L1
L2
L3
L4
L5

Sacrum

Coccyx

GJW

Filum terminale

Cervical plexus
C1
C2
C3
C4
C5
C6
C7
C8

Cervical nerves

T1
T2
T3
T4
T5
T6
T7
T8
T9
T10
T11
T12

Thoracic nerves

Dura mater
Cauda equina

L1
L2
L3
L4
L5

Lumbar nerves

Lumbar plexus

S1
S2
S3
S4
S5

Sacral nerves

Sacral plexus

Coccygeal nerve

CEREBRAL NUCLEI

Lentiform nucleus
Caudate nucleus
— Cerebral nuclei
Thalamus
Amygdaloid nucleus
Substantia nigra (in midbrain)

Corpus striatum
Body of caudate nucleus
Internal capsule
Lentiform nucleus
Putamen
Globus pallidus
Thalamus
Mammillary body
Head of caudate nucleus
Putamen

FUNCTIONAL AREAS OF THE CEREBRAL CORTEX

Precentral gyrus (primary somatic motor area)
Central sulcus
Postcentral gyrus (primary somatic sensory area)
Premotor area
Primary taste area
Prefrontal area
Somatic sensory association area
Visual association area
Broca's area (motor speech area)
Visual cortex
Transverse gyrus
Auditory association area
Primary auditory area
Wernicke's area (sensory speech area)

RETICULAR ACTIVATING SYSTEM

Radiations to cortex
Visual impulses
Reticular formation
Auditory impulses
Projection to spinal cord
Ascending sensory tracts

BASE OF THE BRAIN

ARTERIES
(Circle of Willis)

Anterior cerebral a.

Middle cerebral a.

Internal carotid a.

Posterior communicating a.

Posterior cerebral a.

Superior cerebellar a.

TEMPORAL LOBE

Basilar a.

Internal auditory a.

Anterior inferior cerebellar a.

Vertebral a.

Posterior inferior cerebellar a.

Anterior spinal a.

Posterior cerebral a.

Right lobe of cerebellum removed

CRANIAL NERVES

Olfactory n. (I)

Optic n. (II)

PITUITARY GLAND

Oculomotor n. (III)

Trochlear n. (IV)

Trigeminal n. (V)

Abducens n. (VI)

Facial n. (VII)

Vestibulocochlear n. (VIII)

Glossopharyngeal n. (IX)

Vagus n. (X)

Hypoglossal n. (XII)

Accessory n. (XI)

CEREBELLUM

MEDULLA

BRAINSTEM AND DIENCEPHALON

Intermediate mass

Thalamus

Optic chiasma — Diencephalon

Hypothalamus

Cerebral peduncle

Midbrain

Pons

Medulla oblongata

Olive

Pyramid

Diencephalon

Brain stem

Thalamus

Pineal body — Diencephalon

Superior colliculi

Inferior colliculi — Midbrain

Cerebral peduncle

Superior cerebellar peduncles

Fourth ventricle

Inferior cerebellar peduncles

Middle cerebellar peduncle

Pons

Olive

Medulla oblongata

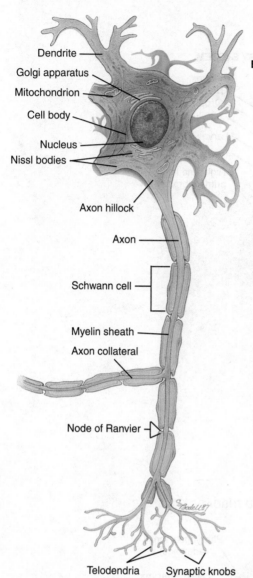

BASIC STRUCTURE OF THE NEURON

Dendrite

Golgi apparatus

Mitochondrion

Cell body

Nucleus

Nissl bodies

Axon hillock

Axon

Schwann cell

Myelin sheath

Axon collateral

Node of Ranvier

Telodendria   Synaptic knobs

MYELINATED AXON

Node of Ranvier

Nucleus of Schwann cell

Myelin sheath

Plasma membrane of axon

Neurilemma (sheath of Schwann cell)

Neurofibrils

RESPIRATORY SYSTEM

ORGANS OF THE RESPIRATORY SYSTEM

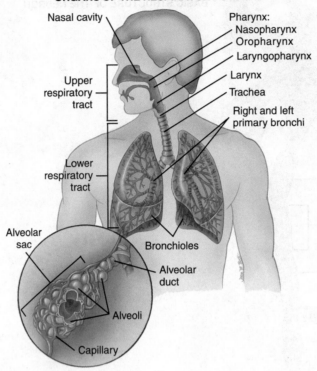

Nasal cavity

Upper respiratory tract

Lower respiratory tract

Pharynx:
Nasopharynx
Oropharynx
Laryngopharynx
Larynx
Trachea
Right and left primary bronchi

Alveolar sac

Bronchioles

Alveolar duct

Alveoli

Capillary

NASAL PASSAGES AND THROAT

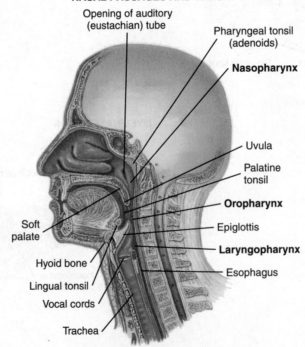

Opening of auditory (eustachian) tube

Pharyngeal tonsil (adenoids)

Nasopharynx

Uvula

Palatine tonsil

Oropharynx

Epiglottis

Laryngopharynx

Esophagus

Soft palate

Hyoid bone

Lingual tonsil

Vocal cords

Trachea

NASAL SEPTUM

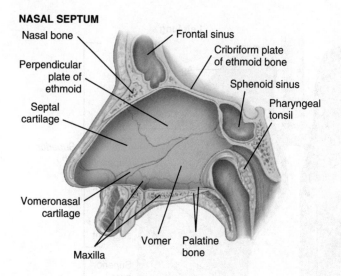

- Nasal bone
- Frontal sinus
- Cribriform plate of ethmoid bone
- Perpendicular plate of ethmoid
- Sphenoid sinus
- Septal cartilage
- Pharyngeal tonsil
- Vomeronasal cartilage
- Maxilla
- Vomer
- Palatine bone

NASAL CAVITY

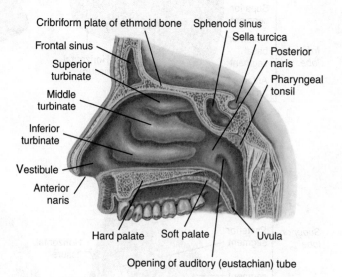

- Cribriform plate of ethmoid bone
- Sphenoid sinus
- Frontal sinus
- Sella turcica
- Superior turbinate
- Posterior naris
- Middle turbinate
- Pharyngeal tonsil
- Inferior turbinate
- Vestibule
- Anterior naris
- Hard palate
- Soft palate
- Uvula
- Opening of auditory (eustachian) tube

BONES OF THE NASAL CAVITY

- Frontal bone
- Crista galli
- Cribriform plate
- Frontal sinus
- Olfactory foramina
- Nasal bone
- Sphenoidal sinus
- Perpendicular plate of ethmoid bone
- Septal cartilage
- Sphenoid bone
- Greater alar cartilage
- Vomer
- Anterior nasal spine
- Horizontal plate of palatine bone
- Incisive canal
- Palatine process of maxilla
- Central incisor

LUNGS

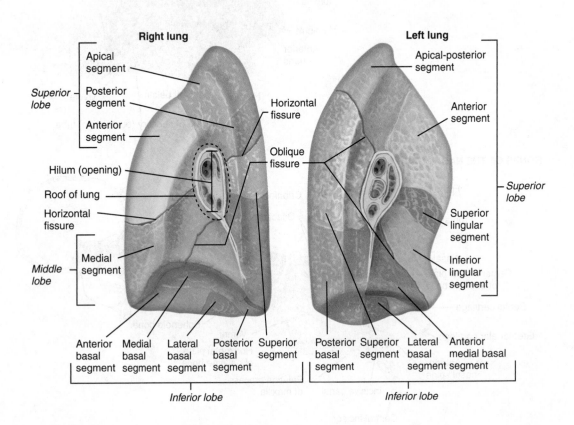

LARYNX AND UPPER TRACHEA

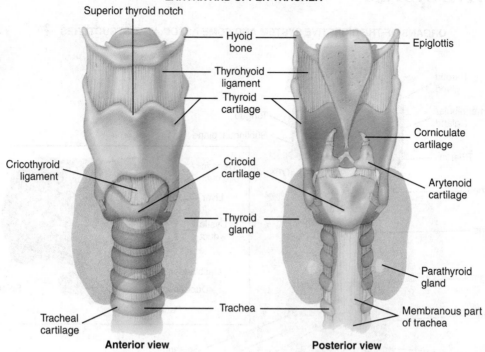

Superior thyroid notch
Hyoid bone
Thyrohyoid ligament
Thyroid cartilage
Cricothyroid ligament
Cricoid cartilage
Thyroid gland
Tracheal cartilage
Trachea

Anterior view

Epiglottis
Corniculate cartilage
Arytenoid cartilage
Parathyroid gland
Membranous part of trachea

Posterior view

GAS-EXCHANGE STRUCTURES OF THE LUNG

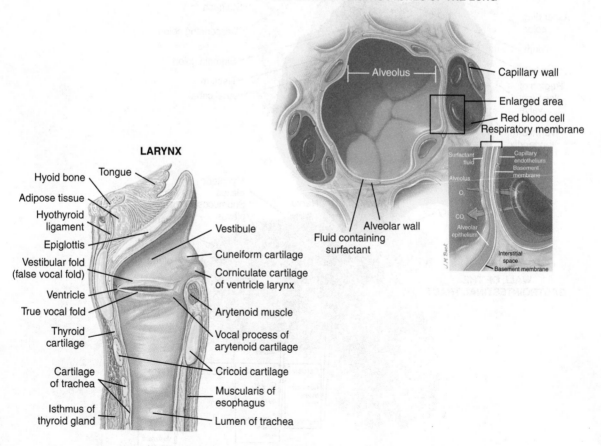

Alveolus
Capillary wall
Enlarged area
Red blood cell
Respiratory membrane
Alveolar wall
Fluid containing surfactant

Surfactant fluid
Capillary endothelium
Basement membrane
Alveolus
O_2
CO_2
Alveolar epithelium
Interstitial space
Basement membrane

LARYNX

Hyoid bone
Adipose tissue
Hyothyroid ligament
Epiglottis
Vestibular fold (false vocal fold)
Ventricle
True vocal fold
Thyroid cartilage
Cartilage of trachea
Isthmus of thyroid gland
Tongue
Vestibule
Cuneiform cartilage
Corniculate cartilage of ventricle larynx
Arytenoid muscle
Vocal process of arytenoid cartilage
Cricoid cartilage
Muscularis of esophagus
Lumen of trachea

DIGESTIVE SYSTEM

ORGANS OF THE DIGESTIVE SYSTEM AND SOME ASSOCIATED STRUCTURES

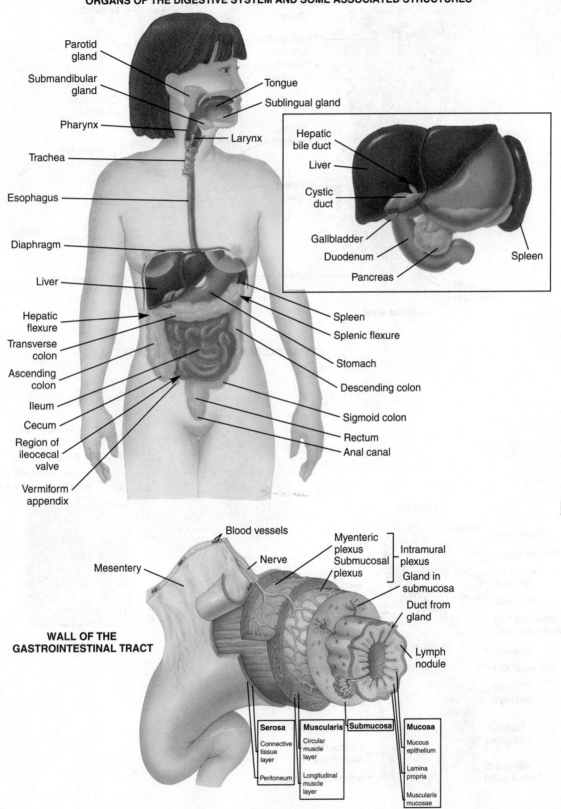

Parotid gland

Submandibular gland

Pharynx

Trachea

Esophagus

Diaphragm

Liver

Hepatic flexure

Transverse colon

Ascending colon

Ileum

Cecum

Region of ileocecal valve

Vermiform appendix

Tongue

Sublingual gland

Larynx

Hepatic bile duct

Liver

Cystic duct

Gallbladder

Duodenum

Pancreas

Spleen

Spleen

Splenic flexure

Stomach

Descending colon

Sigmoid colon

Rectum

Anal canal

Blood vessels

Mesentery

Nerve

Myenteric plexus

Submucosal plexus

Intramural plexus

Gland in submucosa

Duct from gland

Lymph nodule

WALL OF THE GASTROINTESTINAL TRACT

Serosa	**Muscularis**	**Submucosa**	**Mucosa**
Connective tissue layer	Circular muscle layer		Mucous epithelium
Peritoneum	Longitudinal muscle layer		Lamina propria
			Muscularis mucosae

A-32

LOCATION OF THE SALIVARY GLANDS

Parotid duct

Parotid gland

Sternocleidomastoid muscle

Buccinator muscle

Masseter muscle

Mandible (cut)

Submandibular duct (Wharton's duct)

Submandibular gland

Tongue

Frenulum of tongue

Minor sublingual ducts

Major sublingual ducts

Sublingual gland

Mandible (cut)

Mylohyoid muscle

Digastric muscle

Left portion of mandible has been removed

SOURCES OF INTESTINAL SECRETIONS
Bile from the bladder, pancreatic juice from the exocrine pancreas, and mucus secretion from Brunner's glands in the duodenal wall.

Stomach

Cystic duct

Common hepatic duct

Gallbladder neck

Gallbladder

Pancreas (tail)

Spleen

Common bile duct

Villi

Brunner's glands

Ampulla

Duodenum

Pancreas (head)

Pancreatic duct

A-33

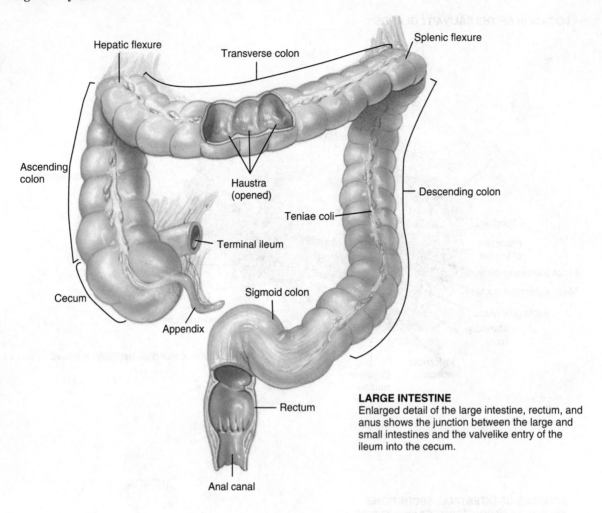

Hepatic flexure

Transverse colon

Splenic flexure

Ascending colon

Haustra (opened)

Descending colon

Teniae coli

Terminal ileum

Cecum

Sigmoid colon

Appendix

Rectum

LARGE INTESTINE
Enlarged detail of the large intestine, rectum, and anus shows the junction between the large and small intestines and the valvelike entry of the ileum into the cecum.

Anal canal

Teniae coli

Haustra

CECUM AND TERMINAL ILEUM

Ascending colon

Ileocecal valve

Terminal portion of ileum

Cecum

Orifice to appendix

Appendix

REPRODUCTIVE SYSTEM

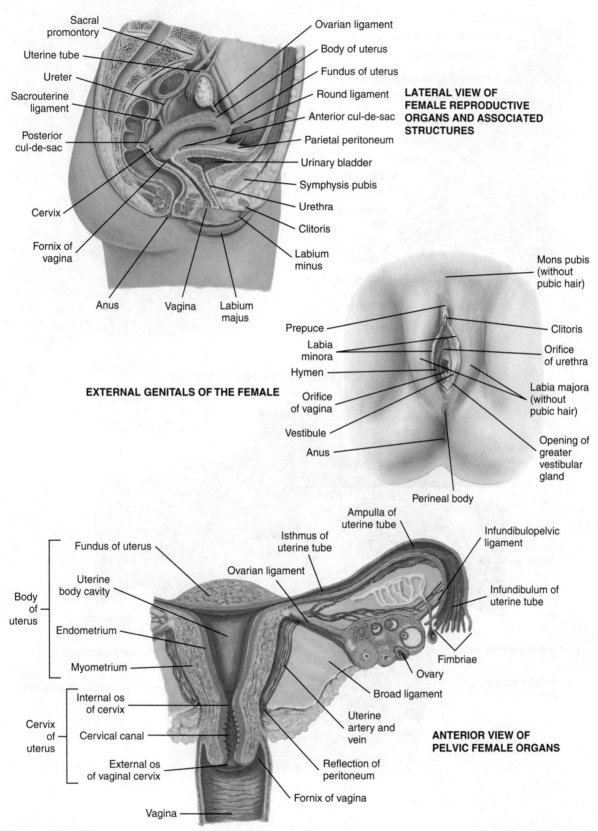

LATERAL VIEW OF FEMALE REPRODUCTIVE ORGANS AND ASSOCIATED STRUCTURES

Sacral promontory
Uterine tube
Ureter
Sacrouterine ligament
Posterior cul-de-sac
Cervix
Fornix of vagina
Anus
Vagina
Labium majus

Ovarian ligament
Body of uterus
Fundus of uterus
Round ligament
Anterior cul-de-sac
Parietal peritoneum
Urinary bladder
Symphysis pubis
Urethra
Clitoris
Labium minus

EXTERNAL GENITALS OF THE FEMALE

Prepuce
Labia minora
Hymen
Orifice of vagina
Vestibule
Anus

Mons pubis (without pubic hair)
Clitoris
Orifice of urethra
Labia majora (without pubic hair)
Opening of greater vestibular gland
Perineal body

ANTERIOR VIEW OF PELVIC FEMALE ORGANS

Fundus of uterus
Uterine body cavity
Body of uterus
Endometrium
Myometrium
Internal os of cervix
Cervix of uterus
Cervical canal
External os of vaginal cervix
Vagina

Ovarian ligament
Isthmus of uterine tube
Ampulla of uterine tube
Infundibulopelvic ligament
Infundibulum of uterine tube
Fimbriae
Ovary
Broad ligament
Uterine artery and vein
Reflection of peritoneum
Fornix of vagina

A-35

FEMALE BREAST

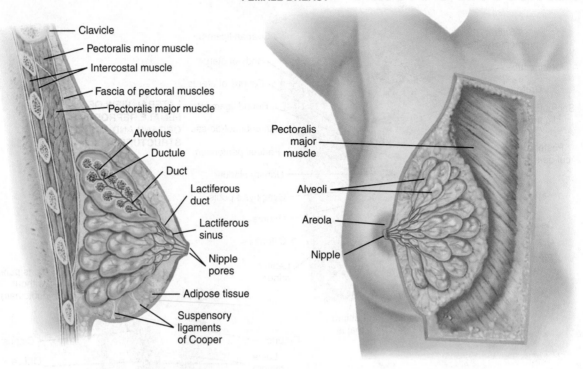

Clavicle
Pectoralis minor muscle
Intercostal muscle
Fascia of pectoral muscles
Pectoralis major muscle
Alveolus
Ductule
Duct
Lactiferous duct
Lactiferous sinus
Nipple pores
Adipose tissue
Suspensory ligaments of Cooper

Pectoralis major muscle
Alveoli
Areola
Nipple

LYMPHATIC SYSTEM AND THE FEMALE BREAST

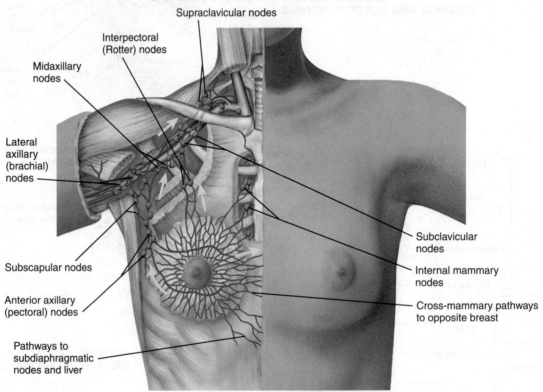

Supraclavicular nodes
Interpectoral (Rotter) nodes
Midaxillary nodes
Lateral axillary (brachial) nodes
Subscapular nodes
Anterior axillary (pectoral) nodes
Pathways to subdiaphragmatic nodes and liver
Subclavicular nodes
Internal mammary nodes
Cross-mammary pathways to opposite breast

MALE REPRODUCTIVE ORGANS AND
ASSOCIATED STRUCTURES

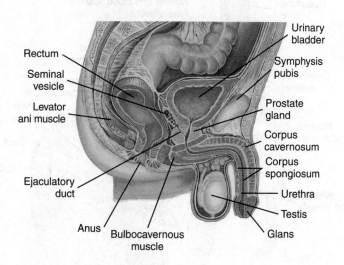

Rectum

Seminal
vesicle

Levator
ani muscle

Ejaculatory
duct

Anus   Bulbocavernous
muscle

Urinary
bladder

Symphysis
pubis

Prostate
gland

Corpus
cavernosum

Corpus
spongiosum

Urethra

Testis

Glans

EXTERNAL GENITALS OF
THE MALE

Location of
symphysis pubis

Urogenital
triangle

Location of
ischial tuberosity

Anal
triangle

Anus

Location of
coccyx

TUBULES OF THE TESTIS AND EPIDIDYMUS

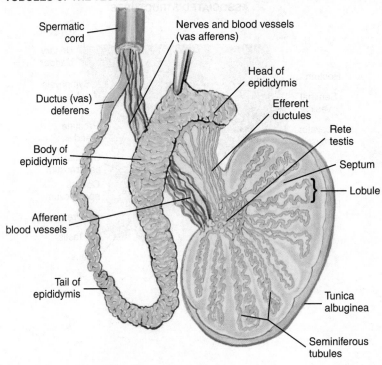

Spermatic cord

Nerves and blood vessels (vas afferens)

Head of epididymis

Efferent ductules

Ductus (vas) deferens

Rete testis

Body of epididymis

Septum

Lobule

Afferent blood vessels

Tail of epididymis

Tunica albuginea

Seminiferous tubules

ANTERIOR VIEW OF MALE REPRODUCTIVE STRUCTURES

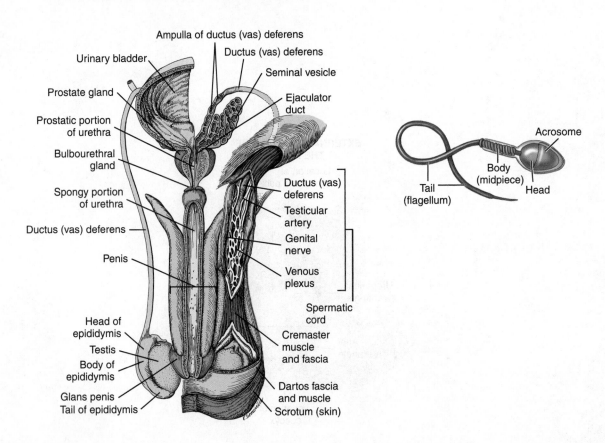

Ampulla of ductus (vas) deferens

Urinary bladder

Ductus (vas) deferens

Prostate gland

Seminal vesicle

Prostatic portion of urethra

Ejaculator duct

Bulbourethral gland

Ductus (vas) deferens

Spongy portion of urethra

Testicular artery

Ductus (vas) deferens

Genital nerve

Penis

Venous plexus

Spermatic cord

Head of epididymis

Cremaster muscle and fascia

Testis

Body of epididymis

Glans penis

Dartos fascia and muscle

Tail of epididymis

Scrotum (skin)

Acrosome

Body (midpiece)

Tail (flagellum)

Head

URINARY SYSTEM

URINARY SYSTEM AND SOME ASSOCIATED STRUCTURES

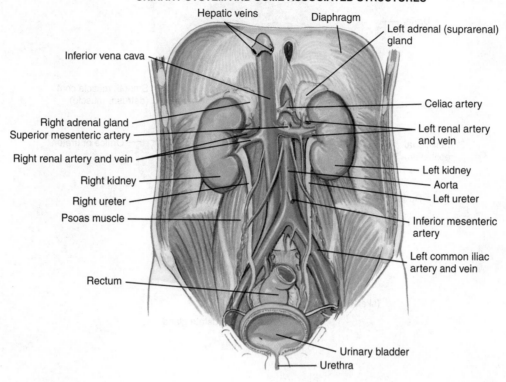

Hepatic veins
Diaphragm
Left adrenal (suprarenal) gland
Inferior vena cava
Celiac artery
Right adrenal gland
Superior mesenteric artery
Left renal artery and vein
Right renal artery and vein
Right kidney
Left kidney
Right ureter
Aorta
Left ureter
Psoas muscle
Inferior mesenteric artery
Left common iliac artery and vein
Rectum
Urinary bladder
Urethra

Vertebra
Renal artery
Muscle
Renal capsule
Kidney
Renal fat pad
Renal vein
Abdominal aorta
Inferior vena cava
Peritoneum
Peritoneal cavity
Body wall

BLADDER

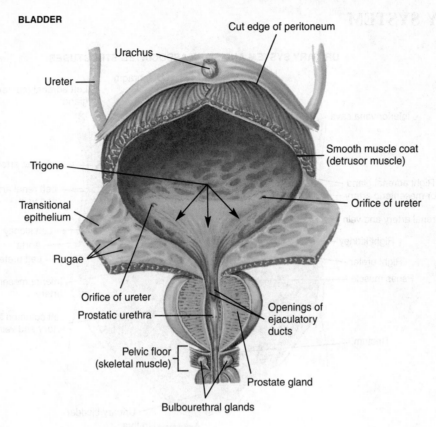

Urachus

Cut edge of peritoneum

Ureter

Trigone

Smooth muscle coat
(detrusor muscle)

Transitional
epithelium

Orifice of ureter

Rugae

Orifice of ureter

Openings of
ejaculatory
ducts

Prostatic urethra

Pelvic floor
(skeletal muscle)

Prostate gland

Bulbourethral glands

INTERNAL STRUCTURE OF THE KIDNEY

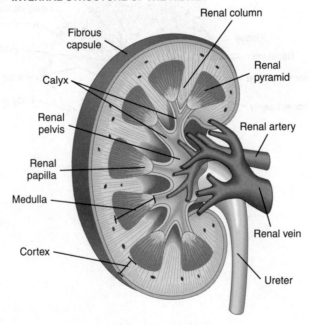

Renal column

Fibrous
capsule

Calyx

Renal
pyramid

Renal
pelvis

Renal artery

Renal
papilla

Medulla

Renal vein

Cortex

Ureter

NEPHRON

Proximal
convoluted
tubule

Renal
corpuscle [Bowman's capsule
Glomerulus

Efferent arteriole

Juxtaglomerular
apparatus

Afferent
arteriole

Peritubular
capillaries

Distal
convoluted
tubule

Interlobular artery
and vein

Arcuate artery
and vein

Peritubular
capillaries
(vasa recta)

Collecting tubule

Ascending
limb of
Henle's loop

Descending
limb of
Henle's loop

SPECIAL SENSES

GROSS ANATOMY OF THE EAR

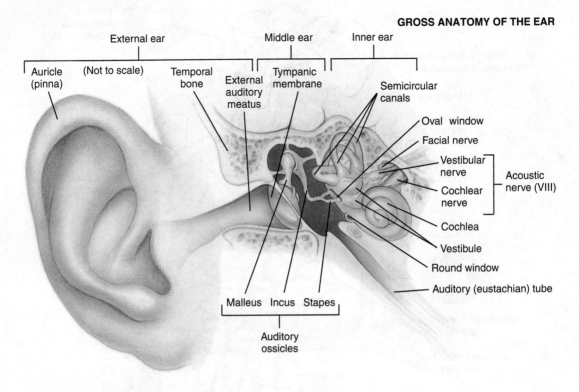

External ear

Middle ear

Inner ear

Auricle (pinna)

(Not to scale)

Temporal bone

External auditory meatus

Tympanic membrane

Semicircular canals

Oval window

Facial nerve

Vestibular nerve

Cochlear nerve

Acoustic nerve (VIII)

Cochlea

Vestibule

Round window

Auditory (eustachian) tube

Malleus   Incus   Stapes

Auditory ossicles

STRUCTURE OF THE SKIN

Hair shaft

Openings of sweat ducts

Stratum corneum

Stratum granulosum

Epidermis

Stratum spinosum

Stratum germinativum

Stratum basale

Dermis

Dermal papilla

Meissner corpuscle

Subcutaneous layer (hypodermis)

Sebaceous (oil gland)

Hair follicle

Papilla of hair

Sweat gland

Cutaneous nerve

Pacinian corpuscle

Arrector pili muscle

A-42

CROSS-SECTIONAL VIEW OF THE EYE

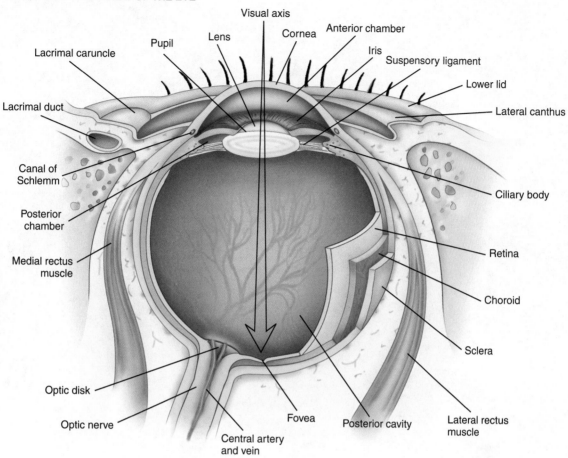

Visual axis

Lacrimal caruncle

Pupil

Lens

Cornea

Anterior chamber

Iris

Suspensory ligament

Lower lid

Lateral canthus

Lacrimal duct

Canal of Schlemm

Posterior chamber

Medial rectus muscle

Ciliary body

Retina

Choroid

Sclera

Optic disk

Optic nerve

Central artery and vein

Fovea

Posterior cavity

Lateral rectus muscle

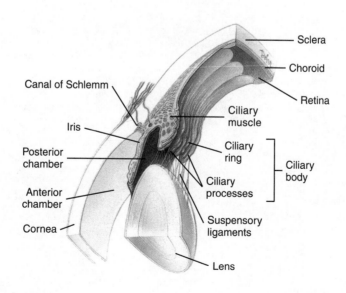

Canal of Schlemm

Iris

Posterior chamber

Anterior chamber

Cornea

Sclera

Choroid

Retina

Ciliary muscle

Ciliary ring

Ciliary body

Ciliary processes

Suspensory ligaments

Lens

a, symbol for **arterial blood,** as in PaO$_2$.

A, **1.** abbreviation for **accommodation. 2.** symbol for alveolar gas. **3.** abbreviation for **ampere. 4.** abbreviation for **anterior. 5.** abbreviation for **atomic weight (mass). 6.** abbreviation for **axial. 7.** symbol for **mass number. 8.** abbreviation for **absolute (temperature). 9.** symbol for **arterial. 10.** symbol for **anesthesia.**

Α, α. See **alpha.**

Å, symbol for **angstrom,** a unit for distance. 1Å = 10^{-10} m.

a-, **1.** a prefix meaning "before" from Latin, *ante.* **2.** a prefix meaning "without," "away from," "not," from Greek *a.*

A68, symbol for a protein found in the brain tissue of Alzheimer's disease patients. It is also found in the developing normal brains of fetuses and infants but begins to disappear by the age of 2 years. It is a major subunit of paired helical filaments and derivatized forms of tau. See also **tau protein.**

AA, **1.** abbreviation for **achievement age. 2.** abbreviation for **Alcoholics Anonymous. 3.** abbreviation for **amplitude of accommodation. 4.** abbreviation for **anesthesiologist's assistant. 5.** abbreviation for **amino acid. 6.** abbreviation for **anterior apical. 7.** abbreviation for **aortic arch. 8.** abbreviation for arm-ankle (pulse rate).

āa, a̅a̅, AA, (in prescriptions) abbreviation for *ana,* indicating an equal amount of each ingredient to be compounded.

AAA, **1.** abbreviation for *American Association of Anatomists.* **2.** abbreviation for **acquired aplastic anemia. 3.** abbreviation for **abdominal aortic aneurysm.**

AAAI, abbreviation for **American Academy of Allergy and Immunology.**

AACE, abbreviation for *American Association of Clinical Endocrinologists.*

AACN, **1.** abbreviation for **American Association of Colleges of Nursing. 2.** abbreviation for **American Association of Critical Care Nurses.**

AAFP, abbreviation for *American Academy of Family Physicians.*

AAI, abbreviation for **ankle-arm index.** See **ankle-brachial index.**

AAIN, abbreviation for **American Association of Industrial Nurses.**

AAL, abbreviation for **anterior axillary line.**

AAMC, abbreviation for **American Association of Medical Colleges.**

AAMI, abbreviation for **Association for the Advancement of Medical Instrumentation.**

AAN, abbreviation for **American Academy of Nursing.**

AANA, abbreviation for **American Association of Nurse Anesthetists.**

AANN, **1.** abbreviation for **American Association of Neuroscience Nurses. 2.** abbreviation for **American Association of Neurological Nurses.**

AAOHN, abbreviation for *American Association of Occupational Health Nurses.*

AAO-HNS, abbreviation for *American Academy of Otolaryngology-Head and Neck Surgery.*

AAOMS, abbreviation for *American Association of Oral and Maxillofacial Surgeons.*

AAPA, abbreviation for **American Academy of Physicians' Assistants.**

AAPB, abbreviation for **American Association of Pathologists and Bacteriologists.**

AAPMR, abbreviation for **American Academy of Physical Medicine and Rehabilitation.**

Aaron's sign [Charles D. Aaron, American physician, 1866–1951], a diagnostic sign in appendicitis indicated by pain or distress when pressure is applied over McBurney's point in the epigastric region. See also **McBurney's point.**

AARP, abbreviation for **American Association of Retired Persons.**

Aarskog syndrome /ärs'kog/ [Dagfinn Charles Aarskog, Norwegian pediatrician, b. 1928], an X-linked syndrome characterized by ocular hypertelorism, anteverted nostrils, broad upper lip, peculiar scrotal "shawl" above the penis, and small hands. Also called **faciodigitogenital syndrome, faciogenital dysplasia.**

AART, abbreviation for **American Association for Respiratory Therapy.**

Aase syndrome /äz/ [Jon Morton Aase, American pediatrician, b. 1936], a familial syndrome characterized by mild growth retardation, hypoplastic anemia, variable leukocytopenia, triphalangeal thumbs, narrow shoulders, and late closure of fontanels, and occasionally by cleft lip, cleft palate, retinopathy, and web neck. A recessive mode of inheritance has been suggested.

AAUP, abbreviation for **American Association of University Professors.**

AAV, abbreviation for **adenoassociated virus.**

Ab, abbreviation for **antibody.**

ab-, abs-, a prefix meaning 'from, off, away from': *abstract, abnormal.*

abacavir, an antiviral, it is a nucleoside reverse transcriptase inhibitor.

■ INDICATIONS: It is prescribed in combination with other antiretroviral agents for HIV-1 infection.

■ CONTRAINDICATIONS: Known hypersensitivity to this drug prohibits its use.

■ ADVERSE EFFECTS: Hypersensitivity reactions occur in approximately 5% of patients, and can be fatal. Other life-threatening adverse effects include granulocytopenia, anemia, fatal hypersensitivity reactions, and lactic acidosis. Common side effects include fever, headache, malaise, insomnia, nausea, vomiting, diarrhea, anorexia, and rash.

abacterial /ab'aktir'ē·əl/, any atmosphere or condition free of bacteria; literally, without bacteria.

abaissement /ä'bāsmäN'/ [Fr, a lowering], **1.** a falling or depressing. **2.** (in ophthalmology) the displacement of a lens.

abalienation /abāl'yənā'shən/, a state of physical deterioration or mental decay. —**abalienate,** *v.,* **abalienated,** *adj.*

Ab amyloid, an abnormal peptide, varying from 40 to 43 amino acids in length and found in aggregates in the cerebrovascular walls and the cores of the plaques in Alzheimer's disease. It is derived from a large transmembrane glycoprotein, amyloid precursor protein. It is postulated to be neurotoxic.

A band, the area between two I bands of a sarcomere, marked by partial overlapping of actin and myosin filaments and appearing dark.

abandonment of care /əban'dənment/, (in law) wrongful cessation of the provision of care to a patient, usually by a physician or a nurse. Unilateral termination of care without the patient's consent or knowledge.

abapical /abap'əkəl/, opposite the apex.

abarognosis /aber'agnō'sis/ [Gk, *a*, not, *baros*, weight, *gnosis*, knowledge], an inability to judge or compare the weight of objects, particularly those held in the hand.

abarthrosis. See **synovial joint.**

abarticular /ab'ärtik'yŏŏlər/, **1.** pertaining to a condition that does not affect a joint. **2.** pertaining to a site or structure remote from a joint.

abarticular gout [L, *ab*, away from, *articulus*, joint], gout that affects structures other than joints, such as ligaments.

abarticulation /ab'ärtik'yəlā'shən/, **1.** dislocation of a joint. **2.** a synovial joint.

abasia /əbā'zhə/ [Gk, *a, basis*, not step], the inability to walk, caused by lack of motor coordination. —**abasic, abatic,** *adj.*

abasia-astasia. See **astasia-abasia.**

abate /əbāt'/ [ME, *abaten*, to beat down], to decrease or reduce in severity or degree.

abatement /əbāt'mənt/, a decrease in severity of symptoms.

abatic, pertaining to an inability to walk.

abaxial /abak'sē·əl/ [L, *ab, axis* from axle], **1.** pertaining to a position outside the axis of a body or structure. **2.** pertaining to a position at the opposite extremity of a structure.

Abbe-Estlander operation /ab'ē·est'-/ [Robert Abbé, American surgeon, 1851–1928; Jakob A. Estlander, Finnish surgeon, 1831–1881], a surgical procedure that transfers a full-thickness section of one oral lip to the other lip, using an arterial pedicle for ensuring survival of a graft.

Abbé-Zeiss apparatus /äbā'tsīs'/ [Ernst K. Abbé, German physicist, 1840–1905; Carl Zeiss, German optician, 1816–1885], an apparatus for calculating the number of blood cells in a measured amount of blood. See also **hemacytometer.**

Abbokinase, a trademark for a plasminogen activator (urokinase).

Abbott-Miller tube. See **Miller-Abbott tube.**

Abbott pump, a trademark for a small portable pump that can be adjusted and finely calibrated to deliver precise amounts of medication in solution through an IV infusion set. It is similar to a Harvard pump, but the flow rate may be increased or decreased by smaller increments. See also **Harvard pump.**

ABC, 1. abbreviation for airway, breathing, circulation. **2.** abbreviation for **aspiration biopsy cytology.**

abciximab /ab-sik'sĭ-mab/, a human-murine monoclonal antibody Fab fragment that inhibits the aggregation of platelets, used in prevention of thrombosis in percutaneous transluminal coronary angioplasty, administered by intravenous infusion.

■ INDICATIONS: It is prescribed as an adjunct to percutaneous transluminal coronary angioplasty or atherectomy.

■ CONTRAINDICATIONS: The drug should not be given to patients with active internal bleeding, recent GI or urinary bleeding of significance, history of stroke, thrombocytopenia, or recent major surgery.

■ ADVERSE EFFECTS: The side effects most often reported include bleeding, thrombocytopenia, pulmonary edema, atrioventricular block, and atrial fibrillation.

Abdellah, Faye Glenn, [b.1919], a nursing theorist who introduced a typology of 21 nursing problems in 1960 in *Patient-Centered Approaches to Nursing.* The concepts of nursing, nursing problems, and the problem-solving process are central to Abdellah's work. The typology is divided into three areas: (1) the physical, sociological, and emotional needs of the patient; (2) the types of interpersonal relationships between the nurse and the patient; and (3) the common elements of patient care. It was formulated in terms of nursing-centered services that can be used to determine the patient's needs and to teach and evaluate nursing students. It was based on systematic research studies. The typology provided a scientific body of knowledge unique to nursing, making it possible to move away from the medical model of educating nurses. The nursing diagnosis classification system may be considered an outgrowth of Abdellah's typology.

abdomen /ab'dəmən, abdō'mən/ [L, belly], the portion of the body between the thorax and the pelvis. The abdominal cavity is lined by the peritoneum; contains the inferior portion of the esophagus, the stomach, the intestines, the liver, the spleen, the pancreas, and other organs; and is bounded by the diaphragm and the pelvis. Also called (*informal*) **belly.** See also **abdominal regions.** —**abdominal** /abdom'-/, *adj.*

abdominal actinomycosis. See **actinomycosis.**

abdominal adhesion /abdom'inəl/, the binding together of tissue surfaces of abdominal organs, usually involving the intestines and causing obstruction. The condition may result from trauma or inflammation and may form after abdominal surgery. The patient experiences abdominal distension, pain, nausea, vomiting, and increased pulse rate. Surgery may be required.

abdominal aorta, the portion of the descending aorta that passes from the aortic hiatus of the diaphragm into the abdomen, descending ventral to the vertebral column, and ending at the fourth lumbar vertebra, where it divides into the two common iliac arteries. It supplies blood to abdominal structures, such as the testes, ovaries, kidneys, and stomach. Its branches are the celiac, superior mesenteric, inferior mesenteric, middle suprarenal, renal, testicular, ovarian, inferior phrenic, lumbar, middle sacral, and common iliac arteries. See also **descending aorta.** Compare **thoracic aorta.**

abdominal aortic aneurysm, a common type of aneurysm, found in the abdominal aorta, usually in an area of severe atherosclerosis.

abdominal aortography, a radiographic study of the abdominal aorta after the introduction of a contrast medium through a catheter in the femoral artery.

abdominal aponeurosis, the conjoined sheetlike tendons of the oblique and transverse skeletal muscles of the abdomen.

abdominal bandage, a broad absorbent gauze or other material commonly used after abdominal surgery.

abdominal binder, a bandage or elasticized wrap that is applied around the lower part of the torso to support the abdomen. It is sometimes applied after abdominal surgery to decrease discomfort, thereby increasing a patient's ability to begin ambulatory activities and accelerating convalescence.

abdominal breathing, a pattern of inhalation and exhalation in which most of the ventilatory work is done with the abdominal muscles. The contractile force of the abdomen is used to elevate the diaphragm. See also **diaphragmatic breathing.**

Abdominal aortic aneurysm
(Mace and Kowalczyk, 2004/courtesy Riverside Methodist Hospitals)

abdominal cavity, the space within the abdominal walls between the diaphragm and the pelvic area, containing the liver, stomach, intestines, spleen, gallbladder, kidneys, and associated tissues and blood and lymph vessels.

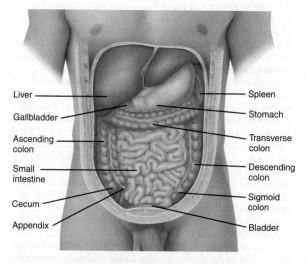

Liver
Gallbladder
Ascending colon
Small intestine
Cecum
Appendix

Spleen
Stomach
Transverse colon
Descending colon
Sigmoid colon
Bladder

Abdominal cavity *(Seidel et al, 2003)*

abdominal decompression, an obstetric technique to reduce pressure on the abdomen during the first stage of labor. The abdomen is enclosed in a chamber that permits surrounding pressure to be controlled. The technique is no longer used.

abdominal delivery, the delivery of a child through a surgical incision in the abdomen. See **cesarean section.**

abdominal examination, the physical assessment of a patient's abdomen by visual inspection and the use of auscultation, percussion, and palpation. Visual inspection of the normally oval shape of the abdominal surface while the patient is supine may reveal abnormal surface features indicating effects of disease, surgery, or injury. Subsurface tumors, fluid accumulation, or hypertrophy of the liver or spleen may be observed as an abnormal surface feature. Auscultation may reveal vascular sounds that provide information about arterial disorders such as aortic aneurysms as well as bowel sounds that are indicative of intestinal function. In the pregnant patient, auscultation can detect fetal heartbeat and blood circulation in the placenta. Percussion involves gently striking the abdominal wall at various points to produce sounds. The sounds help detect the condition of internal organs. In palpation, indirect exploration of the abdomen is performed by using the examiner's sense of touch to detect areas of tenderness or rigidity, muscle tone and skin condition, and shapes and sizes of subsurface organs or masses.

abdominal fistula, an abnormal passage from an abdominal organ to the surface of the abdomen. In a colostomy, a passage from the bowel to an opening on the surface of the abdomen is created surgically.

abdominal gestation, the implantation of a fertilized ovum outside the uterus but within the peritoneal cavity. See also **ectopic pregnancy.**

abdominalgia /abdom'ənal'jə/ [L, *abdomen,* belly; Gk, *algos,* pain], a pain in the abdomen.

abdominal girth, the circumference of the abdomen, usually measured at the umbilicus.

abdominal hernia, a hernia in which a loop of bowel protrudes through the abdominal musculature, often through the site of an old surgical scar that has stretched and thinned. Also called **ventral hernia.** See also **hernia.**

abdominal hysterectomy, the removal of the uterus through the abdominal wall. Also called **abdominohysterectomy.**

abdominal inguinal ring, an opening of the inguinal canal on the abdominal wall, through which the male spermatic cord and the female round ligament pass. The deep abdominal inguinal ring is marked by an oval depression on the deep aspect of the anterior abdominal wall, just above the inguinal ligament. The superficial abdominal inguinal ring is a triangle-shaped opening in the aponeurosis of the external oblique muscle.

abdominal muscles, the set of muscles that make up the ventral abdominal wall, including the external oblique (*obliquus externus abdominis*), internal oblique (*obliquus internus abdominis*), transversalis (*transversus abdominis*), rectus abdominis, and pyramidalis. Broad and thin, the external oblique muscle is the largest and most superficial of the abdominal muscles; it is situated in the lateral and ventral walls of the abdomen. The internal oblique muscle is also situated in the lateral and ventral walls of the abdomen, but is smaller and thinner. The *transversus abdominis* is the most internal of the flat muscles of the abdomen. The *rectus abdominis* is a long, flat muscle that runs the entire length of the front of the abdomen. The *pyramidalis* is a small triangular muscle at the bottom front of the abdomen. The abdominal muscles compress the abdominal contents during urination, defecation, vomiting, parturition, and forced expiration.

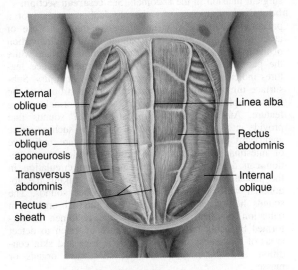

Abdominal muscles *(Seidel et al, 2003)*

Labels on figure: External oblique, External oblique aponeurosis, Transversus abdominis, Rectus sheath, Linea alba, Rectus abdominis, Internal oblique

abdominal nephrectomy [L, *abdominis,* belly; Gk, *nephr,* kidney, *ektomē,* cutting out], the surgical removal of a kidney through an abdominal incision.

abdominal pain, acute or chronic, localized or diffuse pain in the abdominal cavity. Abdominal pain is a significant symptom because its cause may require immediate surgical or medical intervention. The most common causes of severe abdominal pain are inflammation, perforation of an intraabdominal structure, circulatory obstruction, intestinal or ureteral obstruction, intestinal cramping, or rupture of an organ located within the abdomen. Specific conditions include appendicitis, perforated gastric ulcer, strangulated hernia, superior mesenteric arterial thrombosis, diverticulitis, and small and large bowel obstruction. Differential diagnosis of the cause of acute abdominal pain requires its localization and characterization by means of light and deep palpation, auscultation, percussion, and abdominal, rectal, or pelvic examination. Direct physical examination may be supplemented by various laboratory and radiologic examinations. Aspiration of peritoneal fluid (paracentesis) for bacteriologic and chemical evaluation is sometimes indicated. Conditions producing acute abdominal pain that may require surgery include appendicitis, acute or severe and chronic diverticulitis, acute and chronic cholecystitis, cholelithiasis, acute pancreatitis, perforation of a peptic ulcer, various intestinal obstructions, abdominal aortic aneurysms, and trauma affecting any of the abdominal organs. Gynecologic causes of acute abdominal pain that may require surgery include acute pelvic inflammatory disease, ruptured ovarian cyst, and ectopic pregnancy. Abdominal pain associated with pregnancy may be caused by the weight of the enlarged uterus; rotation, stretching, or compression of the round ligament; or squeezing or displacement of the bowel. In addition, uterine contractions associated with premature labor may produce severe abdominal pain. Chronic abdominal pain may be

functional or may result from overeating or excessive air swallowing (aerophagia). When symptoms are recurrent, an organic cause is considered. Organic sources of abdominal pain include peptic ulcer, hiatal hernia, gastritis, chronic cholecystitis and cholelithiasis, chronic pancreatitis, pancreatic carcinoma, chronic diverticulitis, intermittent low-grade intestinal obstruction, and functional indigestion. Some systemic conditions may cause abdominal pain. Examples include systemic lupus erythematosus, lead poisoning, hypercalcemia, sickle cell anemia, diabetic acidosis, porphyria, tabes dorsalis, and black widow spider poisoning.

abdominal paracentesis [L, *abdominis,* belly; Gk, *para,* near, *kentesis,* puncturing], the surgical puncturing of the abdominal cavity to remove fluid for diagnosis or treatment.

abdominal pregnancy, an extrauterine pregnancy in which the conceptus develops in the abdominal cavity after being extruded from the fimbriated end of the fallopian tube or through a defect in the tube or uterus. The placenta may implant on the abdominal or visceral peritoneum. Abdominal pregnancy may be suspected when the abdomen has enlarged but the uterus has remained small for the length of gestation. Abdominal pregnancies constitute approximately 2% of ectopic pregnancies and approximately 0.01% of all pregnancies. The condition results in perinatal death of the fetus in most cases, maternal death in approximately 6%. Because of its rarity, the condition may be unsuspected, and diagnosis is often delayed. Ultrasound or x-ray visualization showing gas in the maternal bowel below the fetus is diagnostic of the condition. Surgical removal of the placenta, sac, and embryo or fetus is necessary if attached to the posterior part of the tube, ovary, broad ligament and uterus. The procedure is often complicated by massive bleeding, and, because the placenta tends to adhere firmly to the peritoneum and to the bowel, complete removal is seldom possible. Allowing it to be absorbed presents fewer problems. Postoperative sequelae may include retained placental tissue, infection, continued bleeding, and sterility.

abdominal pressure, See **intraabdominal pressure.**

abdominal pulse, the pulse of the abdominal aorta.

abdominal quadrant, any of four topographic areas of the abdomen divided by two imaginary lines, one vertical and one horizontal, intersecting at the umbilicus. The divisions are the left upper quadrant (LUQ), the left lower quadrant (LLQ), the right upper quadrant (RUQ), and the right lower quadrant (RLQ).

abdominal reflex, a superficial neurologic reflex obtained by firmly stroking the skin of the abdomen. It normally results in a brisk contraction of abdominal muscles in which the umbilicus moves toward the site of the stimulus. This reflex is lost in diseases of the pyramidal tract. See also **superficial reflex.**

abdominal regions, the nine topographic subdivisions of the abdomen, determined by four imaginary lines, in a tic-tac-toe pattern, imposed over the anterior surface. The upper horizontal line passes along the level of the cartilages of the ninth rib; the lower along the iliac crests. The two vertical lines extend on each side of the body from the cartilage of the eighth rib to the center of the inguinal ligament. The lines divide the abdomen into three upper, three middle, and three lower zones: right hypochondriac, epigastric, and left hypochondriac regions (upper zones); right lateral (lumbar), umbilical, and left lateral (lumbar) regions (middle zones); right inguinal (iliac), pubic (hypogastric), and left inguinal (iliac) regions (lower zones).

abdominal salpingectomy, a salpingectomy done through an incision in the abdomen. Also called **celiosalpingectomy, laparosalpingectomy.**

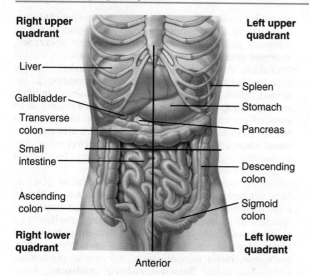

Abdominal quadrants *(Harkreader and Hogan, 2004)*

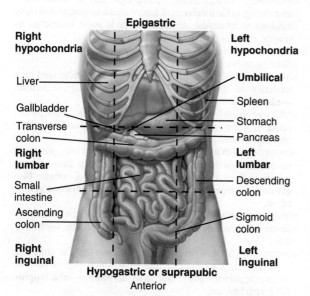

Abdominal regions *(Harkreader and Hogan, 2004)*

abdominal salpingotomy, a salpingotomy done through an incision in the abdominal wall.

abdominal splinting, a rigid contraction of the abdominal wall muscles. It usually occurs as an involuntary reaction to the pain of a visceral disease or disorder or postoperative discomfort. Abdominal splinting, in turn, may result in hypoventilation and respiratory complications. Also called **guarding.**

abdominal sponge [L, *abdominis,* belly; Gk, *spongia,* sponge], a special type of gauze pad used as an absorbent and covering for the viscera. See also **sponge.**

abdominal surgery, any operation that involves an incision into the abdomen. To prepare for surgery, laboratory, radiographic, and cardiac tests and consultations may be done. Immediately before surgery, body hair is clipped and skin is cleansed from the nipple line to the pubis. Food and fluids by mouth are withheld for up to 6 hours or more before surgery. After surgery the nurse ensures that the airway is patent and vital signs are stable, checks tubes and catheters, connects drainage tubes to collection containers, and checks the dressing for excessive bleeding or drainage, and records fluid intake and output. The patient is turned and is helped to breathe deeply every hour and, if secretions are present, to cough. Medication is given as needed for pain relief. Some kinds of abdominal surgery are **appendectomy, cholecystectomy, gastrectomy, herniorrhaphy, laparotomy.** See also **acute abdomen.**

abdominal tenaculum. See **tenaculum.**

abdominal testis, an undescended testis located in the abdominal cavity.

abdominal ultrasound test, an ultrasound test that provides accurate visualization of the abdominal aorta, liver, gallbladder, pancreas, bile ducts, kidneys, ureters, and bladder. This test is used to diagnose and locate cysts, tumors, calculi, and malformations; to document the progression of various diseases; and to guide the insertion of instruments during surgical procedures.

abdominal wound, a break in the continuity of the abdominal wall. A wound that exposes or penetrates the viscera raises the danger of infection or peritonitis.

abdomino- /abdom′inō-/, a combining form meaning 'abdomen': *abdominoscopy, abdominovesical.*

abdominocardiac reflex /-kär′dē·ək/, an immediate, involuntary response of the heart to stimulation of the abdominal viscera. The reflex is mediated through the vagus nerve.

abdominocentesis. See **paracentesis.**

abdominocyesis /abdom′inōsī·ē′sis/, an abdominal pregnancy.

abdominocystic. See **abdominovesical.**

abdominogenital /-jen′itəl/, pertaining to the abdomen and reproductive system.

abdominohysterectomy. See **abdominal hysterectomy.**

abdominohysterotomy /-his′tərot′əmē/, hysterotomy through an abdominal incision. See **hysterotomy.**

abdominopelvic cavity /-pel′vik/, the space between the diaphragm and the groin. There is no structurally distinct separation between the abdomen and pelvic regions.

abdominoperineal /-per′inē′əl/, pertaining to the abdomen and the perineum, including the pelvic area, female vulva and anus, and male anus and scrotum.

abdominoplasty, a surgical procedure to tighten the abdominal muscles. Also called **tummy tuck.**

abdominoscopy /abdom′inos′kəpē/ [L, *abdomen;* Gk, *skopein,* to view], a procedure for examining the contents of the peritoneum in which an electrically illuminated tubular device is passed through a trocar into the abdominal cavity. Also called **peritoneoscopy.** See also **endoscopy, laparoscopy.**

abdominoscrotal /-skrō′təl/, pertaining to the abdomen and scrotum.

abdominothoracic arch /-thôras′ik/, the boundary between the thorax and the abdomen.

abdominovaginal /-vaj′inəl/, pertaining to the abdomen and vagina.

abdominovesical /-ves′ikəl/, pertaining to the abdomen and bladder. Also **abdominocystic.**

ABD pad, a multilayered absorbent dressing used after abdominal surgery.

abducens /abdoo′sənz/ [L, drawing away], pertaining to a movement away from the median line of the body.

abducens muscle, the extraocular lateral rectus muscle that moves the eyeball outward.

abducens nerve [L, *abducere,* to take away], either of the paired sixth cranial nerves. It arises in the pons near the fourth ventricle, leaves the brainstem between the medulla oblongata and pons, and passes through the cavernous sinus and the superior orbital fissure. It controls the lateral rectus muscle, turning the eye outward. Also called abducent nerve, **nervus abducens, sixth cranial nerve.**

Lateral rectus muscle (cut)

Abducens nerve

Abducens nerve

abduct /abdukt′/, to move away from an axis of the body.

abduction [L, *abducere,* to take away], movement of a limb away from the body. Compare **adduction.**

abduction boots, a pair of orthopedic casts for the lower extremities, available in both short-leg and long-leg configurations, with a bar incorporated at ankle level to provide hip abduction. Abduction boots are used for postoperative positioning and immobilization after hip adductor releases with total hip arthroplasty or hip prosthesis implantation. They also promote proper positioning during healing after surgical repair of the lower extremities.

abductor /abduk′tər/ [L, *abducere*], a muscle that draws a body part away from the midline or axis, or one part from another. Compare **adductor.**

abembryonic /ab′embrē·on′ik/, opposite the position of the embryo.

Abernethy's sarcoma /ab′ərnē′thēz/ [John Abernethy, British surgeon, 1764–1831], a malignant neoplasm of fat cells, usually occurring on the trunk.

aberrancy. See **aberrant ventricular conduction.**

aberrant /aber′ənt/, [L, *aberrare,* to wander], **1.** pertaining to a wandering from the usual or expected course, such as various ducts, nerves, vessels in the body, or cardiac conduction. **2.** (in botany and zoology) pertaining to an abnormal individual, such as certain atypical members of a species.

aberrant conduction. See **aberrant ventricular conduction.**

aberrant goiter, an enlargement of a supernumerary or ectopic thyroid gland.

aberrant ventricular conduction (AVC), the temporary abnormal intraventricular conduction of a supraventricular impulse. It is usually associated with an increase in the duration of the QRS complex to more than 120 msec. This conduction pattern is fairly common after a very premature atrial beat and during the paroxysmal supraventricular tachy-

cardia that is caused by orthodromic circus movement tachycardia (using the atrioventricular node intergradely and an accessory pathway retrogradely). Also called **aberrancy, aberrant conduction, ventricular aberration.**

aberration /ab′ərā′shən/, [L, *aberrare,* to wander], **1.** any departure from the usual course or normal condition. **2.** abnormal growth or development. **3.** (in psychology) an illogical and unreasonable thought or belief, often leading to an unsound mental state. **4.** (in genetics) any change in the number or structure of the chromosomes. See also **chromosomal aberration. 5.** (in optics) any imperfect image formation blurring caused by unequal refraction or focalization of light rays through a lens.

abetalipoproteinemia /əbā′təlip′ōprō′tinē′mē·ə/ [Gk, *a, beta,* not beta, *lipos,* fat, *proteios,* first rank, *haima,* blood], a group of rare inherited disorders of fat metabolism, characterized by absence of apoprotein B-100 and manifested by acanthocytosis, low or absent serum beta-lipoproteins, and hypocholesterolemia. In severe cases steatorrhea, ataxia, nystagmus, motor incoordination, and retinitis pigmentosa occur. Also called **Bassen-Kornzweig syndrome** /-kôrn′zwīg/.

abeyance /əbā′əns/, [Fr], a temporary state of inaction or temporary interruption of function.

abfraction /ab-frak′shun/, pathologic loss of tooth structure owing to biomechanical forces (flexion, compression, or tension) or chemical degradation. It is most visible as V-shaped notches in the cervical area of a tooth.

ABG, abbreviation for **arterial blood gas.**

ABI, abbreviation for **ankle-brachial index.**

abient /ab′ē·ənt/ [L, *abire,* to go away], characterized by a tendency to move away from stimuli. Compare **adient. —abience,** *n.*

ability /əbil′itē/, the capacity to act in a specified way because of the possession of appropriate skills and mental or physical fitness.

abiogenesis /ab′ē·ōjen′əsis/ [Gk, *a + bios,* not life, *genein,* to produce], spontaneous generation, the idea that life can originate from inorganic, inanimate matter. Compare **biogenesis. -abiogenetic,** *adj.* Also called **spontaneous generation.**

abiosis /ab′ē·ō′sis/ [Gk, *a + bios* not life], a nonviable condition or a situation that is incompatible with life. **—abiotic,** *adj.*

abiotrophy /ab′ē·ot′rəfē/ [Gk, *a + bios + trophe* nutrition, growth], degeneration or loss of function that is not due to any apparent injury. See also **atrophy. —abiotrophic** /ab′ē·ətrō′fik/, *adj.*

ablastemic /ab′lastem′ik/, nongerminal or not germinating.

ablate /ablāt′/ [L, *ab + latus,* carried away], to cut away or remove, as in ablation.

ablation /ablā′shən/, [L, *ab + latus,* carried away], **1.** an amputation, an excision of any part of the body, or a removal of a growth or harmful substance. **2.** reduction by melting.

ablatio placentae. See **abruptio placentae.**

ABLB test, abbreviation for **alternate binaural loudness balance test.**

-able, -ible, a suffix indicating 'ability or capacity': *intractable, flexible.*

ablepharia /ab′ləfer′ē·ə/, a defect characterized by partial or total absence of the eyelids.

ablepsia /əblep′sē·ə/ [Gk, *a + blepein,* not to see], the condition of being blind. Also called **ablepsy.**

abluent, pertaining to the ability of a substance, such as detergent, to cleanse or wash away.

ablution /abloo′shən/ [L, abluere, wash away], **1.** the act of washing or bathing. **2.** the act of cleaning the body.

ABMS, abbreviation for *American Board of Medical Specialties.*

abnerval current /abnur'vəl/ [L, *ab,* from; Gk, *neuron,* nerve], an electrical current that passes from a nerve to and through muscle.

abneural /abnŏŏr'əl/, away from the central nervous system or the neural axis.

abnormal behavior /abnôr'məl/, [L, *ab* + *norma,* away from rule], behavior that deviates from what is commonly accepted by a group or society. See also **behavior disorder.**

abnormality /ab'nôrmal'itē/ [L, *ab,* away from, *norma,* the rule], a condition that differs from the usual cultural or scientifically accepted norms.

abnormal psychology, the study of any behavior that deviates from culturally accepted norms.

abnormal tooth mobility, excessive movement of a tooth within its socket as a result of injury or disease in the supporting tissues.

ABO blood group, a system for classifying human blood based on the antigenic components of red blood cells and their corresponding antibodies. The ABO blood group is identified by the presence or absence of two different antigens, A and B, on the surface of the red blood cell. The four blood types in this grouping, A, B, AB, and O, are determined by and named for these antigens. Type AB indicates the presence of both antigens; type O the absence of both. Corresponding antibodies, anti-A and anti-B agglutinins, can be found in the plasma of type O blood. The plasma components of type A and type B blood are, respectively, devoid of anti-A and anti-B agglutinins; both agglutinins are absent from type AB blood plasma. In addition to its significant role in transfusion therapy and transplantation, the ABO blood grouping contributes to forensic medicine, to genetics, and, together with the less important blood groups, to anthropology and legal medicine. See also **blood group, Rh factor, transfusion.**

aboiement /ä'bô·ämäN'/, an involuntary making of abnormal, animal-like sounds, such as barking. Aboiement may be a clinical sign of Gilles de la Tourette's syndrome.

abort /əbôrt'/ [L, *ab,* away from, *oriri,* to be born], **1.** to deliver a nonviable fetus; to miscarry. See also **spontaneous abortion. 2.** to terminate a pregnancy before the fetus has developed enough to live outside the uterus. See also **induced abortion. 3.** to terminate in the early stages or to discontinue before completion, as to arrest the usual course of a disease, to stop growth and development, or to halt a project.

aborted systole, a contraction of the heart that is usually weak and is not associated with a radial pulse.

abortifacient /əbôr'tifā'shənt/, **1.** causing abortion. **2.** any agent that causes abortion.

abortion /əbor'shən/ [L, *ab* + *oriri*], the spontaneous or induced termination of pregnancy before the fetus has developed to the stage of viability. Kinds of abortion include **habitual abortion, infected abortion, septic abortion, threatened abortion, voluntary abortion.** See also **complete abortion, elective abortion, incomplete abortion, induced abortion, medical abortion, missed abortion, spontaneous abortion, therapeutic abortion.**

abortionist, a person who performs abortions.

abortion on demand, a concept promoted by prochoice health advocates that it is the right of a pregnant woman to have an abortion performed at her request. That right may be limited by time of gestation, or it may pertain to any period of gestation.

abortion pill. See **mifepristone.**

abortive infection /əbôr'tiv/, an infection in which some or all viral components have been synthesized, but no infective virus is produced. The situation may result from an infection with defective viruses or because the host cell is nonpermissive and prohibits replication of the particular virus.

abortus /əbôr'təs/, any incompletely developed fetus that results from an abortion, particularly one weighing less than 500 g.

abortus fever, a form of brucellosis, the only one endemic to North America. It is caused by *Brucella abortus,* an organism so named because it causes abortion in cows. Infection in humans results from the ingesting of contaminated milk or milk products from cows infected with *B. abortus,* from handling infected meat, or from skin contact with the excreta of living infected animals. A prolonged course of combination antibiotic therapy is required: doxycycline and a parenteral aminoglycoside followed by oral therapy with doxycycline and rifampin. Also called **Rio Grande fever.** See also **brucellosis.**

abouchement /ä'bōōshmäN'/ [Fr, a tube connection], the junction of a small blood vessel with a large blood vessel.

aboulia. See **abulia.**

above-elbow (AE) amputation, an amputation of the upper limb between the elbow and the shoulder. A short amputation (near the shoulder) results in the loss of shoulder rotation. After a long amputation (just above the elbow) the patient should retain good shoulder function. Also called **AE amputation.**

above-knee amputation. See **transfemoral amputation.**

ABP, abbreviation for **arterial blood pressure.**

ABPM, abbreviation for **ambulatory blood pressure monitoring.**

ABR, abbreviation for **auditory brainstem response.**

abrachia /əbrā'kē·ə/ [Gk, *a* + *brachion,* without arm], the absence of arms. —**abrachial,** *adj.*

abrachiocephalia. See **acephalobrachia.**

abrade /əbrād'/, to remove the epidermis, usually by scraping or rubbing.

abrasion /əbrā'zhən/ [L, *abradere,* to scrape off], a scraping, or rubbing away of a surface, such as skin or teeth, by friction. Abrasion may be the result of trauma, such as a skinned knee; of therapy, as in dermabrasion of the skin for removal of scar tissue; or of normal function, such as the wearing down of a tooth by mastication. Compare **laceration.** See also **bruxism, friction burn.** —**abrade,** *v.,* **abrasive,** *adj.*

Abrasion of the skin
(Kumar, Abbas, and Fausto, 2005)

abrasion arthroplasty, arthroplasty with eburnation of one surface with a bur, which induces bleeding and fibrocartilaginous repair tissue to form a new articular surface. It is done in patients who cannot tolerate other arthroplasty procedures, such as after a first procedure has failed.

abrasion layer, a protective covering of gelatin enclosing an emulsion on x-ray film. Also called **overcoat**.

abrasive, 1. pertaining to a substance that can grind or wear down another substance. **2.** an object or surface that can cause an abrasion.

abreact /ab′rē·akt′/, **1.** to release a repressed emotion. **2.** to work off by catharsis effects of a repressed disagreeable experience. **3.** to mentally relive or bring into consciousness repressed experiences.

abreaction /ab′rē·ak′shən/ [L, *ab*, from, *re*, again, *agere*, to act], an emotional release resulting from mentally reliving or bringing into consciousness, through the process of catharsis, a long-repressed, painful experience. See also **catharsis**.

abrosia /əbrō′zhə/ [Gk, fasting], a condition caused by fasting or abstaining from food. See also **anorexia**.

abruption [L, *ab*, away from, *rumpere*, rupture], a sudden breaking off or tearing apart.

abruptio placentae [L, *ab*, away from, *rumpere*, to rupture], separation of the placenta implanted in normal position in a pregnancy of 20 weeks or more or during labor before delivery of the fetus. It occurs in approximately 1 in 200 births, and, because it often results in severe hemorrhage, it is a significant cause of maternal and fetal mortality. Hypertension and preeclampsia are associated with increased rates of occurrence; in many cases, however, there is no explanation. Complete separation causes immediate death of the fetus. Bleeding from the site of separation causes abdominal pain, uterine tenderness, and tetanic uterine contraction. Bleeding may be concealed within the uterus or may be evident externally, sometimes as sudden massive hemorrhage. In severe cases, shock and death can result in minutes. Cesarean section must be performed immediately and rapidly. Extensive extravasation of blood within the uterine wall may deplete fibrinogen, prolong clotting time, bring about intractable bleeding, lead to disseminated intravascular coagulation, and, by damaging the uterine musculature, prevent the uterus from contracting well after delivery. Hysterectomy may be necessary to prevent exsanguination. Partial separation may cause little bleeding and may not interfere with fetal oxygenation. If the pregnancy is near term, labor may be permitted or induced by amniotomy. A premature pregnancy may be allowed to continue under close observation of the mother at bed rest. The nurse must be alert to the possibility that bleeding is present but concealed internally and that if all the blood can escape, there may be little pain. Also called **ablatio placentae, accidental hemorrhage, placental abruption**. Compare **placenta previa**. See also **Couvelaire uterus**.

abscess /ab′səs/ [L, *abscedere*, to go away], **1.** a cavity containing pus and surrounded by inflamed tissue, formed as a result of suppuration in a localized infection (characteristically, a staphylococcal infection). Healing usually occurs when an abscess drains or is incised. If an abscess is deep in tissue, drainage is done by means of a sinus tract that connects it to the surface. In a sterile abscess, the contents are not the result of pyogenic bacteria. **2. dental abscess,** an abscess that develops anywhere along the root length of a tooth. It is usually characterized by pain caused by the pressure of pus against the nerve tissue, redness caused by blood accumulation, and swelling caused by the suppuration.

Dental abscess *(Stone and Gorbach, 2000)*

abscess of liver. See **liver abscess**.

abscissa /absis′ə/ [L, *ab*, away; *scindere*, to cut], a point on a horizontal Cartesian coordinate plane measured from the *y*- (or vertical) axis running perpendicular to the plane, or *x*-axis.

abscission /absish′ən/ [L, *abscinere*, to cut away], the process of cutting away, as in corneal abscission, removal of the prominence of the cornea.

Partial separation
(concealed hemorrhage)

Partial separation
(apparent hemorrhage)

Complete separation
(concealed hemorrhage)

Abruptio placentae

absconsio /abskon'shō/ [L, *ab,* away from, *condo,* hidden], a cavity or fossa.

abscopal /abskō'pəl/, pertaining to the effect of irradiated tissue on remote tissue not exposed to radiation.

absence seizure, an epileptic seizure characterized by a sudden, momentary loss of consciousness. Occasionally it is accompanied by minor myoclonus of the neck or upper extremities, frequent blinking, slight symmetric twitching of the face, or loss of muscle tone. The seizures usually occur many times a day without a warning aura and are most frequent in children and adolescents, especially at puberty. The patient experiencing a typical seizure has a vacant facial expression and ceases all voluntary motor activity; with the rapid return of consciousness, the patient may resume conversation at the point of interruption without realizing what occurred. During and between seizures, the patient's electroencephalogram shows 3-Hz spike-and-wave discharges. Anticonvulsant drugs used to prevent absence seizures include ethosuximide, trimethadione, and valproic acid. Also called **absentia epileptica, petit mal seizure.** See also **epilepsy.**

absenteeism /ab'səntē'izəm/, (for health or related reasons) absence from work. Absenteeism varies according to job assignments, with professional and managerial personnel taking average annual sick leave of 4 days, whereas unskilled workers claim an average of 18 days sick leave during the year. Surveys also indicate that fewer than 10% of workers account for nearly 50% of all absenteeism. The most common causes of absenteeism include influenza and occupationally related skin diseases.

absentia epileptica. See **absence seizure.**

absent without leave (AWOL) /ā'wôl/ [L, *absentia*], a term used to describe a patient who departs from a psychiatric facility without authorization.

abs feb, abbreviation for *absente febre,* a Latin phrase meaning in the absence of fever.

Absidia /absid'ē·ə/, a genus of fungi belonging to the class Phycomycetes. Several species have been found to cause infections of otosclerosis and pulmonary and general mycosis in humans. *A. ramosa* is found on decaying plants and baked goods and can cause mucormycosis. Other pathogenic species cause diseases in livestock.

***Absidia* species** *(Mahon and Manuselis, 2000)*

absolute, unconditional, unrestricted, or independent of arbitrary standards.

absolute agraphia [L, *absolutus,* set loose; Gk, *a,* not, *graphein,* to write], a complete inability to write caused by a central nervous system lesion. The person is unable to write even the letters of the alphabet. See also **agraphia.**

absolute alcohol, a clear, colorless, highly hygroscopic liquid with a burning taste, containing at least 99.5 ethyl alcohol by volume. Also called **dehydrated alcohol.**

absolute cephalopelvic disproportion. See **cephalopelvic disproportion.**

absolute discharge /ab'səlōōt/ [L, *absolutus,* set free], a final and complete termination of the patient's relationship with a care-giving agency.

absolute glaucoma /ab'səlōō't/ [L, *abolutus* + Gk, *cataract*], complete blindness in which a glaucoma-induced increase in intraocular pressure results in permanent vision loss. The optic disc is white and deeply excavated, and the pupil is usually widely dilated and immobile. Also called absolutum glaucoma, **glaucoma consummatum.**

absolute growth, the total increase in size of an organism or a particular organ or part, such as the limbs, head, or trunk.

absolute humidity, the actual mass or content of water in a measured volume of air. It is usually expressed in grams per cubic meter or pounds per cubic foot or cubic yard.

absolute neutrophil count (ANC), the number of neutrophils in a milliliter of blood, having a reference value of approximately 1500–7700 per µL. The ANC is a measure of a person's immune status. Generally, if the count is above 1000 the person may safely mingle with other people or undergo chemotherapy, while a count below 500 indicates that a person is at high risk for infection and should be kept away from those with infectious diseases.

absolute refractory period. See **refractory period.**

absolute temperature, temperature that is measured from a base of absolute zero on the Kelvin scale or the Rankine scale.

absolute threshold [L, *absolutus,* set loose; AS, *therscold*], **1.** the lowest point at which a stimulus can be perceived. **2.** pertaining to millivolts of electrical charge determined by ion fluctuations or movement across cell membranes that result in nerve or muscle stimulation.

absolute zero, the temperature at which all molecular activity except vibration ceases. It is a theoretical value derived by calculations and projections from experiments with the behavior of gases at extremely low temperatures. On the Celcius scale, absolute zero is estimated to be equal to −273° C. On the Fahrenheit scale, the equivalent temperature is calculated at -460° F.

absorb /absôrb', əbzôrb'/ [L, *absorbere,* to swallow], **1.** the act of drinking in, wholly engulfing, assimilating, or taking up various substances; for example, the tissues of the intestines absorb fluids. **2.** the energy transferred to tissues by radiation, such as an absorbed dose of radioactivity.

absorbable cotton, oxidized cellulose.

absorbable gauze /əbsôr'bəbəl/, a material, produced from oxidized cellulose, that can be absorbed. It is applied directly to tissue to stop bleeding.

absorbable surgical suture [L, *absorbere,* to suck up; Gk, *cheirourgos,* surgery; L, *sutura*], a suture made from material that can be completely digested (by enzyme activity) or hydrolyzed (by reaction with water in tissue fluids to breakdown).

absorbance /əbsôr'bəns/, the degree of absorption of light or other radiant energy by a medium that is exposed to the energy. It is expressed as the logarithm of the ratio of energy transmitted through a vacuum to the energy transmitted through the medium. For solutions, it is the logarithm of the ratio of energy transmitted through pure solvent to the energy transmitted through solution. Absorbance varies with factors such as wavelength, solution concentration, and path length.

absorbed dose, the energy imparted by ionizing radiation per unit mass of irradiated material at the place of interest. The SI unit of absorbed dose is the gray, which is 1 J/kg and equals 100 rad.

absorbefacient /absôr′bifā′shənt/ [L, *absorbere*, to suck up, + *facere*, to make], **1.** any agent that promotes or enhances absorption. **2.** causing or enhancing absorption.

absorbent /absôr′bənt/ [L, *absorbere*, to suck up], **1.** capable of attracting and absorbing substances into itself. **2.** a product or substance that can absorb liquids or gases.

absorbent dressing, a dressing of any material applied to a wound or incision to absorb secretions.

absorbent gauze, a fabric or pad with various forms, weights, and uses. It may be a rolled, single-layered fine fabric for spiral bandages, or it may be a thick, multilayered pad for a sterile pressure dressing. There may also be an adhesive backing.

absorbent point. See **paper point.**

absorption /absôrp′shən/ [L, *absorptio*], **1.** the incorporation of matter by other matter through chemical, molecular, or physical action, such as the dissolving of a gas in a liquid or the taking up of a liquid by a porous solid. **2.** (in physiology) the passage of substances across and into tissues, such as the passage of digested food molecules into intestinal cells or the passage of liquids into kidney tubules. Kinds of absorption are **agglutinin absorption, cutaneous absorption, external absorption, intestinal absorption, parenteral absorption, pathologic absorption. 3.** (in radiology) the process of absorbing radiant energy by living or nonliving matter with which the radiation interacts.

Absorption of sodium, glucose, and amino acids
(Thibodeau and Patton, 2003)

absorption coefficient, the factor by which the intensity of electromagnetic energy decreases as it interacts with a unit thickness of an absorbing material. It is usually expressed per unit thickness.

absorption rate constant, a value describing how much drug is absorbed per unit of time.

absorption spectrum, a plot of percent transmittance, absorbance, logarithm of absorbance, or absorptivity of a compound as a function of wavelength, wave number, or frequency of radiation.

absorptivity /ab′sôrptiv′itē/, absorbance at a particular wavelength divided by the product of the concentration of a substance and the sample path length.

abstinence /ab′stinəns/, voluntarily avoiding a substance, such as food or alcohol, or refraining from the performance of an act, such as sexual intercourse.

abstinence syndrome [L, *abstinere*, to hold back; Gk, *syn,* together, *dromos,* course], the physical and psychological withdrawal symptoms experienced by a chemically dependent person who is suddenly deprived of a regular intake of alcohol or other addictive substance.

abstract /ab′strakt, abstrakt′/ [L, *abstrahere*, to drag away], **1.** a condensed summary of a scientific article, literary piece, or address. **2.** to collect data such as from a medical record. **3.** A preparation containing the soluble principles of a medication concentration mixed with lactose. **4.** difficult to understand due to lack of practicality.

abstraction /abstrak′shən/ [L, *abstrahere*, to drag away], a condition in which all or part of the dental arch is farther from the Frankfurt horizontal plane than normal.

abstract thinking, the final, most complex stage in the development of cognitive thinking, in which thought is characterized by adaptability, flexibility, and the use of concepts and generalizations. Problem solving is accomplished by drawing logical conclusions from a set of observations, such as making hypotheses and testing them. This type of thinking is developed by 12 to 15 years of age, usually after some degree of education. In psychiatry, many disorders are characterized by the inability to think abstractly. Compare **concrete thinking, syncretic thinking.**

abulia /əbōō′lyə/ [Gk, *a* + *boule,* without will], a loss of the ability or reduced capacity to exhibit initiative or to make decisions. Also spelled **aboulia.**

abuse /abyōōs′/, [L, *abuti,* to waste, abusus, using up] **1.** improper use of equipment, a substance, or a service, such as a drug or program, either intentionally or unintentionally. See also **substance abuse. 2.** to physically or verbally attack or injure. An example is **child abuse.**

abuse cessation, a nursing outcome from the Nursing Outcomes Classification (NOC) defined as evidence that the victim is no longer abused. See also **Nursing Outcomes Classification.**

abused person [Fr, *abuser,* to disuse, L, *persona,* a role played], an individual who has been harmed or maltreated emtionally, verbally, sexually, or physically, by another person or by a situation.

abuse of the elderly. See **elder abuse.**

abuse protection, a nursing outcome from the Nursing Outcomes Classification (NOC) as protection of self or dependent others from abuse. See also **Nursing Outcomes Classification.**

abuse protection support, a nursing intervention from the Nursing Interventions Classification (NIC) defined as identification of high-risk, dependent relationships and actions to prevent further infliction of physical or emotional harm. See also **Nursing Interventions Classification.**

abuse protection support: child, a nursing intervention from the Nursing Interventions Classification (NIC) defined as identification of high-risk, dependent child relationships and actions to prevent possible or further infliction of physical, sexual, or emotional harm or neglect of basic necessities of life. See also **Nursing Interventions Classification.**

abuse protection support: domestic partner, a nursing intervention from the Nursing Interventions Classification (NIC) defined as identification of high-risk, dependent domestic relationships and actions to prevent possible or further infliction of physical, sexual, or emotional harm, or junctional tissue, with or without retrograde atrial conduction.

accelerated respiration, an abnormally rapid rate of breathing, usually more than 25 breaths per minute. See also **tachypnea.**

acceleration /aksel′ərā′shən/ [L, *accelerare,* to quicken], an increase in the speed or velocity of an object or reaction. Compare **deceleration. —accelerator,** *n.*

acceleration-deceleration injury, injury resulting from a collision between a body part and another object or body part while both are in motion.

acceleration phase, (in obstetrics) the first period of active labor, stage I, characterized by an increased rate of dilation of the cervical canal as charted on a Friedman curve.

accelerator /aksel′ərā′tər/ [L, *accelerare,* to quicken], **1.** a nerve or muscle that increases the rate of performance of some function. **2.** an agent or apparatus that is used to increase the rate at which a substance acts or a function proceeds.

accelerator urinae. See **bulbocavernosus.**

accentuation /aksen′chōō·ā′shən/ [L, *accentus,* accent], an increase in distinctness or loudness, as in heart sounds.

acceptable daily intake (ADI), the maximum amount of any substance that can be safely ingested by a human. Ingestion that exceeds this amount may cause toxic effects.

acceptance: health status, a nursing outcome from the Nursing Outcomes Classification (NOC) defined as reconciliation to health circumstances. See also **Nursing Outcomes Classification.**

acceptance of individuality /aksep′təns/, (in psychiatry) an index of family health in which differentiation or individuation is a valued goal.

acceptance of separation, an indicator of mental well-being in which a loss is mourned in a healthy manner. It indicates higher level of adaptability.

acceptor /aksep′tər/, [L, *accipere,* to receive], **1.** an organism that receives from another person or organism living tissue, such as transfused blood or a transplanted organ. **2.** a substance or compound that combines with, or accepts, a part of another substance or compound, such as an atom, an electron, or an electron pair. Compare **donor.**

access /ak′ses/, a means of approach, such as the space needed for the manipulation of dental or surgical instruments. An example is vascular access in hemodialysis.

access cavity [L, *accedere,* to approach], a coronal opening to the center of a tooth, required for effective cleaning, shaping, and filling of the pulp canal and chamber during endodontic or root canal therapy.

accessory /akses′ərē/, [L, *accessonis,* appendage], **1.** a supplementary, desirable but not necessary, used chiefly for convenience or for safety, such as the electric elevator mechanisms for hospital beds. **2.** a structure that serves one of the main anatomic systems, such as the accessory sex organs in men and women; the accessory organs of the skin; the hair; the nails; and the skin glands. **3.** one who aids in perpetrating a crime.

accessory chromosome. See **monosome.**

accessory diaphragm, a congenital defect in which a second diaphragm or portion of a diaphragm develops in the chest. It is usually found on the right side and is oriented upward and backward to the posterior chest wall. It may be separated from the true diaphragm by a lobe of a lung.

accessory gland, glandular tissue that contributes in a secondary way to the function of a similar gland, which may be nearby or some distance away.

accessory ligament [L, *accessus,* extra, *ligare,* to bind], a

ligament that helps strengthen a union between two bones, even though it is not part of a joint capsule.

accessory movement, a joint movement that is necessary for a full range of motion but is not under direct voluntary control. Examples include rotation and gliding motions.

accessory muscle, a relatively rare anatomic duplication of a muscle that may appear anywhere in the muscular system. The most common sign associated with an accessory muscle is the appearance of a soft-tissue mass. Differential diagnosis without surgical intervention and exploration is difficult because of the similar appearance of some tumors or soft-tissue masses, such as ganglia. The appearance of the soft-tissue mass associated with an accessory muscle may be transient, or it may be constant, depending on the location of the accessory muscle in relation to motion. In many individuals with accessory muscles, specific treatment is not indicated unless the accessory muscle interferes with normal function.

accessory muscles of respiration, muscles of the neck, back, and abdomen that may assist the diaphragm and the internal and external intercostal muscles in respiration, especially in some breathing disorders or during exercise. Often elevated effort of breathing contributes to **barrel chest** over time.

accessory nasal sinuses [L, *accessus,* extra, *nasus,* nose, *sinus,* hollow], the paranasal sinuses that occur as hollows within the skull but open into the nasal cavity and are lined with a mucous membrane that is continuous with the nasal mucous membrane.

accessory nerve, either of a pair of cranial nerves essential for speech, swallowing, and certain movements of the head and shoulders. Each nerve has a cranial and a spinal portion, communicates with certain cervical nerves, and connects to the nucleus ambiguus of the brain. Also called **eleventh nerve, nervus accessorius, spinal accessory nerve.**

Evaluating the accessory nerve *(Swartz, 2002)*

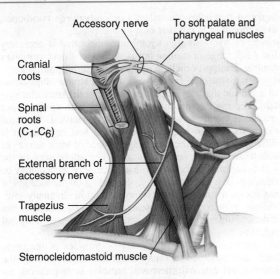

Accessory nerve — To soft palate and pharyngeal muscles

Cranial roots

Spinal roots (C₁-C₆)

External branch of accessory nerve

Trapezius muscle

Sternocleidomastoid muscle

Accessory nerve

accessory organ, an organ or other distinct collection of tissues that contributes to the function of another similar organ, such as the ocular muscles and eyelids, which contribute to the function of the eye.

accessory pancreas [L, *accessus,* extra; Gk, *pan,* all, *kreas,* flesh], small clusters of pancreas cells detached from the pancreas and sometimes found in the wall of the stomach or intestines.

accessory pancreatic duct, a small duct opening into the pancreatic duct or duodenum near the mouth of the common bile duct.

accessory pathway, an abnormal conduction path between an atrium and a ventricle. Ventricular activation via an accessory pathway slows initial ventricular contraction, producing preexcitation and the delta wave of Wolff-Parkinson-White syndrome. The delta wave shortens the P-R interval, and broadens the QRS complex. The most common associated arrhythmias are paroxysmal supraventricular tachycardia and atrial fibrillation. Patients may be cured by transvenous radiofrequency ablation of the accessory pathway or treated medically.

accessory phrenic nerve, the nerve that joins the phrenic nerve at the root of the neck or in the thorax, forming a loop around the subclavian vein. It may arise from the nerve to the subclavius or from the fifth cervical nerve. Compare **phrenic nerve.**

accessory placenta [L, *accessionis,* a thing added, *placenta,* flat cake], a small placenta that may develop attached to the main placenta by umbilical blood vessels. Also called **succenturiate placenta.**

accessory root canal, a lateral branching of the pulp canal in a tooth, usually occurring in the apical third of the root.

accessory sign, a sign that is not typical or characteristic of a particular disease.

accessory sinus of the nose. See **paranasal sinus.**

accessory spleen [L, *accessus,* extra; Gk, *splen*], small nodules of spleen tissue that may occur in the gastrosplenic ligament, greater omentum, or other visceral sites.

accessory thymus [L, *accessus,* extra; Gk, *thymos,* thymelike], a nodule of thymus tissue that is isolated from the gland.

accessory tooth, a supernumerary tooth that does not resemble a normal tooth in size, shape, or position.

access time, the amount of time required for a computer to retrieve data from its disk drive.

ACCH, abbreviation for **Association for the Care of Children's Health.**

accident /ak′sidənt/ [L, *accidere,* to happen], any unexpected or unplanned event that may result in death, injury, property damage, or a combination of serious effects. The victim may or may not be directly involved in the cause of the accident. Accidents frequently are the result of both physical and mental factors that can result in unsafe operating systems at work, home, or other sites.

accidental hemorrhage. See **abruptio placentae.**

accident-prone, describing a person who experiences accidents and accompanying injuries at a much greater than average rate.

acclimate /əklī′mit, ak′limāt/ [L, *ad,* toward; Gk, *klima,* region], to adjust physiologically to a different climate or environment, or to changes in altitude or temperature. Also **acclimatize** /əklī′mətīz′/. —**acclimation, acclimatization,** *n.*

acclimatization to heat [L, *ad,* toward; Gk, *klima,* region], a process whereby the body adapts to warmer environmental temperatures.

accommodation (A, acc, Acc) /əkom′ədā′shən/ [L, *accommodatio,* adjustment], **1.** the state or process of adapting or adjusting one thing or set of things to another. **2.** the continuous process or effort of the individual to adapt or adjust to surroundings to maintain a state of homeostasis, both physiologically and psychologically. **3.** the adjustment of the eye to variations in distance. See also **accommodation reflex. 4.** (in sociology) the reciprocal reconciliation of conflicts between individuals or groups concerning habits and customs, usually through a process of compromise, arbitration, or negotiation. Also called **adjustment.** Compare **adaptation.**

accommodation reflex, an adjustment of the eyes for near vision, consisting of pupillary constriction, convergence of the eyes, and increased convexity of the lens. Also called **ciliary reflex.** See also **light reflex.**

accommodative strabismus /əkom′ədā′tiv/ [L, *accommodatio,* adjustment; Gk, *strabismos,* squint], **1.** strabismus resulting from abnormal demand on accommodation, such as convergent strabismus due to uncorrected hyperopia or divergent strabismus due to uncorrected myopia. **2.** strabismus resulting from the act of accommodation in association with a high AC/A ratio.

accomplishment quotient /əkom′plishmənt/, a numeric evaluation of a person's achievement age compared with mental age, expressed as a ratio multiplied by 100. See also **achievement quotient, intelligence quotient.**

accountability /əkoun′təbil′itē/, being accountable or responsible for the moral and legal requirements of proper patient care.

accreditation /əkred′itā′shən/, a process whereby a professional association or nongovernmental agency grants recognition to a school or healthcare institution for demonstrated ability to meet predetermined criteria, such as the accreditation of hospitals by the Joint Commission on Accreditation of Healthcare Organizations or of nursing schools by the NLNAC. Compare **certification.**

accrementition /ak′rəmentish′ən/, growth or increase in size by the addition of similar tissue or material, as in cellular division, simple fission, budding, or gemmation.

accrete. See **accretion.**

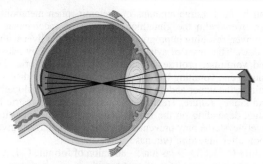

Distant image: lens is flattened

Close image: lens is rounded

Accommodation reflex *(Thibodeau and Patton, 2003)*

accretio cordis /əkrē´shē·ō/ [L, *accrescere,* to increase, *cordis,* heart], an abnormal condition in which the pericardium adheres to a structure around the heart.

accretion /əkrē´shən/ [L, *accrescere,* to increase], **1.** growth by the addition of material similar to that already present. **2.** the adherence or growing together of parts that are normally separated. **3.** an accumulation of foreign material, especially within a cavity. —**accrete,** *v.,* **accretive,** *adj.*

acculturation /əkul´chərā´shən/, **1.** the process of adopting the cultural traits or social patterns of a different population group. **2.** the modification of culture of a group due to association with another group.

accumulated dose equivalent /əkyōō´myələ´tid/, an estimate of an individual's absorbed dose of radiation over a lifetime, expressed in rem. Occupationally exposed persons are allowed no more than 5 rem per year, or 1 rem times age at any time during the person's lifetime. See also **rem.**

accuracy /ak´yərəsē´/, the extent to which a measurement is close to the true value.

accurate empathy /ak´yərit/, a communication technique used by a nurse to convey an understanding of the patient's feelings and experiences.

Accurbron, a trademark for a bronchodilator (theophylline).

Accutane, a trademark for an antiacne agent (isotretinoin).

AC/DC, slang term for a person who is both heterosexual and homosexual. See also **bisexual.**

ACE, abbreviation for **angiotensin-converting enzyme.**

Ace bandage, a trademark for a woven elastic bandage.

acebutolol /as´əbōō´təlol/, a beta-adrenergic blocking agent.

■ INDICATIONS: It is prescribed in the treatment of hypertension, angina pectoris, ventricular arrhythmias, and other cardiovascular disorders.

■ CONTRAINDICATIONS: The drug should not be given to patients with asthma, persistent severe bradycardia, second- and third-degree heart block, overt cardiac failure, cardiogenic shock, or peripheral vascular disease. Generally not recommended during pregnancy.

■ ADVERSE EFFECTS: The most common side effects include fatigue, bradycardia, bronchospasm, flatulence, hypotension, muscle/joint pains, nausea, constipation, diarrhea, headache, skin rashes, dizziness, and insomnia.

acedia /əsē´dē·ə/ [Gk, *akedia,* apathy], a condition of listlessness and a form of melancholy, marked by indifference and sluggish mental processes.

ACE inhibitor. See **angiotensin-converting enzyme (ACE) inhibitor.**

acellular /āsel´yə lər/, without cells.

acentric /āsen´trik/ [Gk, *a, kentron,* not center], **1.** having no center. **2.** (in genetics) describing a chromosome fragment that has no centromere.

acentric occlusion. See **eccentric occlusion.**

-aceous /-ā´shəs/, a suffix meaning "having the appearance of" or "like" something specified: *foliaceous, testaceous.*

ACEP, abbreviation for **American College of Emergency Physicians.**

acephal-, acephalo-, a combining form meaning 'having no head': *acephalobrachia, acephaly.*

acephalia, congenital absence of the head.

acephalism. See **acephalia.**

acephalobrachia /asef´əlōbrā´kē·ə/ [Gk, *a* + *kephale,* without head, *brachion,* arm], a congenital anomaly in which a fetus lacks both arms and a head. Also called **abrachiocephalia.**

acephalocardia /-kär´dē·ə/ [Gk, *a,* not, *kephale,* head, *cardia,* heart], congenital absence of both head and heart.

acephalus /əsef´ələs/ [Gk, *a,* not, *kephale,* head], a headless fetus.

acephaly /əsef´əlē/ [Gk, *a, kephale,* without head], a congenital defect in which the head is absent or not properly developed. Also called **acephalia** /as´əfā´lē·ə/, **acephalism** /əsef´əliz´əm/. —**acephalic,** *adj.*

acerola /as´ərō´lə/, a small, cherrylike fruit of the genus *Malpighia* that grows in tropical climates. It is a richer source of vitamin C than any other known fruit. Also called **Barbados cherry.**

acesulfame-K /as´əsul´fām/, a synthetic noncaloric sweetener marketed under the trademark Sunnette. It is approximately 200 times sweeter than sucrose. Heat does not affect its sweetening ability, an advantage over aspartame. Also called **acesulfame potassium.**

acet, abbreviation for an acetate carboxylate anion. Also abbreviated as OAc.

acet-, a combining form meaning 'vinegar': *acetoin, acetyl.*

acetabula. See **acetabulum.**

acetabular /as´ətab´yələr/ [L, *acetabulum,* little saucer], pertaining to the acetabulum, the cup-shaped hip socket into which the head of the femur is set.

acetabular angle, the angle between the acetabular line and Hilgenreiner's line, normally between 27° and 30° in the neonatal hip. It is used in the radiographic assessment of developmental dysplasia of the hip. Also called **acetabular index.**

acetabular index. See **acetabular angle.**

acetabular line, a line following the slope of the acetabulum that is used in radiographic assessment of the hip joint. With Hilgenreiner's line it forms the **acetabular angle.**

acetabular notch, an indentation in the margin of the acetabulum, the cup-shaped socket of the hip bone.

acetabuloplasty /as′ətab′yəlōplas′ tē/, plastic surgery performed to reshape the acetabulum.

acetabulum pl. **acetabula** /as′ətab′yələm/ [L, vinegar cup], the large, cup-shaped cavity at the juncture and lateral surface of the ilium, the ischium, and the pubis, in which the ball-shaped head of the femur articulates.

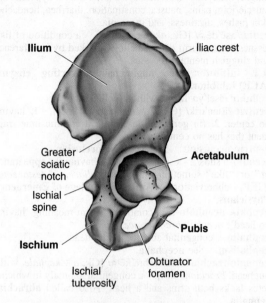

Ilium

Iliac crest

Greater
sciatic
notch

Acetabulum

Ischial
spine

Pubis

Ischium

Obturator
foramen

Ischial
tuberosity

Acetabelum (Herlihy and Maebius, 2003)

acetal, **1.** a colorless liquid, C_2H_4 $(OC_2H_5)_2$, sometimes used as a hypnotic. Also called **diethyl acetal. 2.** any compound with the general formula $R_2C(OR)_2$ or $RCH(OR)_2$, in which R indicates an alkyl or aryl group.

acetaldehyde (CH_3CHO) /as′ətəldē′hīd/, a colorless, volatile liquid aldehyde with a pungent odor produced by the oxidation of ethyl alcohol. Its systematic (IUPAC) name is ethanal. In the human body, acetaldehyde is produced in the liver by the action of alcohol dehydrogenase and other enzymes. It is used commercially in the manufacture of acetic acid and various aromas and flavors. Exposure to high levels of acetaldehyde can result in headache, corneal injury, rhinitis, and respiratory disorders.

acetaminophen /əset′əmin′əfin/, an analgesic and antipyretic drug used in many nonprescription pain relievers. It has no antiinflammatory properties. It may be used in combination with other products which do not contain additional acetaminophen.

■ INDICATIONS: It is often recommended for treatment of mild to moderate pain and fever.

■ CONTRAINDICATION: Known hypersensitivity to acetaminophen prohibits its use. It should not be used in the presence of liver disease.

■ ADVERSE EFFECTS: Among the most serious adverse reactions are anaphylaxis, hepatotoxicity, and hemolytic anemia. Overdosage can result in fatal cyanosis and hepatic necrosis.

acetaminophen poisoning, a toxic reaction to the ingestion of excessive doses of acetaminophen. Dosages exceeding 140 mg/kg can produce liver failure, and larger doses

can be fatal. Large amounts of acetaminophen metabolites can overwhelm the glutathione-detoxifying mechanism of the liver, resulting in progressive necrosis of the liver within 5 days. The onset of symptoms may be marked by nausea and vomiting, profuse sweating, pallor, and oliguria. The nausea and vomiting increase, accompanied by jaundice and pain in the upper abdomen, hypoglycemia, encephalopathy, and kidney failure. Treatment requires emesis or gastric lavage, depending on the length of time since the ingestion. Acetylcysteine may prevent extensive liver damage if given soon after ingestion (via nasogastric tube).

acetate ($CH_3CO_2^-$) /as′itāt/, an anion of formula $C_2H_3O_2$. It is the conjugate base of acetic acid.

acetate kinase, an enzyme that catalyzes the transfer of a phosphate group from adenosine triphosphate to acetate. Also called **acetokinase** /as′ətōkī′nās/.

acetaZOLAMIDE /as′ətəzō′ləmīd/, a carbonic anhydrase inhibitor diuretic agent.

■ INDICATIONS: It is prescribed for the treatment for glaucoma and edema, and as an adjunctive agent for the treatment of refractory epilepsy, and acute mountain sickness.

■ CONTRAINDICATIONS: Hyponatremia, hypokalemia, severe liver or kidney disease or dysfunction, Addison's disease, or known hypersensitivity to this drug or other sulfonamides prohibits its use.

■ ADVERSE EFFECTS: Among the most serious adverse reactions are anorexia and depression, particularly in the elderly; acidosis; hyperuricemia; and crystalluria. Paresthesias, GI disturbances, and lethargy are common.

Acetest, a trademark for a product used to test for the presence of abnormal quantities of acetone in the urine of patients with diabetes mellitus or other metabolic disorders. A large quantity of acetone causes a rapid change in the color of the Acetest tablet. See also **acidosis, ketone bodies.**

acetic /əsē′tik, əset′ik/ [L, acetum, vinegar], pertaining to substances having the sour properties of vinegar or acetic acid; also, to chemical compounds possessing the radical, CH_3CO—.

acetic acid ($HC_2H_3O_2$), a clear, colorless, pungent liquid that is miscible with water, alcohol, glycerin, and ether and that constitutes 3% to 5% of vinegar. Acetic acid is produced commercially by the reaction of methyl alcohol with carbon monoxide in the presence of a catalyst, or it may be obtained from ethyl alcohol by the action of many aerobic bacteria. Various concentrations are used in the manufacture of plastics, dyes, insecticides, cellulose acetate, photographic chemicals, and pharmaceutic preparations, including vaginal jellies and antimicrobial solutions for the treatment of superficial infections of the external auditory canal. Also called **ethanoic acid.**

acetic fermentation, the production of acetic acid or vinegar from a weak alcoholic solution.

acetoacetic acid /as′ətō·əsē′tik, əsē′tō-/, a colorless, oily keto acid produced by the metabolism of lipids and pyruvates. It is excreted in trace amounts in normal urine and in elevated levels in diabetes mellitus, especially in ketoacidosis. Acetoacetic acid is also increased during starvation as a result of incomplete oxidation of fatty acids. Soluble in water, alcohol, and ether, acetoacetic acid decomposes at temperatures below 100° C to acetone and carbon dioxide. Also called **acetone carboxylic acid** /kär′boksil′ik/, **acetylacetic acid** /əsē′tiləsē′tik, as′ətil-/, **beta-ketobutyric acid** /bet′əkē′tōbyōotir′ik/, **diacetic acid** /dī·əsē′tik/.

acetoHEXAMIDE /-hek′səmīd/, a sulfonylurea oral antidiabetic.

■ INDICATION: It may be prescribed in the treatment of type 2 diabetes mellitus.

■ CONTRAINDICATIONS: Its use is prohibited as sole therapy in type I diabetes, diabetic ketoacidosis, severe liver or kidney dysfunction, or known hypersensitivity to this drug or to other sulfonylureas.

■ ADVERSE EFFECTS: Among the most serious adverse reactions are blood dyscrasias, hypoglycemia, and allergic reactions. GI disturbances are common.

acetohydroxamic acid /as′ĕ-to-hi′droks-am′ik/, an inhibitor of bacterial urease used in prophylaxis and treatment of struvite kidney stones whose formation is favored by urease-producing bacteria and as an adjunct in treatment of urinary tract infections caused by urease-producing bacteria. It is administered orally.

acetokinase. See **acetate kinase.**

acetol kinase, an enzyme that catalyzes the transfer of a phosphate group from adenosine triphosphate to hydroxyacetone.

acetonaemia. See **ketonemia.**

acetone /as′ətōn/, a colorless, aromatic, volatile liquid ketone body found in small amounts in normal urine and in larger quantities in the urine of diabetics experiencing ketoacidosis or starvation is also called 2-propanone. It is one of the group of compounds called ketones. Commercially prepared acetone is used to clean the skin before injections, but prolonged exposure to the compound can be irritating. It also has many varied industrial uses.

acetone bodies. See **ketone bodies.**

acetone carboxylic acid. See **acetoacetic acid.**

acetone in urine test, a test for the presence of dimethylketone in the urine of patients, used as a laboratory indication of ketosis and the severity of diabetes mellitus. Chemically treated test paper strips or sticks are exposed to urine. If acetone is present in the urine as the result of incomplete breakdown of fatty and amino acids in the body, the test strips change color. A similar test uses a compound added directly to a urine sample.

acetonide grouping, an acetone-based ketal, or ketone-alcohol derivative, present in some corticosteroid drugs, such as fluocinolone acetonide.

acetonuria /as′ətōnŏŏr′ē·ə/, the presence of acetone and diacetic bodies in the urine. See also **ketoaciduria.**

acetophenetidin. See **phenacetin.**

acetyl (CH₃CO), a monovalent radical associated with derivatives of acetic acid. It is sometimes abbreviated **Ac.**

acetylacetic acid. See **acetoacetic acid.**

acetylcholine (ACh) /as′ətilkō′lēn, əsē′til-/, a direct-acting cholinergic neurotransmitter agent widely distributed in body tissues, with a primary function of mediating synaptic activity of the nervous system and skeletal muscles. Its half-life and duration of activity are short because it is rapidly destroyed by acetylcholinesterase. Its activity also can be blocked by atropine at junctions of nerve fibers with glands and smooth muscle tissue. It is a stimulant of the vagus and parasympathetic nervous system and functions as a vasodilator and cardiac depressant. Acetylcholine is used therapeutically as an adjunct to eye surgery and has limited benefits in certain circulatory disorders because of its short half-life.

acetylcholinesterase (AChE) /-kō′lines′tərās/, an enzyme present at endings of voluntary nerves and parasympathetic involuntary nerves and autonomic nerve ganglia. It inactivates and prevents accumulation of the neurotransmitter acetylcholine released during nerve impulse transmission by hydrolyzing the substance to choline and acetate. The action reduces or prevents excessive firing of neurons at neuromuscular junctions.

acetylcoenzyme A /əsē′til·kō·en′zīm, as′ətil-/, a biomolecule that carries an activated form of the 2-carbon acetyl unit that is found in the course of several important metabolic processes. The formation of acetylcoenzyme A is the critical intermediate step between anaerobic glycolysis and the citric acid cycle. Also called **acetyl-CoA.** See also **citric acid cycle, tricarboxylic acid cycle.**

acetylcysteine /-sis′tēn/, a mucolytic and acetaminophen antidote.

■ INDICATIONS: It is prescribed in the treatment of chronic pulmonary disease, acute bronchopulmonary disease, atelectasis resulting from mucous obstruction, and acetaminophen poisoning.

■ CONTRAINDICATION: Known sensitivity to this drug prohibits its use.

■ ADVERSE EFFECTS: Among the most serious adverse reactions are stomatitis, nausea, rhinorrhea, and bronchospasm.

acetylsalicylic acid. See **aspirin.**

acetylsalicylic acid poisoning /əsē′təlsal′isil′ik, as′itəl-/, toxic effects of overdosage of the commonly used antipyretic and analgesic drug, aspirin. Early symptoms of overdosage include dizziness, ringing in the ears, changes in body temperature, GI discomfort, and hyperventilation. Severe poisoning is marked by respiratory alkalosis, which may lead to metabolic acidosis. Children and the elderly are particularly vulnerable to the potential toxic effects of salicylates. See also **Reye's syndrome, salicylate poisoning.**

acetyltransferase /-trans′fərās/, any of several enzymes that transfer acetyl groups from one compound to another. See also **acetylcoenzyme A.**

ace wrap/dressing, a trademark for elastized wrap. See **elastic bandage.**

ACG, abbreviation for **apexcardiography.**

ACh, abbreviation for **acetylcholine.**

ACH, abbreviation for **adrenocortical hormone.**

achalasia /ak′əlā′zhə/ [Gk, *a + chalasis*, without relaxation], an abnormal condition characterized by inability of a muscle to relax (cardiospasm), particularly the lower esophageal sphincter. Compare **corkscrew esophagus.** See also **dysphagia.**

Advanced stage esophageal achalasia
(Phipps, Sands, and Marek, 1999)

Achard-Thiers syndrome /äsh′ärtērz′/ [Emile C. Achard, French physician, 1860–1941; Joseph Thiers, French physician, b. 1885], a hormonal disorder seen in postmenopausal women with diabetes, characterized by growth of body hair in a masculine distribution. Treatment includes mechanical removal or bleaching of excess hair and hormonal therapy to correct endocrine imbalances related to systemic disease. See also **hirsutism.**

ache /āk/ [OE, *acan,* to hurt], **1.** a pain characterized by persistence, dullness, and, usually, moderate intensity. An ache may be localized, as a stomach ache, headache, bone ache; or a general ache, as in the myalgia that accompanies a viral infection or a persistent fever. **2.** to suffer from a dull, persistent pain of moderate intensity.

AChE, abbreviation for **acetylcholinesterase.**

acheiria /əkī′rē·ə/ [Gk, *a,* not, *cheir,* hand], congenital absence of one or both hands.

acheiropody /ak′īrop′ədē/ [Gk, *a,* not, *cheir,* hand, *pous,* foot], absence of hands and feet.

achievement age /əchēv′mənt/, the level of a person's educational development as measured by an achievement test and compared with the normal score for chronologic age. Compare **mental age.** See also **developmental age.**

achievement quotient (AQ), a numeric expression of a person's achievement age, determined by various achievement tests, divided by the chronologic age and expressed as a multiple of 100. Compare **intelligence quotient.** See also **accomplishment quotient.**

achievement test, a standardized test for the measurement and comparison of knowledge or proficiency in various fields of vocational or academic study. Compare **aptitude test, intelligence test, personality test, psychologic test.**

Achilles jerk. See **Achilles tendon reflex.**

Achilles tendon /əkil′ēz/ [*Achilles,* Greek mythologic hero], the common distal tendon of the soleus and gastrocnemius muscles of the leg. It is the thickest and strongest tendon in the body and connects triceps surae muscle to the heel bone. In an adult it is about 15 cm long. The tendon becomes contracted about 4 cm above the heel and flares out again to insert into the calcaneus. Also called **tendo calcaneus.**

Achilles tendon *(Thibodeau and Patton, 2003)*

Achilles tendon reflex, a deep tendon reflex consisting of plantar flexion of the foot when a sharp tap is given directly to the tendon of the gastrocnemius muscle at the back of the ankle. This reflex is often absent in people with peripheral neuropathies or diabetes. A sluggish return of the flexed foot may occur in patients with hypothyroidism. A hyperactive reflex may be caused by hyperthyroidism or by pyramidal tract disease. Also called **Achilles jerk, ankle reflex.** See also **deep tendon reflex.**

Elicitation of the Achilles tendon reflex
(Barkauskas, Baumann, and Darling-Fisher, 2002)

achiral, pertaining to the absence of chirality in a compound, as in stereochemical isomers.

achlorhydria /ā′klôrhī′drē·ə/ [Gk,*a* + *chloros,* not green, *hydor,* water], an abnormal condition characterized by the absence of hydrochloric acid in gastric secretions. Achlorhydria occurs most commonly in atrophy of the gastric mucosa, gastric carcinoma, and pernicious anemia. It is also found in severe iron deficiency anemia. Malignancy is expected when achlorhydria is seen in combination with gastric ulceration. Protein digestion is severely impaired in patients with achlorhydria, but overall digestion in the alimentary tract is relatively normal, because trypsin and other enzymes of the pancreas and small intestine are not affected. See also **achylia, pernicious anemia. —achlorhydric,** *adj.*

achloropsia /ā′klôrop′sē·ə/ [Gk, *a,* not, *chloros,* green, *opsis,* vision], an inability to see green; green blindness.

acholia /akō′lē·ə/ [Gk, *a* + *chole,* without bile], **1.** the absence or decrease of bile secretion. **2.** any condition that suppresses the flow of bile into the small intestine. **—acholic,** *adj.*

acholuria /ak′əlōōr′ē·ə/, [Gk, *a* + *chole,* without bile, *ouron,* urine], the absence or lack of bile pigments in the urine as occurs in some forms of jaundice.

achondrogenesis /ākon′drōjen′əsis/, a form of dwarfism characterized by gross limb shortening and hydropic head and trunk. It is transmitted by an autosomal recessive gene.

achondroplasia /ākon′drōplā′zhə/ [Gk, *a* + *chondros,* without cartilage, *plassein,* to form], a disorder of the growth of cartilage in the epiphyses of the long bones and skull. It results in premature ossification, permanent limitation of skeletal development, and dwarfism typified by protruding forehead and short, thick arms and legs on a normal trunk. Onset is in fetal life. Familial achondroplasia is inherited as an autosomal dominant gene; the chance is 50% that an offspring of an affected parent will be affected. The majority of affected individuals die during gestation or the first year of life. The minority that survive have relatively normal longevity. There is no treatment other than orthopedic surgery. Antenatal diagnosis is possible. Also called **chondrodystrophy, fetal rickets.**

achondroplastic dwarf /-plas'tik/, the most common type of dwarf, characterized by disproportionately short limbs, a normal-sized trunk, large head with a depressed nasal bridge and small face, stubby hands, and lordosis. The condition results from an inherited defect in bone-forming tissue and is often associated with other defects or abnormalities, although there is usually no involvement of the central nervous system and intelligence is normal. See also **achondroplasia.**

achroma /akrō'mə/ [Gk, *a,* without, *chroma,* color], lack of color.

achromatic, **1.** free of color. **2.** color blind. **3.** a substance not colored by common staining agents.

achromatic lens /ak'rəmat'ik/ [Gk, *a,* without, *chroma,* color; L, *lens*], a lens in which the focal lengths for red and blue colors of the spectrum are the same, refracting light without decomposing it into its component colors.

achromatic vision. See **color blindness.**

achromatocyte. See **achromocyte.**

achromatopsia. See **color blindness.**

achromia /akrō'mēə/ [Gk, *a* + *chroma,* without color], the absence or loss of normal skin pigment.

Achromobacter /akrō'mōbak'tər/, a genus of gram-negative, rod-shaped, flagellated bacteria that do not form pigment on agar. Most species in the genus are saprophytic, nonpathogenic organisms found in water, soil, or the human digestive tract.

achromocyte /ākrō'məsīt/, a sickle-shaped, abnormally pale erythrocyte. Also called **achromatocyte.**

Achromycin V, a trademark for an antibiotic (tetracycline hydrochloride).

achylia /ākī'lē-ə/ [Gk, *a, chylos,* not juice], an absence or severe deficiency of hydrochloric acid and pepsinogen (pepsin) in the stomach. This condition may also occur in the pancreas when the exocrine portion of that gland fails to produce digestive enzymes. Also called **achylosis.** See also **achlorhydria.**

achylous /əkī'ləs/, **1.** pertaining to a lack of gastric juice or other digestive secretions. **2.** pertaining to a lack of chyle.

acicular /əsik'yələr/ [L, *aciculus,* little needle], needle-shaped, such as certain leaves and crystals.

acid /as'id/, [L, *acidus,* sour], **1.** a compound that yields hydrogen ions when dissociated in aqueous solution (Arrhenius definition) or acts as a hydrogen ion donor (Brönsted definition) or acts as an electron pair acceptor (Lewis definition). Acids turn blue litmus red, have a sour taste, and react with bases to form salts. Acids have chemical properties essentially opposite to those of bases. See also **alkali.** **2.** *slang.* lysergic acid diethylamide (LSD). **3.** sour or bitter to the taste. See also **lysergide.**

acid-, a prefix meaning 'sour, bitter, acid': *acidemia, acidophil.*

acidaemia. See **acidemia.**

acidalbumin, a substance formed by the action of mild acid solutions on albumin. Also called **metaprotein.**

acidaminuria. See **aminoaciduria.**

acid-base balance, a condition existing when the net rate at which the body produces acids or bases equals the net rate at which acids or bases are excreted. The result of acid-base balance is a stable concentration of hydrogen ions in body fluids. See also **acid, base.**

acid-base management, a nursing intervention from the Nursing Interventions Classification (NIC) defined as promotion of acid-base balance and prevention of complications resulting from acid-base imbalance. See also **Nursing Interventions Classification.**

acid-base management: metabolic acidosis, a nursing intervention from the Nursing Interventions Classification (NIC) defined as promotion of acid-base balance and prevention of complications resulting from serum HCO_3 levels lower than desired. See also **Nursing Interventions Classification.**

acid-base management: metabolic alkalosis, a nursing intervention from the Nursing Interventions Classification (NIC) defined as promotion of acid-base balance and prevention of complications resulting from serum HCO_3 levels higher than desired. See also **Nursing Interventions Classification.**

acid-base management: respiratory acidosis, a nursing intervention from the Nursing Interventions Classification (NIC) defined as promotion of acid-base balance and prevention of complications resulting from serum pCO_2 levels higher than desired. See also **Nursing Interventions Classification.**

acid-base management: respiratory alkalosis, a nursing intervention from the Nursing Interventions Classification (NIC) defined as promotion of acid-base balance and prevention of complications resulting from serum pCO_2 levels lower than desired. See also **Nursing Interventions Classification.**

acid-base metabolism, the metabolic processes that maintain the balance of acids and bases essential in regulating the composition of body fluids. Acids release hydrogen ions, and bases accept them; the concentration of hydrogen ions present in a solution governs whether it is acid, alkali, or neutral. Hydrogen ions in water are measured on a pH scale of 0.0 to 14.0, with a reading of 7.0 indicating neutral at 25° C. Above 7.0, the solution is alkaline; below 7.0, it is acid. Blood is slightly alkaline, ranging from 7.35 to 7.45. Metabolic buffer systems within the body maintain this ratio, and, when the ratio is upset, either acidosis or alkalosis results. Acidosis may be caused by diarrhea, vomiting, uremia, diabetes mellitus, and the action of certain drugs. Alkalosis may be caused by overingestion of alkaline drugs, loss of chloride in gastric vomitus, and the action of certain diuretic drugs. See also **acid-base balance, acidosis, alkalosis, pH.**

acid-base monitoring, a nursing intervention from the Nursing Interventions Classification (NIC) defined as collection and analysis of patient data to regulate acid-base balance. See also **Nursing Interventions Classification.**

acid bath, a bath taken in water containing a mineral acid to help reduce excessive sweating.

acid burn, damage to tissue caused by exposure to an acid. The severity of the burn is determined by the strength of the acid and the duration and extent of exposure. Emergency treatment includes irrigating the affected area with large amounts of water. Compare **alkali burn.**

acid dust, an accumulation of highly acidic particles of dust. Such substances accumulate in the atmosphere and account for much of the smog hanging over large metropolitan areas. Many respiratory illnesses, such as lung cancer and asthma, may be aggravated or caused by such dust. See also **acid rain.**

acid dyspepsia, a digestive disorder associated with excessive stomach acidity. It occurs in peptic ulcer disease and gallbladder disease.

acidemia /as'idē'mē·ə/, decreased pH status of the blood or abnormal acidity in the blood. Specific types are denoted by prefixes: *lactacidemia, lipacidemia*. Also spelled **acidaemia**.

acid etching, etching of dental enamel with an acid to roughen the surface, increase retention of resin sealant, and promote mechanical retention.

acid-fast bacillus (AFB), a type of bacillus that resists decolorizing by acid after accepting a stain. Examples include *Mycobacterium tuberculosis* and *M. leprae*.

acid-fast stain, a method of staining used in bacteriology in which a smear on a slide is treated with carbol-fuchsin stain or auramine-rhodamine stain, decolorized with acid alcohol, and counterstained with methylene blue or potassium permanganate to identify acid-fast bacteria. Acid-fast organisms resist decolorization and appear red or yellow against a dark background when viewed under a microscope. The stain may be performed on any clinical specimen but is most commonly used in examining sputum for *Mycobacterium tuberculosis*, an acid-fast bacillus. See also **Ziehl-Neelsen test**.

Acid-fast stain of *Mycobacterium tuberculosis*
(Murray et al, 1998)

acid flush, a runoff of precipitation with a high acid content, as may occur during thaws in various parts of the world. Acid flushes may pollute rivers and reservoirs, killing fish and endangering the natural balance of the ecosystem. See also **acid rain**.

acidify /asid'əfī/, **1.** to make a substance acidic, as through the addition of an acid. **2.** to become acidic. Compare **alkalinize**.

acidity /asid'itē/ [L, *acidus*, sour], the degree of sourness, sharpness of taste, or ability of a chemical to yield hydrogen ions in an aqueous solution.

acidity of the stomach, the degree of gastric acid in the stomach. The acidity varies during any 24-hour period but averages a pH of 0.9 to 1.5. The main source of stomach acidity is hydrochloric acid secreted by gastric glands of the stomach.

acid mist, mist containing a high concentration of acid or particles of any toxic chemical, such as carbon tetrachloride or silicon tetrachloride. Such chemicals are often used by industry and stored in tanks that may leak their contents into residential areas, becoming especially dangerous if the toxic substance mixes with fog. Inhalation of acid mists may irritate the mucous membranes, the eyes, and the respiratory tract and seriously upset the chemical balances of the body. See also **acid rain**.

acid mucopolysaccharide, a major chemical constituent of ground substance in the dermis.

acidophil /as'idōfil, əsid'əfil/ [L, *acidus* + Gk, *philein*, to love], **1.** a cell or cell constituent with an affinity for acid dyes. **2.** an organism that thrives in an acid medium. —**acidophilic**, *adj.*

acidophilic adenoma, a tumor of the pituitary gland characterized by cells that can be stained red with an acid dye. Gigantism and acromegaly can be caused by an acidophilic adenoma. Also called **eosinophilic adenoma**.

acidophilus milk /as'idof'ələs/, milk inoculated with cultures of *Lactobacillus acidophilus*, used in various enteric disorders to change the bacterial flora of the GI tract.

acidosis /as'idō'sis/ [L, *acidus* + Gk, *osis*, condition], an abnormal increase in hydrogen ion concentration in the body, resulting from an accumulation of an acid or the loss of a base. It is indicated by a blood pH below the normal range (7.35 to 7.45). The various forms of acidosis are named for their cause; for example, renal tubular acidosis results from failure of the kidney to secrete hydrogen ions or reabsorb bicarbonate ions, respiratory acidosis results from respiratory retention of CO_2, and diabetic acidosis results from an accumulation of ketones associated with lack of insulin. Treatment depends on diagnosis of the underlying abnormality and concurrent correction of the acid-base imbalance. Compare **alkalosis**. —**acidotic**, *adj.*

acidosis dialysis, a type of metabolic acidosis that may develop when contaminating bacteria alter the pH of the dialysis bath.

acidotic, pertaining to acidosis, either depletion of base or accumulation of acid.

acid phosphatase, an enzyme found in the kidneys, serum, semen, and prostate gland. It is elevated in serum in cancers of the prostate and in trauma. Normal concentrations in serum are 0 to 1.1 Bodansky U/ml. See also **alkaline phosphatase**.

acid phosphatase test, a blood test used primarily to diagnose end-stage prostatic carcinoma and to monitor the efficacy of treatment.

acid poisoning, a toxic condition caused by the ingestion of a toxic acid agent such as hydrochloric, nitric, phosphoric, or sulfuric acid, some of which are ingredients in common household cleaning compounds. Compare **alkali poisoning**.

acid rain, the precipitation of moisture, as rain, with high acidity caused by release into the atmosphere of pollutants from industry, motor vehicle exhaust, and other sources. Acid precipitation with a pH of 5.6 or lower is blamed by various authorities for numerous human health problems, fish kills, and the destruction of timber. Also called **acid precipitation, acid snow**.

acid rebound, a condition of hypersecretion of gastric acid that may occur after the initial buffering effect of an antacid. It occurs most noticeably when antacids containing calcium carbonate are used.

acid salt, a salt that is formed from an acid with two or more bases by only partial replacement of hydrogen ions from the related acid, leaving some degree of acidity. An example is sodium bicarbonate, which is also identified as sodium acid carbonate or sodium hydrogen carbonate.

acid snow. See **acid rain**.

acid therapy, a method for removing warts that uses plaster patches impregnated with acid, such as 40% salicylic acid, or with acid drops, such as 5% to 16.7% salicylic and lactic acids in flexible collodion. The application is made every 12 to 24 hours for 2 to 4 weeks. Acid therapy is not usually recommended for body areas that perspire heavily or that are likely to become wet or for exposed body parts where the patches would detract from the patient's appearance.

acidulous /əsid′yələs/, slightly acidic or sour.

aciduria [L, *acidus* + Gk, *ouron,* urine], the presence of acid in the urine. The condition may be caused by a diet rich in meat proteins or certain fruits, a medication used to treat a urinary tract disorder, an inborn error of metabolism, or ketoacidosis.

acinar adenocarcinoma. See **acinic cell adenocarcinoma.**

acinar cell /as′inər/ [L, *acinus,* grape], a cell of the tiny lobules of a compound gland or similar saclike structure such as an alveolus.

Acinetobacter /as′inē′təbak′tər/, a genus of nonmotile, aerobic bacteria of the family Neisseriaceae that often occurs in clinical specimens. The bacterium contains gram-negative or gram-variable cocci and does not produce spores. It grows on regular medium without serum and is oxidase negative and catalase positive. It is mainly found in water, and its disease activity is opportunistic.

acini. See **acinus.**

acinic cell adenocarcinoma /asin′ik/ [L, *acinus,* grape], an uncommon low-grade malignant neoplasm that develops in the secreting cells of racemose glands, especially the salivary glands. The tumor consists of cells with clear or slightly granular cytoplasm and small eccentric dark nuclei. Also called **acinar adenocarcinoma, acinous adenocarcinoma.**

Acinic cell carcinoma *(Skarin, 2003)*

aciniform /asin′ifôrm/ [L, *acinus,* grape; *forma,* shape], shaped like a cluster of grapes. The term refers particularly to glandular tissue.

acinitis /as′ini′tis/, any inflammation of the tiny, grape-shaped portions of certain glands.

acinotubular gland /as′inōt(y)oōb′yələr/ [grape-shaped], a gland in which the acini are tube-shaped.

acinous adenocarcinoma. See **acinic cell adenocarcinoma.**

acinus *pl.* **acini** /as′inəs/ [L, grape], **1.** any small saclike structure, particularly one found in a gland. **2.** a subdivision of the lung consisting of the tissue distal to a terminal bronchiole. Also called **alveolus.**

acitretin /as′e-tret′in/, a second generation retinoid used in treatment of severe psoriasis. It is administered orally.

A.C. joint, abbreviation for *acromioclavicular joint.* See **acromioclavicular articulation.**

Aclovate, a trademark for a topical corticosteroid (alclometasone dipropionate).

ACLS, abbreviation for **advanced cardiac life support.**

ACMC, abbreviation for **Association of Canadian Medical Colleges.**

acme /ak′mē/, [Gk, *akme,* point], the peak or highest point, such as the peak of intensity of a uterine contraction during labor or the peak of perfection.

acne /ak′nē/, /ak′nē/, a disease of the skin common where sebaceous glands are numerous (face, upper back, and chest). Characteristic lesions include open (blackhead) and closed (whitehead) comedones, inflammatory papules, pustules, and nodules. It seems to result from thickening of the follicular opening, increased sebum production, the presence of bacteria, and the host's inflammatory response. Treatment includes the use of topical and oral antibiotics, topical and oral retinoids, benzoyl peroxide, salicylic, and azelaic acid. Kinds of acne include **acne conglobata, chloracne,** and **acne fulminans.** A common form is **acne vulgaris.** See also **comedo.**

acne atrophica /atrof′ikə/, a skin disorder characterized by small scars or pits left by an earlier occurrence of acne vulgaris.

acne cachecticorum, an eruption or irritation of the skin that may occur in patients who are very weak and debilitated. It is characterized by soft, mildly infiltrated pustular lesions.

acne conglobata /kong′glōbā′tə/, a severe form of acne with abscess, cyst, scar, and keloid formation. It may affect the lower back, buttocks, and thighs, as well as the face and chest. It affects more males than females. Also called **cystic acne.**

acneform /ak′nifôrm/, resembling acne. Also **acneiform** /aknē′əfôrm/.

acneform drug eruption, any of various skin reactions to a drug characterized by papules and pustules resembling acne.

acne fulminans, a form of severe nodular acne characterized by inflamed nodules and plaques that can result in skin ulcers and severe scarring. The condition mainly affects teenage boys and may be accompanied by fever, arthritis, and blood disorders.

acnegenic /ak′nijen′ik/ [Gk, *akme* + *genein,* to produce], causing or producing acne.

acneiform. See **acneform.**

acne keloid [Gk, *akme,* point, *kelis,* spot, *eidos,* form], excessive scar tissue that has developed at the site of an acne lesion.

acne medicamentosa, any type of acne resulting from a reaction to medication, such as to a steroid or the salt of a halogen. Also called **drug-induced acne.**

acne necrotica miliaris, a rare, chronic type of pruritic, pustular folliculitis of the scalp, occurring mostly in adults and characterized by tiny pustules, probably a pyoderma or tuberculid. Also called **acne varioliformis.**

acne neonatorum, a skin condition of newborns caused by sebaceous gland hyperplasia and characterized by the localized formation of grouped comedones on the nose, cheeks, and forehead.

acne papulosa, a common skin condition in which comedones develop moderately inflamed papules. It is considered a papular form of acne vulgaris.

acne pustulosa, a form of acne in which the predominant lesions are pustular and may result in scarring.

acne rosacea. See **rosacea.**

Acne neonatorum *(Zitelli and Davis, 1997)*

acne urticaria /ur′tiker′ē·ə/, a form of acne marked by papules that are predominantly edematous and wheallike and that have been aggravated by scratching.

acne varioliformis. See **acne necrotica miliaris.**

acne vulgaris. See **acne.**

Acne vulgaris on the forehead *(Callen et al, 2000)*

ACNM, abbreviation for *American College of Nurse-Midwives.*

ACOG, abbreviation for **American College of Obstetricians and Gynecologists.**

acognosia /ak′og·nō′zhə/, a knowledge of remedies.

acorea /ā′kôrē′ə/ [Gk, *a*, without, *kore*, pupil], an absence of the pupil of the eye.

acoria /akôr′ē·ə/ [Gk, *a*, without, *koros*, satiety], a condition characterized by constant hunger and eating, even when the appetite is small.

Acne vulgaris on the lower face *(Callen et al, 2000)*

acorn-tipped catheter, a flexible catheter with an acorn-shaped tip used in various diagnostic procedures, especially in urology.

acous-, acus-, acust-, acousto-, combining form meaning 'hearing': *acoustic, acousma.*

-acousia, -acusia, -acusis, -akusis, suffix meaning a '(specified) condition of the hearing.'

acousma *pl.* **acousmas, acousmata** /əkooz′mə/, [Gk, *akousma,* something heard], a hallucinatory impression of strange sounds.

acoustic /əkoo̅s′tik/ [Gk, *akouein,* to hear], pertaining to sound or hearing. Also **acoustical.**

-acoustic, -acoustical, **1.** a suffix meaning 'the hearing organs': *entacoustic, otacoustic.* **2.** a suffix meaning 'amplified sound waves': *microcoustic, stethacoustic.*

acoustic apparatus, the various components of the sense of hearing. See also **internal ear, cochlea, organ of Corti.**

acoustic cavitation, a potential biologic effect of ultrasonography, marked by large-amplitude oscillations of microscopic gas bubbles. As normally used, ultrasound pulses are too short to cause acoustic cavitation in human tissues.

acoustic center, the portion of the brain, in the temporal lobe of the cerebrum, in which the sense of hearing is located. Also called **auditory cortex.**

acoustic hair cell. See **auditory hair.**

acoustic-immittance audiometry, an audiologic testing used to evaluate the status of the outer and middle ears and of the acoustic reflex arc. It includes tympanometry, static-compliance testing, and acoustic reflex measures.

acoustic impedance, interference with the passage of sound waves by objects in the path of those waves. It equals the velocity of sound in a medium times the density of the medium. The acoustic impedance of bone may be nearly five times as great as that of blood. Testing of middle ear acoustic impedance is part of audiologic evaluation batteries used to detect middle ear problems.

acoustic meatus [Gk, *akoustikos,* hearing; L, *meatus,* a passage], the external or internal canal of the ear.

acoustic microscope, a microscope in which the object being viewed is scanned with sound waves and its image reconstructed with light waves. Acoustic microscopes produce excellent resolution of the objects being studied and allow close examination of cells and tissues without staining or damaging the specimen.

acoustic nerve. See **vestibulocochlear nerve.**

acoustic neuroma, a benign unilateral or bilateral tumor that develops from the eighth cranial (vestibulocochlear) nerve and grows within the auditory canal. Depending on the location and size of the lesion, tinnitus, progressive hearing loss, headache, facial numbness, papilledema, dizziness, and an unsteady gait may result. Paresis and difficulty in speaking and swallowing may occur in the later stage. Also called **acoustic neurilemmoma, acoustic neurinoma, acoustic neurofibroma.**

Acoustic neuroma
(Kumar, Abbas, and Fausto, 2005/courtesy Dr. K.M. Earle)

acoustic reflex, contraction of the stapedius and tensor tympani muscles in the middle ear in response to a loud sound. The muscle contractions pull the stapes out of the oval window and thus protects the inner ear from damage caused by loud noise. The **acoustic reflex threshold** is the lowest level of sound that will elicit an acoustic reflex and is in the range of 85 to 90 dB hearing level in individuals with normal hearing. Acoustic reflexes are usually elevated or absent in cases of conductive or neural hearing loss and present at normal or lower levels in the case of cochlear (inner ear) hearing loss.

acoustics /əkoos'tiks/ [Gk, *akoustikos,* hearing], the science of sound.

acoustic shadow, in an ultrasound image, the absence of echoes produced by the presence of dense material, such as calculi, which impede the transmission of sound waves. It is often used to detect gallstones.

acoustic trauma, a sudden loss of hearing, partial or complete, caused by an extremely loud noise, a severe blow to the head, or other trauma. The greatest loss of hearing occurs at 4000 Hz. It may be temporary or permanent. Compare **noise-induced hearing loss.**

acoustooptics /əkoos'tō·op'tiks/, a field of physics that studies the generation of light waves by ultra-high-frequency sound waves. Knowledge gained by such study is applied chiefly in the transmission of information by acoustooptic devices.

ACP, 1. abbreviation for *American College of Pathologists.* **2.** abbreviation for **American College of Physicians. 3.** abbreviation for **American College of Prosthodontists.**

acquired /əkwī'ərd/ [L, *acquirere,* to obtain], pertaining to a characteristic, condition, or disease originating after birth, not caused by hereditary or developmental factors but by a reaction to environmental influences outside of the organism. An example is acquired immunity. Compare **congenital, familial, hereditary.**

acquired cystic kidney disease, the development of cysts in a formerly noncystic kidney during end-stage renal disease.

acquired epileptic aphasia. See **Landau-Kleffner syndrome.**

acquired hypogammaglobulinemia [L, *acquirere,* to obtain; Gk, *hypo,* a deficiency, *gamma,* third letter of Greek alphabet; L, *globulus,* small globe; Gk, *haima,* blood], an acquired deficiency of the gamma globulin blood fraction. See also **hypogammaglobulinemia.**

acquired immunity, any form of immunity that is not innate and is obtained during life. It may be naturally or artificially acquired and actively or passively induced. **Naturally acquired immunity** is obtained by the development of antibodies resulting from an attack of infectious disease or by the transmission of antibodies from the mother through the placenta to the fetus or to the infant through colostrum and breast milk. **Artificially acquired immunity** is obtained by vaccination or by the injection of immune globulin. Compare **natural immunity.** See also **active immunity, passive immunity.**

acquired immunodeficiency syndrome (AIDS), a syndrome involving a defect in cell-mediated immunity that has a long incubation period, follows a protracted and debilitating course, is manifested by various opportunistic infections, and without treatment has a poor prognosis. The disorder originally was found in homosexual men and IV drug users but now occurs increasingly among heterosexual men and women and children of those with the disease. More than 1 million cases of AIDS have appeared in the United States, where in the 1990s it was the leading cause of death among men between 25 and 44 years of age and the fourth leading cause of death among women of the same age group. A total of 36.1 million cases of AIDS, including 16.5 million women and 1.4 million children younger than 15 years of age, are estimated worldwide by 2001. An estimated 21.5 million had died from the epidemic by the end of 2000. The disease is particularly prevalent in sub-Saharan Africa, where the estimated number of cases in 2001 exceeded 24 million, including 12.9 million women and 1 million children under 15 years of age.

■ OBSERVATIONS: AIDS is caused by either of two varieties of the human immunodeficiency virus, designated HIV-1 and HIV-2. HIV is a retrovirus that attracts and kills CD4+ lymphocytes (T helper cells), weakening the immune system's ability to prevent infection. The virus may also invade macrophages, in which it replicates freely, undetected by the immune system. HIV is not spread by casual contact but rather by sexual intercourse or exposure to contaminated blood, semen, breast milk, or other body fluids of infected persons. A patient may be diagnosed as having AIDS if he or she is infected with HIV, has a CD4+ count below 200 to 500/ml, and exhibits one or more of the following signs and symptoms: extreme fatigue, intermittent fever, night sweats, chills, lymphadenopathy, enlarged spleen, anorexia and consequent weight loss, severe diarrhea, apathy, and depression. As the disease progresses, characteristics are a general failure to thrive, anergy, and any of a variety of recurring infections, most commonly *Pneumocystis* pneumonia, tuberculosis, meningitis, and encephalitis caused by aspergillosis, candidiasis, cryptococcosis, cytomegalovirus, toxoplasmosis, or herpes simplex. Some patients with AIDS are susceptible to malignant neoplasms, especially Kaposi's sarcoma, Burkitt's lymphoma, and non-Hodgkin's lymphoma, that both cause and result from immunodeficiency. Psychological complications of AIDS may include chronic anxiety, depression, substance dependence, organic mental disorders, and suicidal ideation.

■ INTERVENTIONS: Treatment consists primarily of chronic symptom management and combined chemotherapy to counteract the opportunistic infections. There is no known cure for AIDS. Drugs used in the treatment of AIDS include reverse transcriptase inhibitors, such as zidovudine and didanosine, which interfere with the virus' ability to synthesize DNA within host cells, and protease inhibitors, such as ritonavir and indinavir, which cause the production of noninfectious HIV particles. These drugs are given in combinations (often called *cocktails*); one commonly used combination is made up of two reverse transcriptase inhibitors and a potent protease inhibitor. Vaccines routinely recommended for AIDS include those directed against pneumococcal influenza, hepatitis B, and general childhood infections, as well as infections that may be endemic in countries where the patient may travel, such as typhoid and yellow fever.

■ NURSING CONSIDERATIONS: Nursing care of the patient with AIDS varies with the patient's symptoms. These may include dyspnea, nutritional wasting, fatigue, pain, and incontinence. Intervention is directed at providing education to prevent the spread of disease and infection, promoting self-care and optimal nutrition, and providing emotional support for patients and their families. Patients with tumors, hematologic abnormalities, and infections require routine treatment for those disorders concurrently with care for their HIV-related complaints. See also **AIDS-dementia complex, AIDS-wasting syndrome, CD4, CD8, gp160, human immunodeficiency virus, retrovirus.**

acquired pellicle, an acellular film composed of salivary glycoproteins that closely and firmly adheres to the oral cavity. It is distinct from plaque, which is cellular and loosely adhered to the teeth until calcified into calculus. Acquired pellicle that has become discolored as a result of poor oral hygiene is called brown pellicle. Compare **bacterial plaque.**

acquired reflex. See **conditioned reflex.**

acquired sterility [L, *acquirere,* to obtain, *sterilis,* barren], the failure to conceive after once bearing a child. Also called **one-child sterility, secondary infertility.**

acquired trait [L, *acquirere,* to obtain + *trahere,* to draw], a physical characteristic that is not inherited but may be an effect of the environment or of a somatic mutation.

ACR, abbreviation for **American College of Radiology.**

acral /ak′rəl/ [Gk, *akron,* extremity], pertaining to an extremity or apex.

acral erythema, erythema localized to the palms and soles, as in hand-foot syndrome.

Acremonium /ak′rĕ-mo′ne-um/, a genus of Fungi Imperfecti of the form-class Hyphomycetes, formerly called *Cephalosporium.* Some species produce cephalosporin antibiotics.

acrid /ak′rid/ [L, *acris,* sharp], sharp or pungent, bitter and unpleasant to the smell or taste.

acridine /ak′ridēn/, a dibenzopyridine compound used in the synthesis of dyes and drugs. Its derivatives include fluorescent yellow dyes and the antiseptic agents acriflavine hydrochloride, acriflavine base, and proflavine.

acridine orange stain, a fluorochrome stain used to detect bacteria and fungi in blood cultures, cerebrospinal fluid, buffy coats and corneal scrapings. The fluorochrome inserts into nuclei acid and fluoresces orange when attached to bacteria or fungi.

acrimony /ak′rəmō′nē/ [L, *acrimonia,* pungency], a quality of bitterness, harshness, or sharpness.

acrivastine /ak′rĭ-vas′tēn/, a non-sedating antihistamine used in treatment of hay fever; administered orally.

■ INDICATIONS: When combined with the decongestant pseudoephedrine hydrochloride, it is prescribed in the treatment of allergic rhinitis.

■ CONTRAINDICATIONS: The drug should not be given to patients with known sensitivity to acrivistane or other alkylamine antihistamines or any components of the formulation. Since pseudoephedrine is a sympathomimetic, the use of this combination is contraindicated in patients using monoamine oxidase inhibitors or in those with severe coronary artery disease or severe hypertension, and in those with renal insufficiency.

■ ADVERSE EFFECTS: The side effects most often reported include somnolence, headache, dizziness, nervousness, insomnia, tachycardia, palpitations, dry mouth, nausea, and muscle weakness.

acro-, a prefix meaning 'extremities': *acrocentric, acrocyanosis.*

acrocentric /ak′rōsen′trik/ [Gk, *akron,* extremity, *kentron,* center], pertaining to a chromosome in which the centromere is located near one of the ends so that the arms of the chromosome are extremely uneven in length. Compare **metacentric, submetacentric, telocentric.**

acrocephalopolysyndactyly [*acrocephaly* + *polysyndactyly*], acrocephaly (see **oxycephaly**) and syndactyly with polydactyly as an additional feature. Four types are distinguished: *type I* is Noack's syndrome, *type II* is Carpenter's syndrome, *type III* is Sakati-Nyhan syndrome, and *type IV* is Goodman syndrome.

acrocephalosyndactylism. See **acrocephalosyndactyly.**

acrocephalosyndactyly /ak′rō·sef′ə·lō·sin·dak′ti·lē/ [*acrocephaly* + *syndactyly*], craniostenosis characterized by acrocephaly and syndactyly; the term is often used alone to denote **Apert's syndrome.** Sometimes, however, Apert's syndrome is designated *acrocephalosyndactyly, type I,* and acrocephalosyndactyly occurring with other anomalies is split into *acrocephalosyndactyly, type III* (**Saethre-Chotzen syndrome),** *acrocephalosyndactyly, type IV* (**Waardenburg's syndrome),** and *acrocephalosyndactyly, type V)* (**Pfeiffer type acrocephalosyndactyly,** which is the same as Noack's syndrome.

acrocephaly. See **oxycephaly.**

acrochordon /ak′rōkôr′don/, a benign, pedunculated growth commonly occurring on the eyelids, neck, axilla, or groin. Also called **skin tag.**

Acrochordon *(Callen et al, 2000)*

acrocyanosis. See **Raynaud's phenomenon.**

acrodermatitis /-dur'məti'tis/ [Gk, *akron* + *derma,* skin, *itis,* inflammation], any eruption of the skin of the hands and feet caused by a parasitic mite belonging to the order Acarina.

acrodermatitis enteropathica /en'tərōpath'ikə/, a rare, chronic disease of infants characterized by vesicles and bullae of the skin and mucous membranes, alopecia, diarrhea, and failure to thrive. An autosomal recessive disorder of zinc malabsorption, the disease may be lethal if not treated. Zinc sulfate is usually prescribed.

Acrokeratosis verruciformis (du Vivier, 1993)

Acrodermatis enteropathica (Callen et al, 2000)

acrodermatitis papulosa infantum. See **Gianotti-Crosti syndrome.**

acrodynia /ak'rōdin'ē·ə/ [Gk, *akron* + *odyne,* pain], a disease that occurs in infants and young children. Symptoms include edema, pruritus, generalized skin rash, pink coloration of the extremities and scarlet coloration of the cheeks and nose, swollen, painful extremities, cold and clammy skin, profuse sweating, digestive disturbances, photophobia, polyneuritis, extreme irritability alternating with periods of listlessness and apathy, and failure to thrive. Mercury poisoning is strongly implicated. Also called **erythredema polyneuropathy, Feer's disease, pink disease, Swift's disease.**

acroesthesia /ak'rō·esthē'zhə/ [Gk, *akron,* extremity, *aisthesis,* sensation], a condition of increased sensitivities or pain in the hands or feet.

acrokeratosis verruciformis /ak'rōker'ətō'sis/, a skin disorder characterized by the appearance of flat wartlike lesions on the dorsum of the hands and feet and occasionally on the wrists, forearms, and knees. It is an inherited disease, transmitted as a dominant trait.

acrokinesis /-kīnē'sis/ [Gk, *akron,* extremity, *kinesis,* motion], a state in which the limbs possess an abnormally wide range of motion.

acromegalia. See **acromegaly.**

acromegalic eunuchoidism /-məgal'ik/, a rare disorder characterized by genital atrophy and development of female secondary sex characteristics occurring in men with advanced acromegaly caused by a tumor in the anterior pituitary gland. Initially the gonadal function of the anterior lobe may be stimulated, but with the growth of the tumor the patient may become impotent; lose facial, axillary, and pubic hair; and acquire soft skin and a feminine distribution of fat. Also called **retrograde infantilism.**

acromegaly /ak'rəmeg'əlē/, [Gk, *akron* + *megas,* great], a chronic metabolic condition in adults caused by over secretion of growth hormones. It is characterized by gradual, marked soft tissue enlargement and widening and thickening of skeletal bones in the face, jaw, hands, and feet. Complications from increased growth hormone levels include atherosclerosis, hypertension, hyperglycemia, airway obstruction, and cardiomyopathy. Treatment normally includes radiation pharmacological agents, or surgery, often involving partial resection of the pituitary gland. Also called **acromegalia.** Compare **gigantism.** See also **adenohypophysis, growth hormone.** —**acromegalic,** *adj.*

Acromegaly
(Seidel et al, 2003/courtesy Gary Wand, MD,
The Johns Hopkins University and Hospital)

acromial. See **acromion.**

acromial process /əkrō′mē·əl/ [Gk, *akron,* extremity, *omos,* shoulder], a flat, triangular lateral extension of the scapula.

acromicria /ak′rəmik′rē·ə/, an anomaly characterized by abnormally small hands and feet. The person may also possess unusually small facial features, such as nose and ears.

acromioclavicular articulation /-mī′ōklavik′yələr/, the gliding joint between the acromial end of the clavicle and the medial margin of the acromion process of the scapula. It forms the highest part of the shoulder. The joint has six ligaments.

acromiocoracoid /-kôr′əkoid/, pertaining to the acromion and coracoid process.

acromiohumeral /-hyoo̅′mərəl/, pertaining to the acromion and the humerus.

acromion /əkrō′mē·ən/ [Gk, *akron* + *omos,* shoulder], the lateral extension of the spine of the scapula, forming the highest point of the shoulder and connecting with the clavicle at a small oval surface in the middle of the spine. It gives attachment to the deltoideus and trapezius muscles. Also called **acromion process.** Compare **coracoid process.** —**acromial,** *adj.*

acromioscapular /-skap′yələr/, pertaining to the acromion and the scapula.

acroosteolysis /ak′rō·os′tē·ol′isis/, an occupational disease that mainly affects people who work with polyvinylchloride (PVC) plastic materials. It is characterized by Raynaud's phenomenon, loss of bone tissue in the hands, and sensitivity to cold temperatures. A nonoccupational form of the disease is believed to be inherited.

acroparesthesia /ak′rōpar′isthē′zhə/ [Gk, *akron* + *para,* near, *aisthesis,* feeling], **1.** an extreme sensitivity at the tips of the extremities of the body, caused by nerve compression in the affected area or by polyneuritis. **2.** a disease characterized by tingling, numbness, and stiffness in the extremities, especially in the fingers, the hands, and the forearms. It sometimes produces pain, skin pallor, or mild cyanosis. The disease occurs in a simple form, which may produce acrocyanosis, and in an angiospastic form, which may produce gangrene.

acrophobia [Gk, *akron* + *phobos,* fear], a pathologic fear or dread of high places that results in extreme anxiety. Therapy attempts to overcome or eliminate the phobic response. See also **obsession, phobia, flooding.**

acrosomal. See **acrosome.**

acrosomal cap, acrosomal head cap. See **acrosome.**

acrosomal reaction /ak′rəsō′məl/, the pattern of various chemical changes that occur in the anterior of the head of the spermatozoon in response to contact with the ovum and that lead to the sperm's penetration and fertilization of the ovum.

acrosome /ak′rəsōm′/ [Gk, *akron* + *soma,* body], the caplike structure surrounding the anterior end of the head of a spermatozoon. It is derived from the Golgi apparatus within the cytoplasm and contains degradative enzymes that function in the penetration of the ovum during fertilization. Also called **acrosomal cap, acrosomal head cap.** See also **acrosomal reaction.** —**acrosomal,** *adj.*

acrotic /əkrot′ik/ [Gk, *a* + *krotos,* not beating], **1.** pertaining to the surface of the body or to the skin glands. **2.** pertaining to an absent or weak pulse.

acryl-, acrylo-, a prefix for terms meaning 'acrylic compound.'

acrylate, an anion, salt, ester, or conjugate base of acrylic acid. Also called **2-propenoate.**

acrylic acid (CH₂COOH) /əkril′ik/, a corrosive liquid used in the production of the plastic materials used in medical and dental procedures. Also called **2-propenoic acid.**

acrylic resin base, a denture base made of acrylic resin.

acrylic resin dental cement, a cement for restoring or repairing damaged teeth. In powder form it contains polymethyl methacrylate, which acts as a filler, plasticizer, and polymerization initiator. In liquid form it contains methyl methacrylate with an inhibitor and an activator.

ACS, **1.** abbreviation for *American Cancer Society.* **2.** abbreviation for *American Chemical Society.* **3.** abbreviation for **American College of Surgeons. 4.** abbreviation for *anodal closing sound.* **5.** abbreviation for **acute confusional state. 6.** abbreviation for *Association of Clinical Scientists.* **7.** abbreviation for abdominal compartment syndrome.

ACSM, abbreviation for *American College of Sports Medicine.*

act-, prefix meaning 'to do, drive, act': *action, activate.*

ACTH, abbreviation for **adrenocorticotropic hormone.**

Acthar, a trademark for adrenocorticotropic hormone injection (ACTH corticotropin).

-actide, combining form designating a synthetic corticotropin.

Actifed, trademark for a fixed-combination drug containing an adrenergic vasoconstrictor (pseudoephedrine hydrochloride) and an antihistamine (triprolidine hydrochloride).

actigraph /ak′tigraf′/, any instrument that records changes in the activity of a substance or an organism and produces a graphic record of the process, such as an electrocardiograph machine, which produces a record of electrical cardiac activity.

actin, a protein forming the thin filaments in muscle fibers that are pulled on by myosin cross-bridges to cause a muscle contraction. Actin is also used by some bacteria for motility by the formation of actin tails. See also **myosin.**

actin-. See **actino-.**

acting out, the expression of intrapsychic conflict or painful emotion through overt behavior that is usually pathologic, defensive, and unconscious and that may be destructive or dangerous. In controlled situations such as psychodrama, Gestalt therapy, or play therapy, such behavior may be therapeutic in that it may serve to reveal to the patient the underlying conflict governing the behavior. See also **transference.**

actinic /aktin′ik/ [Gk, *aktis,* ray], pertaining to radiation, such as sunlight or x-rays.

actinic burn, a burn caused by exposure to sunlight or other source of ultraviolet radiation.

actinic conjunctivitis [Gk, *actis,* ray, + L, *conjunctivus,* connecting; Gk, *itis,* inflammation], an inflammation of the conjunctiva caused by exposure to the ultraviolet radiation (UV) of sunlight or other UV sources, such as acetylene torches, therapeutic lamps (sun lamps), and klieg lights. Also called **actinic ophthalmia.**

actinic dermatitis, a skin inflammation or rash resulting from exposure to sunlight, x-ray, or atomic particle radiation. Chronic or recurrent actinic dermatitis can predispose to skin cancer. See also **actinic keratosis.**

actinic keratosis, a slowly developing, localized thickening and scaling of the outer layers of the skin as a result of chronic, prolonged exposure to the sun. Treatment of this premalignant lesion includes surgical excision, cryotherapy, and topical chemotherapy. Also called **senile keratosis, senile wart, solar keratosis.**

actinic ophthalmia. See **actinic conjunctivitis.**

actinism, the ability of sunlight or similar forms of radiation to produce chemical changes.

actinium (Ac), a rare, radioactive metallic element. Its atomic number is 89; its atomic mass is 227. It occurs in some ores of uranium.

Actinic keratosis
(Swartz, 2002)

actino-, actin-, prefix meaning 'ray or radiation': *actinocardiogram, actiniform.*

Actinobacillus /ak'tinōbasil'əs/, a genus of small, gram-negative bacillus, with members that are pathogenic for humans and other animals. The species *Actinobacillus actinomycetemcomitans* is the cause of actinomycosis in humans.

Actinobacillus actinomycetemcomitans
(Mahon and Manuselis, 2000)

Actinomyces /ak'tinōmī'sēz/, [Gk, *aktis,* ray, *mykes,* fungus], a genus of anaerobic or facultative anaerobic, gram-positive bacteria. Species that may cause disease in humans, such as *Actinomyces israelii,* are normally present in the mouth and throat. Disease activity is normally limited to periodontal disease. See also **actinomycosis.**

actinomycin A, the first of a group of chromopeptide antibiotic agents derived from soil bacteria. Most are derivatives of phenoxazine and contain actinocin. They are generally active against gram-positive and gram-negative bacteria and some fungi. Because of their cytotoxic properties, they are effective for certain types of neoplasms. See **dactinomycin.**

actinomycin B, an antibiotic antineoplastic agent derived from *Actinomyces antibioticus.*

actinomycin D. See **dactinomycin.**

actinomycosis /ak'tinōmīkō'sis/, a chronic, systemic disease characterized by deep, lumpy abscesses that extrude a thin, granular pus through multiple sinuses. The disease occurs worldwide but is seen most frequently in those who live in rural areas. It is not spread from person to person or from animals to humans. The most common causative organism in humans is *Actinomyces israelii,* a normal inhabitant of the bowel and mouth. Disease occurs after tissue damage, usually in the presence of another infectious organism. It can be diagnosed by microscopic identification of sulfur granules, pathognomonic of *Actinomyces,* in the exudate. There are several forms of actinomycosis. **Orocervicofacial actinomycosis** occurs with the spread of the bacterium into the subcutaneous tissues of the mouth, throat, and neck as a result of dental or tonsillar infection. **Thoracic actinomycosis** may represent proliferation of the organism from cervicofacial abscesses into the esophagus, or it may result from inhalation of the bacterium into the bronchi. **Abdominal actinomycosis** usually follows an acute inflammatory process in the stomach or intestines, such as appendicitis, diverticulum of the large bowel, or a perforation found in the groin or another area that drains exudate into the stomach. A large mass may be palpated, and sinus tracts from abscesses deep in the abdomen may form. **Pelvic actinomycosis** is most commonly associated with intrauterine devices. Central nervous system actinomycosis is a rare cause of brain abscess. **Musculoskeletal actinomycosis** involves subcutaneous tissue, muscle, and bone. **Disseminated actinomycosis** follows hematogenous spread of the infection and may involve the skin, brain, liver, and urogenital system. All forms of actinomycosis are treated with at least 6 weeks of daily injections of penicillin in large doses. Abdominal actinomycosis can be cured in 40% of cases, thoracic actinomycosis in 80%, and orocervicofacial actinomycosis in 90%.

Cervical *actinomycosis* *(Stone and Gorbach, 2000)*

actinotherapy, the use of ultraviolet, other parts of the spectrum of the sun's rays, or x-rays to treat various disorders, particularly skin diseases.

action, activity used to carry out a function or produce an effect.

action current. See **action potential.**

action level, the level of concentration at which an undesirable or toxic component of a food is considered dangerous enough to public health to warrant government prohibition of the sale of that food. The U.S. Food and Drug Administration tests foods for action levels.

action potential, an electrical impulse consisting of a self-propagating series of polarizations and depolarizations, transmitted across the plasma membranes of a nerve fiber during the transmission of a nerve impulse and across the plasma membranes of a muscle cell during contraction or other activity. In the absence of an impulse, the inside is electrically negative and the outside is positive (the resting potential). During the passage of an impulse at any point on the nerve fiber, the inside becomes positive and the outside, negative. Also called **action current.**

action tremor [L, *agere,* to do, *tremor,* shaking], a slight shaking that occurs or is evident during voluntary movements of the upper extremities. Also called **intention tremor.**

Activase, a trademark for a commercial form of tissue plasminogen activator (alteplase recombinant).

activate /ak'təvāt/, [L, *activus,* active], **1.** to induce or prolong an activity or render optimal action. **2.** to treat sewage by using a combination of bacteria and air.

activated charcoal, a general-purpose emergency antidote and a powerful pharmaceutic adsorbent.

■ INDICATIONS: It is prescribed in the treatment of acute poisoning and the control of flatulence.

■ CONTRAINDICATIONS: There are no known contraindications, but activated charcoal is ineffective in poisoning caused by a strong acid or alkali, cyanide, organic solvents, ethanol, methanol, iron, and lithium. It should not be administered to unconscious persons.

■ ADVERSE EFFECTS: There are no known adverse effects.

activated clotting time (ACT) test, a blood test primarily used to measure the effect of heparin as an anticoagulant during cardiac angioplasty, hemodialysis, and cardiopulmonary bypass surgery (CPB). It can also be used to monitor the dose of protamine sulfate required to reverse the effect of heparin. The test measures the time required for whole blood to clot after the addition of particulate activators.

activated 7-dehydrocholesterol. See **vitamin D₃.**

activated partial thromboplastin time (APTT), See **partial thromboplastin time.**

activated prothrombin complex concentrate (APCC), anti-inhibitor coagulant complex.

activated resin. See **self-curing resin.**

activating enzyme, an enzyme that promotes or sustains an activity, such as catalyzing the combining of amino acids to form peptides or proteins.

activation /ak'tivā'shən/, the promotion or production of an activity, such as the generation of a catalyst, protein synthesis, or enzymatic function.

activation energy [L, *activus,* active], the energy required to convert reactants to transition-state species or an activated complex that will spontaneously proceed to products.

activation factor. See **factor XII.**

activator /ak'tivā'tər/, **1.** a substance, force, or device that stimulates activity in another substance or structure, especially a substance that activates an enzyme. **2.** a substance that stimulates the development of an anatomic structure in

the embryo. **3.** an internal secretion of the pancreas. **4.** an apparatus for making substances radioactive, such as a cyclotron or neutron generator. **5.** (in dentistry) a removable orthodontic appliance that functions as a passive transmitter and stimulator of the perioral muscles.

active algolagnia. See **sadism.**

active anaphylaxis [Gk, *ana,* up, *phylaxis,* protection], a condition of hypersensitivity caused by the reaction of the immune system to the injection of a foreign protein. See also **anaphylaxis.**

active assisted exercise [L, *activus*], the movement of the body or any of its parts primarily through the individual's own efforts but accompanied by the aid of a member of the health care team or some device, such as an exercise machine. See also **exercise, passive exercise, range of motion.**

active carrier [OFr, *carier*], a person without signs or symptoms of an infectious disease who carries the causal microorganisms and can transmit the disease to others.

active electrode [Gk, *elektron,* amber, *hodos,* way], an electrode that is applied at a specific point to produce stimulation in a concentrated area in electrotherapy.

active euthanasia, the ending of life by the deliberate administration of drugs.

active exercise, repetitive movement of a part of the body as a result of voluntary contraction and relaxation of the controlling muscles. Compare **passive exercise.** See also **aerobic exercise, anaerobic exercise.**

active expiration [L, *expirare,* to breathe out], forced exhalation, using the abdominal wall, internal intercostal muscles, and diaphragm.

active hyperemia [L, *activus* + Gk, *hyper,* excessive, *haima,* blood], the increased flow of blood into a particular body part.

active immunity, a form of long-term, acquired immunity; it protects the body against a new infection as the result of antibodies that develop naturally after an initial infection or artificially after a vaccination. Compare **passive immunity.** See also **immune response.**

active labor [L, *activus,* active, *labor,* work], the normal progress of the birth process, including uterine contractions, dilation of the cervix, and descent of the fetus into the birth canal.

active listening[1], the act of alert intentional hearing and demonstration of an interest in what a person has to say through verbal signal, nonverbal gestures, and body language.

active listening[2], a nursing intervention from the Nursing Interventions Classification (NIC) defined as attending closely to and attaching significance to a patient's verbal and nonverbal messages. See also **Nursing Interventions Classification.**

active matrix array (AMA), a large-area integrated circuit that consists of millions of identical semiconductor elements and acts as the flat-panel image receptor in digital radiographic and fluoroscopic systems.

active movement, muscular action at a joint as a result of voluntary effort. Compare **passive movement.**

active-passive, (in psychiatry) a concept that characterizes persons as either actively involved in shaping events, such as being proactive, or passively reacting to them, such as being reactive.

active play, any activity from which one derives amusement, entertainment, enjoyment, or satisfaction by taking a participatory rather than a passive role. Children of all age groups engage in various forms of active play, from the exploration of objects and toys by the infant and toddler to the formal games, sports, and hobbies of the older child. Compare **passive play.**

active range of motion (AROM), the range of movement through which a patient can actively (without assistance) move a joint by the adjacent muscles.

active resistance exercise, the movement or exertion of the body or any of its parts performed totally through the individual's own efforts against a resisting force. See also **progressive resistance exercise.**

active resistance training (ART), a conditioning or rehabilitation program designed to enhance a patient's muscular strength, power, and endurance through progressive active resistance exercises and muscle overloading.

active sensitization [L, *agere,* to do, *sentire,* to feel], the condition that results when a specific antigen is injected into a person known to be susceptible. See also **sensitization.**

active site, the place on the surface of an enzyme where its catalytic action occurs.

active specific immunotherapy, a therapy in which a cancer patient is exposed to irradiated tumor cells. The injected cells stimulate the production of antibodies that destroy the tumor cells.

active transport, the movement of materials across the membranes and epithelial layers of a cell by means of chemical activity that allows the cell to admit otherwise impermeable molecules against a concentration gradient. Expediting active transport are carrier molecules within the cell that bind and enclose themselves to incoming molecules. Active transport is the means by which the cell absorbs glucose and other substances needed to sustain life and health. Certain enzymes play a role in active transport, providing a chemical "pump" that typically uses adenosine triphosphate to help move substances through the plasma membrane. Compare **osmosis, passive transport.**

activities of daily living (ADL) /aktiv'itēz/, the activities usually performed in the course of a normal day in the person's life, such as eating, toileting, dressing, bathing, or brushing the teeth. The ability to perform ADL may be compromised by a variety of causes, including chronic illnesses and accidents. The limitation may be temporary or permanent; rehabilitation may involve relearning the skills or learning new ways to accomplish ADL. The goal of health care professionals is to promote the greatest degree of independence for the patient. An ADL checklist is often used before discharge from a hospital. If any activities cannot be adequately performed, arrangements are made with an outside agency, health care professionals, or family members to provide the necessary assistance. See also **Barthel Index.**

Specific elements to consider in activities of daily living training

Feeding:
- Utensil, cup, plate management, and napkin use.
- Tidiness/organization.
- Awareness of swallowing, chewing, or pocketing problems.
- Ability to handle different food consistencies (e.g., finger foods versus soups).
- Mouth care after eating.

Bathing:
- Assembling of items and appropriate equipment.
- Management of caps, lids, sprays, etc.
- Facial cleansers and cosmetic application.
- Shaving foam or soap application versus electric razor.
- Shaving face, underarms, and/or legs.
- Hair care.
- Deodorant application.
- Tooth/denture care.
- Nail care.
- Replacement of care items.
- Location of bath facilities in hospital and home.
- Transfer ability to bathtub or shower.

Dressing:
- Selection of clothing.
- Assembling of clothing.
- Application of underwear.
- Management of fasteners.
- Application of trousers/slacks, belt, or suspenders.
- Management of pullover tops.
- Application of shirt, jacket, dress (front opening), or tie.
- Management of buttons.
- Application of socks or stockings.
- Application of shoes and tying laces.
- Location of dressing activities: bed, sitting or standing.
- Ability to care for and apply glasses, contact lenses, or hearing aid.

Toileting and elimination management:
- Transfer ability.
- Clothing management.
- Cognitive function.
- Bowel and bladder control.
- External devices: assembly, application, removal, and care of equipment.
- Suppository insertion (include preparation of suppository and cleaning of insertion device if used).
- Post toileting hygiene.
- Timing of bowel program (morning or evening).
- Employment/school/home/environment considerations.
- Colostomy or ileal conduit care.
- Performance of bladder management programs.
- Accident management.

Active transport: the sodium-potassium pump
(Thibodeau and Patton, 2003)

Adapted from Mumma CM, ed: *Rehabilitation nursing concepts and practice: a core curriculum,* ed 2, Skokie, Ill, 1987, Rehabilitation Nursing Foundation.

activity, the action of an enzyme on an amount of substrate that is converted to product per unit time under defined conditions.

activity coefficient, a proportionality constant, γ, relating activity, α, to concentration, *c,* expressed in the equation, α = γ*c.*

activity intolerance, a nursing diagnosis accepted by the Fifth National Conference on the Classification of Nursing Diagnoses. Activity intolerance is a state in which an individual has insufficient physiologic or psychologic energy to endure or complete required or desired daily activities. The cause of the condition may be generalized weakness, a sedentary lifestyle, imbalance between oxygen supply and demand, or bed rest or immobility. ■ DEFINING CHARACTERISTICS: The defining characteristics include verbal report of fatigue or weakness, abnormal heart rate or blood pressure response to activity, exertional discomfort or dyspnea, electrocardiographic changes reflecting arrhythmias or ischemia, and changes in skin color or moisture. ■ RELATED FACTORS: The related factors include generalized weakness, sedentary life-style, imbalance between oxygen supply and demand, bed rest or immobility. See also **nursing diagnosis.**

activity intolerance, risk for, a nursing diagnosis accepted by the Seventh National Conference on the Classification of Nursing Diagnoses. Risk for activity intolerance is a state in which an individual is at risk of experiencing insufficient physiologic or psychologic energy to endure or complete required or desired daily activities. ■ RISK FACTORS: Risk factors are a history of previous intolerance, deconditioned status, presence of circulatory or respiratory problems, and inexperience with activity. See also **nursing diagnosis.**

activity theory, a concept proposed by Havighurst and Albrecht, that continuing activities from middle age promotes well-being and satisfaction in aging. Thus older adults who are actively involved in a variety of situations and who establish new roles and relationships are more likely to age with a sense of satisfaction.

activity therapy, a nursing intervention from the Nursing Interventions Classification (NIC) defined as prescription of and assistance with specific physical, cognitive, social, and spiritual activities to increase the range, frequency, or duration of an individual's (or group's) activity. See also **Nursing Interventions Classification.**

activity tolerance[1], the type and amount of exercise a patient may be able to perform without undue exertion or possible injury.

activity tolerance[2], a nursing outcome from the Nursing Outcomes Classification (NOC) defined as responses to energy-consuming body movements involved in required or desired daily activities. See also **Nursing Outcomes Classification.**

actomyosin /ak′təmī′əsin/, the complex consisting of parallel threads of actin and myosin proteins that constitutes muscle fibers. It is responsible for contraction and relaxation of muscle. When a muscle fiber contracts, the two proteins slide past each other, shortening the fiber while increasing its apparent thickness. See also **sliding filaments.**

actual cautery /ak′chōō·əl/ [L, *actus,* act], the application of heat, rather than a chemical substance, in the destruction of tissue.

actual charge, the amount actually charged or billed by a practitioner for a service. The actual charge usually is not the same as that paid for the service by an insurance plan.

actual damages. See **damages.**

actual focal spot. See **focal spot.**

actualize /ak′chōō·əlīz′/, **1.** the act of fulfilling a potential, as by a person who may develop capabilities through experience and education. **2.** to fulfill highest level of human needs based on Maslow's hierarchy of needs.

acu-, combining form meaning 'sharp, clear, needle': *acuity, acupuncture.*

acuity /əkyōō′itē/ [L, *acuere,* to sharpen], the clearness or sharpness of perception, such as visual acuity.

acuminate /ə·kyōō′mi·nāt/, [L, *acuminatus*], **1.** sharp-pointed. **2.** to sharpen something or to make it tapered.

acuminate wart. See **genital wart.**

acupressure[1] /ak′yəpresh′ər/ [L, *acus,* needle, *pressura,* pressure], a therapeutic technique of applying digital pressure in a specified way on designated points on the body to relieve pain, produce anesthesia, or regulate a body function.

acupressure[2], a nursing intervention from the Nursing Interventions Classification (NIC) defined as the application of firm, sustained pressure to special points on the body to decrease pain, produce relaxation, and prevent or reduce nausea. See also **Nursing Interventions Classification.**

acupressure needles, needles inserted near a source of bleeding to help control blood loss. The needles exert pressure on tissues adjacent to the damaged vessel.

acupuncture /ak′yəpunk′chər/, [L, *acus* + *punctura,* puncture], a traditional Chinese method of producing analgesia or altering the function of a body system by inserting fine, wire-thin needles into the skin at specific sites on the body along a series of lines, or channels, called meridians. Acupuncture is highly effective in treating both acute and chronic pain associated with multiple causes. In addition, common conditions are effectively treated, including sinusitis, allergies, tinnitus, sore throats, high blood pressure, gastroesophageal reflex, hyperacidity and peptic ulcer disease, constipation, diarrhea, spastic colon, urinary incontinence, bladder and kidney infection, premenstrual syndrome (PMS), infertility, dysmenorrhea, memory problems, sensory disturbances, depression, anxiety, and other psychologic disorders. See also **moxibustion. —acupuncturist,** *n.*

acupuncture point, one of many discrete points on the skin along the several meridians, or chains of points of the body. Stimulation of any of the various points may induce an increase or decrease in function or sensation in an area or system of the body.

acus /ā′kəs/ [L], any needlelike structure.

-acusis. See **-acousia.**

acute /əkyōōt′/ [L, *acutus,* sharp], **1.** (of a disease or disease symptoms) beginning abruptly with marked intensity or sharpness, then subsiding after a relatively short period. **2.** sharp or severe. Compare **chronic.**

acute abdomen, an abnormal condition characterized by the acute onset of severe pain within the abdominal cavity. An acute abdomen requires immediate evaluation and diagnosis because it may indicate a condition that calls for surgical intervention. Information about the onset, duration, character, location, and symptoms associated with the pain is critical in making an accurate diagnosis. The patient is asked what decreases or increases the pain; constant, increasing pain is generally associated with appendicitis and diverticulitis, whereas intermittent pain is more likely indicative of a bowel obstruction, ureteral calculi, or gallstones. Appendicitis may often be differentiated from a perforated ulcer by the slower onset or development of pain. Although the patient's report of the location of the pain is sometimes misleading because of referral, radiation, or reflection of pain, it may serve to identify a specific organ or system. Factors in the patient's history that are useful in the diagnosis and

Acupuncture sites on a male model *(Swartz, 2002)*

management of an acute abdomen include changes in bowel habits, weight loss, bloody stool, diarrhea, menses, vomiting, clay-colored stool, and previous abdominal surgery. Also called **surgical abdomen.** See also **abdominal pain.**

acute abscess [L, *acutus,* sharp, *abscedere,* to go away], a collection of pus in a body cavity accompanied by localized inflammation, pain, pyrexia, and swelling.

acute air trapping, a condition of bronchiolar obstruction that results in early airway closure and trapping of air distal to the affected bronchiole. Airtrapping can occur in persons with chronic obstructive pulmonary disease or asthma. Persons prone to episodes of acute air trapping learn to control exhalations through pursed-lip breathing.

acute alcoholism, drunkenness or intoxication resulting from excessive consumption of alcoholic beverages. The syndrome is temporary and is characterized by depression of the higher nerve centers, causing impaired motor control, stupor, lack of coordination, and often nausea, dehydration, headache, and other physical symptoms. Compare **chronic alcoholism.** See also **alcoholism.**

acute angle [L, *acutus + angulus*], any angle of less than 90 degrees.

acute anicteric hepatitis [Gk, *a,* without, *ikteros,* jaundice, *hēpar,* liver, *itis,* inflammation], an acute hepatitis that is not accompanied by jaundice.

acute articular rheumatism [L, *articulare,* to divide into joints; Gk, *rheumatismos,* that which flows], a common form of adult rheumatism, possibly associated with a pyogenic infection in the joints. Symptoms include fever and arthritis.

acute ascending myelitis [L, *ascendere,* to go up; Gk, *myelos,* marrow, *itis,* inflammation], a severe inflammation of the spinal cord that extends progressively upward with corresponding interference in nerve functions. See also **myelitis.**

acute ascending spinal paralysis, a severe progressive spinal paralysis that spreads upward toward the brain.

acute atrophic paralysis [Gk, *a, trophe,* without nourishment, *paralyein,* to be palsied], a severe poliomyelitis involving the anterior horns of the spinal cord. It results first in flaccid paralysis of involved muscle groups and later by atrophy of those muscles.

acute bacterial arthritis. See **septic arthritis.**

acute bronchitis. See **bronchitis.**

acute care, a pattern of health care in which a patient is treated for a brief but severe episode of illness, for the sequelae of an accident or other trauma, or during recovery from surgery. Acute care is usually given in a hospital by specialized personnel using complex and sophisticated technical equipment and materials, and it may involve intensive care, critical care, or emergency care. This pattern of care is often necessary for only a short time, unlike chronic care.

acute catarrhal sinusitis [Gk, *kata + rhoia,* flow; L, *sinus,* hollow], an inflammation that involves the nose and sinuses.

acute cervicitis. See **cervicitis.**

acute childhood leukemia, a progressive, malignant disease of the blood-forming tissues. It is characterized by the uncontrolled proliferation of immature leukocytes and their precursors, particularly in the bone marrow, spleen, and lymph nodes. It is the most frequent cancer in children, with a peak onset occurring between 2 and 5 years of age.

■ OBSERVATIONS: Acute leukemia is classified according to cell type: **acute lymphoid leukemia (ALL)** includes lymphatic, lymphocytic, lymphoblastic, and lymphoblastoid types; **acute nonlymphoid leukemia (ANLL)** includes granulocytic, myelocytic, monocytic, myelogenous, monoblastic, and monomyeloblastic types (the myelocytic and monocytic series are abbreviated **AML**). ALL is predominantly a disease of childhood, whereas AML and ANLL occur in all age groups. The traditional classification of leukemia into chronic and acute types is based on duration or expected course of the illness and the relative maturity of the leukemic cells. The exact cause of the disease is unknown, although various factors are implicated, including genetic defects, immune deficiency, viruses, and carcinogenic environmental factors, primarily ionizing radiation. In acute leukemia, large immature leukocytes accumulate rapidly and infiltrate other body tissues, especially the reticuloendothelial system, causing decreased production of erythrocytes and platelets. Neutropenia, anemia, increased susceptibility to infection and hemorrhage, and weakening of the bones with a tendency to fracture also occur. Initial symptoms of the disease include fever; pallor; fatigue; anorexia; secondary infections (usually of the mouth, throat, or lungs); bone, joint, and abdominal pain; subdermal or submucosal hemorrhage; and enlargement of the spleen, liver, and lymph nodes. Onset may be abrupt or may follow a gradual, progressive course. Involvement of the central nervous system may lead to leukemic meningitis. Characteristically, a peripheral blood smear reveals many immature leukocytes. The diagnosis is confirmed by bone marrow aspiration or biopsy and examination, which in ALL reveal a highly elevated number of lymphoblasts with almost complete absence of erythrocytes, granulocytes, and megakaryocytes. The prognosis is poor in untreated cases, and death occurs usually within 6 months after onset of symptoms. Survival rates have dramatically increased in recent years with the use of antileukemic agents in combination regimens. Remission of 5 years or longer occurs in 50% to 70% of children with ALL, with 20% to 30% achieving complete remission. Children with AML have a poorer prognosis, and the remission rate is far less than for ALL.

■ INTERVENTIONS: Treatment of acute leukemia consists of a three-stage process involving the use of chemotherapeutic agents and irradiation. In the first phase (remission induction), complete destruction of all leukemic cells is achieved within a 4- to 6-week period with the use of a combination drug-therapy regimen. The main drugs used in ALL are the corticosteroids, usually three daily oral doses of prednisone; vincristine, administered intravenously once a week; and L-asparaginase, given intramuscularly three times a week for a total of nine doses. Allopurinol, a xanthine-oxidase inhibitor, is usually administered to inhibit uric acid production. Other drugs used in various combination regimens in sequential cycles include methotrexate, 6-mercaptopurine, cyclophosphamide, cytosine arabinoside, hydroxyurea, daunorubicin, and doxorubicin. In children with AML the primary drugs for induction remission are 6-thioguanine, daunomycin, cytosine arabinoside, 5-azacytidine, vincristine, and prednisone. The child is usually hospitalized for part or all of the treatment because of the many side effects of the drugs and the high risk of complications, especially infection and hemorrhage. If severe hemorrhaging occurs and does not respond to local treatment, platelet transfusions may be necessary, and in cases of severe anemia, especially during induction therapy, whole blood or packed red cells may be needed to raise hemoglobin levels. The second stage of treatment involves prophylactic maintenance to prevent leukemic infiltration of the central nervous system. Because chemotherapy drugs do not cross the blood-brain barrier, therapy usually consists of daily high-dose cranial irradiation for about 2 weeks after induction remission and weekly or twice-weekly doses of intrathecal methotrexate, for a total of five or six injections; in some cases only the drug is given. In small children the irradiation is limited to the cranium to prevent retardation of linear growth, but older children may receive craniospinal radiation. Therapy to maintain remission usually begins after the child is discharged from the hospital and consists of various regimens of drugs in combination. A common schedule includes daily oral doses of 6-mercaptopurine and weekly doses of oral methotrexate, intermittent short-term therapy with prednisone and vincristine, and periodic doses of intrathecal methotrexate for prophylaxis against spread to the central nervous system. Complete blood counts are done weekly or monthly, and bone marrow examinations are performed every 3 to 4 months to detect myelosuppression and drug toxicity. Maintenance therapy is discontinued after a period of 2 to 3 years if initial remission is maintained. Continuous treatment beyond 3 years is not advised, as the adverse affects of the medications increase with prolonged use. Relapse occurs in as many as 20% of treated children. If relapse occurs, the child begins the treatment cycle again, usually with prednisone, vincristine, and a combination of other drugs not previously tried. With each relapse the prognosis becomes poorer. Other treatments for prolonging remission include immunotherapy using periodic inoculation with bacille Calmette-Guérin vaccine or bone marrow transplantation, which has been successful in inducing long-term remissions in about 10% to 20% of the cases, especially those with AML or severe, terminal ALL.

■ NURSING CONSIDERATIONS: Nursing care for the child with acute leukemia involves intensive physical and emotional support during all phases of the disease, its diagnosis, and treatment. Foremost is the preparation of the child and parents for the various diagnostic and therapeutic procedures, including venipuncture, bone-marrow aspiration or biopsy,

lumbar puncture, and x-ray treatment. Specific medical and nursing management depends on the particular regimen of drug therapy, although most of the chemotherapeutic agents used in treatment cause myelosuppression that may lead to secondary complications of infection, hemorrhage, and anemia. Overwhelming infection is a major problem and one of the most frequent causes of death. Severe neutropenia indicates increased risk of infection. It may occur during immunosuppressive therapy or after prolonged antibiotic therapy. The most common infectious organisms are viruses, especially varicella, herpes zoster, herpes simplex, measles, mumps, rubella, and poliomyelitis; both gram-positive and gram-negative bacteria, including *Staphylococcus aureus, S. epidermidis,* group-A beta-hemolytic *Streptococcus, Pseudomonas aeruginosa, Escherichia coli, Proteus,* and *Klebsiella;* and various parasites and fungi, especially *Pneumocystis jiroveci* and *Candida albicans.* To prevent infection, the nurse isolates the child as much as possible, screens visitors for active infection, institutes strict aseptic procedures, monitors temperature closely, evaluates possible infection sites (such as needle punctures), encourages adequate nutrition, helps the child to avoid exertion or fatigue, and, at discharge, teaches the child and parents the necessity for avoiding all known sources of infection, primarily the common childhood communicable diseases. Preventive measures to control infection also help decrease the tendency toward hemorrhage. Special attention is given to skin care, oral hygiene, cleanliness of the perineal area, and restriction of activities that could result in accidental injury. A major nursing consideration is the management of the many side effects resulting from drug toxicity and irradiation, including nausea and vomiting, anorexia, oral and rectal ulceration, alopecia, hemorrhagic cystitis, and peripheral neuropathy, including weakness and numbing of the extremities and severe jaw pain. Although corticosteroid treatment usually increases the appetite and produces a euphoric sense of well-being in the child, it also causes moon face, which is reversed with cessation of the steroid therapy. During maintenance therapy, the nurse continues to provide emotional support and guidance, specifically teaching parents which side effects are normal reactions to drugs and which indicate toxicity and require medical attention. In terminal stages of the disease, relief of discomfort and pain becomes the primary focus. Effective measures include careful physical handling of the child, frequent position changes, prevention of pressure on painful areas, and control of annoying environmental factors, such as excessive light and noise. Nonsalicylate analgesics are used as needed, depending on the severity of pain. See also **acute lymphocytic leukemia, acute myelocytic leukemia, leukemia.**

acute cholecystitis. See **cholecystitis.**

acute circulatory failure /sur'kyələtôr'ē/, a drop in cardiac output resulting from cardiac or noncardiac causes and leading to tissue hypoxia. Acute circulatory failure usually happens so rapidly that the body does not have time to adjust to the changes. If not controlled immediately, the condition usually progresses to shock.

acute circumscribed edema [L, *circum,* around, *scribere,* to draw; Gk, *oidema,* swelling], a localized edema, often associated with an inflammatory lesion or process.

acute confusional state, a form of delirium caused by interference with the metabolic or other biochemical processes essential for normal brain functioning. Symptoms may include disturbances in cognition, levels of awareness, short-term memory deficit, retrograde and enterograde amnesia, and orientation, accompanied by restlessness, apprehension, irritability, and apathy. The condition may be asso-

Acute childhood leukemia *(Carr and Rodak, 1999)*

ciated with an acute physiologic state, delirium, toxic psychosis, or acute brain syndrome. An acute stress reaction to new surroundings or new demands is common in adolescence; it generally subsides as the person adjusts.

acute coronary syndrome, a classification encompassing clinical presentations ranging from unstable angina through myocardial infarctions not characterized by alterations in Q waves. The classification sometimes also includes myocardial infarctions characterized by altered Q waves.

acute delirium, an episode of acute organic reaction that is sudden, severe, and transient. See also **delirium.**

acute diarrhea [Gk, *dia + rhein,* to flow], a sudden severe attack of diarrhea.

acute diffuse peritonitis [L, *diffundere,* to pour out; Gk, *peri,* near, *tenein,* to stretch, *itis,* inflammation], an acute widespread attack of peritonitis affecting most of the peritoneum and usually caused by a perforation of an abdominal organ (e.g., stomach or appendix). It is also a complication of peritoneal dialysis. Also called **generalized peritonitis.**

acute disease, a disease characterized by a relatively sudden onset of symptoms that are usually severe. An episode of acute disease results in recovery to a state comparable to the patient's condition of health and activity before the disease, in passage into a chronic phase, or in death. Examples are pneumonia and appendicitis. See also **chronic disease.**

acute disseminated encephalitis. See **acute disseminated encephalomyelitis.**

acute disseminated encephalomyelitis, a form of encephalitis that commonly develops after an acute viral infection, such as measles, apparently as an immune attack on the myelin tissue of the nervous system. Early symptoms may include fever, headache, vomiting, and drowsiness and progress to seizures, coma, and paralysis. Frequently patients who recover experience neurologic disorders. Also called **acute disseminated encephalitis.**

acute diverticulitis, a sudden severe, painful disorder of the intestinal tract, resulting from inflammation of one or more diverticula, or pouches, in the wall of the bowel. The condition is typically diagnosed through x-rays and treated surgically. If left untreated, the inflamed pouches may rupture, spilling fecal matter into the abdominal cavity and causing peritonitis.

acute endarteritis [Gk, *endon,* within, *arteria,* windpipe, *itis,* inflammation], inflammation of the cells lining an artery. It may be caused by an infection or the proliferation of fibrous tissue inside the arterial wall. Also called **endarteritis.**

acute epiglottitis, a severe, rapidly progressing bacterial infection of the upper respiratory tract that occurs in young children, primarily between 2 and 7 years of age. It is characterized by sore throat, croupy stridor, and inflamed epiglottis, which may cause sudden respiratory obstruction and possibly death. The infection is generally caused by *Haemophilus influenzae,* type B, although streptococci may occasionally be the causative agent. Transmission occurs by infection with airborne particles or contact with infected secretions. The diagnosis is made by bacteriologic identification of *H. influenzae,* type B, in a specimen taken from the upper respiratory tract or in the blood. A lateral x-ray film of the neck shows an enlarged epiglottis and distension of the hypopharynx, which distinguishes the condition from croup. Direct visualization of the inflamed, cherry-red epiglottis by depression of the tongue or indirect laryngoscopy is also diagnostic but may produce total acute obstruction and should be attempted only by trained personnel with equipment to establish an airway or to provide respiratory resuscitation, if necessary. Compare **croup.**

■ OBSERVATIONS: The onset of the infection is abrupt, and it progresses rapidly. The first signs—sore throat, hoarseness, fever, and dysphagia—may be followed by an inability to swallow, drooling, varying degrees of dyspnea, inspiratory stridor, marked irritability and apprehension, and a tendency to sit upright and hyperextend the neck to breathe. Difficulty in breathing may progress to severe respiratory distress in minutes or hours. Suprasternal, supraclavicular, intercostal, and subcostal inspiratory retractions may be visible. The hypoxic child appears frightened and anxious; the skin color ranges from pallor to cyanosis.

■ INTERVENTIONS: Establishment of an airway is urgent, either by endotracheal intubation or by tracheostomy. Humidity and oxygen are provided, and airway secretions are drained or suctioned. IV fluids are usually required, and antibiotic therapy is initiated immediately, usually with ceftriaxone, cefuroxime, or ampicillin/sulbactam. Sedatives are contraindicated because of their depressant effect on the respiratory system, and antihistamines and adrenergic drugs are not usually of any therapeutic value. Steroids are useful.

■ NURSING CONSIDERATIONS: The nurse may assist with intubation or tracheostomy once the diagnosis is confirmed. Intensive nursing care is required for a child with acute epiglottitis. The most acute phase of the condition passes within 24 to 48 hours, and intubation is rarely needed beyond 3 to 4 days. As the child responds to therapy, breathing becomes easier; rapid recovery usually occurs so that bed rest and quiet activity to relieve boredom become primary nursing concerns. The infection may spread, causing such complications as otitis media, pneumonia, and bronchiolitis. Complications of the tracheostomy may also develop, including infection, atelectasis, cannula occlusion, tracheal bleeding, granulation, stenosis, and delayed healing of the stoma. Also called **acute epiglottiditis.**

acute erosive gastritis, acute gastritis involving erosions of the full thickness of the stomach mucosa, usually with some degree of hemorrhaging. It may be either localized or diffuse.

acute fatigue, a sudden onset of physical and mental exhaustion or weariness, particularly after a period of mental or physical stress. Physical factors usually include an accumulation of waste products of muscle contractions. Boredom is a common mental factor. Recovery follows a period of rest and restoration of energy sources.

acute febrile neutrophilic dermatosis. See **Sweet's syndrome.**

acute febrile polyneuritis. See **Guillain-Barré syndrome.**

acute fibrinous pericarditis [L, *fibra,* fibrous; Gk, *peri,* near, *kardia,* heart, *itis,* inflammation], acute inflammation of the endothelial cells of the pericardium with fibers extending into the pericardial sac.

Acute fibrinous pericarditis
(Kumar, Cotran, and Robbins, 1997)

acute focal bacterial nephritis. See **pyelonephritis.**

acute gastritis. See **gastritis.**

acute glaucoma. See **glaucoma.**

acute glomerulonephritis. See **postinfectious glomerulonephritis.**

acute goiter [L, *guttur,* throat], a condition of sudden enlargement of the thyroid gland. Clinical manifestations are those of hyperthyroidism.

acute granulocytic leukemia (AGL). See **acute myelocytic leukemia.**

acute hallucinatory paranoia, a form of psychosis in which hallucinations are combined with delusions of paranoia.

acute hallucinosis. See **alcoholic hallucinosis.**

acute hemorrhagic conjunctivitis, a highly contagious eye disease usually caused by enterovirus type 70 but also by coxsackie AZA. The disease is found primarily in densely populated humid areas, particularly the developing countries or places with a large immigrant population. Clinical features include sudden onset of severe ocular pain, blurred vision, photophobia, subconjunctival hemorrhage, chemosis, and profuse watery discharge from the eye. Spontaneous improvement occurs within 2 to 4 days and is complete by 7 to 10 days. Treatment consists of hygienic measures and ophthalmic preparations.

acute hemorrhagic leukoencephalitis. See **acute necrotizing hemorrhagic encephalopathy.**

acute hemorrhagic pancreatitis [Gk, *haima,* blood, *rhegnynei,* to gush, *pan,* all, *kreas,* flesh], a potentially fatal inflammation of the pancreas characterized by bleeding, tissue necrosis, and digestive tract paralysis.

acute hypoxia, a sudden or rapid depletion in available oxygen at the tissue level. The condition may result from asphyxia, airway obstruction, acute hemorrhage, blockage of the alveoli by edema or infectious exudate, or abrupt cardiorespiratory failure. Clinical signs may include hypoventilation or hyperventilation to the point of air hunger and neurologic deficits ranging from headache and confusion to loss of consciousness.

acute idiopathic polyneuritis. See **Guillain-Barré syndrome.**

acute idiopathic thrombocytopenic purpura. See **idiopathic thrombocytopenic purpura.**

acute illness, any illness characterized by signs and symptoms that are of rapid onset and short duration; it may be severe and impair normal functioning.

acute immune disease. See **autoimmunity.**

acute infectious nonbacterial gastroenteritis, former name for *Norwalk virus gastroenteritis.*

acute infectious paralysis [L, *inficere,* to stain; Gk, *paralyein,* to be palsied], **1.** an alternative term for acute anterior poliomyelitis. **2.** infectious polyneuritis.

acute infective hepatitis. See **hepatitis A.**

acute intermittent porphyria (AIP), an autosomal dominant, genetically transmitted metabolic hepatic disorder characterized by acute attacks of neurologic dysfunction that can be started by environmental or endogenous factors. Women are affected more frequently than men, and attacks often are precipitated by starvation or severe dieting, alcohol ingestion, bacterial or viral infections, and a wide range of pharmaceutic products. Any part of the nervous system can be affected, and an initial common effect is mild to severe abdominal pain. Other effects can include tachycardia, hypertension, hyponatremia, peripheral neuropathy, and organic brain dysfunction marked by seizures, coma, hallucinations, and respiratory paralysis. A frequent diagnostic factor is a high level of porphyrin precursors in the urine, which usually increases during periods of acute attacks. Treatment is generally symptomatic, with emphasis on respiratory support, beta blockers, pain control and education of the patient about environmental factors, particularly medications such as barbiturates, that are known to cause an onset of symptoms, and avoidance of alcohol, sunlight, and skin trauma. A high-carbohydrate diet is reported to reduce the risk of acute attacks because glucose tends to block the induction of hepatic gamma-aminolevulinic acid (ALA) synthetase, an enzyme involved in the porphyrias. See also **porphyria.**

acute interstitial nephritis. See **interstitial nephritis.**

acute laryngotracheobronchitis. See **croup.**

acute lichenoid pityriasis. See **Mucha-Habermann disease.**

acute lobar pneumonia, a form of pneumonia characterized by lobar distribution of the consolidation of the serofibrous fluid exuded by the alveoli. The condition results from an infection by a virulent type of *Streptococcus pneumoniae.* Onset is sudden. Symptoms include a pleuritic chest pain, dry cough, and rust-colored sputum.

acute lymphoblastic leukemia. See **acute lymphocytic leukemia.**

acute lymphocytic leukemia (ALL), a hematologic, malignant disease characterized by large numbers of immature cells, lymphoblasts in the bone marrow, circulating blood, lymph nodes, spleen, liver, and other organs. The number of normal blood cells is usually reduced. More than three-fourths of the cases in the United States occur in children, with the greatest number diagnosed between 2 and 5 years of age. The risk of the disease is increased for people with Down syndrome and for siblings of leukemia patients. The disease has a sudden onset and rapid progression marked by fever, pallor, anorexia, fatigue, anemia, hemorrhage, bone pain, splenomegaly, and recurrent infection. Blood and bone marrow studies are used for diagnosis and for determination of the type of proliferating lymphocyte, which may be B cells, T cells (which usually respond poorly to therapy), or null cells that lack T- or B-cell characteristics. Treatment includes intensive combination chemotherapy, therapy for secondary infections and hyperuricemia, irradiation, and intrathecal methotrexate.

Acute lymphocytic leukemia *(Zitelli and Davis, 1997)*

acute lymphoid leukemia (ALL). See **acute childhood leukemia.**

acute mastitis. See **mastitis.**

acute mountain sickness. See **altitude sickness.**

acute myelitis, a sudden, severe inflammation of the spinal cord. See also **acute transverse myelitis, myelitis.**

acute myelocytic leukemia (AML), a malignant neoplasm of blood-forming tissues characterized by the uncontrolled proliferation of immature granular leukocytes that usually have azurophilic Auer rods in their cytoplasm. Typical symptoms are spongy bleeding gums, anemia, fatigue, fever, dyspnea, moderate splenomegaly, joint and bone pains, and repeated infections. AML occurs most frequently in adolescents and young adults. The risk of the disease is increased among people who have been exposed to massive doses of radiation and who have certain blood dyscrasias, such as polycythemia vera, primary thrombocytopenia, and refractory anemia. Variants of AML, in which only one cell line proliferates, are erythroid, eosinophilic, basophilic, monocytic, and megakaryocytic leukemias. The diagnosis is based on blood counts and bone marrow biopsies. Radiotherapy, chemotherapy, biotherapy, and bone marrow transplantation are used, but long remissions resulting from any form of treatment are rare. Also called **acute granulocytic leukemia (AGL), acute myelogenous leukemia, acute nonlymphocytic leukemia (ANLL), myeloid leukemia, splenomedullary leukemia, splenomyelogenous leukemia.** See also **acute childhood leukemia, chronic myelocytic leukemia.**

acute myocardial infarction (AMI) [L, *acutus,* + Gk, *mys,* muscle, *kardia,* heart; L, *infarcire,* to stuff], the early critical stage of necrosis of heart muscle tissue caused by blockage of a coronary artery. It is characterized by elevated S-T segments in the reflecting leads and elevated levels of cardiac enzymes. See also **myocardial infarction.**

acute necrotizing hemorrhagic encephalopathy, a degenerative brain disease, characterized by marked edema, numerous minute hemorrhages, necrosis of blood vessel walls, demyelination of nerve fibers, and infiltration of the meninges with neutrophils, lymphocytes, and histiocytes. Typical signs are severe headache, fever, and vomiting; convulsions may occur, and the patient may rapidly lose consciousness. Treatment consists of decompression by withdrawing cerebrospinal fluids. Also called **acute hemorrhagic leukoencephalitis.**

acute necrotizing ulcerative gingivitis (ANUG), a recurrent periodontal disease of sudden onset that primarily affects the interdental papillae. It is characterized by painful inflammation and ulceration of the gums, leading to the formation of craterlike defects and ulcers. The necrotic tissue appears as a gray membrane that is easily sloughed off. There also may be fever, bone destruction, a fetid odor, and enlarged lymph nodes in the throat and neck. It is usually associated with poor oral hygiene and stress and is most common in conditions in which there is crowding of the teeth and malnutrition. Treatment includes chlorhexidine mouthwashes, antibiotics, analgesics, and dental care. Also called **trench mouth, Vincent's angina, Vincent's infection.** See **gingivitis.**

Acute necrotizing gingivitis *(Eisen and Lynch, 1998)*

acute nephritis, a sudden inflammation of the kidney, characterized by albuminuria and hematuria, but without edema or urine retention. It affects children most commonly and usually involves only a few glomeruli. See also **nephritis.**

acute nicotine poisoning [L, *Nicotiana, potio,* drink], a toxic effect produced by nicotine. Characteristics include burning sensation in the mouth, nausea and vomiting, diarrhea, palpitations, salivation, agitation, respiratory, depression, and convulsions that may lead to death.

acute nongonorrheal vulvitis [L, *non,* not; Gk, *gone,* seed, *rhoia,* flow; L, *vulva,* wrapper; Gk, *itis,* inflammation], an inflammation of the vulva resulting from chafing of the lips of the vulva, accumulation of sebaceous material, atopic reactions, local infections, or other causes that are nonvenereal.

acute nonlymphocytic leukemia (ANLL). See **acute myelocytic leukemia.**

acute nonspecific pericarditis [Gk, *peri,* around, *kardia,* heart, *itis,* inflammation], inflammation of the pericardium, with or without effusion. It often is associated with myocarditis but usually resolves without complications. See also **pericarditis.**

acute pain, severe pain, as may follow surgery or trauma or accompany myocardial infarction or other conditions and diseases. Acute pain occurring in the first 24 to 48 hours after surgery is often difficult to relieve, even with drugs. Some studies show that patients over 50 years of age need less analgesia to relieve acute pain than do younger patients. Another study indicates that 23% of surgical patients, except for orthopedic patients, do not require analgesia. Acute pain in individuals with orthopedic problems originates from the periosteum, the joint surfaces, and the arterial walls. Muscle pain associated with bone surgery results from muscle ischemia rather than muscle tension. Acute abdominal pain often causes the individual involved to lie on one side and draw up the legs in the fetal position. Compare **chronic pain.** See also **pain, pain intervention, pain pathway.**

acute pancreatitis [Gk, *pan,* all, *kreas,* flesh, *itis,* inflammation], a sudden inflammation of the pancreas caused by autodigestion and marked by symptoms of acute abdomen and escape of pancreatic enzymes into the pancreatic tissues. The condition is associated with biliary disease or alcoholism. The autodigestion is caused by premature activation of the digestive enzymes. The disorder can also be of unknown cause. See also **pancreatitis.**

acute paranoid disorder, a psychopathologic condition characterized by persecutory delusional thoughts of rapid onset, quick development, and short duration, usually lasting less than 6 months. The disorder, which rarely becomes chronic, is most commonly seen in persons who have experienced drastic changes in their environment, such as immigrants, refugees, prisoners, military inductees, and, in a less severe form, those leaving home for the first time. See also **brief psychotic reaction.**

acute parapsoriasis. See **Mucha-Habermann disease.**

acute pharyngitis, sudden, severe inflammation of the pharynx. See also **pharyngitis.**

acute pleurisy, inflammation of the pleura, often as a result of lung disease. It is characterized by irritation without recognizable effusion and is localized. See also **pleurisy.**

acute primary myocarditis, **1.** inflammation of the heart muscle most commonly caused by a bacterial infection initiated locally or carried through the bloodstream. **2.** severe inflammation of the heart muscle associated with degeneration of the muscle fibers and release of leukocytes into the interstitial tissues. See also **myocarditis.**

acute promyelocytic leukemia (AProL), a malignancy of the blood-forming tissues, characterized by the proliferation of promyelocytes and blast cells with distinctive Auer rods. Symptoms include severe bleeding and bruises. The patient may also have low fibrinogen level and platelet count. Management of the disease typically requires replacement of coagulation factors and administration of cytotoxic drugs. See **leukemia.**

acute prostatitis [L, *acutus,* sharp; Gk, *prostates,* one standing before, *itis,* inflammation], a sudden, severe inflammation of the prostate. See also **prostate, prostatitis.**

acute psychosis, one of a group of disorders in which ego functioning is either impaired or inhibited. The ability to process reality-based information is diminished and disordered. The cause of the particular disorder may be a known psychological abnormality. In situations where a physiologic abnormality is not recognized, the functional impairment is still clearly present.

acute pyelonephritis. See **pyelonephritis.**

acute pyogenic arthritis, an acute bacterial infection

Acute promyelocytic leukemia *(Carr and Rodak, 1999)*

of one or more joints, caused by trauma or a penetrating wound and occurring most frequently in children. Typical signs are pain, redness, and swelling in the affected joint; muscular spasms in the area; chills; fever; sweating; and leukocytosis. Treatment consists of immobilization of the joint, analgesia, sedation, and IV administration of an antibiotic. If required, the joint may be irrigated with normal saline solution and an antibiotic. Hospitalization is usually required.

acute radial nerve palsy. See **radial nerve palsy.**

acute radiation exposure. See **radiation exposure.**

acute rejection [L, *rejicere,* to throw back], following organ transplantations, the rapid reaction against allograph or xenograph tissue that is incompatible. It often occurs a week after treatment, during which the immune response increases in intensity.

acute renal failure (ARF), renal failure of sudden onset, such as from physical trauma, infection, inflammation, or toxicity. Symptoms include uremia and usually oliguria or anuria, with hyperkalemia and pulmonary edema. Three types are distinguished: prerenal, associated with poor systemic perfusion and decreased renal blood flow, such as with hypovolemic shock or congestive heart failure; intrarenal, associated with disease of the renal parenchyma, such as tubulointerstitial nephritis, acute interstitial nephritis, or nephrotoxicity; and postrenal, resulting from obstruction of urine flow out of the kidneys. See **renal failure.**

acute respiratory distress syndrome. See **adult respiratory distress syndrome.**

acute respiratory failure (ARF) [L, *acutus + respirare,* respiratory, *fallere,* to deceive], a sudden inability of the lungs to maintain normal respiratory function. The condition may be caused by an obstruction in the airways or by failure of the lungs to exchange gases in the alveoli.

acute rheumatic arthritis, arthritis that occurs during the acute phase of rheumatic fever.

acute rhinitis. See **rhinitis.**

acute schizophrenia, a disorder consisting of various degrees of psychosis that is characterized by the sudden onset of personality disorganization. Symptoms include disturbances in thought, mood, and behavior. Positive symptoms include delusions, which may be bizarre in nature; hallucinations, especially auditory; disorganized speech; inappropriate affect; and disorganized behavior. Negative symptoms include flat affect, avolition, alogia, and anhedonia. Episodes appear suddenly in persons whose previous behavior has been relatively normal and are usually of short duration.

Recurrent episodes are common, and in some instances a more chronic type of the disorder may develop. See also **schizoaffective disorder, schizophrenia, schizophreniform disorder.**

acute secondary myocarditis, sudden, severe inflammation of the heart muscle, as a result of a disease of the endocardium or pericardium or a generalized infection. See also **myocarditis.**

acute septic myocarditis [Gk, *septikos*, putrid, *mys*, muscle, *kardia*, heart, *itis*, inflammation], severe inflammation of the myocardium associated with pus formation, necrosis, and abscess formation. See also **myocarditis.**

acute suppurative arthritis [L, *suppurare*, to form pus], a form of arthritis characterized by an invasion of the joint space by pyogenic organisms and the formation of pus in the joint cavity.

acute suppurative sinusitis [L, *acutus*, sharp, *suppurare*, to form pus, *sinus*, hollow; Gk, *itis*, inflammation], a purulent infection of the sinuses. Symptoms are pain over the inflamed area, headache, chills, and fever.

acute tonsillitis [L, *acutus*, sharp, *tonsilla*; Gk, *itis*, inflammation], an inflammation of the tonsil(s) associated with a catarrhal exudate over the tonsil or the discharge of caseous or suppurative material from the tonsil crypts.

acute toxicity, the harmful effect of a toxic agent that manifests itself in seconds, minutes, hours, or days after entering the patient.

acute transverse myelitis, an inflammation of the entire thickness of the spinal cord, affecting both the sensory and motor nerves. It can develop rapidly, accompanied by necrosis and neurologic deficit that commonly persist after recovery. Patients in whom spastic reflexes develop soon after the onset of this disease are more likely to recover. This disorder may result from a variety of causes, such as multiple sclerosis, measles, pneumonia, viral infections and the ingestion of certain toxic agents such as carbon monoxide, lead, and arsenic. Such poisonous substances can destroy the entire circumference of the spinal cord, including the myelin sheaths, the axis cylinders, and the neurons, and can also cause hemorrhage and necrosis. There is no effective treatment, and the prognosis for complete recovery is poor. Nursing care includes frequent assessment of vital signs, vigilance for signs of spinal shock, maintenance of a urinary catheter, and proper skin care.

acute tubular necrosis (ATN), acute renal failure with mild to severe damage or necrosis of tubule cells, usually as a result of either nephrotoxicity, ischemia after major surgery, trauma (see **crush syndrome**), severe hypovolemia, sepsis, or burns. See also **renal failure.**

Ischemic acute tubular necrosis
(Cotran, Kumar, and Collins, 1999)

acute tubulointerstitial nephritis, an early stage of tubulointerstitial nephritis similar to acute pyelonephritis but with involvement further into the renal medulla to involve the tubules.

acute urethral syndrome [Gk, *ourethra*, urethra, *syn*, together, *dromos*, course], a group of pelvic symptoms experienced by women, including dysuria, urinary frequency, urinary tenesmus, lower back pain, and suprapubic aching and cramping. Clinical evidence of a pathogen or other factor to account for the symptoms may be absent, and further testing may be required.

acute vulvar ulcer, a nonvenereal, usually shallow lesion of the vulva, often associated with a febrile illness. Its cause is uncertain. Also called **Lipschütz's disease**.

acyanotic /ā′sī·ənot′ik/ [Gk, *a*, not, *kyanos*, blue], lacking a blue appearance of the skin and mucous membranes. See also **cyanosis.**

acyanotic congenital defect [Gk, *a*, *kyanos*, not blue], a heart defect present at birth that does not produce blue discoloration of the skin and mucous membranes under normal circumstances. However, the condition does increase the load on the pulmonary circulation and may lead to cyanosis, right ventricular failure, or other complications during physical exertion.

acyclovir /əsī′klōvir/, an antiviral agent with activity against herpesvirus types 1 and 2 and varicella zoster virus. Acyclovir is converted by a herpes virus enzyme into a molecule (acyclovir triphosphate) that inhibits the synthesis of deoxyribonucleic acid (DNA) molecules in the virally infected cells, thereby inhibiting viral replication.

■ INDICATIONS: It is prescribed topically in an ointment for the treatment of herpes simplex lesions (cold sores) and both orally and systemically (oral and IV) in other types of herpes infections, including genital herpes, herpes encephalitis, chickenpox (varicella-zoster) and shingles (herpes zoster).

■ CONTRAINDICATION: Known sensitivity to this drug prohibits its use.

■ ADVERSE EFFECTS: After topical use, irritation or pruritus may occur; after systemic use, diaphoresis, headache, and nausea may occur. When it is administered intravenously in the treatment of immunosuppressed patients, there may be pain at the site of the injection and 1%-10% have acute renal failure.

acyesis /ā′sī·ē′sis/, **1.** the absence of pregnancy. **2.** a condition of sterility in women.

acyl /ā′sil/, an organic radical derived from an organic acid by removal of the hydroxyl group from the carboxyl group. It is represented as R—CO—.

acylation /as′ilā′shən/, the incorporation into a molecule of an organic compound of an acyl group, R—CO—.

AD, abbreviation for **Alzheimer's disease.**

ad-, prefix meaning 'to, toward, addition to, or intensification': *adneural, adrenal.*

-ad, suffix meaning 'toward (a specified terminus)': *cephalad.*

a.d., abbreviation for **auris dextra,** or right ear.

A/D, 1. abbreviation for **analog-to-digital. 2.** abbreviation for **anodal duration. 3.** abbreviation for **average deviation.**

ADA, 1. abbreviation for **American Dental Association. 2.** abbreviation for **American Diabetes Association. 3.** abbreviation for **American Dietetic Association. 4.** abbreviation for **adenosine deaminase.**

ADAA, abbreviation for *American Dental Assistants' Association.*

adactyly /ādak′tilē/ [Gk, *a* + *daktylos*, not finger or toe], a congenital defect in which one or more digits of the hand or foot are missing.

Adair-Dighton syndrome [Charles Adair-Dighton, twentieth century British physician]. See **osteogenesis imperfecta.**

Adalat, trademark for a calcium channel blocker (nifedipine).

adalimumab, an antirheumatic immunomodulating agent used to treat patients greater than 18 years of age with moderate to severe rheumatoid arthritis.

adamantinoma, adamantoblastoma. See **ameloblastoma.**

Adam, Evelyn, a Canadian nursing theorist who applied the structure of a conceptual model for nursing in her book, *Être Infirmière* in 1979 (*To Be a Nurse,* 1980). A conceptual model consists of assumptions, beliefs and values, and major units. Adam believes that a theory is useful to more than one discipline, but that a conceptual model for a discipline is useful only to that discipline. Adam developed Virginia Henderson's concepts within Dorothy Johnson's structure of a conceptual model. She describes the goal of nursing as maintaining or restoring the client's independence in the satisfaction of 14 fundamental needs. Each need has biological, physiological, and psychosocial aspects. The nurse has the role of complementing and supplementing the client's strength, knowledge, and will.

ADAMHA, abbreviation for U.S. *Alcohol, Drug Abuse, and Mental Health Administration.*

Adam's apple, *informal,* the bulge at the front of the neck produced by the thyroid cartilage of the larynx. Also called **laryngeal prominence.**

Adams-Stokes syndrome [Robert Adams, Irish surgeon, 1791–1875; William Stokes, Irish physician, 1804–1878], a condition characterized by sudden, recurrent episodes of loss of consciousness caused by incomplete heart block. Seizures may accompany the episodes. Also called **Stokes-Adams syndrome.** See also **infranodal block.**

adapalene /ah-dap'ah-lēn/, a synthetic analogue of retinoic acid used topically in the treatment of acne vulgaris.

adaptation /ad'aptā'shən/ [L, *adaptatio,* act of adapting], a change or response to stress of any kind, such as inflammation of the nasal mucosa in infectious rhinitis or increased crying in a frightened child. Adaptation may be normal, self-protective, and developmental, as when a child learns to talk; it may be all-encompassing, creating further stress, as in polycythemia, which occurs naturally at high altitudes to provide more oxygen-carrying red blood cells but may also lead to thrombosis, venous congestion, or edema. The degree and nature of adaptation shown by a patient are evaluated regularly by the nurse. They constitute a measure of the effectiveness of nursing care, the course of the disease, and the ability of the patient to cope with stress. Compare **accommodation.**

adaptation model, (in nursing) a conceptual framework that focuses on the patient as an adaptive system, one in which nursing intervention is required when a deficit develops in the patient's ability to cope with the internal and external demands of the environment. These demands are classified into four groups: physiologic needs, the need for a positive self-concept, the need to perform social roles, and the need to balance dependence and independence. The nurse assesses the patient's maladaptive response and identifies the kind of demand that is causing the problem. Nursing care is planned to promote adaptive responses to cope successfully with the current stress on the patient's wellbeing. This model, first proposed by Sister Callista Roy, is frequently used as a conceptual framework for programs of nursing education.

adaptation syndrome. See **general adaptation syndrome.**

adaptation to physical disability, a nursing outcome from the Nursing Outcomes Classification (NOC) defined as an adaptive response to a significant functional challenge due to a physical disability.

adapted clothing, clothing that has been modified, such as with taped hook and loop or Velcro fasteners, to permit disabled persons to dress themselves with minimal difficulty.

adapter [L, *adaptatio,* the process of adjusting], a device for joining or connecting two or more parts of a system to enable it to function properly, usually with tubing.

adaptive capacity, decreased intracranial, a nursing diagnosis accepted by the Eleventh National Conference on the Classification of Nursing Diagnoses. Adaptive capacity, decreased: intracranial is a clinical state in which intracranial fluid dynamic mechanisms that normally compensate for increases in intracranial volumes are compromised, resulting in repeated disproportionate increases in intracranial pressure (ICP) in response to a variety of noxious and nonnoxious stimuli.

■ DEFINING CHARACTERISTICS: Major defining characteristics include repeated increases in ICP of greater than 10 mm Hg for more than 5 minutes after any of a variety of external stimuli. Minor defining characteristics include disproportionate increases in ICP after a single environmental or nursing maneuver stimulus; elevated component of P_2 ICP waveform; volume pressure response test variation (volume pressure ratio >2, pressure-volume index <10); baseline ICP equal to or greater than 10 mm Hg; and wide-amplitude ICP elevation.

■ RELATED FACTORS: Factors include brain injuries; sustained increase in ICP ≥G10 to 15 mm Hg; decreased cerebral perfusion pressure ≤H70 mm Hg; and systemic hypotension with intracranial hypertension. See also **nursing diagnosis.**

adaptive device /adap'tiv/ [L, *adaptatio,* process of adapting; OFr, *devise*], any structure, design, instrument, contrivance, or equipment that enables a person with a disability to function independently. Examples include plate guards, grab bars, and transfer boards. Also called **self-help device** or **assistive device.**

adaptive hypertrophy [L, *adaptatio,* process of adapting; Gk, *hyper,* excessive, *trophe,* nourishment], a reactive increase in amount of tissue that compensates for a loss of the same or similar tissue so that function is not impaired.

adaptive response, an appropriate reaction to an environmental demand.

adaptor RNA. See **transfer RNA.**

ADA Seal of Acceptance, an approval given by the American Dental Association to oral care products that are supported by adequate research evidence as to their safety and efficacy.

ADC, abbreviation for **AIDS-dementia complex.**

ADCC, abbreviation for **antibody-dependent cell-mediated cytotoxicity.**

ADC Van Disal /ā'dē'sē'vandī'səl/, a term used as a mnemonic device for recalling the protocol of hospital admission orders. The letters stand for **A**dmission authorization, **D**iagnosis, **C**ondition, **V**ital signs, **A**ctivity, **D**rugs, **I**nstructions, **S**pecial studies, **A**llergies, **L**aboratory tests.

Addams, Jane (1860–1935), an American social reformer. In Chicago in 1889 she founded Hull House, one of the first social settlements in the United States, where volunteers from many disciplines, including nursing, lived and worked in their professions. She played a central role in most of the social reforms of her time and provided an inspiration to those in the nursing profession who were striving to establish high educational standards and better working conditions. She was co-recipient of the Nobel peace prize in 1931.

adder, any of numerous venomous elapid and viperine

snakes. The death adder is found in Australia and New Guinea and the puff adder is found in Africa and Arabia. See also **snakebite.**

addict /ad′ikt/ [L, *addicere,* to devote], a person who has become physiologically or psychologically dependent on a chemical such as alcohol or other drugs to the extent that normal social, occupational, and other responsible life functions are disrupted.

addiction /ədik′shən/, [L, *addicere,* to devote], compulsive, uncontrollable dependence on a chemical substance, habit, or practice to such a degree that either the means of obtaining or ceasing use may cause severe emotional, mental, or physiologic reactions. Compare **habituation.**

addictive personality /ədik′tiv/, a personality marked by traits of compulsive and habitual use of a substance or practice in an attempt to cope with psychic pain engendered by conflict and anxiety.

addisonian anemia. See **pernicious anemia.**

addisonian crisis. See **adrenal crisis.**

addisonism, [Thomas Addison, London physician, 1793–1860], a condition characterized by the physical signs of Addison's disease, although loss of adrenocortical functions is not involved. The signs include increase in bronze pigmentation of the skin and mucous membranes caused by increased melanocyte-stimulating hormone (MSH), as well as general debility.

Addison's crisis. See **adrenal crisis.**

Addison's disease [Thomas Addison], a life-threatening condition caused by partial or complete failure of adrenocortical function, often resulting from autoimmune processes, infection (especially tubercular or fungal), neoplasm, or hemorrhage in the gland. All three general functions of the adrenal cortex (glucocorticoid, mineralocorticoid, and androgenic) are lost. Also called **Addison's syndrome, adrenocortical insufficiency.** See also **adrenal crisis.**

■ OBSERVATIONS: The disease is characterized by increased bronze pigmentation of the skin and mucous membranes; weakness; decreased endurance; anorexia; dehydration; weight loss; GI disturbances; salt cravings; anxiety, depression, and other emotional distress; and decreased tolerance to physical and emotional stress. The person's requirements for glucocorticoid, mineralocorticoid, and salt are increased by stress, as in infection, trauma, and surgical procedures. The onset is usually gradual, over a period of weeks or months. Laboratory tests reveal abnormally low blood concentrations of sodium and glucose, a greater than normal level of serum potassium, and a decreased urinary output of certain steroids. The diagnosis is established if the amount of cortisol in the plasma and steroid in the urine does not increase after stimulation with ACTH.

■ INTERVENTIONS: Treatment includes replacement therapy with glucocorticoid, and mineralocorticoid drugs, an adequate fluid intake, control of sodium and potassium balance, and a diet high in complex carbohydrates and protein. Follow-up care includes continued administration of glucocorticoid drugs.

■ NURSING CONSIDERATIONS: The complications of Addison's disease include high fever, confused behavior, and adrenal crisis (addisonian crisis). With careful management, the patient's resistance to infection, capacity for work, and general well-being can be maintained. Nursing care includes administering corticosteroids and other drugs, observing the patient for signs of abnormal sodium and potassium levels, monitoring body weight and fluid intake and output, and encouraging adequate intake of nutrients. The patient also needs protection against stress while in the hospital and instruction in the importance of avoiding stress at home. The significance of emotional distress, the value of wearing a medical-alert bracelet or tag, the signs of impending crisis, the use of a prepared kit for emergencies, and the importance of scrupulous attention to drug and diet regimens are emphasized before discharge. Discharge teaching also emphasizes the need to take cortisone after meals or with milk to prevent gastric irritation and the development of ulcers.

Addison's disease *(Moll, 1997)*

Addison's keloid. See **morphea.**

Addison's syndrome. See **Addison's disease.**

addition [L, *additio,* something added], a chemical reaction in which two complete molecules combine to form a new product, usually by attachment to carbon atoms at a double or triple bond of one of the molecules.

additive /ad′itiv/, any substance added intentionally or indirectly that becomes a part of the food, pharmaceutical, or other product. Additives may be introduced in growing, processing, packaging, storage, or cooking or other final preparation for consumption.

additive effect [L, *additio,* something added, *effectus*], the combined effect of drugs that, when used in combination, produce an effect that is greater than the sum of their separately measured individual effects.

adducent /ədoo′sənt/, an agent or other stimulus that causes a limb to be drawn toward the median axis of the body, or causes the fingers or toes to move together.

adduct /ədukt′/ [L, *adducere,* to bring to], to move toward the median axis of the body.

adduction /əduk′shən/ [L, *adducere,* to bring to], movement of a limb toward the median axis of the body. Compare **abduction. —adduct,** *v.*

adductor /əduk′tər/, a muscle that draws a part toward the axis or midline of the body. Compare **abductor, tensor.**

adductor brevis, a somewhat triangular muscle in the thigh and one of the five medial femoral muscles. It acts to adduct and rotate the thigh medially and to flex the leg. Compare **adductor longus, adductor magnus, gracilis, pectineus.**

adductor canal, a triangular channel beneath the sartorius muscle and between the adductor longus and vastus medialis

Adductor brevis, adductor longus, and adductor magnus muscles of the anterior thigh
(Thibodeau and Patton, 2003)

through which the femoral vessels and the saphenous nerve pass. Also called **Hunter's canal, subsartorial canal.**

adductor longus, the most superficial of the three adductor muscles of the thigh and one of five medial femoral muscles. It functions to adduct and flex the thigh. Compare **adductor brevis, adductor magnus, gracilis, pectineus.**

adductor magnus, the long, heavy triangular muscle of the medial aspect of the thigh. The adductor magnus acts to adduct the thigh. The proximal portion acts to rotate the thigh medially and to flex it on the hip; the distal portion acts to extend the thigh and rotate it laterally.

adefovir dipivoxil, an antiviral agent used to treat chronic hepatitis B.

aden-. See **adeno-.**

adenalgia /ad′ənal′jə/ [Gk, *aden*, gland, *algos*, pain], pain in any of the glands. Also called **adenodynia** /ad′ənōdin′ē·ə/.

adenectomy /ad′ənek′təmē/ [Gk, *aden* + *ektomē*, excision], the surgical removal of any gland.

Aden fever. See **dengue fever.**

-adenia, suffix meaning '(condition of the) glands': *anadenia, heteradenia.*

adenine /ad′ənin/, a purine base that is a component of DNA, RNA, adenosine monophosphate (AMP), cyclic AMP, adenosine diphosphate (ADP), and adenosine triphosphate (ATP). See **adenosine triphosphate, deoxyribonucleic acid, ribonucleic acid.**

adenine arabinoside. See **vidarabine.**

adenine-D-ribose. See **adenosine.**

adenitis /ad′əni′tis/, an inflammatory condition of a lymph node. Acute adenitis of the cervical lymph nodes may accompany a sore throat and stiff neck, simulating mumps if severe. It is most often related to an oral, pharyngeal, or ear infection. Scarlet fever may cause an acute suppurative cervical adenitis. Swelling of the lymph nodes in the back of the neck is often the result of a scalp infection, insect bite, or infestation by head lice. Inflammation of the lymph nodes of the mesenteric portion of the peritoneum often produces pain and other symptoms similar to those of appendicitis. Mesenteric adenitis may be mistaken for appendicitis, but characteristically mesenteric adenitis is preceded by a respiratory infection, the pain is less localized and less constant than in appendicitis, and it does not increase in severity. Generalized adenitis is a secondary symptom of syphilis. Therapy requires treatment of the primary infection by the administration of antimicrobial agents, application of warm compresses, and, in some cases, when fluctuation is present, incision and drainage. Also called **lymphadenitis.** Compare **acinitis.**

adeno-, aden-, prefix meaning 'gland': *adenocarcinoma, adenectomy.*

adenoacanthoma /ad′ənō·ak′anthō′mə/ [Gk, *aden* + *akantha,* thorn, *oma,* tumor], a neoplasm that may be malignant or benign, derived from glandular tissue with squamous differentiation shown by some of the cells.

adenoameloblastoma *pl.* **adenoameloblastomas, adenoameloblastomat,** /ad′ənō·amel′ōblastō′mə/, a benign tumor of the maxilla or mandible composed of ducts lined with columnar or cuboidal epithelial cells. It develops in tissue that normally gives rise to the teeth, and it most often occurs in young people.

adenoassociated virus (AAV) /ad′ənō-/, a defective virus, belonging to a group of DNA viruses of the *parvoviridae,* that can reproduce only in the presence of adenoviruses. It is not yet known what role, if any, these organisms have in causing disease.

adenocarcinoma *pl.* **adenocarcinomas, adenocarcinomata** /ad′ənōkärsinō′mə/ [Gk, *aden* + *karkinos,* crab, *oma*], any one of a large group of malignant, epithelial cell tumors of the glands. Specific tumors are diagnosed and named by cytologic identification of the tissue affected; for example, an adenocarcinoma of the uterine cervix is characterized by tumor cells resembling the glandular epithelium of the cervix. —**adenocarcinomatous,** *adj.*

Adenocarcinoma *(Damjanov, 2000)*

adenocarcinoma in situ, a localized growth of abnormal glandular tissue that may become malignant. However, the abnormal cells do not extend beyond the basement membrane. It is most common in the endometrium and in the large intestine.

adenocarcinoma of the kidney. See **renal cell carcinoma.**

adenocarcinoma of the lung, a type of bronchogenic carcinoma made up of a discrete mass of cuboidal or columnar cells, generally at the lung periphery. Most of these tumors form glandular structures that contain mucin, although a few lack mucin and are solid. Growth is slow, but there may be early invasion of blood and lymph vessels, with metastases while the primary lesion is still asymptomatic. There are two types of lung adenocarcinomas: **bronchogenic adenocarcinoma** and **bronchioloalveolar carcinoma.**

adenocarcinomatous. See **adenocarcinoma.**

adenocele /ad′ənōsēl′/, a cystic, glandular tumor.

adenochondroma *pl.* **adenochondromas, adenochondromata** /ad'ənōkondrō'mə/ [Gk, *aden* + *chondros,* cartilage, *oma*], a neoplasm of cells derived from glandular and cartilaginous tissues, as a mixed tumor of the salivary glands. Also called **chondroadenoma.**

adenocyst /ad'ənōsist'/ [Gk, *aden* + *kytis,* bag], a benign tumor in which the cells form cysts. A kind of adenocyst is **papillary adenocystoma lymphomatosum.** Also called **adenocystoma.**

adenocystic carcinoma, a malignant neoplasm composed of cords of uniform small epithelial cells arranged in a sievelike pattern around cystic spaces that often contain mucus. The tumor occurs most frequently in the salivary glands, breast, mucous glands of the upper and lower respiratory tract, and, occasionally, in vestibular glands of the vulva. The malignant slow growth tends to spread along nerves, causing neurologic damage. Facial paralysis often results from adenocystic carcinoma of the salivary gland. Bloodborne metastases to bones and liver have been reported. Also called **adenoid cystic carcinoma, adenomyoepithelioma, cribriform carcinoma, cylindroma.**

Adenocystic carcinoma *(Silverberg, DeLellis, and Frable, 1997)*

adenocystoma. See **adenocyst.**
adenodynia. See **adenalgia.**
adenoepithelioma *pl.* **adenoepitheliomas, adenoepitheliomata** /ad'ənō·ep'ithē'lē·ō'mə/ [Gk, *aden* + *epi,* on, *thele* nipple, *oma*], a neoplasm consisting of glandular and epithelial components.
adenofibroma *pl.* **adenofibromas, adenofibromata** /ad'ənōfībrō'mə/ [Gk, *aden* + L, *fibra,* fiber, *oma*], a tumor of the connective tissues that contains glandular elements.
adenofibroma edematodes, a neoplasm consisting of glandular elements and connective tissue in which marked edema is present.
adenofibromata. See **adenofibroma.**
adenohypophysis /ad'ənō'hīpof'isis/ [Gk, *aden* + *hypo,* beneath, *phyein,* to grow], the anterior lobe of the pituitary gland. It secretes growth hormone, thyroid stimulating hormone, adrenocorticotropic hormone, melanocyte stimulating hormone, follicle stimulating hormone, luteinizing hormone, prolactin, beta lipotropin molecules, and endorphins. Releasing hormones from the hypothalamus regulate secretions. Also called **anterior pituitary.**
adenoid /ad'ənoid/ [Gk, *aden* + *eidos,* form], **1.** having a glandular appearance, particularly lymphoid. **2.** adenoids, the pharyngeal tonsils. **—adenoidal,** *adj.*
adenoidal speech, an abnormal manner of speaking caused by hypertrophy of the adenoidal tissue that normally

exists in the nasopharynx of children. It is often characterized by a muted, nasal quality and may be corrected by a natural reduction of the swollen tissues or by surgical excision of the adenoids.
adenoid cystic carcinoma. See **adenocystic carcinoma.**
adenoidectomy /ad'ənoidek'təmē/ [Gk, *aden* + *eidos,* form, *ektomē,* excision], removal of the lymphoid tissue in the nasopharynx. The surgical procedure may be performed because the adenoids are enlarged, chronically infected, or causing obstruction. Normal adenoids may be excised as a prophylactic measure during tonsillectomy. Preoperative procedures usually include a partial thromboplastin time test and for African-American patients a sickle cell preparation test. The operation is performed with general anesthesia in children, but local anesthesia may be used in adults. After removal of the adenoids, bleeding is stemmed with pressure or vessels may be ligated with sutures or electrocoagulation current may be used. Postoperatively, the patient is observed for signs of hemorrhage, and the pulse, blood pressure, and respiration are checked every 15 minutes for the first hour and every 30 minutes for several hours thereafter. See also **tonsillectomy.**
adenoid facies, the dull expression, with open mouth, sometimes seen in children with hypertrophy of the pharyngeal tonsils ("adenoids").
adenoid hyperplasia, a condition of enlarged adenoid glands, especially in children. Enlarged adenoids, often in association with enlarged tonsils, are a frequent cause of recurrent otitis media, sinusitis, conduction hearing loss, and partial respiratory obstruction. Severe obstruction can result in alveolar hypoventilation and pulmonary hypertension with congestive heart failure. Treatment usually consists of surgical removal of the adenoids.
adenoid hypertrophy [Gk, *aden,* gland, *eidos,* form, *hyper,* excessive, *trophe,* nourishment], an enlargement of the pharyngeal tonsil.
adenoiditis /ad'ənoidī'tis/, inflammation of the adenoids or pharyngeal tonsils.
adenoids, small masses of lymphoid tissue forming the pharyngeal tonsils on the posterior wall of the nasopharynx. Also called **pharyngeal tonsils.**
adenoid tissue, the lymphoid tissue that forms the pharyngeal tonsils.
adenoleiomyofibroma *pl.* **adenoleiomyofibromas, adenoleiomyofibromata** /ad'ənōlī'ōmī'ōfībrō'mə/ [Gk, *aden* + *leios,* smooth, *mys,* muscle; L, *fibra,* fiber; Gk, *oma*], a glandular tumor with smooth muscle, connective tissue, and epithelial elements.
adenolipoma *pl.* **adenolipomas, adenolipomata** /ad'ənōlipō'mə/ [Gk, *aden* + *lipos,* fat, *oma*], a neoplasm consisting of elements of glandular and fatty tissue.
adenolipomatosis /ad'ənōlip'ōmətō'sis/, a condition characterized by the growth of adenolipomas in the groin, axilla, and neck.
adenolymphoma. See **papillary adenocystoma lymphomatosum.**
adenoma *pl.* **adenomas, adenomata** /ad'ənō'mə/ [Gk, *aden* + *oma*], a tumor of glandular epithelium in which the cells of the tumor are arranged in a recognizable glandular structure. An adenoma may cause excess secretion by the affected gland, such as acidophilic pituitary adenoma resulting in an excess of growth hormone. Kinds of adenomas include **acidophilic adenoma, basophilic adenoma, fibroadenoma,** and **insulinoma. —adenomatous,** *adj.*
-adenoma, suffix meaning a 'tumor composed of glandular tissue or glandlike in structure': *sarcoadenoma, splenadenoma.*

adenoma sebaceum /sebā'sē·əm/, an abnormal skin condition consisting of multiple wartlike, yellowish red, waxy papules on the face that are not sebaceous, composed chiefly of fibrovascular tissue. The lesions are usually benign. See also **tuberous sclerosis.**

Adenoma sebaceum (du Vivier, 1993)

adenomatoid /ad'ənō'mətoid/ [Gk, *aden* + *oma* + *eidos,* form], resembling a glandular tumor.

adenomatosis /ad'ənōmətō'sis/, an abnormal condition in which hyperplasia or tumor development affects two or more glands, usually the thyroid, adrenals, or pituitary.

adenomatous. See **adenoma.**

adenomatous goiter /ad'ənō'mətəs/, an enlargement of the thyroid gland caused by an adenoma or numerous colloid nodules.

adenomatous polyp [Gk, *aden,* gland, *oma,* tumor, *polys,* many, *pous,* foot], a tumor that develops in glandular tissue. It is characterized by neoplastic changes in epithelium.

adenomatous polyposis coli (APC), a gene associated with **familial adenomatous polyposis (FAP),** an inherited disorder characterized by the development of myriad polyps in the colon, beginning in late adolescence or early adulthood. Untreated, the condition nearly always leads to colon cancer. The gene is located on chromosome 5.

Familial adenomatous polyposis (Goldman et al, 2004)

adenomyoepithelioma. See **adenocystic carcinoma.**

adenomyofibroma *pl.* **adenomyofibromas, adenomyofibromata** /ad'ənōmī'ōfībrō'mə/ [Gk, *aden* + *mys,* muscle; L, *fibra,* fiber; Gk, *oma*], a fibrous tumor that contains glandular and muscular components.

adenomyoma *pl.* **adenomyomas, adenomyomata,** /ad'ənōmī·ō'mə/, a tumor of the endometrium of the uterus characterized by a mass of smooth muscle containing endometrial tissue and glands.

adenomyomatosis /ad'ənōmī'ōmətō'sis/, an abnormal condition characterized by the formation of benign nodules resembling adenomyomas, found in the uterus or in parauterine tissue.

adenomyosarcoma *pl.* **adenomyosarcomas, adenomyosarcomata,** /ad'ənōmī'ōsärkō'mə/, a malignant tumor of soft tissue containing glandular elements and striated muscle.

adenomyosis /ad'ənōmī·ō'sis/, an invasion of the muscular wall of the uterus by the endometrium.

adenopathy /ad'ənop'əthē/ [Gk, *aden* + *pathos,* suffering], an enlargement of any gland. **—adenopathic,** *adj.*

adenopharyngitis /ad'ənōfer'injī'tis/, an inflammation of the adenoid tonsils and the pharynx.

adenosarcoma *pl.* **adenosarcomas, adenosarcomata** /ad'ənōsärkō'mə/ [Gk, *aden* + *sarx,* flesh, *oma*], a malignant glandular tumor of the soft tissues of the body.

adenosarcorhabdomyoma *pl.* **adenosarcorhabdomyomas, adenosarcorhabdomyomata,** /ad'ənōsär'kōrab'dōmīō'mə/, a tumor composed of glandular and connective tissue, and striated muscle elements.

adenosine /əden'əsin, -sēn/, a compound derived from nucleic acid, composed of adenine and a sugar, D-ribose. Adenosine is the major molecular component of the nucleotides adenosine monophosphate, adenosine diphosphate, and adenosine triphosphate and of the nucleic acids deoxyribonucleic acid and ribonucleic acid. Also called **adenine-D-ribose.** See also **adenosine phosphate.**

adenosine 3′,5′-cyclic monophosphate. See **cyclic adenosine monophosphate.**

adenosine deaminase (ADA) /dē·am'inās/, an enzyme that catalyzes the conversion of adenosine to the nucleoside inosine through the removal of an amino group. A deficiency of ADA can lead to **severe combined immunodeficiency syndrome (SCIDS).** See also **adenosine.**

adenosine diphosphate (ADP), a product of the hydrolysis of adenosine triphosphate.

adenosine hydrolase, an enzyme that catalyzes the conversion of adenosine into adenine and ribose.

adenosine kinase, an enzyme in the liver and kidney that catalyzes the transfer of a phosphate group from adenosine triphosphate to produce adenosine diphosphate.

adenosine monophosphate (AMP), an ester, composed of adenine-D-ribose and phosphoric acid, that participates in energy released by working muscle. Also called **adenylic acid.**

adenosine phosphate, a compound consisting of the nucleotide adenosine attached through its ribose group to one, two, or three phosphate units, or phosphoric acid molecules. Kinds of adenosine phosphate, all of which are interconvertible, are **adenosine diphosphate, adenosine monophosphate,** and **adenosine triphosphate.**

adenosine triphosphatase (ATPase), an enzyme in skeletal muscle and other tissues that catalyzes the hydrolysis of adenosine triphosphate to adenosine diphosphate and inorganic phosphate. Among various enzymes in this group, mitochondrial ATPase is involved in obtaining energy for cellular metabolism, and myosin ATPase is involved in muscle contraction.

Adenosine triphosphate in metabolism
(Thibodeau and Patton, 2003)

adenosine triphosphate (ATP), a compound consisting of the nucleotide adenosine attached through its ribose group to three phosphoric acid molecules. Hydrolysis of adenosine triphosphate to adenosine diphosphate releases energy. By coupling a less favorable reaction in the cell with this hydrolysis, the less favorable reaction may proceed, allowing one to think of ATP as the cellular energy currency, especially in muscle.

adenosis /ad'ənō'sis/, **1.** any disease of the glands, especially a lymphatic gland. **2.** an abnormal development or enlargement of glandular tissue.

adenotomy /ad'ənot'əmē/ [Gk, *aden,* gland, *tome,* a cutting], dissection or incision of a gland.

adenotonsillectomy /ad'ənōton'silek'təmē/, surgical removal of the adenoids and tonsils. Compare **tonsillectomy.**

adenovirus /ad'ənōvī'rəs/ [Gk, *aden* + L, *virus,* poison], any one of the 49 medium-sized viruses of the Adenoviridae family, pathogenic to humans, that cause conjunctivitis, upper respiratory infection, cystitis, or GI infection. After the acute and symptomatic period of illness, the virus may persist in a latent stage in the tonsils, adenoids, and other lymphoid tissue. Compare **rhinovirus. —adenoviral,** *adj.*

Adenovirus infection within transitional cells
(Silverberg, DeLellis, and Frable, 1997)

adenylate /əden'ilāt/, a salt or ester of adenylic acid.

adenylate cyclase, an enzyme that initiates the conversion of adenosine triphosphate (ATP) to cyclic adenosine monophosphate (cAMP), a mediator of many physiologic activities.

adenylate kinase, an enzyme in skeletal muscle that makes possible the reaction ATP + AMP = 2ADP. Also called **myokinase.**

adenylic acid. See **adenosine monophosphate.**

adequate and well-controlled studies, clinical and laboratory studies that the sponsors of a new drug are required by law to conduct to demonstrate the truth of the claims made for its effectiveness.

adermia /ədur'mē·ə/ [Gk, *a* + *derma,* without skin], a congenital or acquired skin defect or the absence of skin.

ADH, abbreviation for **antidiuretic hormone.**

ADHA, abbreviation for the **American Dental Hygienists' Association.**

adhere /adhir'/, to stick together or become fastened together, as two surfaces.

adherence /adhir'əns/, **1.** the quality of clinging or being closely attached. **2.** the process in which a person follows rules, guidelines, or standards, especially as a patient follows a prescription and recommendations for a regimen of care.

adherence behavior, a nursing outcome from the Nursing Outcomes Classification (NOC) defined as self-initiated action taken to promote wellness, recovery, and rehabilitation. See also **Nursing Outcomes Classification.**

adherent /adhir'ənt/ [L, *adhaerens,* sticking to], having the tendency to cling, as one substance to the surface of another substance.

adherent pericardium. See **pericardial adhesion.**

adherent placenta [L, *adhaerens,* sticking to, *placenta,* flat cake], a placenta that remains attached to the uterine wall beyond the normal time after birth of the fetus. See also **placenta accreta.**

adhesin /adhē'sin/, a bacterial product that can split proteins. It combines with epithelial cell glycoproteins or glycolipid receptors.

adhesion /adhē'zhən/, [L, *adhaerens,* sticking to], a band of scar tissue that binds anatomic surfaces that normally are separate from each other. Adhesions most commonly form in the abdomen, after abdominal surgery, inflammation, or injury. A loop of intestine may adhere to unhealed areas. Scar tissue constricting the bowel's lumen may cause obstruction, blocking the intestinal flow and causing abdominal pain, nausea and vomiting, and distension. Nasogastric intubation and suction may relieve the symptoms. If the blockage does not resolve spontaneously, surgery to lyse adhesions may be necessary. See also **adhesiotomy, intestinal obstruction.**

adhesiotomy /adhē'sē·ot'əmē/ [L, *adhaerens* + Gk, *temnein* to cut], the surgical dividing or separating of adhesions, usually performed to relieve an intestinal obstruction. Also called **lysis of adhesions.** See also **abdominal surgery.**

adhesive /adhē'siv/ [L, *adhaerens,* sticking to], a quality of a substance that enables it to become attached to another substance.

adhesive capsulitis, shoulder condition characterized by stiffness, pain, and limited range of motion. It most often occurs in midlife and may be associated with shoulder surgery or injury. Also called **frozen shoulder.** See also **capsulitis.**

adhesive pericarditis, a condition characterized by adhesions between the visceral and parietal layers of the pericardium or by adhesions between the pericardium and the mediastinum, diaphragm, or chest wall. Adhesions between the pericardial layers may completely obstruct the pericardial cavity. Adhesive pericarditis may seriously impair normal heart movements.

adhesive peritonitis, an inflammation of the peritoneum, characterized by adhesions between adjacent serous surfaces. This condition may be marked by an exudate of serum, fibrin, cells, and pus, accompanied by abdominal pain and tenderness, vomiting, constipation, and fever.

adhesive phlebitis. See **obliterative phlebitis.**

adhesive plaster. See **adhesive tape.**

adhesive pleurisy, inflammation of the pleura with exudation. It causes obliteration of the pleural space through the fusion of the visceral pleural layer covering the lungs and the parietal layer lining the walls of the thoracic cavity.

adhesive skin traction, one of two kinds of skin traction in which the therapeutic pull of traction weights is applied with adhesive straps that stick to the skin over the body structure involved, especially a fractured bone. Adhesive skin traction is a short-term treatment used only when continuous traction is desired and skin care for the affected area is easily maintained. It is not suitable for clients with fragile skin. Compare **nonadhesive skin traction.**

adhesive tape, a strong fabric material covered on one side with an adhesive. Often water-repellent, it may be used to hold bandages and dressings in place, to immobilize a part, or to exert pressure. Also called **adhesive plaster.**

ADI, abbreviation for **acceptable daily intake.**

adiadochokinesia /ā′dē·ad′əkō′kinē′zhə, ədī′ədō′kō-/, an inability to perform rapidly alternating movements, such as pronation and supination, or elbow flexion and extension. The activity is commonly included in a neurologic examination.

adiaphoresis /ā′dē·əfôrē′sis/, an absence or deficiency of sweat.

adiastole /ā′dī·as′təlē/ [Gk, *a,* not, *dia,* across, *stellein,* to set], the absence or imperceptibility of the diastolic stage of the cardiac cycle. See also **diastole.**

adiathermance /a′dī·əthur′məns/ [Gk, *a + dia,* not across, *therme,* heat], the quality of being unaffected by radiated heat.

adient /ad′ē·ənt/ [L, *adire,* moving toward], characterized by a tendency to move toward rather than away from stimuli. Compare **abient. —adience,** *n.*

Adie's pupil /ā′dēz/ [William J. Adie, English physician, 1886–1935], an abnormal condition of the eyes marked by one pupil that reacts much more slowly to light changes or to accommodation or convergence than the pupil of the other eye. It is considered a pupillary muscle problem. There is no specific treatment. Also called **tonic pupil.**

Adie's syndrome [William J. Adie], the condition of Adie's pupil accompanied by depressed or absent tendon reflexes, particularly the ankle and knee-jerk reflexes. See also **Adie's pupil.**

adip-. See **adipo-.**

adipectomy. See **lipectomy.**

adipic /ədip′ik/ [L, *adeps,* fat], pertaining to fatty tissue.

adipo-, adip-, combining form meaning 'fat': *adipocele, adipogenesis.*

adipocele /ad′ipōsēl′/ [L, *adeps* + Gk, *kele,* hernia], a hernia containing fat or fatty tissue. Also called **lipocele.**

adipocyte /ad′ipōsīt′/, a fat (adipose) cell, potentially containing a large fat vacuole consisting mainly of triglycerides.

adipofibroma *pl.* **adipofibromas, adipofibromata** /ad′ipōfībrō′mə/ [L, *adeps* + *fibra,* fiber; Gk, *oma*], a fibrous neoplasm of the connective tissue with fatty components.

adipokinesis /ad′ipō′kinē′sis/, the mobilization of fat or fatty acids in lipid metabolism.

adipokinin /ad′ipokī′nin/, a hormone of the anterior pituitary that causes mobilization of fat from adipose tissues.

adipometer /ad′ipom′ətər/, an instrument for measuring the thickness of a skin area as a guide to calculating the amount of subcutaneous fat.

adiponecrosis /ad′ipōnikrō′sis/ [L, *adeps* + Gk, *nekros,* dead, *osis* condition], a necrosis of fatty tissue in the body. The condition may be associated with hemorrhagic pancreatitis. **—adiponecrotic,** *adj.*

adiponecrosis subcutanea neonatorum, an abnormal dermatologic condition of the newborn characterized by patchy areas of hardened subcutaneous fatty tissue and a bluish-red discoloration of the overlying skin. The lesions, often a result of manipulation during delivery, spontaneously resolve within a period of days to several weeks without scarring. Also called **pseudosclerema, subcutaneous fat necrosis.**

adiponecrotic. See **adiponecrosis.**

adipose /ad′ipōs/, fatty. Adipose tissue is composed of fat-containing cells arranged in lobules. See also **fat, fatty acid, lipoma.**

adipose capsule [L, *adeps,* fat, *capsula,* little box], a capsule of fatty tissue surrounding the kidney. Also called **renal fat.**

adipose degeneration. See **fatty degeneration.**

adipose tissue [L, *adeps,* fat; OFr, *tissu*], a collection of fat cells. See also **fatty tissue.**

Storage area for fat   Plasma membrane

Nucleus of adipose cell

Adipose tissue (© Ed Reschke/used with permission)

adipose tumor. See **lipoma.**

adiposis dolorosa. See **Dercum's disease.**

adiposogenital dystrophy /ad′ipō′sōjen′itəl/ [L, *adeps* + *genitalis,* generation], a disorder occurring in males, characterized by genital hypoplasia and feminine secondary sex characteristics, including female distribution of fat. It is caused by hypothalamic malfunction or by a tumor in the anterior pituitary gland. Subnormal body temperature, low blood pressure, and reduced blood glucose level are frequently associated with the disorder. Diabetes insipidus also results from hyposecretion of antidiuretic hormone, which causes increased diluted urine output, electrolyte imbalances, and thirst. In addition, involvement of the hypothalamic satiety center may induce overeating and result in pronounced obesity. If a tumor is present, there may be drowsiness and symptoms of increased intracranial pressure (for example, subtle locus of control changes and headache). Treatment may include the administration of testosterone and a weight reduction program, excision or radiologic ablation of a tumor, and replacement of hormones, as necessary. Also called **adiposogenital syndrome, Fröhlich's syndrome.**

adipsia /ādip′sē·ə/ [Gk, *a + dipsa,* not thirst], absence of thirst.

aditus /ad′itəs/ [L, going to], an approach or an entry.

adjunct /ad′jungkt/ [L, *adjungere,* to join], (in health care) an additional substance, treatment, or procedure used for increasing the efficacy or safety of the primary substance, treatment, or procedure or for facilitating its performance. —**adjunctive,** *adj.*

adjunctive group /adjungk'tiv/, a group with specific activities and focuses, such as socialization, perceptual stimulation, sensory stimulation, or reality orientation.

adjunctive psychotherapy, a form of psychotherapy that concentrates on improving a person's general mental and physical well-being without trying to resolve basic emotional problems. Some kinds of adjunctive psychotherapy are **music therapy, occupational therapy, physical therapy,** and **recreational therapy.**

adjunct to anesthesia, one of a number of drugs or techniques used to enhance anesthesia but that are not classified as anesthetics. They may include NSAIDs such as ketorolac, benzodiazephine sedatives, and antiemetics such as H_2 blockers. Each has a use in anesthetic procedures, as well as a therapeutic indication in other aspects of health care. Adjuncts to anesthesia are used before anesthetic as premedications and during anesthesia to augment anesthetic effects. Premedications are given to reduce anxiety, sedate the patient, and reduce oral and respiratory secretions. Opioid analgesics, sedatives and hypnotics, phenothiazines, anticholinergics, and antianxiety agents are common premedications.

adjustable axis face-bow. See **kinematic face-bow.**

adjustable orthodontic band /adjus'təbəl/, a thin metal ring, usually made of stainless steel, equipped with an adjusting screw to allow alteration in size, that is fitted to a tooth and allows the attachment of orthodontic appliances. See also **orthodontic band.**

adjusted death rate. See **standardized death rate.**

adjustment, the changing of something to improve its relationship to something else. See also **accommodation.**

adjustment disorder [L, *adjuxtare,* to bring together], a temporary disorder of varying severity that occurs as an acute reaction to overwhelming stress in persons of any age who have no apparent underlying mental disorders. Symptoms include anxiety, withdrawal, depression, brooding, impulsive outbursts, crying spells, attention-seeking behavior, enuresis, loss of appetite, aches, pains, and muscle spasms. It can be persistent if symptoms continue for six months or more. It can develop in response to an identifiable stressor and result from such situations as separation of an infant from its mother, the birth of a sibling, loss or change of job, death of a loved one, or forced retirement. Symptoms usually recede and eventually disappear as stress diminishes. See also **anxiety disorder.**

adjustment, impaired, a nursing diagnosis accepted by the Seventh National Conference on the Classification of Nursing Diagnoses (revised 1998). Impaired adjustment is a state in which the individual is unable to modify his or her life-style or behavior in a manner consistent with a change in health status.

■ DEFINING CHARACTERISTICS: The defining characteristics include a denial of health status change, a failure to achieve optimal sense of control, a failure to take actions that would prevent further health problems and a demonstration of nonacceptance of health status change.

■ RELATED FACTORS: Related factors include a disability requiring a change in life-style; lack of motivation to change; multiple stressors; absence of social support for changed beliefs and practices; intense emotional state; low state of optimism; negative attitudes towards health behavior; and failure to intend to change behavior. See also **nursing diagnosis.**

adjuvant /ad'jəvənt/ [L, *ad* + *juvare,* to help], **1.** a sub-

stance, especially a drug, added to a prescription to assist in the action of the main ingredient. **2.** (in immunology) a substance added to an antigen that enhances or modifies the antibody response to the antigen. **3.** an additional treatment or therapy.

adjuvant chemotherapy, the use of anticancer drugs after or in combination with another form of cancer treatment, as after apparently complete surgical removal of a cancer. The method is used when there is a significant risk that undetected cancer cells may still be present. Adjuvant chemotherapy is most commonly used in treating breast cancer.

adjuvant radiotherapy, radiotherapy used in addition to surgical resection in the treatment of cancer.

adjuvant therapy, the treatment of a disease with substances that enhance the action of drugs, especially drugs that promote the production of antibodies.

ADL, abbreviation for **activities of daily living.**

adlerian psychology [Alfred Adler, Viennese psychiatrist, 1870–1937], a branch of psychoanalysis that focuses on physical security, sexual satisfaction, and social integration. See also **individual psychology.**

ad lib, abbreviation of the Latin phrase *ad libitum,* meaning to be taken as desired.

ADME, an abbreviation for the time course of drug distribution, representing the terms *absorption, distribution, metabolism,* and *elimination.*

administration of parenteral fluids /admin'istrā'shən/, the IV infusion of various solutions to maintain adequate hydration, restore and/or maintain fluid volume, reestablish lost electrolytes, or provide partial nutrition. See **parenteral.**

■ METHOD: Fluid is administered parenterally through a closed system consisting of a bottle or bag of sterile solution and tubing which has been attached to an intracatheter or butterfly needle that is inserted into a peripheral vein and securely taped to the patient's arm, leg, or scalp. The fluid is infused at a rate appropriate to the client's clinical condition. Five percent dextrose in distilled water may be used to maintain volume and provide nutrients; ascorbic acid and B vitamins are often added to the solution. Five percent dextrose in saline solution plus potassium chloride may be infused to reestablish electrolyte balance, but potassium is contraindicated in renal failure and untreated adrenal insufficiency. A one-sixth molar lactate solution may be administered if sodium is deficient, and an ammonium chloride solution may be administered when chloride must be replaced. Distilled water containing 10% to 20% glucose or fructose may be used to supply carbohydrate, but, because these solutions are hypertonic, additional hydration is needed for proper excretion. Low-molecular-weight dextran is frequently used as a plasma volume expander in treating shock, but it increases bleeding time and is contraindicated in pregnancy and severe renal disease. During parenteral fluid administration, the venipuncture site is observed every 1 to 2 hours for signs of infiltration, which is evidenced by localized swelling, coolness, pallor, and discomfort at the site; for the patient's complaints of pain or discomfort; for the security and comfort of the tape; and for the position of the patient's extremity. The flow rate, level, color, and clarity of the fluid; the label; and the patency of the tubing and needle are checked, and the patient is monitored for signs of dehydration, fever, and signs of circulatory overload, such as headache, tachycardia, elevated blood pressure, weight gain, dyspnea, engorged neck veins, and pulmonary edema. The patient is also monitored for signs and symptoms of phlebitis: redness, warmth, and swelling at the IV site and burning pain along the vein.

■ INTERVENTIONS: Depending on the purpose and patient's specific condition, the nurse may select the necessary equipment, prepare the venipuncture site, check the labels of fluid bottles for content, and perform the venipuncture. During fluid administration, the nurse keeps the system closed, watches the flow rate, records the amount of solution given, and observes the venipuncture site and the patient's general condition. If there are any signs of increased blood volume, the nurse reduces the flow of the infusion until further orders are obtained. The nurse changes the dressing according to institutional protocol and ensures that the patient understands the importance of not disturbing the tubing, of reporting pain or swelling, of avoiding sudden twisting or turning movements of the extremity, and of reporting pain or swelling at the IV site or blood in the IV tubing.

■ OUTCOME CRITERIA: Parenteral fluid therapy is usually uneventful. Patients requiring special attention include infants, elderly patients with circulatory or renal impairment or confusion, and burn patients, whose plasma may shift suddenly from interstitial tissue, causing increased blood volume.

Administration on Aging (AOA), the principal U.S. agency designated to carry out the provisions of the Older Americans Act of 1965. The AOA advises the U.S. Secretary of the Department of Health and Human Services and other federal departments and agencies on the characteristics and needs of older people and develops programs designed to promote their welfare.

admission, 1. the act of being received into a place or class of things. 2. a patient accepted for inpatient service in a hospital. 3. a concession or acknowledgment.

admission care, a nursing intervention from the Nursing Interventions Classification (NIC) defined as facilitating entry of a patient into a health care facility. See also **Nursing Interventions Classification.**

ADN, abbreviation for **Associate Degree in Nursing.**

ad nauseam [L, *ad,* to; Gk, *nausia,* seasickness], to the extent of inducing nausea and vomiting.

adneural /adnŏŏ′əl/, 1. located near or toward a nerve or nerve ending. 2. pertaining to the stage of a nervous disorder in which the symptoms are apparent. Also **adnerval.**

adnexa, *sing.* **adnexus** /adnek′sa/ [L, *adnectere,* to tie together], tissue or structures in the body that are adjacent to or near another, related structure. The ovaries and the uterine tubes are adnexa of the uterus. Also called **annexa.** —**adnexal,** *adj.*

adnexal [L, *adnectere,* to tie together], pertaining to accessory organs or tissues, as in the relationship of the fallopian tubes and uterus.

adnexa oculi, the accessory organs of the eye: the eyelids, lashes, eyebrows, conjunctival sac, lacrimal apparatus, and extrinsic muscles of the eye.

adnexa uteri, the uterine appendages: the ovaries, fallopian tubes, and associated ligaments.

adnexectomy /ad′neksek′təmē/ [Gk, *ektomē,* excision], surgical removal of accessory structures.

adnexitis /ad′neksī′tis/, an inflammation of the adnexal organs of the uterus, such as the ovaries or the fallopian tubes.

adnexopexy /adnek′sōpek′sē/, a surgical procedure in which the fallopian tubes and ovaries are elevated and sutured to the abdominal wall.

adnexus. See **adnexa.**

-adol, combining form designating an analgesic.

adolescence /ad′əles′əns/ [L, *adolescere,* to grow up], 1. the period in development between the onset of puberty and adulthood. It usually begins between 11 and 13 years of age, with the appearance of secondary sex characteristics, and spans the teenage years, terminating at 18 to 20 years of age with the completion of the development of the adult form. During this period the individual undergoes extensive

Superior rectus muscle
Levator palpebrae superioris muscle
Smooth muscle to tarsal plate
Eyebrow
Orbicularis oculi muscle
Superior conjunctival fornix
Palpebral conjunctiva
Tarsal (meibomian) gland
Tarsal plate
Eyelash
Palpebral fissure
Cornea
Bulbar conjunctiva
Inferior conjunctival fornix
Orbicularis oculi muscle
Inferior rectus muscle
Inferior oblique muscle

Adnexa oculi *(Thibodeau and Patton, 2003)*

physical, psychologic, emotional, and personality changes. 2. the state or quality of being adolescent or youthful. See also **postpuberty, prepuberty, psychosexual development, psychosocial development, pubarche.**

adolescent, 1. pertaining to characteristic of adolescence. 2. one in the state or process of adolescence; a teenager.

adolescent vertebral epiphysitis. See **Scheuermann's disease.**

adoption /ədop′shən/, [L, *adoptere,* to choose], a selection and inclusion in an established relationship or a choice of treatment protocol.

ADP, abbreviation for **adenosine diphosphate.**

ADPKD, abbreviation for **autosomal dominant polycystic kidney disease.**

adrenal /ədrē′nəl/ [L, *ad,* to, *ren,* kidney], pertaining to the adrenal, or suprarenal glands, which are located atop the kidneys.

adrenal cortex [L, *ad,* to, *ren,* kidney], the outer and greater portion of the adrenal, or suprarenal, gland, fused with the gland's medulla. It produces mineralocorticoids, androgens, and glucocorticoids, hormones essential to homeostasis.

adrenal cortical carcinoma, a malignant neoplasm of the adrenal cortex that may cause adrenogenital syndrome or Cushing's syndrome. Such tumors vary in size and may occur at any age. Metastases frequently occur in the lungs, liver, and other organs. See also **adrenal virilism, Cushing's syndrome.**

adrenal crisis, an acute, life-threatening state of profound adrenocortical insufficiency in which immediate therapy is required. It is characterized by glucocorticoid deficiency, a drop in extracellular fluid volume, and hyperkalemia. Also called **crisis.** See also **Addison's disease, adrenal cortex.**

■ OBSERVATIONS: Typically, the patient appears to be in shock or coma with a low blood pressure, weakness, and loss of vasomotor tone. The person's medical history may include

Adrenal cortical carcinoma
(Silverberg, DeLellis, and Frable, 1997)

abrupt discontinuation of exogenous steroids or Addison's disease or reveal symptoms indicating its presence. Results of laboratory tests show hyperkalemia and hyponatremia.
■ INTERVENTIONS: An IV isotonic solution of sodium chloride containing a water-soluble glucocorticoid is administered rapidly. Vasopressor agents may be necessary to combat hypotension. If the patient is vomiting, a nasogastric tube is inserted to prevent aspiration and relieve hyperemesis. Total bed rest and monitoring of blood pressure, temperature, and other vital signs are mandatory. After the first critical hours, the patient is followed as for Addison's disease, and corticosteroid dosage is tapered to maintenance levels. Infection and a failure to increase the maintenance glucocorticoid (steroid) dose are common causes of crisis in people who have Addison's disease.
■ NURSING CONSIDERATIONS: Nursing care during adrenal crisis includes eliminating all forms of stimuli, especially loud noises or bright lights. The patient is not moved unless absolutely necessary and is not allowed to perform self-care activities. If the condition is identified and treated promptly, the prognosis is good. Discharge instructions include a reminder to the patient to seek medical attention in any stressful situation, whether physiologic or psychologic, to prevent a recurrence of the crisis.

adrenalectomy /ədrē'nəlek'təmē/, [L, *ad* + *ren* + Gk, *ektomē*, excision], the total or partial surgical resection of one or both adrenal glands. It is performed to reduce the excessive secretion of adrenal hormones caused by an adrenal tumor or a malignancy of the breast or prostate. The incision is made under the twelfth rib in the rear flank area with the patient under general anesthesia. Preoperative laboratory tests include electrolytes, fasting blood glucose, glucose tolerance, and fluid states and adrenergic and blockade if needed. Hemodynamic monitoring and preoperative steroid replacement are needed. Before surgery a nasogastric tube may be inserted. Careful intraoperative positioning is necessary for the patient with Cushing's syndrome because of osteoporosis, fragile bone, and muscle wasting. In patients with pheochromocytoma, intraoperative manipulation of an adrenal tumor can cause a surge of catecholamines, resulting in a blood pressure increase. Postoperative care focuses on maintaining blood pressure with vasopressors or vasodilators as needed, giving replacement doses of corticosteroids,

and monitoring fluid and electrolyte status. When both glands are removed, the maintenance dosage of steroids continues for life. Stress and fatigue must be avoided. See also **Addison's disease, Cushing's syndrome, pheochromocytoma.**

adrenal gland, either of two secretory organs perched atop the kidneys and surrounded by the protective fat capsule of the kidneys. Each consists of two parts having independent functions: the cortex and the medulla. The adrenal cortex, in response to adrenocorticotropic hormone secreted by the anterior pituitary, secretes cortisol and androgens. Adrenal androgens serve as precursors that are converted by the liver to testosterone and estrogens. Renin from the kidney controls adrenal cortical production of aldosterone. The adrenal medulla manufactures the catecholamines epinephrine and norepinephrine. Also called **suprarenal gland.**

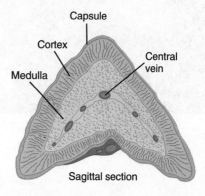

Adrenal gland *(Black and Hawks, 2005)*

Adrenalin, trademark for an adrenergic (epinephrine).
adrenaline. See **epinephrine.**
adrenal insufficiency [L, *ad*, to, *ren*, kidney, *in*, not, *sufficere*, to suffice], a condition in which the adrenal gland is unable to produce adequate amounts of cortical hormones. See also **Addison's disease.**
adrenalism /ah-dren'al-izm/, any disorder of adrenal function, whether of decreased or of heightened function.
adrenalize /ədrē'nəliz/, to stimulate or excite.
adrenal medulla, the inner portion of the adrenal gland. Adrenal medulla cells secrete epinephrine and norepinephrine when stimulated by the sympathetic division of the autonomic nervous system. See also **adrenal cortex.**
adrenal virilism, a condition characterized by hypersecretion of adrenal androgens, resulting in somatic masculinization. Excessive production of the hormone may be caused by a virilizing adrenal tumor, congenital adrenal hyperplasia, or an inborn deficiency of enzymes required to transform endogenous androgenic steroids to glucocorticoids. Girls born with adrenogenitalism may be pseudohermaphroditic with clitoral enlargement and labial fusion in infancy and later have low vocal pitch, acne, amenorrhea, and masculine distribution of hair and muscle development. Boys with congenital adrenogenitalism show precocious development of the penis, the prostate, and pubic and axillary hair; but their testes remain small and immature because negative feedback from the high level of adrenal androgens prevents the normal pubertal increase in pituitary gonadotropin. Children with the disorder are unusually tall, but their epiphyses close

prematurely, and as adults they are abnormally short. Virilizing tumors are more common or more frequently diagnosed in women. The tumors usually occur between 30 and 40 years of age but may arise later, after menopause. Signs of the tumor in women include hirsutism, amenorrhea, oily skin, ovarian changes, muscular hypertrophy, and atrophy of the uterus and breasts. Treatment may involve tumor resection, cortisol administration, and cosmetic surgical procedures. Electrolytic hair removal may be indicated. Also called **adrenogenital syndrome.** See also **congenital adrenal hyperplasia, pseudohermaphroditism, virilization.**

Adrenal virilism *(Fletcher, 2000)*

adrenarche /ad'rinär'kē/ [L, *ad* + *ren* + Gk, *arche,* beginning], the intensified activity in the adrenal cortex that occurs at about 8 years of age and increases the elaboration of various hormones, especially androgens.

adrenergic /ad'rinur'jik/ [L, *ad* + *ren;* Gk, *ergon,* work], pertaining to sympathetic nerve fibers of the autonomic nervous system that liberate norepinephrine at a synapse where a nerve impulse passes. Compare **cholinergic.** See also **sympathomimetic.**

adrenergic blocking agent. See **antiadrenergic.**

adrenergic bronchodilator, a drug that acts on the beta-2 sympathetic nervous system receptors to relax bronchial smooth muscle cells. Examples include drugs that contain epinephrine, ephedrine, isoproterenol, or albuterol.

adrenergic drug. See **sympathomimetic.**

adrenergic fibers, nerve fibers of the autonomic nervous system that release the neurotransmitter norepinephrine and, in some areas, dopamine. Most postganglionic sympathetic nerve fibers are of this type.

adrenergic receptor [L, *ad* + *ren,* kidney; Gk, *ergon,* work; L, *recipere,* to receive], a site in a sympathetic effector cell that reacts to adrenergic stimulation. Two types of adrenergic receptors are recognized: **alpha-adrenergic,** which act in response to sympathomimetic stimuli, and **beta-adrenergic,** which block sympathomimetic activity. In general, stimulation of alpha receptors is excitatory of the function of the host organ or tissue, and stimulation of the beta receptors is inhibitory.

-adrenia, combining form meaning '(degree or condition of) adrenal activity': *anadrenia, hypadrenia.*

adrenocortical /-kôr'tikəl/ [L, *ad* + *ren* + *cortex,* bark], pertaining to the outer or superficial portion of the adrenal gland.

adrenocortical cytomegaly, abnormal enlargement of cells in the outer layer of the adrenal cortex.

adrenocortical hormone (ACH) [L, *ad,* to, *ren,* kidney, *cortex,* bark; Gk, *hormaein,* to set in motion], any of the hormones secreted by the cortex of the adrenal gland, including the glucocorticoids, mineralocorticoids, and androgens.

adrenocorticotrophic hormone. See **adrenocorticotropic hormone.**

adrenocorticotropic /ədrē′nōkôr′tikōtrop′ik/ [L, *ad* + *ren* + *cortex,* bark; Gk, *trope,* a turning], pertaining to stimulation of the adrenal cortex. Also **adrenocorticotrophic** /-trof′ik/.

adrenocorticotropic hormone (ACTH), a hormone of the anterior pituitary gland that stimulates the growth of the adrenal gland cortex and the synthesis and secretion of corticosteroids. ACTH secretion, regulated by corticotropin releasing hormone (CRH) from the hypothalamus, increases in response to a low level of circulating cortisol and to stress, fever, acute hypoglycemia, and major surgery. Under normal conditions a diurnal rhythm occurs in ACTH secretion, with an increase beginning after the first few hours of sleep and reaching a peak at the time a person awakens and a low in the evening. ACTH may be used in the treatment of rheumatoid arthritis, multiple sclerosis, and myasthenia. Normal ranges are from 15 to 100 pg/ml or 10 to 80 ng/L in the morning to less than 50 pg/ml or 50 ng/L in the evening. Normal values vary by laboratory. Also called **adrenocorticotrophic hormone, corticotropin.**

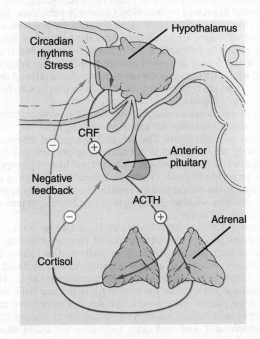

Feedback mechanism of ACTH *(Zitelli and Davis, 1997)*

adrenocorticotropic hormone test, a blood test used to study the anterior pituitary gland's functioning by measuring cortisol levels. The test is used to diagnose Cushing's syndrome and Addison's disease, which are characterized by overproduction and underproduction of cortisol, respectively.

adrenocorticotropin /-trop'in/, the adrenocorticotropic hormone (**ACTH**) secreted by the anterior pituitary gland that stimulates secretion of corticosteroid hormones by the adrenal cortex.

adrenodoxin /ədrē'nōdok'sin/, a nonheme iron protein, produced by the adrenal glands, that participates in the transfer of electrons within animal cells.

adrenogenital syndrome. See **adrenal virilism.**

adrenoleukodystrophy (ALD), a rare hereditary neonatal/childhood metabolic disease that is transmitted as a recessive sex-linked trait and affects mainly males. It is characterized by adrenal atrophy and widespread cerebral demyelination, producing progressive mental deterioration, aphasia, apraxia, eventual blindness, and quadriplegia. In the neonate form prognosis is poor, with death occurring usually in 1 to 5 years. The childhood form may be chronic and treatable for a few years with a special diet. ALD was formerly classified under Schilder's disease.

adrenomegaly /-meg'əlē/ [L, *ad* + *ren* + Gk, *megaly*, large], an abnormal enlargement of one or both adrenal glands.

adrenomimetic /-mimet'ik/, mimicking the functions of the adrenal hormones.

adrenotropic /-trop'ik/, having a stimulating effect on the adrenal glands.

Adriamycin RDF, trademark for an antibiotic antineoplastic agent (doxorubicin hydrochloride).

adromia /ədrō'mē·ə/ [Gk, *a* + *dromos,* not course], the absence of the conductive capacity of any nerve that normally innervates a muscle.

Adrucil, trademark for an antineoplastic (fluorouracil).

ADRV, abbreviation for **adult rotavirus.**

ADS, abbreviation for **antidiuretic substance.**

Adson-Brown forceps, a thumb forceps similar to the Adson forceps, having fine teeth at the tip, used for grasping delicate tissue. Also called **Brown-Adson forceps.**

Adson forceps, a small thumb forceps having a fine tip, with or without teeth.

Adson's maneuver [Alfred W. Adson, American surgeon, 1887–1951], a test for the thoracic outlet syndrome. It is performed with the patient sitting with hands on the thighs. The examiner palpates both radial pulses as the patient takes a deep breath and holds it while extending the neck and turning the head toward the affected side. If the radial pulse on the affected side is significantly diminished or there is numbness or tingling in the hand, the result is regarded as positive. Also called **Adson's test.**

adsorb, to attract and hold other material on the surface.

adsorbent /adsôr'bənt/, a substance, such as activated charcoal, that takes up another by the process of adsorption, as by the attachment of one substance to the surface of the other.

adsorption /adsôrp'shən/ [L, *ad* + *sorbere,* to suck in], a natural process whereby molecules of a gas or liquid adhere to the surface of a solid. The phenomenon depends on an assortment of factors such as surface tension and electrical charges. Many biologic reactions involve adsorption. In chemistry, adsorption is the principle on which chromatography is based and which allows for the separation of a mixture into component fractions for qualitative analysis. See also **chromatography.**

ADT, abbreviation for *Accepted Dental Therapeutics,* a journal published by the Council on Dental Therapeutics of the American Dental Association.

adult /ədult', ad'ult/ [L, *adultus,* grown up], **1.** one who is fully developed and matured and who has attained the intellectual capacity and the emotional and psychologic sta-

bility characteristic of a mature person. **2.** a person who has reached full legal age. Compare **child. 3.** any fully grown and mature organism.

adult celiac disease. See **celiac disease.**

adult ceroid-lipofuscinosis. See **Kufs' disease.**

adult day-care center, a facility for the supervised care of older adults, providing such activities as meals and socialization one or more days a week during specified daytime hours. The participants, primarily persons with physical and/or mental problems who need socialization, physical assistance, and/or psychological assistance, return to their homes each evening. The program is often used as respite by family members caring for an older person who cannot be left alone safely in the home.

adult ego state, (in psychiatry) a part of the self that analyzes and solves problems, using information received from the parent ego and child ego states. It is assumed to be fully developed in a normal individual at the age of 12. The term is used in transactional analysis.

adulteration /ədul'tərā'shən/ [L, *adulterare,* to defile], the debasement or dilution of the purity of any substance, process, or activity by the addition of extraneous material.

adult hemoglobin. See **hemoglobin A.**

adulthood, the phase of development characterized by physical and mental maturity.

adult nurse practitioner, a registered nurse who has received additional education in the primary health care of adults. The additional education may be obtained through a master's degree program or a nondegree-granting continuing education certificate program.

adult-onset diabetes. See **type 2 diabetes mellitus.**

adult polycystic disease. See **polycystic kidney disease.**

adult respiratory distress syndrome (ARDS), severe pulmonary congestion characterized by diffuse injury to alveolar-capillary membranes. Fulminating sepsis, especially when gram-negative bacteria are involved, is the most common cause. ARDS may occur after trauma; near-drowning; aspiration of gastric acid; paraquat ingestion; inhalation of corrosive chemicals, such as chlorine, ammonia, or phosgene; or use of certain drugs, including barbiturates, chlordiazepoxide, heroin, methadone, propoxyphene, and salicylates. Other causes include diabetic ketoacidosis, fungal infections, high altitude, pancreatitis, tuberculosis, and uremia. Also called **acute respiratory distress syndrome, congestive atelectasis, hemorrhagic lung, noncardiogenic pulmonary edema, pump lung, shock lung, stiff lung, wet lung.**

■ OBSERVATIONS: Signs and symptoms of ARDS include breathlessness, dyspnea, tachypnea, adventitious breath sounds, hypoxemia, and decreased lung compliance. Changes occurring within the lung include damage to the alveolar-capillary membranes, leakage of plasma proteins into the alveoli, dilution of surfactant, cessation of surfactant production, hemorrhage, interstitial edema, impaired gas exchange, and ventilation-perfusion abnormalities.

■ INTERVENTIONS: Treatment includes establishing an airway, administering oxygen, improving the underlying condition, removing the cause of ARDS, suctioning the respiratory passages as necessary, and reducing oxygen consumption. When ventilation cannot be maintained and there is evidence of a rising $PaCO_2$, mechanical ventilation is necessary. PEEP is widely used in the treatment of ARDS. All interventions for ARDS are supportive; there is no cure.

■ NURSING CONSIDERATIONS: The patient with ARDS requires constant and meticulous care, reassurance, and observation for changes in respiratory function and adequacy, including signs of hypercapnia, hypoxemia, especially confusion, skin flushing, and behavior changes such as agitation and restlessness. Increasing hypoxia may be signaled by tachycardia, elevated blood pressure, increased peripheral resistance, and fulminant respiratory failure. If PEEP is being used, the patient is carefully observed for a sudden disappearance of breath sounds accompanied by signs of respiratory distress—an indication that pneumothorax may be present. Respiratory therapy, sterile suction techniques, and position changes are continued as necessary. The patient's weight is measured frequently, chest x-ray films are evaluated, and bacteriologic cultures of secretions are analyzed for the causative organism. Throughout treatment, ventilation is carefully monitored through analysis of arterial blood gases. According to *Lewis Med Surgery,* 6th edition, this has a 50% mortality rate.

Adult respiratory distress syndrome: diffuse alveolar damage
(Kumar, Cotran, and Robbins, 1997)

adult rickets. See **osteomalacia.**
adult rotavirus (ADRV), a form of rotavirus that causes severe diarrhea in adults. The virus resembles the usual rotavirus and its genome, but it is not antigenically related and does not react against rotavirus antibodies. ADRV antibodies have been found in adults in China and Australia. See also **rotavirus.**
advanced cardiac life support (ACLS), emergency medical procedures in which basic life support efforts of cardiopulmonary resuscitation are augmented by establishment of an IV fluid line, possible defibrillation, drug administration, control of cardiac arrhythmias, endotracheal intubation, and use of ventilation equipment.
advance directive [Fr, *avancer,* to move forward; L, *dirigere,* to direct], an advance declaration by a person of treatment preferences if he or she is unable to communicate his or her wishes. See **durable power of attorney for health care, living will.**
advanced life support (ALS), a higher level of emergency medical care, usually provided by EMT-intermediates or paramedics. Typically ALS includes invasive techniques such as IV therapy, intubation, and/or drug administration.
advanced practice nurse (APN), a registered nurse having education beyond the basic nursing education and certified by a nationally recognized professional organization in a nursing specialty, or meeting other criteria established by a Board of Nursing. The Board of Nursing

establishes rules specifying which professional nursing organization certifications can be recognized for advanced practice nurses and sets requirements of education, training, and experience. Designations recognized as advanced practical nursing include clinical nurse specialist, nurse practitioner, certified registered nurse anesthetist, and certified nurse-midwife.
advancement /advans'/, [Fr, *avancer,* to move forward], a surgical technique in which a muscle or tendon is detached and then reattached at an advanced point.
adventitia /ad'ventish'ə/ [L, *adventitius,* coming from abroad], the outermost layer, composed of connective tissue with elastic and collagenous fibers, of an artery or other structure.
adventitious [L, *adventitius,* from outside sources], **1.** pertaining to an accidental condition or an arbitrary action. **2.** not hereditary. **3.** occurring at an inappropriate place, such as a coating on an artery.
adventitious bursa, an abnormal bursa that develops as a response to friction or pressure.
adventitious crisis, a rare accidental and unexpected tragedy that may affect an entire community or population, such as an earthquake, flood, or airplane crash. In addition to injuries, loss of life, and property damage, an adventitious crisis often results in long-term psychologic effects.
adventitious cyst. See **pseudocyst.**
adventitious sound, a breath sound that is not normally heard, such as a crackle, gurgle, rhonchus, or wheeze. It may be superimposed on normal breath sounds.
adverse drug effect /advurs', ad'vers/, an unintended reaction to a drug administered at normal dosage.
adverse drug reaction, any unintended effect on the body as a result of the usage of therapeutic drugs, drugs of abuse, or the interaction of two or more pharmacologically active agents. Also called **drug reaction.**
adverse reaction, any harmful, unintended effect of a medication, diagnostic test, or therapeutic intervention.
advocacy /ad'vəkas'ē/, **1.** a process whereby a nurse provides a patient with the information to make certain decisions. **2.** a method by which patients, their families, attorneys, health professionals, and citizen groups can work together to develop programs that ensure the availability of high-quality health care for a community. **3.** pleading a cause on behalf of another, such as a nurse pleading for better care of a patient.
adynamia /ad'inā'mē-ə/ [Gk, *a* + *dynamis,* not strength], lack of physical strength resulting from a pathologic condition. See also **asthenia. —adynamic,** *adj.*
adynamia episodica hereditaria, a condition seen in infancy, characterized by periodic muscle weakness and episodes of flaccid paralysis. It is inherited as an autosomal dominant trait. Also called **hyperkalemic periodic paralysis.**
adynamic. See **adynamia.**
adynamic fever, an elevated temperature with a feeble pulse, and cool, moist skin. Also called **asthenic fever.**
adynamic ileus. See **ileus, paralytic ileus.**
AE amputation. See **above-elbow amputation.**
AEC syndrome. See **Hay-Wells syndrome.**
AED, abbreviation for **automated external defibrillator.**
Aedes /ā·ē'dēz/ [Gk, *aedes,* unpleasant], a genus of mosquito, prevalent in tropical and subtropical regions. Several species are capable of transmitting pathogenic organisms to humans, including dengue, equine encephalitis, St. Louis encephalitis, tularemia, and yellow fever.

Abnormal (adventitious) lung sounds

Type	Physiology	Auscultation	Sound	Possible condition
Crackles	Air passing through fluid in small airways, or sudden opening of deflated weakened airways	More commonly heard during inspiration	Fine high-pitched or coarse low-pitched popping sounds that are short and discontinuous	Pneumonia, heart failure, atelectasis, emphysema
Rhonchi	Large airway obstructed by fluid	Heard commonly during expiration	Low-pitched continuous snoring sound	Chronic obstructive pulmonary disease (COPD), bronchospasm, pneumonia
Wheezes	Air passing through narrowed airways	Can be heard throughout inspiration and expiration	High-pitched whistling sound	Airway obstruction, bronchospasm as in asthma, COPD
Pleural friction rub	Rubbing of inflamed pleura	May occur throughout respiratory cycle, heard best at base of lung at end of expiration	Scratching, grating, rubbing, creaking	Inflamed pleura, pulmonary infarction

From Phipps WJ et al: *Medical-surgical nursing: health and illness perspectives,* ed 7, St Louis, 2003, Mosby.

-aemia. See **-emia.**

aequator. See **equator.**

aer-. See **aero-.**

aerate /er′āt/ [Gk, *aer,* air], to charge a substance or a structure with air, carbon dioxide, or oxygen.

aeration [Gk, *aer,* air], **1.** exchange of carbon dioxide for oxygen by blood in the lungs. **2.** the process of exposing a tissue or fluid to air or artificially charging it with oxygen or another gas, such as carbon dioxide.

aero-, aer-, combining form meaning 'air or gas': *aerobe, aerate.*

Aerobacter aerogenes. See *Enterobacter cloacae.*

aerobe /er′ōb/, [Gk, *aer* + *bios,* life], a microorganism that is able to live, and grow, in the presence of free oxygen. An aerobe may be **facultative** or **obligate.** Compare **anaerobe, microaerophile.**

aerobic /erō′bik/, **1.** pertaining to the presence of air or oxygen. **2.** able to live and function in the presence of free oxygen. **3.** requiring oxygen for the maintenance of life. **4.** chemical requiring the presence of oxygen.

aerobic capacity, the maximum amout of physiologic work that an individual can do as measured by oxygen consumption. It is determined by combination of aging and cardiovascular conditioning and is associated with the efficiency of oxygen extraction in the tissue.

aerobic exercise, any physical exercise that requires additional effort by the heart and lungs to meet the skeletal muscles' increased demand for oxygen. Aerobic exercise increases the breathing rate and ultimately raises heart and lung efficiency. Prolonged aerobic exercise (at least 20 minutes three times per week) is recommended for the maintenance of a healthy cardiovascular system. Examples of aerobic exercise include running, jogging, swimming, and vigorous dancing or cycling. Also called **aerobics.** See also **active exercise, passive exercise.**

aerobic glycolysis. See **glycolysis.**

aerobics. See **aerobic exercise.**

AeroBid /ār′o-bid′/, trademark for preparations of flunisolide, an antiinflammatory agent administered by inhalation to treat asthma.

aerodermectasia. See **subcutaneous emphysema.**

aerodontalgia /er′ōdontal′jə/ [Gk, *aer* + *odous,* tooth, *algos,* pain], a painful sensation in the teeth caused by a change in atmospheric pressure, as may occur at high altitudes.

aerodynamics, the study of air or other gases in motion or of bodies moving in air.

aerodynamic size, pertaining to the behavior of various aerosol particle sizes and densities.

aeroembolism. See **air embolism.**

Aeromonas /er′ōmō′nəs/, a genus of pathogenic rod-shaped gram-negative bacteria found in fresh and salt water and also soil and sewage. Various species affect fish and animals as well as humans, causing wound infections and gastroenteritis.

aerophagy /erof′əjē/ [Gk, *aer* + *phagein,* to eat], the swallowing of air, usually followed by belching, gastric distress, and flatulence. Also called **aerophagia** /er′ōfā′jē·ə/.

aerosinusitis /er′ōsī′nəsī′tis/ [Gk, *aer* + L, *sinus,* curve; Gk. *itis*], inflammation, edema, or hemorrhage of the frontal sinuses, caused by expansion of air within the sinuses when barometric pressure is decreased, as in aircraft at high altitudes. Also called **barosinusitis.**

aerosol /er′əsol′/ [Gk, *aer*; L, *solutus,* dissolved], **1.** nebulized particles suspended in a gas or air. **2.** a pressurized gas containing a finely nebulized medication for inhalation therapy. **3.** a pressurized gas containing a nebulized chemical agent for sterilizing the air of a room.

aerosol bronchodilator therapy, the use of drugs that relax the respiratory tract smooth muscle tissue when administered as tiny droplets or a mist to be inhaled.

aerosol therapy, use of an aerosol for respiratory care in the treatment of bronchopulmonary disease. The major purpose of this is the delivery of medications or humidity or both to the mucosa of the respiratory tract and pulmonary alveoli. Agents delivered by aerosol therapy may act in a number of ways: to relieve spasm of the bronchial muscles and reduce edema of the mucous membranes, to render bronchial secretions liquid so that they are more easily removed, to humidify the respiratory tract, and to administer antibiotics locally by depositing them in the respiratory tract.

aerospace medicine /er′ōspās′/, a branch of medicine concerned with the physiologic and psychologic effects of living and working in an artificial environment beyond the atmospheric and gravitational forces of the earth. The stress of extraterrestrial travel requiring long periods of weightlessness is a major concern. See also **aviation medicine.**

aerotherapy /er′ōther′əpē/, the use of air in treating disease, as in hyperbaric oxygen treatments.

aerotitis /er′ətī′tis/ [Gk, *aer* + *otikos*, ear, *itis*], an inflammation of the ear caused by changes in atmospheric pressure. Also called **barotitis.**

aerotitis media, inflammation or bleeding in the middle ear caused by a difference between the air pressure in the middle ear and that of the atmosphere, as occurs in sudden changes in altitude, in scuba diving, and in hyperbaric chambers. Symptoms are pain, tinnitus, diminished hearing, and vertigo. Also called **barotitis media.**

Æsculapius /es′kyōōlā′pē·əs/, the ancient Greek god of medicine. According to legend, Æculapius, the son of Apollo, was trained by the centaur Chiron in the art of healing; he became so proficient that he not only cured sick patients but also restored the dead to life. Because Zeus feared that Æsculapius could help humans escape death altogether, he killed the healer with a bolt of lightning. Later, Æsculapius was raised to the stature of a god and was worshipped also by the Romans, who believed he could prevent pestilence. Serpents were regarded as sacred by Æsculapius, and he is symbolized in modern medicine by a staff with a serpent entwined about it. See **staff of Æsculapius.**

aesthesia. See **esthesia.**

-aesthesia, -esthesia, suffix meaning '(condition of) feeling, perception, or sensation': *allaesthesia, hypercrysaesthesia.*

-aesthetic. See **-esthetic.**

aesthetics. See **esthetics.**

aesthetic surgery. See **cosmetic surgery.**

AF, 1. abbreviation for **atrial fibrillation. 2.** abbreviation for **atrial flutter.**

af-. See **ad-.**

AFB, abbreviation for **acid-fast bacillus.**

afebrile /āfē′bril, āfeb′ril/ [Gk, *a* + *febris*, not fever], without fever.

affect /əfekt′/ [L, *affectus* influence], an outward, observable manifestation of a person's expressed feelings or emotions, such as flat, blunted, bland, or bright. —**affective,** *adj.*

affection /əfek′shən/ [L, *affectus*, influence], **1.** an emotional state expressed as by a warm or caring feeling toward another individual. **2.** a disease process affecting all or a part of the human body.

affective /əfek′tiv/ [L, *affectus*], pertaining to emotion, mood, or feeling.

affective disorder. See **mood disorder.**

affective intimacy, a measure of well-being in a family group that focuses on whether members feel close to one another yet do not lose their individuality.

affective learning, the acquisition of behaviors involved in expressing feelings in attitudes, appreciations, and values.

affective melancholia [L, *affectus*, influence; Gk, *melas*, black, *chole*, bile], a form of severe depression characterized by a lack of interest in normally pleasant activities. The condition may occur in the depressed phase of a bipolar disorder.

affective psychosis, a psychologic reaction in which the ego's functioning is impaired and the primary clinical feature is a severe disorder of mood or emotions.

affect memory, a particular emotionally expressed feeling that recurs whenever a significant experience is recalled.

afferent /af′ərənt/ [L, *ad* + *ferre*, to carry], proceeding toward a center, as applied to arteries, veins, lymphatics, and nerves. Compare **efferent.**

afferent glomerular arteriole. See **vas afferens.**

afferent nerves [L, *ad* + *ferre*, to bear, *nervus*], nerve fibers that transmit impulses from the periphery toward the central nervous system.

afferent pathway [L, *ad* + *ferre*, to bear; AS, *paeth* + *weg*], the course or route taken, usually by a linkage of neurons, from the periphery of the body toward the center.

afferent tract [L, *ad* + *ferre*, to bear, *tractus*], a pathway for nerve impulses traveling inward or toward the brain, the center of an organ, or another body structure. Also called **ascending tract.**

affidavit /af′idā′vit/ [L, he has pledged], a written statement that is sworn to before a notary public or an officer of the court.

affiliated hospital /əfil′ē·ā′tid/ [L, *ad* + *filius*, to son], a hospital that is associated to some degree with a medical school, other health profession, a health program, or other health care institution.

affinity /əfin′itē/ [L, *affinis*, related], the measure of the binding strength of the antibody-antigen reaction.

affirmation [L, *affirmare*, to make firm], (in psychology) autosuggestion, the point at which a tendency toward positive reaction or belief is observed by the therapist.

affirmative defense /əfur′mətiv/ [L, *affirmare*, to make firm], (in law) a denial of guilt or wrongdoing based on new evidence rather than on simple denial of a charge, as a plea of immunity according to a good Samaritan law. The defendant bears the burden of proof in an affirmative defense.

afflux /af′luks/ [L, *affluere*, to flow], the sudden flow of blood or other liquid to a part of the body.

affusion /afyōō′zhən/ [L, *affundere*, to pour out], a form of therapy in which water is sprinkled or poured over the body or a particular body part. It is used for pyrexia or other disease conditions.

afibrinogenemia /afī′brinō′jenē′mē·ə/ [Gk, *a*, not; L, *fibra*, fiber; Gk, *genein*, to produce, *haima*, blood], a relative lack or absence of fibrinogen in the blood. It may be the result of a primary, congenital blood dyscrasia or acquired, as in disseminated intravascular coagulation. Also spelled **afibrinogenaemia.**

aflatoxins /af′lātok′sins/ [Gk, *a*, not; L, *flavus*, yellow; Gk, *toxikon*, poison], a group of carcinogenic and toxic factors produced by *Aspergillus flavus* food molds. The mycotoxins cause liver necrosis and liver cancer in laboratory animals and are believed to be responsible for a high incidence of liver cancer among people in tropical regions of Africa and Asia who may consume moldy grains, peanuts, or other *Aspergillus*-contaminated foods. See *Aspergillus.*

AFO, abbreviation for **ankle-foot orthosis.**

AFP, abbreviation for **alpha-fetoprotein.**

African lymphoma. See **Burkitt's lymphoma.**

African relapsing fever. See **Dutton's relapsing fever.**

African sleeping sickness. See **African trypanosomiasis.**

African tick fever. See **relapsing fever.**

African tick typhus, a rickettsial infection transmitted by ixodid ticks and characterized by fever, chills, maculopapular rash, headache, myalgia, arthralgias, and swollen lymph nodes. At the onset of the infection, a local lesion called tache noire, a buttonlike ulcer with a black center, appears at the site of the tick bite. The rash usually begins on the forearms and spreads over the rest of the body. The fever may persist into the second week, but death or complications are rare.

African trypanosomiasis, a disease caused by the parasite *Trypanosoma brucei gambiense* (West African or Gambian trypanosomiasis) or *T. brucei rhodesiense* (East African or Rhodesian trypanosomiasis), transmitted to humans by the bite of the tsetse fly. African trypanosomiasis occurs only in the savannahs and woodlands of central and east Africa, where tsetse flies are found. The disease progresses through two phases: Stage 1 is marked by fever, lymphadenopathy, splenomegaly, and myocarditis. Stage 2 is marked by symptoms of central nervous system involvement, including lethargy, sleepiness, headache, convulsions, and coma. The disease is fatal unless treated, though it may be years before the patient reaches the neurologic phase. Antimicrobial medications specific for the treatment of trypanosomiasis (suramin, pentamidine, organic arsenicals difluoromethylorthinine and eflornithine) are available in the United States only from the Centers for Disease Control and Prevention. Kinds of African trypanosomiasis are **Gambian trypanosomiasis** and **Rhodesian trypanosomiasis.** Also called **African sleeping sickness, sleeping sickness.** See also **trypanosomiasis, tsetse fly.**

African trypanosomiasis: parasites in blood
(Kumar, Abbas, and Fausto, 2005)

Afrin, trademark for an adrenergic vasoconstrictor (oxymetazoline hydrochloride).

afterbirth [AS, *aefter* + ME, *burth*], the placenta, the amnion, the chorion, and some amniotic fluid, blood, and blood clots expelled from the uterus after childbirth.

aftercare [AS, *aefter* + *caru*], health care offered a patient after discharge from a hospital or other health care facility. The patient may require a certain amount of medical or nursing attention for a health problem that no longer demands inpatient status.

afterdepolarization /-dēpō′lərizā′shən/, a membrane potential depolarization that follows an action potential. In cardiac muscles, it may be early (during phases 2 and 3 of the action potential) or delayed (during phase 4) and it is thought to cause atrial and ventricular tachycardia, especially in the setting of a long Q-T interval or digitalis toxicity. Also called **afterpotential.**

aftereffect, a physical or psychologic effect that continues after the stimulus is removed.

afterimage, a visual sensation that continues after the stimulus ends. The image may appear in colors complementary to those of the stimulus.

afterload [AS, *aefter* + ME *lod*], the load, or resistance, against which the left ventricle must eject its volume of blood during contraction. The resistance is produced by the volume of blood already in the vascular system and by the constriction of the vessel walls.

afterloading, a technique in which an unloaded applicator or needle is placed within a patient at the time of an operative procedure and subsequently loaded with a radioactive source. The loading is done under controlled conditions in which health care personnel are protected against radiation exposure. See also **remote afterloading.**

aftermovement, an involuntary muscle contraction that causes a continued movement of a limb after a strong exertion against resistance has stopped. It is often demonstrated in abduction of the arm. Also called **Kohnstamm's phenomenon, rebound effect.**

afterpains [AS, *aefter* + Gk, *poine,* penalty], contractions of the uterus common during the first days after delivery. They tend to be strongest in nursing mothers during breastfeeding, in multiparas, after the birth of large babies, and when the uterus has been overdistended. They usually resolve spontaneously but may require analgesia. The nurse may reassure the mother that afterpains are normal and prove that the uterus is contracting as it should.

afterperception, the apparent perception of a stimulus that continues after the stimulus is removed.

afterpotential. See **afterdepolarization.**

afterpotential wave /-pəten′shəl/, either of two smaller waves, positive or negative, that follow the main spike potential wave of a nerve impulse, as recorded on an oscillograph tracing of an action potential that propagates along a nerve fiber.

Ag, symbol for the element **silver.**

ag-. See **ad-.**

AGA, abbreviation for **appropriate for gestational age.**

against medical advice (ama), a phrase pertaining to a client's decision to discontinue a therapy despite the advice of medical professionals.

agalactia /ā′gəlak′shə/ [Gk *a* + *gala,* not milk], the inability of the mother to secrete enough milk to breastfeed an infant after childbirth.

agamete /āgam′ēt/ [Gk *a* + *gamos* not marriage], **1.** any of the unicellular organisms, such as bacteria and protozoa, that reproduce asexually by multiple fission instead of producing gametes. **2.** any asexual reproductive cell, such as a spore or merozoite, that forms a new organism without fusion with another gamete. See also **fungus. —agametic, agamous,** *adj.*

agametic /āgəmē′tik/, asexual; without recognizable sex organs or gametes. Also called **agamous** /ag′əmos/.

agamic /āgam′ik/, reproducing asexually, without the union of gametes; asexual.

agammaglobulinemia /agam′əglob′yoōlinē′mē·ə/ [Gk *a* + *gamma,* not gamma (third letter of Greek alphabet); L, *globulus,* small sphere; Gk, *haima,* blood], the absence of the serum immunoglobulin gamma globulin, associated with an increased susceptibility to infection. The condition may be transient, congenital, or acquired. The transient form is common in infancy before 6 weeks of age, when the infant becomes able to synthesize the immunoglobulin. The congenital form is rare and sex-linked, affecting male children; it results in decreased production of antibodies. The acquired form usually occurs in malignant diseases such as leukemia, myeloma, or lymphoma. Also spelled **agammaglobulinaemia.** See also **Bruton's agammaglobulinemia, immune gamma globulin.**

agamogenesis /əgam′ōjen′əsis/ [Gk, *a* + *gamos,* not marriage, *genein,* to produce], asexual reproduction, as by budding, simple fission of cells, or parthenogenesis. **—agamocytogenic, agamogenetic, agamogenic, agamogonic,** *adj.*

agamont. See **schizont.**

agamous. See **agametic.**

aganglionic megacolon. See **Hirschsprung's disease.**

aganglionosis /əgang′lē·ənō′sis/ [Gk, *a,* not, *gagglion,* knot, *osis,* condition], absence of parasympathetic ganglion cells in the myenteric plexus, a diagnostic sign of congenital megacolon.

agar-agar /a′gärə′gär/ [Malay], a dried hydrophilic, colloidal product obtained from certain species of red algae. Because it is unaffected by bacterial enzymes, it is widely used as the basic ingredient in solid culture media in bacteriology. Agar-agar is also used as a suspending medium, as an emulsifying agent, and as a bulk laxative. Also called **agar.**

agarose /ag′ärōs/, an essentially neutral fraction of agar used as a medium in electrophoresis, particularly for separation of serum proteins, hemoglobin variants, and lipoprotein fractions.

agastria /əgas′trē·ə/ [Gk, *a + gaster,* without stomach], the absence of a stomach.

agastric /āgas′trik/ [Gk, *a + gaster,* without stomach], pertaining to lack of a stomach or digestive tract.

AGC, abbreviation for *absolute granulocyte count.*

age [L, *aetus*], **1.** a stage of development at which the body has arrived, as measured by physical and laboratory standards to what is normal for a male or female of the same chronologic span of life. See also **mental age. 2.** to grow old.

age 30 transition, (in psychiatry) a period between 28 and 33 years of age when an individual may reevaluate the choices made in his or her twenties.

aged /ājd/, a state of having grown older or more mature than others of the population group.

ageism /ā′jizəm/ [L, *aetas,* lifetime], an attitude that discriminates, separates, stigmatizes, or otherwise disadvantages older adults on the basis of chronologic age.

agency [L, *agere,* to do], **1.** (in law) a relationship between two parties in which one authorizes the other to act in his or her behalf as agent. It usually implies a contractual arrangement between two parties managed by a third party, the agent. **2.** the business of any power or firm empowered to act for another.

Agency for Healthcare Research and Quality (AHRQ), a governmental agency of the U.S. Department of Health and Human Services. Its mission is to support research "to improve the outcomes and quality of health care, reduce its costs, address patient safety and medical errors, and broaden access to effective service." The agency systematically develops statements and recommendations to help individuals, institutions, and agencies make better decisions about health care based on research that provides evidence-based information. It publishes scientific information for other agencies and organizations on which to base clinical guidelines, performance measures, and other quality improvement tools through its evidence-based practice centers, outcomes research findings for clinicians, and technology reviews. It provides access to scientific evidence, recommendations on clinical preventive services, and information on how to implement recommended preventive services in clinical practice. Copies of the reports may be obtained free from the Publications Clearinghouse by calling 1-800-358-9295 or consulting the agency's web site at http://www.ahcpr.gov. The agency was formerly called the Agency for Health Care Policy and Research.

Agency for Toxic Substances and Disease Registry (ATSDR), an agency of the U.S. Department of Health and Human Services, charged with performing specific functions concerning the effect on public health of hazardous substances in the environment. These functions include public health assessments of waste sites, health consultations concerning specific hazardous substances, health surveillance and registries, emergency responses to release of hazardous substances, applied research in support of public health assessments, information development and dissemination, and education and training concerning hazardous substances.

agenesia. See **agenesis.**

agenesia corticalis /ā′jenē′zhə/ [Gk, *a + genein,* not to produce; L, cortex], the failure of the cortical cells of the brain, especially the pyramidal cells, to develop in the embryo, resulting in infantile cerebral paralysis and severe mental retardation.

agenesis /ājen′əsis/ [Gk, *a + genein,* not to produce], **1.** congenital absence of an organ or part, usually caused by a lack of primordial tissue and failure of development in the embryo. **2.** impotence or sterility. Also called **agenesia.** Compare **dysgenesis. —agenic,** *adj.*

agenetic fracture /ā′jenet′ik/, a spontaneous fracture caused by an imperfect bone development.

agenic. See **agenesis.**

ageniocephaly /ājen′ē·ōsef′əlē/ [Gk, *a + genein,* not to produce, *kephale,* head], a form of otocephaly in which the brain, cranial vault, and sense organs are intact but the lower jaw is malformed. Also called **ageniocephalia. —ageniocephalic, ageniocephalous,** *adj.*

agenitalism /ājen′itəliz′əm/, any condition caused by the lack of sex hormones and the absence or malfunction of the ovaries or testes.

agenosomia /əjen′əsō′mē·ə/, a congenital malformation characterized by the absence or defective formation of the genitals and protrusion of the intestines through an incompletely developed abdominal wall.

agenosomus /əjen′əsō′məs/ [Gk, *a + genein,* not to produce, *soma,* body], a fetus with agenosomia.

agent [L, *agere,* to do], (in law) a party authorized to act on behalf of another and to give the other an account of such actions.

Agent Orange, a U.S. military code name for a mixture of two herbicides, 2,4-D and 2,4,5-T, used as a defoliant in Southeast Asia during the 1960s conflict in Vietnam. The herbicides were unintentionally contaminated with the highly toxic chemical dioxin, which is believed to be a cause of cancer and birth defects in animals and established as a cause of chloracne and porphyria cutanea tarda in humans. See **dioxin.**

age of consent, (in medical jurisprudence) the age at which an individual is legally free to act as an adult, without parental permission for such activities as marriage or sexual intercourse or giving permission for medical treatment or surgery. The specific age of consent varies from 13 to 21, according to local laws.

age of majority, the age at which a person is considered to be an adult in the eyes of the law.

age-specific, data in which the age of the individual is significant for epidemiologic or statistical purposes.

ageusia /əgyoo′sē·ə/ [Gk, *a+ geusis,* without taste], a loss or impairment of the sense of taste. Also called **ageustia, gustatory anesthesia.**

agger /ag′ər, aj′ər/, a small protuberance or eminence of tissue, such as the curved elevation above the atrium of the nose.

agglomerate /əglom′ərāt/ [L, *glomus,* a ball], to collect or gather into a mass, ball, or cluster.

agglomeration [L, *agglomerare,* to gather into a ball], a mass or cluster of individual units.

agglutinant /əgloo′tənənt/ [L, *agglutinare,* to glue],

something that causes adhesion, such as a circulating antibody that is stimulated by the presence of an antigen to adhere to it.

agglutination /əgloo'tinā'shən/ [L, *agglutinare,* to glue], the clumping together of cells as a result of interaction with specific antibodies called agglutinins. Agglutinins are used in blood typing and in identifying or estimating the strength of immunoglobulins or immune sera. See also **agglutinin, blood typing, precipitin.**

Latex agglutination (Conlon and Snydman, 2000)

agglutination-inhibition test, a serologic technique useful in testing for certain unknown soluble antigens. The unknown antigen is mixed with a known agglutinin. If there is a reaction, the agglutinin can no longer adhere to the cells or particles that carry its corresponding antigen, and the unknown antigen is thus identified. One type of pregnancy test is based on agglutination inhibition.

agglutination reaction, formation of an aggregate on mixing soluble antibody with particulate antigen molecules in an aqueous medium; the visible aggregates are formed when specific antibody crosslinks the antigens.

agglutination titer, the highest dilution of a serum that will produce clumping of cells or particulate antigens. It is a measure of the concentration of specific antibodies in the serum.

agglutinin /əgloo'tinin/, an antibody that interacts with antigens, resulting in agglutination. Usually multivalent, agglutinins act on insoluble antigens in stable suspension to form a cross-linking lattice that may clump or precipitate. Compare **precipitin.** See also **agglutination, blood typing, hemagglutination.**

agglutinin absorption, the removal from immune serum of antibody by treatment with homologous antigen, followed by centrifugation and separation of the antigen-antibody complex.

agglutinogen /ag'lootin'əjin/ [L, *agglutinare* + Gk, *genein,* to produce], any antigenic substance that causes agglutination (clumping together of cells) by the production of agglutinin.

aggregate /ag'rəgāt/ [L, *ad* + *gregare,* to gather together], the total of a group of substances or components making up a mass or complex. Data on individual patients can be aggregated to allow conclusions about the patient population to be made.

aggregate anaphylaxis, an exaggerated immune reaction of immediate hypersensitivity induced by an antigen that forms a soluble antigen-antibody complex.

aggregation /ag'rəgā'shən/ [L, *ad* + *gregare,* to gather together], an accumulation of substances, objects, or individuals, as in the clumping of blood cells or the clustering of clients with the same disorder.

aggression /əgresh'ən/ [L, *aggressio,* to attack], a forceful behavior, action, or attitude that is expressed physically, verbally, or symbolically. It may arise from innate drives or occur as a defensive mechanism, often resulting from a threatened ego. It is manifested by either constructive or destructive acts directed toward oneself or against others. Kinds of aggression are **constructive aggression, destructive aggression,** and **inward aggression.**

aggression control, a nursing outcome from the Nursing Outcomes Classification (NOC) defined as self-restraint of assaultive, combative, or destructive behavior toward others. See also **Nursing Outcomes Classification.**

aggressive infantile fibromatosis, an uncommon condition, present at birth or developing during infancy or childhood, characterized by fast-growing, firm, painless, single or multiple nodules involving subcutaneous tissue, muscle, fascia, and tendons and seen anywhere on the body; tumors are locally invasive but do not metastasize and have a high tendency to recur after excision.

aggressive personality /əgres'iv/, a personality with behavior patterns characterized by irritability, impulsivity, destructiveness, or violence in response to frustration.

aggressive-radical therapy, (in psychiatry) a form of therapy that introduces the political and social viewpoints of the therapist into the therapeutic process. Proponents of this technique believe that making all values explicit, sometimes through actual didactic input, enables the patient to view the solution of an emotional conflict and the raising of political consciousness as one and the same.

aging [L, *aetas,* lifetime], the process of growing old, biological aging results in part from a failure of body cells to function normally or to produce new body cells to replace those that are dead or malfunctioning. Normal cell function may be lost through infectious disease, malnutrition, exposure to environmental hazards, or genetic influences. Among body cells that exhibit early signs of aging are those that normally cease dividing after reaching maturity. Sociological and psychological theories of aging seek to explain the other influences on aging caused by the environment, engagement, personality, and non-biological influences. See also **assessment of the aging patient.**

Aging changes affecting cognition and perception

Decreased brain weight
Diminished enzyme activity
Slowed reflexes
Decreased sensory receptors for temperature, pain, and tactile discrimination
Weakening of interneuron connections
Increased response time
Chronic hypoxia

From Phipps WJ et al: *Medical-surgical nursing: health and illness perspectives,* ed 7, St Louis, 2003, Mosby.

agitated /aj'ətā'təd/ [L, *agitare,* to shake], describing a condition of psychomotor excitement characterized by purposeless, restless activity. Pacing, talking, crying, and laughing sometimes are characteristic and may serve to release nervous tension associated with anxiety, fear, or other mental stress. **—agitate,** *v.,* **agitation,** *n.*

agitated depression, a severe depressive disorder characterized by severe anxiety accompanied by continuous physical restlessness, and, frequently, somatic symptoms. Psychomotor agitation is prominent. Delusions may also be present, as well as depression with psychotic features. See also **depression.**

agitation, a state of chronic restlessness and increased psychomotor activity that is generally observed as an expression of emotional tension.

agitographia /aj′itōgraf′ē·ə/ [L, *agitare* + Gk, *graphein,* to write], a condition characterized by abnormally rapid writing in which words or parts of words are unconsciously omitted. The condition is commonly associated with agitophasia.

agitophasia /aj′itōfā′zhə/ [L, *agitare* + Gk, *phasis,* speech], a condition characterized by abnormally rapid speech in which words, sounds, or syllables are unconsciously omitted, slurred, or distorted. The condition is commonly associated with agitographia. Also called **agitolalia.**

Agkistrodon /ag-kis′trŏ-don/, a genus of venomous pit vipers. *A. contortrix* is the copperhead and *A. piscivorus* is the water moccasin. See also **snakebite.**

aglossia /əglos′ē·ə/ [Gk, *a* + *glossa,* without tongue], congenital absence of the tongue.

aglycemia /ā′glīsē′mē·ə/ [Gk, *a, glykis,* not sweet, *haima,* blood], an absence of blood glucose.

agnathia /ag-nath′ē·ə/ [Gk, *a, gnathos,* not jaw], a developmental defect characterized by total or partial absence of the lower jaw. Also called **agnathy** /ag′nəthē/. Compare **synotia.** See also **otocephaly. —agnathous,** *adj.*

agnathocephalia, agnathocephalic, agnathocephalous. See **agnathocephaly.**

agnathocephalus /ag-nath′əsef′ələs/, a fetus with agnathocephaly.

agnathocephaly /ag-nath′əsef′əlē/ [Gk, *a* + *gnathos* + *kephale,* head], a congenital malformation characterized by the absence of the lower jaw, defective formation of the mouth, and placement of the eyes low on the face with fusion or approximation of the zygomas and the ears. Also called **agnathocephalia.** See also **otocephaly. —agnathocephalic, agnathocephalous,** *adj.*

agnathus /ag-nath′əs/ [Gk, *a* + *gnathos,* without jaw], a fetus with agnathia.

agnathy. See **agnathia.**

AgNO₃, the chemical formula for silver nitrate.

agnogenic myeloid metaplasia. See **myeloid metaplasia.**

agnosia /ag-nō′zhə/, [Gk, *a* + *gnosis,* not knowledge], total or partial loss of the ability to recognize familiar objects or persons through sensory stimuli as a result of organic brain damage dementia. The condition may affect any of the senses and is classified accordingly as auditory, visual, olfactory, gustatory, or tactile agnosia. Also called **agnosis.** See also **autotopagnosia.**

-agnosia, -agnosis, suffix meaning '(condition of the) loss of the faculty to perceive': *autotopagnosia, paragnosia.*

-agogue, -agog, suffix meaning an 'agent promoting the expulsion of a (specified) substance': *lymphagogue, uragogue.*

agonal /ag′ənəl/ [Gk, *agon,* struggle], pertaining to death and dying.

agonal respiration. See **Cheyne-Stokes respiration.**

agonal thrombus, a mass of blood platelets, fibrin, clotting factors, and cellular elements that forms in the heart of a dying patient.

agonist /ag′ənist/ [Gk, *agon,* struggle], **1.** a contracting muscle whose contraction is opposed by another muscle (an antagonist). **2.** a drug or other substance having a specific cellular affinity that produces a predictable response.

agony /ag′ənē/ [Gk, *agon*], severe physical or emotional anguish or distress, as in pain.

agoraphobia /ag′ərə-/ [Gk, *agora,* marketplace, *phobos,* fear], an anxiety disorder characterized by a fear of being in an open, crowded, or public place, such as a field, tunnel, bridge, congested street, or busy department store, where escape is perceived as difficult or help not available in case of sudden incapacitation.

-agra, suffix meaning a 'pain or painful seizure': *cardiagra, trachelagra.*

agranular endoplasmic reticulum. See **endoplasmic reticulum.**

agranulocyte /āgran′yoolōsīt′/ [Gk, *a,* not; L, *granulum,* small grain; Gk, *kytos,* cell], any leukocyte that does not contain predominant cytoplasmic granules, such as a monocyte or lymphocyte. Compare **granulocyte.** See also **leukocyte.**

Agranulocyte *(Carr and Rodak, 1999)*

agranulocytic /-si′tik/ [Gk, *a,* not, *granule, kytos,* cell], pertaining to a white blood cell that, when stained, shows no granules in its cytoplasm.

agranulocytosis /āgran′yoŏlō′sītō′sis/, a severe reduction in the number of white blood cells (basophils, eosinophils, and neutrophils). Neutropenia results, whereby the body is severely depleted in its ability to defend itself. Fever, prostration, and bleeding ulcers of the rectum, mouth, and vagina may be present. The acute disease may be an adverse reaction to a medication or the result of radiation therapy or chemotherapy.

agranulosis. See **agranulocytosis.**

agraphesthesia. See **graphanesthesia.**

agraphia /āgraf′ē·ə/ [Gk, *a, graphein,* not to write], a loss of the ability to write, resulting from injury to the language center in the cerebral cortex. Compare **dysgraphia. —agraphic,** *adj.*

A:G ratio, the ratio of protein albumin to globulin in the blood serum. On the basis of differential solubility with neutral salt solution the normal values are 3.5 to 5 g/dl for albumin and 2.5 to 4 g/dl for globulin.

agrimony, an herb found in Asia, Europe, and the United States.

■ USES: This herb is used for mild diarrhea, gastroenteritis, intestinal mucus secretion, inflammation of the mouth and throat, cuts and scrapes, and amenorrhea; insufficient reliable information to assess its effectiveness.

■ CONTRAINDICATIONS: Agrimony is not recommended during pregnancy and lactation, in children, or in those with known hypersensitivity to this plant or roses.

Agrobacterium, an environmental gram-negative bacilli. *A. tumefaciens* has been implicated in nosocomial urinary tract infections, peritonitis, wound infections, prosthetic valve endocarditis, and sepsis.

agrypnia. See **insomnia.**

agrypnocoma /agrip′nōkō′mə/ [Gk, *agrypnos,* sleepless], a coma in which there is some degree of wakefulness. The condition may be manifested by extreme lethargy or drowsiness accompanied by delirium.

agrypnotic /ag′ripnot′ik/, **1.** insomniac. **2.** medication or other substance that prevents sleep. **3.** causing wakefulness.

AGS, 1. abbreviation for *American Geriatrics Society.* **2.** abbreviation for adrenogenital syndrome.

agyria /əjī′rē·ə/, a cerebral cortex abnormality in which the gyri are poorly developed. The cortical tissue is reduced, leading to severe mental retardation. Also called **lissencephaly.**

AHA, abbreviation for **American Hospital Association.**

"aha" reaction /ähä′/, (in psychology) a sudden realization or inspiration, experienced especially during creative thinking. Some psychologists associate great scientific discoveries and artistic inspirations with this reaction, which is not necessarily related to intelligence. The term has apparently replaced **"aha" experience,** formerly used by psychologists, especially those of the Gestalt school, to label experiences in which an individual utters "Aha!" during a moment of revelation.

AHCPR, abbreviation for **Agency for Health Care Policy and Research.**

AHF, abbreviation for **antihemophilic factor.**

AHH, abbreviation for **aryl hydrocarbon hydroxylase.**

AHIMA, abbreviation for *American Health Information Management Association.*

AHRQ, abbreviation for *Agency for Healthcare Research and Quality.*

Ahumada-del Castillo syndrome /ä′hoomä′dädel′kästē′yō/ [Juan Carlos Ahumada; E.B. del Castillo; twentieth-century Argentine physicians], a form of secondary amenorrhea that may be associated with a pituitary gland tumor. It is characterized by both galactorrhea and amenorrhea in the absence of a pregnancy.

AI, 1. abbreviation for **artificial intelligence. 2.** abbreviation for **artificial insemination.**

AICC, abbreviation for **anti-inhibitor coagulant complex.**

AICD, abbreviation for **automatic implanted cardioverter defibrillator.**

aid, assistance given a person who is ill, injured, or otherwise unable to cope with normal demands of life.

AID, abbreviation for **artificial insemination by donor.**

AIDS /ādz/, abbreviation for **acquired immunodeficiency syndrome.**

AIDS-associated retinopathy. See **HIV-associated retinopathy.**

AIDS cholangiopathy, bile duct disease seen complicating the acquired immunodeficiency syndrome. The most common effect is primary sclerosing cholangitis; some patients also have sphincter of Oddi dysfunction.

AIDS-dementia complex (ADC), a neurologic effect of encephalitis or brain inflammation experienced by nearly one-third of all patients with acquired immunodeficiency syndrome (AIDS). The condition is characterized by memory loss and by varying levels and forms of dementia. It may be caused by the destruction of brain neurons by the AIDS virus, as autopsies indicate that the density of the neurons may be 40% lower in AIDS patients than in persons who have not had AIDS. Also called **AIDS-related dementia.**

AIDS nephropathy, former name for HIV-associated nephropathy.

AIDS-related complex. See **AIDS-wasting syndrome.**

AIDS serology test (AIDS screen, HIV antibody test, Western blot test, ELISA), a test used to detect the antibody to the human immunodeficiency virus (HIV), which causes AIDS. Home testing kits are now available in addition to the tests performed by health care providers.

AIDS-wasting syndrome, a syndrome associated with progressed acquired immunodeficiency syndrome (AIDS). Signs and symptoms may include weight loss, fever, malaise, lethargy, oral thrush, and immunologic abnormalities characteristic of AIDS. Formerly called **AIDS-related complex (ARC).**

AIH, abbreviation for **artificial insemination husband.**

AILD, abbreviation for **angioimmunoblastic lymphadenopathy with dysproteinemia.**

ailment [OE, *eglan*], any disease, physical disorder, or complaint, generally of a chronic, acute, or mild nature.

ainhum. See **autoamputation.**

air [Gk, *aer*], the colorless, odorless gaseous mixture constituting the earth's atmosphere. It consists of 78% nitrogen; 20% oxygen; almost 1% argon; small amounts of carbon dioxide, hydrogen, and ozone; traces of helium, krypton, neon, and xenon; and varying amounts of water vapor.

air abrasion, a type of microabrasion in which a jet of air blows tiny particles against the tooth or cavity surface.

air bath, the exposure of the naked body to warm air for therapeutic purposes. Also called **balneum pneumaticum.**

airborne contaminants, materials in the atmosphere that can affect the health of persons in the same or nearby environments. Particularly vulnerable are tissues of the upper respiratory tract and lungs, including the terminal bronchioles and alveoli. The effects depend in part on the solubility of the inhaled matter. Inhaled contaminants may cause tissue damage, tissue reaction, disease, or physical obstruction. Some airborne contaminants, such as carbon monoxide gas, may have little or no direct effect on the lungs but can be absorbed into the bloodstream and carried to other organs or damage the blood itself. Biologically inert gases may dilute the atmospheric oxygen below the normal blood saturation value, thereby disturbing cellular respiration.

airborne precautions, safeguards designed to reduce the risk of airborne transmission of infectious agents. Airborne droplet nuclei consist of small-particle residue (5 mm or smaller in size) of evaporated droplets that may remain suspended in the air for long periods of time. Airborne transmission occurs by dissemination of either airborne droplet nuclei or dust particles containing the infectious agent. Microorganisms carried in this manner can be widely dispersed by air currents and may become inhaled or deposited on a susceptible host from the source patient. Special air handling and ventilation are required to prevent airborne transmission. Airborne precautions apply to patients known or suspected to have serious illnesses that are transmitted by airborne droplet nuclei. Examples include measles, varicella-zoster virus infections, legionella, disseminated zoster, and tuberculosis. See also **standard precautions, transmission-based precautions.**

aircast splint. See **air splint.**

air compressor, a mechanical device that compresses air for storage and is used in handpieces and other air-driven medical and dental tools.

air embolism, the abnormal presence of air in the cardiovascular system, resulting in obstruction of blood flow. Air embolism may occur if a large quantity of air is inadvertently introduced by injection, as during IV therapy or surgery, or by trauma, as a puncture wound. Also called **aeroembolism.** See also **decompression sickness, embolus, gas embolism.**

air encephalography. See **encephalography.**

air entrainment, the movement of room air into the chamber of a jet nebulizer used to treat respiratory diseases. Air entrainment increases the rate of nebulization and the amount of liquid administered per unit of time.

airflow pattern, the pattern of movement of respiratory gases through the respiratory tract. The pattern is affected by such factors as gas density and viscosity.

air fluidization, the process of blowing temperature-controlled air through a collection of microspheres to create a fluidlike movement. The technique is used in special mattresses designed to reduce pressure against a patient's skin. See also **air-fluidized bed.**

air-fluidized bed, a bed with body support provided by thousands of tiny soda-lime glass beads suspended by pressurized temperature-controlled air. The patient rests on a polyester filter sheet that covers the beads. The special bed is designed for use by patients with posterior pressure ulcers or at risk for pressure ulcers or posterior grafts, burns, or donor areas. Pressure against the skin surface of the patient is less than capillary filling pressure. The improved capillary blood flow to the skin speeds the growth of granulation tissue.

air hunger, a form of respiratory distress characterized by gasping, labored breathing, or dyspnea.

airplane splint a splint used to immobilize a shoulder during healing from injury, such as a fractured humerus. The splint holds the arm in an abducted position at or below shoulder level, with the elbow bent. It extends to the waist and may be made of plastic or wire, or it may be supported by a plaster body.

air pollution [L, *polluere,* to defile], contamination of the air by noxious fumes, aromas, or toxic chemicals.

air pump, a pump that forces air into or out of a cavity or chamber.

air sac, a small, terminal cavity in the lung, consisting of the alveoli connected to one terminal bronchiole.

air sickness, a form of motion sickness caused by air travel and, in some cases, by traveling on land at high elevations. Symptoms usually include nausea and vomiting and are sometimes accompanied by headache or drowsiness. See also **motion sickness.**

air spaces, the alveolar ducts, alveolar sacs, and alveoli of the respiratory system.

air splint, a device for temporarily immobilizing fractured or otherwise injured extremities. It consists of an inflatable cylinder that can be closed at both ends and becomes rigid when filled with air under pressure. Also called **aircast splint.**

air swallowing, the intake of air into the digestive system, usually involuntary and during eating, drinking, or chewing gum. Air swallowing may also be an effect of anxious behavior. The problem occurs commonly in infants as a result of faulty feeding methods.

air thermometer, a thermometer using air as its expansible medium. See also **thermometer.**

airway [Gk, *aer* + AS, *weg,* way], **1.** a tubular passage for movement of air into and out of the lung. An airway with a diameter greater than 2 mm is defined as a large, or central, airway such as mainstream bronchi; one smaller than 2 mm is called a small, or peripheral, airway such as terminal bronchitis. **2.** a respiratory anesthesia device. **3.** an oropharyngeal tube used for mouth-to-mouth resuscitation.

airway clearance, ineffective, a nursing diagnosis accepted by the Fourth National Conference on the Classification of Nursing Diagnoses (revised 1998). Ineffective airway clearance is a state in which an individual is unable to clear secretions or obstructions from the respiratory tract to maintain a clear airway.

■ DEFINING CHARACTERISTICS: The defining characteristics are abnormal breath sounds (crackles, gurgles, wheezes); cough, ineffective or absent; sputum; report of chest congestion; dyspnea; diminished breath sounds; orthopnea; cyanosis; difficulty vocalizing; wide-eyed changes in respiratory rate and rhythm; and restlessness.

■ RELATED FACTORS: Related factors include environmental elements, such as smoking, smoke inhalation, and secondhand smoke. Other related factors include airway spasm, retained secretions, excessive mucus, presence of an artificial airway, a foreign body in the airway, secretions in the bronchi, exudate in the alveoli, neuromuscular dysfunction, hyperplasia of the bronchial walls, chronic obstructive pulmonary disease, infection, asthma, and allergic airways. See also **nursing diagnosis.**

airway conductance, the instantaneous rate of gas flow in the airway per unit of pressure difference between the mouth, nose, or other airway opening and the alveoli. It is the reciprocal of airway resistance and is indicated by the symbol G_{aw}.

airway division, one of the 18 segments of the bronchopulmonary system. The segments are usually numbered from

Air fluidized bed (© Hill-Rom Services, Inc./used with permission)

1 to 10 for the right lung, which has three lobes, and from 1 to 8 for the left lung, which has two lobes.

airway insertion and stabilization, a nursing intervention from the Nursing Interventions Classification (NIC) defined as insertion or assisting with insertion and stabilization of an artificial airway. See also **Nursing Interventions Classification.**

airway management, a nursing intervention from the Nursing Interventions Classification (NIC) defined as facilitation of patency of air passages. See also **Nursing Interventions Classification.**

airway obstruction, a mechanical impediment to the delivery of air to the lungs or to the absorption of oxygen in the lungs.

■ OBSERVATIONS: If the obstruction is minor, as in sinusitis or pharyngitis, the person is able to breathe, but not normally. If the obstruction is acute, the person may grasp the neck, gasp, become cyanotic, and lose consciousness.

■ INTERVENTIONS: Acute airway obstruction requires rapid intervention to save the person's life. In cases of obstruction caused by a bolus of food, a collection of mucus, or a foreign body, the object may be removed manually, by suction, or with the Heimlich maneuver. Obstruction caused by an inflammatory or allergic reaction may be treated with bronchodilating drugs, corticosteroids, intubation, and administration of oxygen. An emergency tracheotomy may be required if the obstruction cannot be mechanically or pharmacologically relieved within a few minutes.

■ NURSING CONSIDERATIONS: The patient is usually very apprehensive and may physically resist assistance. Medical help is summoned, and emergency care is begun and includes removing the obstruction, administering oxygen, and performing cardiopulmonary resuscitation, if necessary. See also **aspiration, cardiopulmonary resuscitation, Heimlich maneuver.**

airway resistance, a measure of the impedance to airflow through the bronchopulmonary system. It is the reciprocal of airway conductance and is indicated by the symbol R_{aw}.

airway suctioning, a nursing intervention from the Nursing Interventions Classification (NIC) defined as removal of airway secretions by inserting a suction catheter into the patient's oral airway and/or trachea. See also **Nursing Interventions Classification.**

AIUM, abbreviation for *American Institute of Ultrasound in Medicine.*

AK, abbreviation for *above the knee,* referring to amputations, amputees, prostheses, and orthoses.

AK amputation. See **transfemoral amputation.**

akaryocyte /āker′ē·əsīt′/ [Gk, *a,* not, *karyon,* kernel], a cell without a nucleus, such as an erythrocyte.

akathisia /ak′əthē′zhə/ [Gk, *a* + *kathizein,* not to sit], a pathologic condition characterized by restlessness and agitation, such as an inability to sit still. —**akathisiac,** *adj.*

akeratosis /āker′ətō′sis/, a skin condition in which there is a lack of horny tissue in the epidermis.

akinesia /ā′kinē′zhə, ā′kīnē′zhə/ [Gk, *a, kinesis,* without movement], an abnormal state of motor and psychic hypoactivity or muscular paralysis. Also called akinesis. —**akinetic,** *adj.*

akinesthesia /ākin′esthē′zhə/, a loss of the sense of movement.

akinetic /ā′kinet′ik/ [Gk, *a, kinesis*], without movement, pertaining to a loss of ability to move a part or all of the body.

akinetic apraxia, the inability to perform a spontaneous movement. See also **apraxia.**

akinetic mutism, a state of apparent alertness in which a person is unable or refuses to move or to make sounds, resulting from neurologic or psychologic disturbance.

akinetic seizure, a type of seizure disorder observed in children. It is a brief, generalized seizure in which the child suddenly falls to the ground.

Akineton, trademark for a peripheral anticholinergic (biperiden hydrochloride).

-akusis. See **-acousia.**

Al, symbol for the element **aluminum.**

-al, suffix designating a compound containing a member of the aldehyde group: *chloral, ethanal.*

-al, -ale, suffix meaning "characterized by" or "pertaining to": *appendiceal, meningeal.*

ala *pl.* **alae** /ā′lə/ [L, wing], **1.** any winglike structure. **2.** the axilla.

Ala, abbreviation for the amino acid **alanine.**

ALA, abbreviation for **aminolevulinic acid.**

ala auris, the auricle of the ear.

ala cerebelli /ser′əbel′ī/, the ala of the central lobule of the cerebellum.

ala cinerea /sinir′ē·ə/, the triangular area on the floor of the fourth ventricle of the brain from which the autonomic fibers of the vagus nerve arise.

alactasia. See **lactase deficiency.**

Alagille syndrome /ä·lä·zhēl′/ [Daniel Alagille, French pediatrician, b. 1925], an autosomal dominant syndrome of neonatal jaundice, cholestasis with peripheral pulmonic stenosis, and occasionally septal defects or patent ductus arteriosus, resulting from low numbers or absence of intrahepatic bile ducts; it is characterized by unusual facies and ocular, vertebral, and nervous system abnormalities.

ala nasi /nā′sī/, the outer flaring cartilaginous wall of each nostril.

alanine (Ala) /al′ənin/, a nonessential amino acid found in many food protein sources as well as in the body. It is degraded in the liver to produce important biomolecules such as pyruvate and glutamate. Its carbon skeleton also can be used as an energy source. See also **amino acid, protein.**

Chemical structure of alanine

alanine aminotransferase (ALT), an enzyme normally present in the serum and tissues of the body, especially the tissues of the liver. This enzyme catalyzes the transfer of an amino group from *l*-alanine to alpha-ketoglutarate, forming pyruvate and 1-glutamate. The reaction is reversible. The enzyme is released into the serum as a result of tissue injury and increases in persons with acute liver damage. Normal findings are 5-35 IU/L. Also called **alanine transferase.** Previously called **serum glutamic pyruvic transaminase.** Compare **aspartate aminotransferase.**

alanine aminotransferase test (ALT or SGPT), a blood test that measures levels of ALT, an enzyme found predominantly in the liver. Elevated levels of ALT are highly specific in indicating hepatocellular disease.

alanine transferase, 1. an intracellur enzyme in amino acid and carbohydrate metabolism. 2. found in high concentration in brain, liver, and muscle. An increased level indicates necrosis or disease in these tissues. See also **alanine aminotransferase (ALT).**

Al-Anon, an international organization that offers guidance, counseling, and support for the relatives, friends, and associates of alcoholics. See also **Alcoholics Anonymous.**

ala of the ethmoid, a small projection on each side of the crista galli of the ethmoid bone. Each ala fits into a corresponding depression of the frontal bone.

ala of the ilium, the upper flaring portion of the iliac bone.

ala of the sacrum, the flat extension of bone on each side of the sacrum.

alar /ā′lär/ [L, *ala*, wing], pertaining to a winglike structure, such as the shoulder.

ALARA, 1. an abbreviation for *as low as reasonably achievable.* 2. acronym for *as low as reasonably achievable.* It refers to the principle that all radiation exposure, both to patients and to radiologic personnel, should be minimized in diagnostic imaging.

alar lamina [L, *ala*, wing, *lamina*, thin plate], the posterolateral area of the embryonic neural tube through which sensory nerves enter.

alar ligament, one of a pair of ligaments that connect the axis to the occipital bone and limit rotation of the cranium. Also called **check ligament, odontoid ligament.** Compare **membrana tectoria.**

alarm reaction, the first stage of the general adaptation syndrome. It is characterized by the release of ACTH by the pituitary gland and of epinephrine by the medulla of the adrenal gland, which cause increased blood glucose levels and faster respirations, increasing the oxygen level of the blood. These actions provide the body with increased energy to deal with a stressful situation. See also **general adaptation syndrome, stress.**

alar process [L, *ala*, wing, *processus*], a projection of the cribriform plate of the ethmoid bone articulating with the frontal bone.

alaryngeal speech /ā′lä·rin′je·əl spēch/ [Gk, *a*, without + *larynx*; ME, *speche*], a method of speech used after laryngectomy, with sound produced by vibration of the column of air in the esophagus against the sphincter between the esophagus and pharynx. Also called **esophageal speech.**

alastrim /al′əstrim/ [Port, *alastrar,* to spread], a mild form of smallpox, with little rash. It is thought to be caused by a weak strain of *Poxvirus variolae.* Unlike smallpox, alastrim is rarely fatal. Also called **Cuban itch, milkpox, variola minor.** See also **smallpox.**

Alateen, an international organization that offers guidance, counseling, and support for the children of alcoholics. See also **Alcoholics Anonymous.**

alatrofloxacin /ah-lat′ro-flok′sah-sin/, a broad-spectrum antibacterial that is the prodrug of trovafloxacin, to which it is rapidly converted after IV infusion; used in the form of the mesylate salt.

alatrofloxacin/trovafloxacin, a quinolone antibiotic.

■ INDICATIONS: This drug is used to treat nosocomial pneumonia, community-acquired pneumonia, chronic bronchitis, acute sinusitis, complicated intra-abdominal infections, skin and skin structure infections, urinary tract infections, chronic

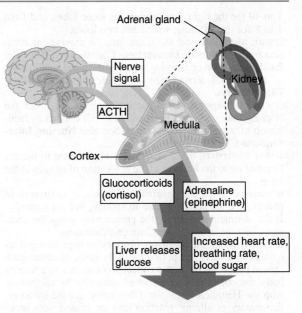

Alarm reaction *(Thibodeau and Patton, 2003)*

bacterial prostatitis, urethral gonorrhea in males, pelvic inflammatory disease, and cervicitis caused by susceptible organisms.

■ CONTRAINDICATIONS: Known hypersensitivity to quinolones, seizure disorders, cerebral atherosclerosis, and photosensitivity prohibit the use of this drug.

■ ADVERSE EFFECTS: Life-threatening side effects include pseudomembranous colitis. Other adverse effects include headache, dizziness, insomnia, anxiety, nausea, flatulence, vomiting, diarrhea, abdominal pain, vaginitis, crystalluria, rash, pruritus, and photosensitivity.

ala vomeris /vō′məris/, an extension of bone on each side of the upper border of the vomer.

alb-, prefix meaning "white": *albumin.*

alba /al′bə/, literally, "white," as in *linea alba.* white substance on the brain.

albedo /albē′dō/ [L, *albus,* white], a whiteness, particularly as a surface reflection.

albendazole /al-ben′dah-zōl/, a broad-spectrum anthelmintic used against many parasites, including in treatment of hydatid disease and cysticercosis.

Albers-Schönberg disease /-shœn′burg, -shōn′-/ [Heinrich E. Albers-Schönberg, Hamburg radiologist, 1865–1921], a form of osteopetrosis characterized by marblelike calcification of bones. The condition, often discovered by chance during x-ray examination, is transmitted as an autosomal dominant trait. See also **osteopetrosis.**

Albert's disease [Eduard Albert, Austrian surgeon, 1841–1900], an inflammation of the bursa that lies between the Achilles tendon and the calcaneus. It is most frequently caused by injury but may also result from the wearing of poorly fitted shoes, increased strain on the tendon, or rheumatoid arthritis. Treatment includes intrabursal injection of corticosteroid with lidocaine and warm compresses. If treatment is delayed, the inflammation may cause erosion of the calcaneus. Also called **anterior Achilles bursitis,** *Swediaur's d.*

albicans /al'bikənz/ [L, *albus,* white],   white or whitish. See also **corpus albicans.**

albinism /al'biniz'əm/,   a congenital hereditary condition characterized by partial or total lack of melanin pigment in the body. Total albinos have pale skin that does not tan, white hair, pink eyes, nystagmus, astigmatism, and photophobia. Albinos are prone to severe sunburn, actinic dermatitis, and skin cancer. Compare **piebald, vitiligo.**

White hair and pale skin in albinism
(Zitelli and Davis, 1997)

Pale fundus in albinism *(Zitelli and Davis, 1997)*

Albini's nodules /äl·be'nēz/ [Giuseppe Albini, Italian physiologist, 1827–1911],   gray nodules the size of small grains, sometimes seen on the free edges of the atrioventricular valves of infants; they are remains of fetal structures.

albino /albī'nō/ [L, *albus,* white],   an individual with a marked deficiency of pigment in the eyes, hair, and skin. Because of a lack of eye pigment, the choroid is vulnerable to adverse effects of sunlight frequently resulting in photophobia, astigmatism, and other visual disorders. Lack of skin pigment predisposes the individual to skin cancer.

albinuria /al'binŏŏr'ē·ə/,   white or colorless urine.

Albl's ring,   a calcified ring-shaped shadow visible on a radiograph of an aneurysm of a cerebral artery.

Albright's hereditary osteodystrophy /awl'brīts/ [Fuller Albright, American physician and endocrinologist, 1900–1969],   See **pseudohypoparathyroidism.**

Albright's syndrome /ôl'brīts/ [Fuller Albright, Boston physician, 1900–1969],   a disorder characterized by fibrous dysplasia of bone, isolated brown macules on the skin, and endocrine dysfunction. It causes precocious puberty in girls but not in boys. The bone lesions are reddish gray, gritty fibromas containing areas of coarse fiber that may be con-fined to one bone or occur in several, frequently causing deformities, pain, and pathologic fractures. Treatment may involve osteotomy, curettage, and bone grafts. Also called Albright-McCune-Sternberg syndrome, **osteitis fibrosa disseminata.**

Albright's syndrome
(du Vivier, 1993/courtesy Dr. David Atherton)

albumin /albyoo'min/ [L, *albus,* white],   a water-soluble, heat-coagulable protein. Various albumins are found in practically all animal tissues and in many plant tissues. Determination of the levels and kinds of albumin in urine, blood, and other body tissues is the basis of a number of laboratory diagnostic tests.

albumin A,   a blood serum constituent that gathers in cancer cells and is deficient in circulation in cancer patients.

albuminaturia,   urine that contains high level of albumin salts and has a low specific gravity.

albumin/creatinine ratio,   the ratio of albumin to creatinine in the urine, calculated as a measure of albuminuria.

albumin (human),   a plasma-volume expander.

■ INDICATIONS: It is prescribed in the treatment of hypoproteinemia, hyperbilirubinemia, and hypovolemic shock.

■ CONTRAINDICATIONS: Severe anemia, cardiac failure, or allergic reaction to albumin prohibits its use.

■ ADVERSE EFFECTS: Among the most serious adverse reactions are chills, hypertension, fever, and urticaria.

albumin microspheres sonicated,   microbubbles, mean size 2 to 4.5 mm, created by heat treatment and sonication of diluted human albumin in the presence of octafluoropropane gas; injected intravenously as a diagnostic adjunct in echocardiography.

albuminous liver.   See **amyloid liver.**

albumin test [L, *albus,* white],   any of several tests for the presence of albumin, a class of simple proteins, in the urine, a common sign of renal or chronic disease. One type of albumin test depends on the change in color of a chemically treated strip of paper in the presence of albumin.

-albuminuria,   suffix meaning a '(specified) condition characterized by excess serum proteins in the urine': *noctalbuminuria, pseudalbuminuria.*

albuminuria,   presence of albumin in the urine. See also **proteinuria.**

albuterol,   a beta-2 receptor adrenergic agent.

■ INDICATION: It is prescribed in the treatment of bronchospasm in patients with reversible obstructive airway disease, including asthma.

■ CONTRAINDICATION: Known sensitivity to this drug prohibits its use.

■ ADVERSE EFFECTS: Among the most serious adverse reactions are tachycardia, insomnia, dizziness, and hypertension.

alcalase, an enzyme found in certain laundry detergents. It is a cause of enzymatic detergent asthma.

alclometasone /al-klo-met'ah-sōn'/, a synthetic corticosteroid used topically in the dipropionate form for the relief of inflammation and pruritus.

alclometasone dipropionate, a topical corticosteroid.

■ INDICATIONS: It is prescribed for the relief of symptoms of inflammation and pruritus of corticosteroid-responsive dermatoses.

■ CONTRAINDICATIONS: It is contraindicated in patients with hypersensitivity to the drug. Children may absorb proportionally greater amounts of the drug per area of skin surface and should be treated with the smallest amount of the drug needed.

■ ADVERSE EFFECTS: Among adverse reactions are burning, stinging, and itching.

Alcock's canal [Benjamin Alcock, Irish anatomist, b. 1801], a canal formed by the obturator internus muscle and the obturator fascia through which the pudendal nerve and vessels pass. Also called **pudendal canal.**

alcohol /al'kəhôl/ [Ar *alkohl* subtle essence], **1.** a preparation containing at least 92.3% and not more than 93.8% by weight of ethyl alcohol, used as a topical antiseptic and solvent. **2.** a clear, colorless, volatile liquid that is miscible with water, chloroform, or ether, obtained by the fermentation of carbohydrates with yeast. **3.** a compound derived from a hydrocarbon by replacing one or more hydrogen atoms with an equal number of hydroxyl (OH) groups. Depending on the number of hydroxyl groups, alcohols are classified as monohydric, dihydric, trihydric.

alcohol bath, a procedure for decreasing an elevated body temperature. It is not widely used because of the drying effect of alcohol. A tepid solution of 25% to 50% alcohol in water is sponged lightly on each limb, then on the trunk; the person is turned only once from supine to prone position if possible and then back again. Some sources recommend placing a hot-water bottle at the feet and a cold compress on the head to accelerate heat loss through vasodilation, to promote the comfort of the patient during the procedure, and to reduce the temperature of the circulation to the brain.

Alcohol, Drug Abuse, and Mental Health Administration (ADAMHA), an agency of the U.S. Department of Health and Human Services with three components—the National Institute on Alcohol Abuse and Alcoholism, the National Institute on Drug Abuse, and the National Institute of Mental Health. It conducts and supports research on the biologic, psychologic, epidemiologic, and behavioral aspects of alcoholism, drug abuse, and mental health and illness.

alcoholic, **1.** pertaining to alcohol or its effects on other substances. **2.** a person who has developed a dependency on alcohol through abuse of the substance.

alcoholic ataxia [Ar, *alkohl,* essence; Gk, *ataxia,* disorder], a loss of coordination in performing voluntary movements associated with peripheral neuritis as a result of alcoholism. A similar form of ataxia may occur with neuritis resulting from other toxic agents.

alcoholic blackout, a form of amnesia in which a person has no memory of what occurred during a period of alcohol abuse.

alcoholic cardiomyopathy [Ar, *alkohl,* essence; Gk, *kardia,* heart, *mys,* muscle, *pathos,* disease], a cardiac disease associated with alcohol abuse and characterized by an enlarged heart and low cardiac output. Treatment consists of abstinence from alcohol and results in marked reduction in heart size in over 50% of patients.

alcoholic cirrhosis. See **Laënnec's cirrhosis.**

alcoholic coma [Ar, *alkohl* + Gk, *koma,* deep sleep], a state of unconsciousness that results from severe alcoholic intoxication.

alcoholic dementia [Ar, *alkohl* + L, *de,* away, *mens,* mind], a deterioration of normal cognitive and intellectual functions associated with long-term alcohol abuse.

alcoholic dyspepsia, a digestive disorder characterized by abdominal discomfort and provoked by the consumption of alcohol.

alcoholic fermentation, the conversion of carbohydrates to ethyl alcohol.

alcoholic hallucinosis, a form of alcoholic psychosis characterized primarily by auditory hallucinations occuring in a clear sensorium, abject fear, and persecutory delusions. The condition develops in acute alcoholism as withdrawal symptoms shortly after stopping or reducing prolonged and heavy alcohol intake, usually within 48 hours. Also called **acute hallucinosis.** See also **alcoholic psychosis, hallucinosis.**

alcoholic hepatitis, acute toxic liver injury associated with excess ethanol consumption. It is characterized by necrosis, polymorphonuclear inflammation, and in many instances Mallory bodies.

Alcoholic hepatitis *(Kumar, Cotran, and Robbins, 2003)*

alcoholic hepatopathy, liver disease resulting from alcoholism, progressing in time to fibrosis and cirrhosis.

alcoholic ketoacidosis, the fall in blood pH (acidosis) sometimes seen in alcoholics and associated with a rise in serum ketone bodies (acetone, beta-hydroxybutyric acid, and acetoacetic acid).

alcoholic neuropathy. See **alcoholic paralysis.**

alcoholic-nutritional cerebellar degeneration, a sudden, severe incoordination in the lower extremity characteristic of poorly nourished alcoholics. The patient walks, if at all, with anataxic or wide-based gait. Cerebellar tumors, multiple sclerosis, and other neurologic disorders are characterized by similar motor impairments. Treatment consists of improved nutrition, abstinence from alcohol, and physical therapy. See also **alcoholism.**

alcoholic paralysis [Ar, *alkohl,* essence; Gk, *paralyein,* to be palsied], a paralysis affecting the peripheral nerves as a result of alcohol consumption. Also called **alcoholic neuropathy.**

alcoholic psychosis, any of a group of severe mental disorders in which the ego's functioning is impaired, such as pathologic intoxication, delirium tremens, Korsakoff's psychosis, and acute hallucinosis. It is characterized by brain damage or dysfunction that results from excessive alcohol use.

Alcoholics Anonymous (AA), an international nonprofit organization, founded in 1935, consisting of abstinent alcoholics whose purpose is to stay sober and help others recover from the disease of alcoholism through a 12-step program, including group support, shared experiences, and faith in a higher power. The AA program, which emphasizes both medical and religious resources for help in overcoming alcoholism, consists of attending meetings and coping with abstinence "one day at a time." Meetings are held at convenient times in factories, schools, churches, hospitals, and other community buildings. Similar groups who work with the children, relatives, friends, and associates of alcoholics are **Al-Anon** and **Alateen.**

alcoholic trance, a state of automatism resulting from ethanol intoxication.

alcoholism /al'kəhôliz'əm/, the extreme dependence on excessive amounts of alcohol, associated with a cumulative pattern of deviant behaviors. Alcoholism is a chronic illness with a slow, insidious onset, which may occur at any age. The cause is unknown, but cultural and psychosocial factors are suspect, and families of alcoholics have a higher incidence of alcoholism.

■ OBSERVATIONS: The most frequent medical consequences of alcoholism are central nervous system depression and cirrhosis of the liver. The severity of each may be greater in the absence of food intake. Alcoholic patients also may suffer from alcoholic gastritis, peripheral neuropathies, auditory hallucinations, and cardiac problems. Abrupt withdrawal of alcohol in addiction causes weakness, sweating, and hyperreflexia. The severe form of alcohol withdrawal is called **delirium tremens.**

■ INTERVENTIONS: Extreme caution should be used in administering drugs to the alcoholic patient because of the possibility of additive central nervous system depression and toxicity caused by inability of the liver to metabolize the drugs. Treatment of alcoholism consists of psychotherapy (especially group therapy, by organizations like Alcoholics Anonymous), or administration of drugs such as disulfiram that cause an aversion to alcohol. See also **acute alcoholism, Alcoholics Anonymous, chronic alcoholism, delirium tremens.**

alcohol poisoning, poisoning caused by the ingestion of any of several alcohols, of which ethyl, isopropyl, and methyl are the most common. Ethyl alcohol (ethanol) is found in beverages, hairspray, and mouthwashes. Ordinarily, it is lethal only if large quantities are ingested in a brief period. Isopropyl (rubbing) alcohol is more toxic. Methyl alcohol (methanol) is extremely poisonous: in addition to nausea, vomiting, and abdominal pain, it may cause blindness; death may follow the consumption of only 2 ounces. Treatment for alcohol poisoning may include gastric lavage and other supportive interventions.

alcohol withdrawal syndrome, the clinical symptoms associated with cessation of alcohol consumption. These may include tremor, hallucinations, autonomic nervous system dysfunction, and seizures.

alcuronium /al-ku-ro'ne-um/, a nondepolarizing skeletal muscle relaxant used in general anesthesia for surgical procedures; used in the form of the chloride salt.

ALD, abbreviation for **adrenoleukodystrophy.**

Aldactazide, trademark for a fixed-combination drug containing a potassium-wasting diuretic (hydrochlorothiazide) and a potassium-sparing diuretic (spironolactone).

Aldactone, trademark for a potassium-sparing diuretic (spironolactone).

aldehyde /al'dəhīd'/ [Ar, *alkohl* + L, *dehydrogenatum,* dehydrogenated], any of a large category of organic compounds derived from oxidation of a corresponding primary alcohol, as in the conversion of ethyl alcohol to acetaldehyde, also known as ethanal. Each aldehyde is characterized by a carbonyl group (—CO—) attached directly to a hydrogen (—CHO) in its formula, and can be converted into a corresponding acid by oxidation, as in the conversion of acetaldehyde to acetic acid.

Aldoclor, trademark for a fixed-combination antihypertensive drug containing chlorothiazide, a diuretic, and methyldopa, an antihypertensive.

aldolase /al'dəlās/, enzymes found in muscle tissue that catalyze the step in anaerobic glycolysis involving the breakdown of fructose 1,6-biphosphate to glyceraldehyde 3-phosphate (GAP). The enzyme can also catalyze the reverse reaction. Normal adult findings are 3 to 8.2 Sibley-Lehninger U/dl or 22 to 59 mU at 37° C. See also **glycolysis.**

aldolase test, a blood test that is most useful in indicating muscular or hepatic cellular injury or disease. It measures levels of aldolase, an enzyme that exists throughout most body tissues and that is used in the breakdown of glucose.

Aldomet, trademark for an antihypertensive (methyldopa).

Aldoril, trademark for a fixed-combination drug containing a potassium-wasting diuretic (hydrochlorothiazide) and an antihypertensive (methyldopa).

aldose /al'dōs/, the chemical form of monosaccharides in which the carbonyl group is an aldehyde.

aldosterone /al'dōstərōn', aldos'tərōn/, a mineralocorticoid steroid hormone produced by the adrenal cortex with action in the renal tubule to retain sodium, conserve water by reabsorption, and increase potassium excretion or increase of urinary excretion of potassium.

aldosterone test, a blood or 24-hour urine test used to diagnose hyperaldosteronism, which is associated with primary or secondary aldosteronism. Primary aldosteronism involves a tumor of the adrenal cortex or bilateral adrenal nodular hyperplasia, while secondary aldosteronism is associated with a variety of nonadrenal conditions, converting glycogen into lactic acid.

aldosteronism /al'dōstərō'nizəm, aldos'-/, a condition characterized by hypersecretion of aldosterone, occurring as a primary disease of the adrenal cortex or, more often, as a secondary disorder in response to various extraadrenal pathologic processes. Primary aldosteronism, also called **Conn's syndrome,** may be caused by adrenal hyperplasia or by an aldosterone-secreting adenoma. Secondary aldosteronism is associated with increased plasma renin activity and may be induced by the nephrotic syndrome, hepatic cirrhosis, idiopathic edema, congestive heart failure, trauma, burns, or other kinds of stress. Hypersecretion of aldosterone promotes sodium retention and potassium excretion, leading to increased blood volume and blood pressure. The electrolyte imbalance in aldosteronism usually causes increased thirst and urination. Treatment of primary aldosteronism caused by a tumor may include surgical resection and chemotherapy with the adrenal cytotoxic agent mitotane. Spironolactone, an aldosterone antagonist, or amiloride, a diuretic that blocks potassium excretion and sodium resorption, are frequently used to treat symptoms of aldosteronism. Also called **hyperaldosteronism.**

■ OBSERVATIONS: In many cases the only manifestation of

Conn's syndrome is a mild to moderate hypertension. Other signs and symptoms include episodic weakness, fatigue, paresthesia, polyuria, polydipsia, and nocturia. Glycosuria, hyperglycemia, and personality disturbances are occasionally manifested. Lab tests may show decreased plasma renin activity (measured after restricted sodium and/or diuretic therapy), increased aldosterone levels (measured after sodium loading), normal blood chemistry or increased sodium and decreased potassium levels. An adrenal CT scan may be used to detect the presence of adenoma.

■ INTERVENTIONS: Treatment includes regular monitoring and control of blood pressure and hypokalemia with spironolactone, amiloride, or angiotensin-converting enzyme (ACE) inhibitors. A low sodium diet, cessation of tobacco use, weight reduction (if indicated), and regular exercise are also advised. A unilateral adrenalectomy is performed if an adenoma or carcinoma is present.

■ NURSING CONSIDERATIONS: Nurses need to focus on blood pressure monitoring and education. Instruction is needed in use of and expected side effects of medications, such as gynecomastia, menstrual irregularities, and reduced libido with spironolactone. Dietary management (low sodium) should be addressed and a regular exercise regimen established and monitored. Counseling or referrals should be made for those who use tobacco products. The patient and a family member should be taught to monitor blood pressure levels on a regular basis.

aldosteronoma pl. **aldosteronomas, aldosteronomata,** /al'dōstir'əno'mə/, an aldosterone-secreting adenoma of the adrenal cortex that is usually small and occurs more frequently in the left than the right adrenal gland. Hyperaldosteronism with salt retention, expansion of the extracellular fluid volume, and increased blood pressure may occur.

-aldrate, suffix designating an antacid aluminum salt.

alemtuzumab /al'em-tuz'u-mab'/, a recombinant, DNA-derived, humanized monoclonal antibody directed against the CD antigen CD52; administered intravenously as an antineoplastic in the treatment of B-cell chronic lymphocytic leukemia.

alendronate, a bone-resorption inhibitor.

■ INDICATIONS: This drug is used to treat osteoporosis in postmenopausal women and Paget's disease.

■ CONTRAINDICATIONS: Known hypersensitivity to biphosphonates prohibits the use of this drug.

■ ADVERSE EFFECTS: Side effects of this drug include anemia, hypokalemia, hypomagnesemia, hypophosphatemia, abdominal pain, anorexia, constipation, nausea, vomiting, bone pain, hypertension, urinary tract infection, and fluid overload.

Aleppo boil. See **oriental sore.**

alertness [Fr, alerte], a condition of being mentally quick, active, and keenly aware of the environment.

aleukemia, an acute form of leukemia characterized by a diminished total white cell content in the peripheral blood supply, accompanied by a loss of normal bone marrow function. Also spelled **aleukaemia.**

aleukemic leukemia /ā'lookē'mik/, a type of leukemia in which the total leukocyte count remains within normal limits and few abnormal forms appear in the peripheral blood. Diagnosis requires bone marrow biopsy. Also called **aleukocythemic leukemia, subleukemic leukemia.** See also **leukemia.**

aleukemic myelosis. See **myeloid metaplasia.**

aleukia /āloo'kē-ə/ [Gk, a + leukos, not white], a marked reduction in or complete absence of white blood cells or blood platelets. Compare **leukopenia, thrombocytopenia.** See also **aplastic anemia.**

aleukocythemic leukemia. See **aleukemic leukemia.**

aleukocytosis /āloo'kōsītō'sis/, an extreme decrease or absence of leukocytes in the blood.

Alexander's deafness, congenital deafness caused by cochlear aplasia involving chiefly the organ of Corti and adjacent ganglion cells of the basal coil of the cochlea; high-frequency hearing loss results.

Alexander's disease /al'eg·zan'dərz/ [W. Stewart Alexander, English pathologist, 20th century], an infantile form of leukodystrophy, characterized by collection of eosinophilic material at the surface of the brain and around its blood vessels, resulting in brain enlargement.

Alexander technique [Frederick Matthias Alexander, Australian actor, 1869–1955, who developed and taught the technique], a bodywork technique that uses psychophysical reeducation to correct dysfunctional habits of posture and movement, based on the principle that human movement is most fluid when the head leads and the spine follows to improve postural balance, coordination, and breathing function; relieve stress and chronic pain; and improve general well-being.

alexandrite laser, a laser whose active medium is alexandrite doped with chromium, emitting light in the mid-infrared spectrum and tunable between 701 and 826 nm and used usually at 755 nm; used for hair removal and other dermatologic procedures.

alexia /əlek'sē-ə/ [Gk, a, lexis, not speech], an inability to comprehend written words. See also **word blindness.** Compare **dyslexia.** —**alexic,** adj.

alexic /əlek'sik/ [Gk, a, without, lexis, speech], pertaining to alexia.

alexithymia /əlek'sithī'mē-ə, -thim'ē-ə/, an inability to experience and communicate feelings consciously.

alfa. See **alpha.**

alfacalcidol /al'fah-kal'sĭ-dol/, a synthetic analogue of calcitriol, to which it is converted in the liver; used in the treatment of hypocalcemia, hypophosphatemia, rickets, and osteodystrophy associated with various medical conditions, including chronic renal failure and hypoparathyroidism; administered orally or intravenously.

alfalfa, an herb that is grown throughout the world.

■ USES: This herb is used for poor appetite, hay fever and asthma, and high cholesterol. It may also be used as a nutrient source.

■ CONTRAINDICATIONS: Alfalfa is not recommended during pregnancy and lactation, in children, in persons using blood thinners, or in those with known hypersensitivity to this product.

alfuzosin, an antiadrenergic agent used to treat symptoms of benign prostatic hyperplasia.

ALG, abbreviation for antilymphocyte globulin. See **antilymphocyte serum.**

alg-. See **algesi-.**

alga pl. **algae** /al'gə/ [L, seaweed], any of a large group of mostly photosynthetic protists. Many species of algae are found worldwide in fresh water, in salt water, and on land. —**algal,** adj.

algesi-, alg-, alge-, algo-, prefix meaning 'pain': algesia, algophobia.

-algesia, suffix meaning '(condition of) sensitivity to pain': asphalgesia, hyperthermalgesia.

-algesic, suffix meaning 'sensitivity to pain': analgesic, paralgesic.

-algia, -algy, suffix meaning 'pain, painful condition': epigastralgia, uteralgia.

-algic, suffix meaning 'pain': cardialgic, tibialgic.

algid /al'jid/ [L, algere, to be cold], chilly or cold.

algid malaria [L, *algere*, to be cold], a stage of malaria caused by the protozoan *Plasmodium falciparum*. It is characterized by coldness of the skin, profound weakness, and severe diarrhea. See also **falciparum malaria, malaria.**

alginate /al′ji·nāt/, a salt of alginic acid, extracted from marine kelp. The calcium, sodium, and ammonium alginates have been used in foam, cloth, and gauze for absorbent surgical dressings. Soluble alginates, such as those of sodium, potassium, or magnesium, form a viscous sol that can be changed into a gel by a chemical reaction with compounds such as calcium sulfate; this makes them useful as materials for taking dental impressions.

algo-. See **algesi-.**

algodystrophy /al′gōdis′trəfē/, a painful wasting of the muscles of the hands, often accompanied by tenderness and a loss of bone calcium. The condition may begin in the hand or in the shoulder and spread over the entire limb, causing contractures, edema, and cyanosis of the skin. It may be associated with injury, heart disease, stroke, or a viral infection.

algolagnia /al′gōlag′nē·ə/ [Gk, *algos*, pain, *lagneia*, lust], a form of sexual perversion characterized by sadism or masochism. See also **sadism, sadomasochism.**

algologist /algol′əjist/, **1.** a person who specializes in the study of or the treatment of pain. **2.** also called **phycologist.** a person who specializes in the study of algae.

algology, 1. the branch of medicine that is concerned with the study of pain. **2.** the branch of science that is concerned with algae. Also called **phycology.**

algophobia [Gk, *algos*, pain, *phobos*, fear], an anxiety disorder characterized by an abnormal, pervasive fear of experiencing pain or of witnessing pain in others.

algor [L, cold], the sensation of cold or a chill, particularly in the first stage of a fever.

algorithm /al′gərith′əm/, **1.** a step-by-step procedure for the solution to a problem by a computer, using specific mathematic or logical operations. Compare **heuristic. 2.** an explicit protocol with well-defined rules to be followed in solving a health care problem.

algor mortis, the reduction in body temperature and accompanying loss of skin elasticity that occur after death. Also called **death chill.**

algospasm /al′gōspaz′əm/, an acute, painful spasm of the muscles.

aliasing, an artifact that is caused by undersampling of signal data in diagnostic imaging.

Alice in Wonderland syndrome, perceptual distortions of space and size, as experienced by the character Alice in the Lewis Carroll story. Similar hallucinogenic experiences have been reported by individuals using drugs of abuse and by patients with certain neurologic diseases.

alien /āl′yən/ [L, *alienare*, to estrange], strange, unusual, or foreign.

alienate /al′yənāt/ [L, *alienare*], to cause a withdrawal or transference of affection, or detachment.

alienation /āl′yənā′shən/ [L, *alienare*, to estrange], the act or state of being estranged or isolated. See also **depersonalization.**

alignment /əlīn′mənt/ [Fr, *aligner*, to put in a straight line], **1.** the arrangement of a group of points or objects along a line. **2.** the placing or maintaining of body structures in their proper anatomic positions, such as straightening the teeth or repairing a fractured bone. Also spelled **alinement.**

aliment [L, *alimentum*, to nourish], nutrition.

alimentary /al′əmen′tərē/ [L, *alimentum*, nourishment], pertaining to food or nourishment and to the digestive organs.

alimentary bolus. See **bolus,** def. 1.

alimentary canal. See **digestive tract.**

alimentary duct, the thoracic duct of the lymphatic system.

alimentary system [L, *alimentum*, nourishment; Gk, *systema*], the digestive system.

alimentary tract. See **digestive tract.**

alimentation, nourishment. See also **feeding.**

alinement. See **alignment.**

aliphatic /al′ifat′ik/ [Gk, *aleiphar*, oil], pertaining to fat or oil, specifically to those hydrocarbon compounds that are open chains of carbon atoms, such as the fatty acids, rather than aromatic ring structures. Aliphatic compounds do not have conjugated unsaturated cyclic structures as are found in the aromatic compounds benzene or naphthalene, etc.

aliphatic acid, an acid containing a hydrocarbon fragment derived from a nonaromatic hydrocarbon.

aliphatic alcohol, an alcohol containing a hydrocarbon fragment derived from a fatty, nonaromatic hydrocarbon. Examples include ethyl alcohol and isopropyl alcohol, both of which have fat-solvent properties as well as bactericidal effects.

-alis, suffix meaning "pertaining to" something specified.

alitretinoin, a second-generation retinoid.

■ INDICATIONS: It is used to treat the cutaneous lesions seen in Kaposi's sarcoma.

■ CONTRAINDICATIONS: Known hypersensitivity and pregnancy prohibit this drug's use.

■ ADVERSE EFFECTS: Side effects include rash, stinging, warmth, redness, erythema, blistering, crusting, peeling, contact dermatitis, and pain at the site of application.

alkalemia [Ar, *al + galiy*, wood ash; Gk, *haima*, blood], a condition of increased pH of the blood, above the normal range of 7.35 to 7.45. Also spelled alkalaemia.

alkali /al′kəlī/ [Ar, *al + galiy*, wood ash], a compound with the chemical characteristics of a base. Usually used with reference to hydroxides of Group I metals and ammonium. Alkalis combine with fatty acids to form soaps, turn red litmus blue, and enter into reactions with carbon dioxide that form water-soluble carbonates. See also **acid, base. —alkaline,** *adj.* **alkalinity,** *n.*

alkali burn, damage to tissue caused by exposure to an alkaline compound like lye. Treatment includes washing the area with copious amounts of water to remove the chemical. It takes much more water to irrigate an alkali burn than to irrigate an acid burn. The victim is immediately taken to a medical facility for assessment of tissue damage. Compare **acid burn.**

-alkaline, suffix meaning 'alkali': *subalkaline.*

alkaline ash /al′kəlīn/, residue in the urine having a pH higher than 7.0.

alkaline ash–producing foods, foods that may be ingested to produce an alkaline pH in the urine, thereby reducing the incidence of acidic urinary calculi, or that may be avoided to reduce the incidence of alkaline calculi. Some foods that result in alkaline ash are milk, cream, buttermilk, fruit (except prunes, plums, and cranberries), vegetables (except corn and lentils), almonds, chestnuts, coconuts, and olives.

alkaline bath, a bath taken in water containing sodium bicarbonate, used especially for skin disorders.

alkaline phosphatase, an enzyme present in all tissues and in high concentration in bone, the kidneys, the intestine, bile ducts, plasma, and teeth. It may be elevated in the serum in some diseases of the bone and liver and in some other illnesses. The normal concentrations of this enzyme in the serum of adults are 1.5 to 4.5 Bodansky units; in children, 5 to 14 Bodansky units. See also **Bodansky unit.**

alkaline phosphatase test (ALP), a blood test used to determine a variety of liver and bone disorders such as extrahepatic and intrahepatic obstructive biliary disease, cirrhosis, hepatic tumors, hepatotoxic drugs, hepatitis, osteoblastic metastatic tumors, Paget's disease, rheumatoid arthritis, and hyperparathyroidism.

alkaline reflux gastritis, chronic gastritis caused by reflux of alkaline intestinal contents after partial gastrectomy.

alkaline reserve, an additional amount of sodium bicarbonate the body produces to maintain a normal arterial blood pH (7.35 to 7.45) when the carbon dioxide level increases as a result of hypoventilation. The alkaline reserve is maintained by the kidneys, which control excretion of bicarbonate ions in the urine.

alkalinity /al'kəlin'itē/, pertaining to the acid-base relationship of any solution that has a lower concentration of hydrogen ions or a higher concentration of hydroxide ions than pure water, which is an arbitrarily neutral standard with a pH of 7.0 at 25° C.

alkalinize /al'kəlinīz/, **1.** to make a substance alkaline, as through the addition of a base. **2.** to become alkaline. Also called **alkalize** /al'kəlīz/. Compare **acidify.**

alkali poisoning, a toxic condition caused by the ingestion of an alkaline agent like liquid ammonia, lye, and some detergent powders. Compare **acid poisoning.**

alkali reserves [Ar, *al + galiy,* the wood ashes, + L, *reservare,* to save], the volume of carbon dioxide or carbonates at standard temperature and pressure in 100 mL of blood plasma. The principal buffer in blood is bicarbonate, which represents most of the alkali reserve. Hemoglobin phosphates and additional bases also act as buffers. If the alkali reserve is low, acidosis exists. If the alkali reserve is high, alkalosis exists.

alkalize. See **alkalinize.**

alkaloid /al'kəloid/ [Ar, *al + galiy* + Gk, *eidos,* form], any of a large group of nitrogen-containing organic compounds produced by plants, including many pharmacologically active substances, such as atropine, caffeine, cocaine, morphine, nicotine, and quinine.

alkalosis /al'kəlō'sis/ [Ar, *al + galiy* + Gk, *osis,* condition], an abnormal condition of body fluids, characterized by a tendency toward a blood pH level greater than 7.45, as from an excess of alkaline bicarbonate or a deficiency of acid. Respiratory alkalosis may be caused by hyperventilation, resulting from an excess loss of carbon dioxide and a carbonic acid deficit. Metabolic alkalosis may result from an excess intake or retention of bicarbonate, loss of gastric acid in vomiting, potassium depletion, or any stimulus that increases the rate of sodium-hydrogen exchange. When a buffer system, such as carbon dioxide retention or bicarbonate excretion, prevents a shift in pH, it is labeled compensating alkalosis. Treatment of uncompensated alkalosis involves correction of dehydration and various ionic deficits to restore the normal acid-base balance in which the ratio of carbonic acid to bicarbonate is 20:1. Compare **acidosis.**

alkane, a saturated aliphatic hydrocarbon containing no double or triple bonds in the carbon chain, such as propane. Also called **paraffin.**

alkaptonuria /alkap'tōnŏŏr'ē·ə/ [Ar, *al + galiy* + Gk, *haptein* to possess, *ouron* urine], a rare inherited disorder marked by the excretion of large amounts of homogentistic acid in the urine, which is the result of incomplete metabolism of the amino acids tyrosine and phenylal. Presence of the acid is indicated by darkening of urine on standing or when alkinated and the dark staining of didneision limes. See also **ochronosis. —alkaptonuric,** *adj.*

Alkaptonuria *(Moll, 1997)*

alkene /al'kēn/, an unsaturated aliphatic hydrocarbon containing one double bond in the carbon chain, such as ethylene (ethene). Also called **olefin.**

Alkeran, trademark for an alkylating antineoplastic agent (melphalan).

alkyl /al'kil/, a hydrocarbon fragment derived from an alkane by the removal of one of the hydrogen atoms.

alkylamine /al'kiləmīn'/, an amine in which an alkyl group replaces one to three of the hydrogen atoms that are attached to the nitrogen atom of ammonia, such as methylamine (amino-methane).

alkylating agent /al'kilā'ting/, any substance that contains an alkyl radical and is capable of replacing a free hydrogen atom in an organic compound, or one that acts by a similar mechanism. This type of chemical reaction results in interference with mitosis and cell division, especially in rapidly proliferating tissue. They are radiometric in that their action is similar to that of irradiation. The agents are useful in the treatment of cancer. Agents include cyclophosphamide. Adverse effects include nausea, vomiting, alopecia, and anemia.

alkylation, a chemical reaction in which an alkyl group is transferred from an alkylating agent. When such organic reactions occur with a biologically significant cellular constituent such as deoxyribonucleic acid (DNA), they result in interference with mitosis and cell division.

ALL, abbreviation for **acute lymphocytic leukemia.** See also **acute childhood leukemia.**

all-. See **allo-.**

allachesthesia /al'əkesthē'zhə/ [Gk, *allache,* elsewhere], a defect of touch sensation in which a stimulus is perceived to be at a point distant from where it is actually applied.

allanto-, combining form meaning 'allantois': *allantotoxicon.*

allantoic. See **allantois.**

allantoidoangiopagus /al'əntoi'dō·an'jē·op'əgəs/ [Gk, *allantoeides,* sausagelike, *angeion,* vessel, *pagos,* fixed], conjoined monozygotic twin fetuses of unequal size that are united by the vessels of the umbilical cord. Also called **omphaloangiopagus.** See also **omphalosite. —allantoidoangiopagous,** *adj.*

allantoin /əlan'tō·in/, a chemical compound (5-ureidohydantoin), $C_4H_6N_4O_3$, that occurs as a white crystallizable substance found in many plants and in the allantoic and amniotic fluids and fetal urine of primates. It is also present in the urine of mammals other than primates as a product of purine metabolism. The substance, which can be produced synthetically by the oxidation of uric acid, was once used to promote tissue growth in the treatment of suppurating wounds and ulcers.

allantois /əlan'tois/ [Gk, *allas,* sausage, *eidos,* form], a tubular extension of the endoderm of the yolk sac that extends with the allantoic vessels into the body stalk of the embryo. In human embryos, allantoic vessels become the umbilical vessels and the chorionic villi. See also **body stalk, umbilical cord. —allantoic** /al'əntō'ik/ *adj.*

allele /əlēl'/, **1.** one of two or more alternative forms of a gene that occupy corresponding loci on homologous chromosomes. Each allele encodes a phenotypic feature or a certain inherited characteristic. An individual normally has two alleles for each gene, one contributed by the mother and one by the father. If both alleles are the same, the individual is homozygous. If the alleles are different, the individual is heterozygous. In heterozygous individuals, one of the alleles is usually dominant, and the other is recessive. In humans, for example, the allele for brown eyes is dominant, and the allele for blue eyes is recessive. **2.** also called **allelomorph** /əlēl'əmôrf'/. One of two or more contrasting characteristics transmitted by alternative forms of a gene. **—allelic,** *adj.*

allelo-, combining form meaning 'another': *allelocatalysis, allelomorph.*

allelomorph. See **allele.**

Allen-Doisy test [Edgar Allen, U.S. endocrinologist, 1892–1943; Edward Doisy, U.S. biochemist and Nobel laureate, 1893–1986], a bioassay test for estrogen and gonadotropins in which ovariectomized mice are injected with an estrogenic substance. The appearance of cornified cells on vaginal smears is regarded as a positive finding.

Allen test, a test for the patency of the radial artery after insertion of an indwelling monitoring catheter. The patient's hand is formed into a fist while the nurse compresses the ulnar artery. Compression continues while the fist is opened. If blood perfusion through the radial artery is adequate, the hand should flush and resume normal pinkish coloration.

allergen /al'ərjin/ [Gk, *allos,* other, *ergein,* to work, *genein,* to produce], an environmental substance that can produce a hypersensitive allergic reaction in the body but may not be intrinsically harmful. Common allergens include pollen, animal dander, house dust, feathers, and various foods. Studies indicate that one of six Americans is hypersensitive to one or more allergens. Methods to identify specific allergens affecting individuals include the patch test, the scratch test, the radioallergosorbent (RAST) test, and the Prausnitz-Küstner (PK) test. **—allergenic,** *adj.* See also **allergic reaction, allergy.**

allergenic /al'ərjen'ik/, provoking allergic reactions.

allergenic extract, a protein-containing extract purified from a substance to which a person may be sensitive. The extract, may be used for diagnosis or for desensitization therapy.

allergic /əlur'jik/, **1.** pertaining to allergy. **2.** having an allergy.

allergic alveolitis. See **diffuse hypersensitivity pneumonia.**

allergic arthritis, appearance of symptoms of arthritis such as swollen joints after the ingestion of allergenic foods or medications.

allergic asthma, a form of asthma caused by exposure of the bronchial mucosa to an inhaled airborne antigen. The antigen causes the production of antibodies that bind to mast cells in the bronchial tree. The mast cells then release histamine, which stimulates contraction of bronchial smooth muscle and causes mucosal edema. Hyposensitization treat-

Radial and ulnar arteries occluded

Pressure released on ulnar artery

Allen test *(Phipps et al, 2003)*

ments are more effective for pollen sensitivity than for allergies to house dust, animal dander, mold, and insects. Psychologic factors may provoke asthma attacks in bronchi already sensitized by antigens. Medication, including immunotherapy, can help relieve allergy symptoms. Often a diurnal pattern of histamine release occurs, causing variable degrees of bronchospasm at different times of the day. Also called **atopic asthma, extrinsic asthma.** See also **asthma, asthma in children, asthmatic eosinophilia, status asthmaticus.**

allergic bronchopulmonary aspergillosis, a form of aspergillosis that occurs in asthmatics when the fungus *Aspergillus fumigatus,* growing within the bronchial lumen, causes a type I or type III hypersensitivity reaction. The characteristics of the condition are similar to those of asthma, including dyspnea and wheezing. Chest examination and pulmonary function tests may reveal airway obstruction. Serologic tests usually reveal precipitating antibodies to *A. fumigatus.* Bacteriologic and microscopic examination of sputum may reveal *A. fumigatus* in addition to Charcot-Leyden crystals. Eosinophilia is usually also present. Compare **aspergillosis.**

allergic conjunctivitis, inflammation of the conjunctiva caused by an allergy. Common allergens that cause this condition are pollen, grass, topical medications, air pollutants, occupational irritants, and smoke. It is bilateral, usually starts before puberty, and commonly recurs in a seasonal pattern for about 10 years.

■ OBSERVATIONS: The common signs include itching, burning and swelling around the eyes and excessive tearing. Eosinophils predominate in stained blood smears. Diagnosis is usually based on the results of cultures and sensitivity tests to identify the causative allergen.

■ INTERVENTIONS: Oral antihistamines and vasoconstrictor and corticosteroid eyedrops, such as prednisone acetate are typically prescribed.

■ NURSING CONSIDERATIONS: Cold compresses may be administered. Also called **redeye.** See also **conjunctivitis.**

allergic contact dermatitis. See **allergic dermatitis.**

allergic coryza, acute rhinitis caused by exposure to any allergen to which the person is hypersensitive.

allergic dermatitis [Ger, *allergie,* reaction; Gk, *derma,* skin, *itis,* inflammation], an acute, cell-mediated inflammatory response of an area of skin after exposure of that area to a contact allergen to which the patient is hypersensitive. Such allergens include dyes, perfumes, poison ivy, certain chemicals, and metals. Also called **allergic contact dermatitis.**

Allergic dermatitis from poison ivy
(Goldstein and Goldstein, 1997)

allergic interstitial nephritis, acute interstitial nephritis that is part of an allergic reaction, such as to medication.

allergic interstitial pneumonitis. See **diffuse hypersensitivity pneumonia.**

allergic proctitis, in children, allergic gastroenteropathy having its focus in the rectum. In adults, rectal irritation may be caused by chemicals in the rectum, such as after medical procedures or anal intercourse.

allergic purpura [Gk, *allos,* other, *ergein,* to work; L, *purpura,* purple], a chronic disorder of the skin associated with urticaria, erythema, asthma, and rheumatic joint swellings. Unlike in other forms of purpura, platelet count, bleeding time, and blood coagulation are normal.

allergic reaction, an unfavorable physiologic response to an allergen to which a person has previously been exposed and to which the person has developed antibodies. The response may be characterized by a variety of symptoms including urticaria, eczema, dyspnea, bronchospasm, diarrhea, rhinitis, sinusitis, laryngospasm, and anaphylaxis. Allergic reactions may be immediate or delayed. Eosinophilia is usually present and is revealed in the differential white blood cell count.

allergic response: localized, a nursing outcome from the Nursing Outcomes Classification (NOC) defined as the severity of localized hypersensitive immune response to a specific environmental (exogenous) antigen.

allergic response: systemic, a nursing outcome from the Nursing Outcomes Classification (NOC) defined as the severity of systemic hypersensitive immune response to a specific environmental (exogenous) antigen.

allergic rhinitis, inflammation of the nasal passages, usually associated with watery nasal discharge and itching of the nose and eyes, caused by a localized sensitivity reaction to an allergen, such as house dust, animal dander, or pollen. The condition may be seasonal, as in hay fever, or perennial, as in allergy to dust or animals. Treatment may include the local, systemic, or topical administration of antihistamines or steroids, avoidance of the antigen, and hyposensitization by injections of diluted antigen in gradually increasing amounts.

Allergic rhinitis: view through fiberoptic rhinoscope
(Zitelli and Davis, 1997)

allergic vasculitis, an inflammatory condition of the blood vessels that is induced by allergens, such as iodides, penicillin, sulfonamides, and thioureas. It is characterized by itching, malaise, and a slight fever and by the presence of papules, vesicles, urticarial wheals, or small ulcers on the skin.

Allergic vasculitis *(du Vivier, 1993/courtesy St. Mary's Hospital)*

allergist /al′ərjist/, a physician who specializes in the diagnosis and treatment of allergic disorders.

allergy /al′ərjē/ [Gk, *allos,* other, *ergein,* to work], a hypersensitive reaction to common, often intrinsically harmless substances most of which are environmental. More than 20 million Americans have allergic reactions to airborne or inhaled allergens, such as cigarette smoke, house dust, and pollens. Symptoms of mild allergies, such as those associated with rhinitis, conjunctivitis, and urticaria, can be suppressed by antihistamines with glucocorticoids administered as supplements to primary therapy. Severe allergic reactions, such as anaphylaxis and angioneurotic edema of the glottis, can cause systemic shock and death and commonly require immediate therapy with subcutaneous epinephrine or IV steroids, such as dexamethasone sodium phosphate. See also **allergic reaction, allergy testing.**

allergy blood test, a blood test used to measure serum immunoglobulin E (IgE), which is an effective method of diagnosing allergy and of specifically identifying the allergen. This test can be helpful when results of an allergy skin test are questionable, when the allergen is not available in a form for dermal injection, when the allergen may incite an anaphylactic reaction if injected into the patient, or when skin testing is particularly difficult (i.e., in infants, or patients with dermographia or widespread skin disease).

allergy management, a nursing intervention from the Nursing Interventions Classification (NIC) defined as identification, treatment, and prevention of allergic responses to food, medications, insect bites, contrast material, blood, or other substances. See also **Nursing Interventions Classification.**

allergy skin test, a skin test used to detect allergic reactions. Properly performed, it is considered the most convenient and least expensive test for detecting such reactions. The test involves injecting an allergen into the skin and then evaluating the wheal (swelling) and flare (redness) responses that follow.

allergy testing, any one of the various procedures used in identifying the specific allergens that afflict a patient. Such tests are helpful in prescribing treatment to prevent allergic reactions or to reduce their severity. The most common is skin testing, which exposes the patient to small quantities of the suspected allergens. Positive reactions usually occur within 20 minutes as varying degrees of erythema. Factors considered in performing allergy tests include the medical history of the patient, the allergy history, the environment, and the diet. Individuals to be tested are usually instructed to discontinue the use of any antihistamines at least 24 hours before the test, because these drugs can interfere with normal test responses. The most common kinds of allergy testing are the **intradermal, scratch, patch, conjunctival, Prausnitz-Küstner (PK), radioallergosorbent (RAST),** and **use** tests.

allesthesia /al'esthē'zha/, a referred pain or other sensation that is perceived at a remote site on the same or opposite side of the body stimulated. Also called **alloesthesia.**

all fours position, the sixth stage in the Rood system of ontogenetic motor patterns. In this stage, the lower trunk and lower extremities are brought into a co-contraction pattern while stretching of the trunk and limb girdles develops co-contractions of the trunk flexors and extensors.

allicin /al'i·sin/ [*Allium,* the genus of garlic], an oily substance extracted from garlic, having antibacterial activity.

allied health personnel. See **paramedical personnel.**

alligator forceps, 1. a forceps with heavy teeth and a double clamp, used in orthopedic surgery. **2.** a forceps with long, thin, angular handles and interlocking teeth. Also called alligator clamp.

Allis forceps, curved forceps with serrated edges, used for grasping tissues. Also called Allis clamps.

allo-, all-, combining form meaning 'differing from the normal, reversal, or referring to another': *allopathy, allergic.*

alloantigen /al'ō·an'tijen/ [Gk, *allos,* other], an isoantigen; a substance present in some members of a species which stimulates production of antibodies in other members of the species. An example is blood group antigens.

allodiploid /al'ōdip'loid/ [Gk, *allos,* other, *diploos,* double, *eidos,* form], **1.** an individual, organism, strain, or cell that has two genetically distinct sets of chromosomes derived from different ancestral species, as occurs in hybridization. **2.** pertaining to such an individual, organism, strain, or cell. Also called allodiploidic. Compare **autopolyploid.**

allodiploidy /al'ōdip'loidē/, the state or condition of having two genetically distinct sets of chromosomes derived from different ancestral species.

alloeroticism, alloerotism. See **heteroeroticism.**

alloesthesia. See **allesthesia.**

allogamy. See **cross fertilization.**

allogeneic. See **allogenic.**

allogenic /al'ōjen'ik/ [Gk, *allos* + *genein,* to produce], **1.** (in genetics) denoting an individual or cell type that is from the same species but genetically distinct. **2.** (in transplantation biology) denoting tissues, particularly stem cells from either bone marrow or peripheral blood, that are from the same species but antigenically distinct; homologous. Compare **syngeneic, xenogeneic.**

allograft /al'əgraft/ [Gk, *allos,* other + *graphion,* stylus], a graft of tissue between two genetically dissimilar individuals of the same species, such as a tissue transplant between two humans who are not identical twins. Tissues commonly used for allografts include cornea, cartilage, bone, artery, and cadaver skin stored in a skin-tissue bank. Also called homogenous graft, **homograft, homologous graft.** Compare **autograft, isograft, xenograft.** See also **graft.**

allohexaploid, allohexaploidic. See **allopolyploid.**

allokeratoplasty /al'ōker'ətoplas'tē/, the repair of a cornea with synthetic transparent material.

allometric. See **allometry.**

allometric growth, the increase in size of different organs or parts of an organism at various rates. Also called **heterauxesis.** Compare **isometric growth.** See also **allometry.**

allometron /əlom'itron/, a quantitative change in the proportional relationship of the parts of an organism as a result of evolution.

allometry /əlom'itrē/ [Gk, *allos* + *metron,* measure], the measurement and study of the changes in proportions of the various parts of an organism in relation to the growth of the whole or of such changes in within a series of related organisms. See also **allometric growth. —allometric,** *adj.*

allomorphism /al'ōmôr'fizəm/ [Gk, *allos,* other, *morphe,* form], **1.** a change in crystalline form without a change in chemical composition. **2.** a change in the shape of a group of cells caused by pressure or other physical factors.

allopathic physician /al'ōpath'ik/, a physician who treats disease and injury with active interventions, such as medical and surgical treatment, intended to bring about effects opposite of those produced by the disease or injury. Almost all practicing physicians in the United States are allopathic. Compare **chiropractic, homeopathy, osteopathy.**

allopathy /əlop'əthē/ [Gk, *allos* + *pathos,* suffering], a system of medical therapy in which a disease or an abnormal condition is treated by creating an environment that is antagonistic to the disease or condition; for example, an antibiotic toxic to a pathogenic organism is given to treat an infection.

allopentaploid, allopentaploidic. See **allopolyploid.**

alloplast /al'ōplast/ [Gk, *allos,* other, *plassein,* to mold], a graft made of plastic, metal, or other material foreign to the human body.

alloplastic /al'ō·plas'tik/, **1.** pertaining to or characterized by alloplasty. **2.** pertaining to an alloplast.

alloplastic maneuver [Gk, *allos* + *plassein,* to mold], (in psychology) a process that is part of adaptation, involving an adjustment or change in the external environment. Compare **autoplastic maneuver.**

alloplasty /al'ōplas'tē/ [Gk, *allos,* other, *plassein,* to mold], plastic surgery in which materials foreign to the human body are implanted.

alloploid, alloploidic. See **allodiploid, allopolyploid.**

alloploidy. See **allodiploidy, allopolyploidy.**

allopolyploid /al′əpol′iploid/ [Gk, *allos* + *polyplous*, many times, *eidos* form], **1.** an individual, organism, strain, or cell that has more than two genetically distinct sets of chromosomes derived from two or more different ancestral species, as occurs in hybridization. Such individuals are referred to as allotriploid, allotetraploid, allopentaploid, allohexaploid, and so on, depending on the number of haploid sets of chromosomes they contain. **2.** pertaining to such an individual, organism, strain, or cell. Also **allopolyploidic.** See also **mosaic.** Compare **autopolyploid.**

allopolyploidy /al′əpol′iploi′dē/, the state or condition of having more than two genetically distinct sets of chromosomes derived from two or more different ancestral species. See also **mosaic.** Compare **autopolyploidy.**

allopurinol /al′əpyoor′ənôl/, a xanthine oxidase inhibitor uricosuric agent.

■ INDICATIONS: It is prescribed in the treatment of gout and other hyperuricemic conditions.

■ CONTRAINDICATIONS: It is not prescribed for children (except those with hyperuricemia resulting from malignancy), lactating mothers, or people suffering an acute attack of gout. Known hypersensitivity to this drug prohibits its use.

■ ADVERSE EFFECTS: Among the most serious adverse reactions are blood dyscrasias and severe rashes and other allergic reactions. GI and ophthalmologic disturbances also may occur.

allorhythmia /al′ōrith′mē′ə/, an irregular heart rhythm that occurs repeatedly.

all-or-none law, **1.** the principle in neurophysiology stating that a stimulus must be strong enough to reach threshold to trigger a nerve impulse. Once theshold is achieved, the entire impulse is discharged. A weak stimulus will not produce a weak reaction. **2.** the principle that the heart muscle, under any stimulus above a threshold level, will respond either with a maximal strength contraction or not at all. Also called **Bowditch's law.**

allostatic load, term coined as a more precise alternative to the term *stress,* used to refer to environmental challenges that cause an organism to begin efforts to maintain stability (allostasis).

allosteric sites /al′ōster′ik/ [Gk, *allos* + *stereos,* solid], the sites, other than the active site or sites, of an enzyme that bind regulatory molecules.

allotetraploid, allotetraploidic. See **allopolyploid.**

allotransplantation, transplantation of an allograft. See **allograft.**

allotrio-, prefix meaning 'strange or foreign': *allotriodontia.*

allotriodontia /əlot′rē·ōdon′shə/, **1.** the development of a tooth in an abnormal location, such as in a dermoid tumor. **2.** the transplantation of teeth from one individual to another.

allotriploid, allotriploidic. See **allopolyploid.**

allotropic, **1.** pertaining to a substance that is changed by digestion to retain some of its nutritive value. **2.** pertaining to an element that may exist in two or more forms at the atomic level, such as carbon in the diamond, graphite, and buckminsterfullerene forms.

allowable charge /əlou′əbəl/, the maximum amount that a third party, usually an insurance company, will reimburse a provider for a specific service.

allowable costs, components of an institution's costs that are reimbursable as determined by a payment formula. In general, costs of services not considered to be reasonable or necessary to the proper provision of health services are excluded from allowable costs.

allowable dose. See **accumulated dose equivalent.**

allowable error, the amount of error that can be tolerated without invalidating the medical usefulness of the analytic result. Allowable error is defined as having a 95% limit of analytic error; only 1 sample in 20 can have an error greater than this limit.

alloxan /əlok′san/, an oxidation product of uric acid that is found in the human intestine in diarrhea. Alloxan has been used to produce diabetes in experimental animals by destroying the insulin-secreting islet cells of the pancreas.

alloy /al′oi/ [Fr, *aloyer,* to combine metals], a mixture of two or more metals or of substances with metallic properties. Most alloys are formed by mixing molten metals that dissolve in each other. A number of alloys have medical applications, such as those used for prostheses and in dental amalgams. See **amalgam.**

almond oil, an oil expressed from the kernels of the fruit of the sweet almond tree, *Prunus amygdalus,* which is native to the Mediterranean region. The fixed oil is a demulcent and mildly laxative. Bitter almond oil is a volatile oil that contains lethal prussic acid.

almotriptan /al′mo-trip′tan/, a selective serotonin receptor agonist used as the malate salt in the acute treatment of a migraine; administered orally.

aloe, a succulent found throughout the world.

■ USES: Aloe vera gel is used externally for minor burns, skin irritations, minor wounds, frostbite, and radiation-caused injuries. Internally, it is used to heal intestinal inflammation and ulcers, and as a digestive aid to stimulate bile secretion.

■ CONTRAINDICATIONS: *Topically:* Hypersensitivity to this plant, garlic, onions, or tulips prohibits the use of aloe. Aloe also should not be used on deep wounds. *Internally:* The dried juice is contraindicated during pregnancy and lactation, in children less than 12 years of age, and in those with kidney or cardiac disease or bowel obstruction. This product should not be used long-term.

alopecia /al′əpē′shə/, [Gk, *alopex,* fox mange], partial or complete lack of hair resulting from normal aging, endocrine disorder, drug reaction, anticancer medication, or skin disease. Kinds of alopecia include **alopecia areata, alopecia totalis, alopecia universalis, androgenic alopecia, male pattern, premature alopecia,** alopecie and scarring.

alopecia areata /er′ē·ā′tə/, a disease of unknown cause in which sudden well-defined bald patches occur. The bald areas are usually round or oval and located on the head and other hairy parts of the body with characteristic "exclamation point" formation by the hair at the end that leaves the scalp not clear. The condition is usually self-limited and often clears completely within 6 to 12 months without treatment. Recurrences are common. Compare **alopecia totalis, alopecia universalis.**

alopecia congenitalis, congenital baldness in which there may be partial or complete absence of hair at birth.

alopecia neurotica, loss of hair, usually occurring at one site, after a disease or injury involving the nervous system.

alopecia prematura, baldness that occurs early in life, beginning as early as late adolescence.

alopecia senilis, a form of natural hair loss that affects older persons.

alopecia totalis, an uncommon condition characterized by the loss of all the hair on the scalp. The cause is unknown, and the baldness is usually permanent. No treatment is known. Compare **alopecia areata, alopecia universalis.**

alopecia toxica, a form of hair loss attributed to a febrile illness.

Alopecia areata
*(Barkauskas, Baumann, and Darling-Fisher, 1998/
courtesy American Academy of Dermatology and Institute
for Dermatologic Communication and Education)*

Alopecia totalis *(Hordinsky, Sawaya, and Scher, 2000)*

alopecia universalis, a total loss of hair on all parts of the body. The condition is occasionally an extension of alopecia areata. Compare **alopecia areata, alopecia totalis.**

alpha /al'fə/, A, α, the first letter of the Greek alphabet. It is commonly used as a scientific notation, as in denoting the position of an atom in a molecule, identifying a nuclear particle, or designating a particular physiologic rhythm. For example, it is used in chemical nomenclature to distinguish one variation in a chemical compound from others.

alpha-adrenergic. See **adrenergic receptor.**

alpha-adrenergic blocking agent. See **antiadrenergic.**

alpha-adrenergic receptor. See **alpha receptor.**

alpha alcoholism, a mild form of alcoholism in which the dependence is psychologic rather than physical. The person may consume alcohol in excessive amounts to relieve physical pain or psychologic distress but is usually able to retain control when the distress subsides and can cease use of alcohol voluntarily.

alpha-aminoisovalerianic acid. See **valine.**

alpha$_1$-antitrypsin [Gk, *anti,* against, trypsin], a plasma protein produced in the liver that inhibits the action of proteolytic enzymes such as trypsin. Deficiencies are associated with hepatitis in children and panacinar emphysema in adults. The latter is an inherited condition.

Alpha$_1$-antitrypsin deficiency
*(Kumar, Abbas, and Fausto, 2005/
courtesy Dr. I Wanless, Toronto Hospital)*

alpha$_1$-antitrypsin test, a blood test administered to individuals with a family history of emphysema, since a familial tendency to have a deficiency of this antienzyme exists. A similar deficiency also exists in children with cirrhosis and other liver diseases.

alpha cell [Gk, *alpha,* first letter of the Greek alphabet; L, *cella,* storeroom], one of a class of cells located in the anterior lobe of the pituitary gland or in the pancreatic islets. Alpha cells in the pancreas produce glucagon, which raises the level of glucose in the blood.

alpha chain disease. See **immunoproliferative small intestine disease.**

alpha error. See **type I error.**

alpha feedback, alpha biofeedback.

alpha-fetoprotein (AFP), a protein normally synthesized by the liver, yolk sac, and GI tract of a human fetus, but it may be found at an elevated level in the sera of adults having certain malignancies. AFP measurements in amniotic fluid are used for early diagnosis of fetal neural tube defects, such as spina bifida and anencephaly. Elevated serum levels may be present in ataxia-telangiectasia, hereditary tyrosinemia, cirrhosis, alcoholic hepatitis, hepatocellular carcinoma, and viral hepatitis. Although not a specific marker for malignancies, AFP may be used to monitor effectiveness of surgical and chemotherapeutic management of hepatomas and germ cell neoplasms.

alpha-fetoprotein test (AFP), a blood test used to assist in diagnosing certain neoplastic conditions, such as hepatoma, some tumors and teratomas, Hodgkin's disease, lymphoma, and renal cell carcinoma. Elevated AFP levels also may indicate cirrhosis, chronic active hepatitis, and neural tube defects in the fetus.

alpha-fucosidase, a lysosomal enzyme that catalyzes the hydrolysis of fucosides. A deficiency of this enzyme is a cause of fucosidosis.

alpha-galactosidase, an enzyme that catalyzes the conversion of alpha-D-galactoside to D-galactose.

alpha-globulins, one of a group of serum proteins classified as alpha, beta, or gamma on the basis of their electrophoretic mobility. Alpha-globulins have the greatest negative charge.

alpha-glucosidase inhibitor, any of a group of oral antihyperglycemic agents that act by competitive inhibition of a-glucosidase, delaying intestinal carbohydrate absorption and lessening postprandial increases in glucose levels.

alpha hemolysis, the development of a greenish zone around a bacterial colony growing on blood-agar medium, characteristic of pneumococci and certain streptococci and caused by the partial decomposition of hemoglobin. Compare **beta hemolysis.**

alpha-hydroxypropionic acid. See **lactic acid.**

alpha$_2$-interferon /in'tərfir'on/, a protein molecule effective in controlling the spread of common colds caused by rhinoviruses. It is administered as a nasal spray.

alpha-methyldopa. See **methyldopa.**

alphanumeric, data in the form of letters A-Z and numerals 0-9. The characters, which also may include punctuation marks, are used commonly in computer programming to code applications.

alpha particle, a particle emitted from an atom during one kind of radioactive decay. It consists of two protons and two neutrons, the equivalent of a helium nucleus. Ordinarily, alpha particles are a weak form of radiation with a short range and are not considered hazardous unless inhaled or ingested.

alpha$_1$-proteinase inhibitor, alpha$_1$-antitrypsin.

alpha receptor, any of the postulated adrenergic components of receptor tissues that respond to norepinephrine and to various blocking agents. The activation of the alpha receptors causes such physiologic responses as increased peripheral vascular resistance, dilation of the pupils, and contraction of pilomotor muscles. Also called **alpha-adrenergic receptor.** Compare **beta receptor.**

alpha redistribution phase, a period after IV administration of a drug when the blood level begins to fall from its peak. It is caused primarily by redistribution of the drug throughout the body.

alpha rhythm. See **alpha wave.**

alpha state, a condition of relaxed, peaceful wakefulness devoid of concentration and sensory stimulation. It is characterized by the alpha rhythm of brain wave activity, as recorded by an electroencephalograph, and is accompanied by feelings of tranquility and a lack of tension and anxiety. Biofeedback training and meditation techniques are used to achieve this state. See also **EEG.**

Alpha Tau Delta /al'fə tou' del'tə/, a national fraternity of professional nurses.

alpha-thalassemia [Gk, *thalassa,* sea + *haema,* blood], thalassemia caused by decreased rate of synthesis of the alpha chains of hemoglobin. The homozygous form is incompatible with life, the stillborn infant displaying severe hydrops fetalis; the heterozygous form may be asymptomatic or marked by mild anemia.

alpha-tocopherol. See **vitamin E.**

alphavirus /al'favi'rəs/, any of a group of very small togaviruses consisting of a single molecule of single-stranded ribonucleic acid (RNA) within a lipoprotein capsule. Many alphaviruses multiply in the cytoplasm of cells of arthropods and are transmitted to humans through insect bites, such as that causing equine encephalitis, Semiliki Forest virus. See also **encephalitis, togaviruses.**

alpha wave, one of the four types of brain waves, characterized by a relatively high voltage or amplitude and a frequency of 8 to 13 Hz. Alpha waves are the "relaxed waves" of the brain and constitute the majority of waves recorded by electroencephalograms registering the activity of the parietal and the occipital lobes and the posterior parts of the temporal lobes when the individual is awake but nonattentive and relaxed, with the eyes closed. Opening and closing the eyes affect the patterns of the alpha waves and the beta waves. Also called **alpha rhythm, Berger wave.** Compare **beta wave, delta wave, theta wave.**

Alport's syndrome [A.C. Alport, South African physician, 1880–1959], a form of hereditary nephritis with symptoms of glomerulonephritis, hematuria, progressive sensorineural hearing loss, and occasional ocular disorders such as cataracts, drusen, and lenticonus. The trait is transmitted most often through females, who are often asymptomatic. In males kidney impairment tends to develop in the third decade; death from renal complications occurs in middle age. Treatment is directed toward relief of uremia or other kidney disorders. Kidney transplantation and dialysis are sometimes successful.

alprazolam /alpraz'əlam/, a benzodiazepine antianxiety agent.
■ INDICATIONS: It is prescribed in the treatment of anxiety disorders or the short-term relief of the symptoms of anxiety.
■ CONTRAINDICATIONS: Acute narrow-angle glaucoma or known sensitivity to this drug or other benzodiazepines prohibits its use. It is contraindicated with ketoconazole and itraconazole. Pregnancy is also a contraindication.
■ ADVERSE EFFECTS: Among the most serious adverse reactions are drowsiness, lightheadedness, and tolerance or physical dependence.

alprostadil, a proprietary form of prostaglandin E$_1$ used to treat erectile dysfunction and (temporarily) to maintain the patency of the ductus arteriosus in certain neonates.
■ INDICATIONS: It is recommended as palliative therapy for neonates awaiting surgery to correct congenital heart defects, such as tetralogy of Fallot and tricuspid atresia.
■ CONTRAINDICATIONS: It is contraindicated in respiratory distress syndrome and in cases of known hypersensitivity. This drug is contraindicated in pregnant patients.
■ ADVERSE EFFECTS: The most common adverse effects are apnea, fever, seizures, cerebral bleeding, flushing, bradycardia, and hypertension.

ALS, **1.** abbreviation for **advanced life support.** See **Emergency Medical Technician-Advanced Life Support (EMT-ALS). 2.** abbreviation for **amyotrophic lateral sclerosis.**

Alström's syndrome [Carl A. Alström, twentieth century geneticist], an inherited disease characterized by multiple system resistance to hormones. Clinical features include retinal degeneration leading to childhood blindness, insulin-resistant diabetes mellitus, infantile obesity, nerve deafness, baldness, hyperuricemia, and hypertriglyceridemia. Males may also have high plasma gonadotropin levels and hypogonadism. The condition is transmitted through an autosomal recessive gene.

ALT, abbreviation for **alanine aminotransferase.** Also called serum glutamate, pyruvate transaminase (SGPT).

alteration, change.

altered mucous membrane, impaired, a nursing diagnosis accepted by the Fifth National Conference on the Classification of Nursing Diagnoses. The condition is defined as a state in which an individual experiences disruptions in the tissue layers of the oral cavity.
■ DEFINING CHARACTERISTICS: Defining characteristics include oral pain or discomfort, coated tongue, xerostomia (dry mouth), stomatitis, oral lesions or ulcers, lack of or decreased salivation, leukoplakia, edema, hyperemia, oral

plaque, desquamation, vesicles, hemorrhagic gingivitis, carious teeth, and halitosis.

■ RELATED FACTORS: Related factors include pathologic condition of the oral cavity caused by radiation to head or neck, dehydration, chemical trauma (including acidic foods, drugs, noxious agents, and alcohol), mechanical trauma (such as ill-fitting dentures, braces, endotracheal or nasogastric tubes, and surgery in the oral cavity), taking nothing by mouth for more than 24 hours, ineffective oral hygiene, mouth breathing, malnutrition, infection, lack of or decreased salivation, and medication. See also **nursing diagnosis.**

altered state of consciousness (ASC) [L, *alter,* other], any state of awareness that differs from the normal awareness of a conscious person. Altered states of consciousness have been achieved, especially in Eastern cultures, by many individuals using various techniques, such as prolonged fasting, deep breathing, whirling, and chanting. Researchers now recognize that such practices can affect body chemistry and help induce the desired state. Experiments suggest that telepathy, mystical experiences, clairvoyance, and other altered states of consciousness may be subconscious capabilities in most individuals and can be used to improve health and help fight disease.

alteregoism /ôl′tərē′gō·iz′əm/, an altruistic feeling for an individual who is similar to or in a similar situation as oneself.

alternans /ôl′tərnənz/ [L, *alternare,* to alternate], a regular heart rhythm that causes the pulse to alternate between strong beats and weak beats (pulsus alternans).

alternate binaural loudness balance (ABLB) test, comparison of the intensity levels at which a given pure tone sounds equally loud to the normal ear and the ear with hearing loss; done to determine recruitment with unilateral sensorineural loss.

alternate generation /ôl′tərnit/ [L, *alter,* other of two], a type of reproduction in which a sexual generation alternates with one or more asexual generations, as in many plants and simple animals. Also called **alternation of generations.**

alternating current (AC) /ôl′tərnā′ting/, an electric current that reverses direction, according to a consistent sinusoidal pattern. Compare **direct current.** See also **current.**

alternating mydriasis, a visual disorder in which there is abnormal dilation of the pupils that affects the left and right eyes alternately. See also **mydriasis.**

alternating pulse. See **pulsus alternans.**

alternation, the recurrent, successive occurrence of two functions or phases, as when a nerve fiber responds to every other stimulus, or when a heart produces an irregular beat with every other cardiac cycle.

alternation of generations. See **alternate generation.**

alternation rules, (in psychology) the sociolinguistic rules that establish options available to a person when he or she is speaking to someone else. The rules are influenced by social categories, such as kinship, sex, status, age, and type of interpersonal relationship.

alternative inheritance /ôltur′nətiv/, the acquisition of all genetic traits and conditions from one parent, as in self-pollinating plants and self-fertilizing animals.

alternative medicine, any of the systems of medical diagnosis and treatment differing in technique from that of the allopathic practitioner's use of drugs and surgery to treat disease and injury. Examples include faith healing, homeopathy, Indian Ayurvedic medicine, acupuncture, aroma therapy, and therapeutic touch.

alternative pathway of complement activation, a process of antigen-antibody interaction in which activation of the C3 step occurs without prior activation of C1, C4, and

C2. The initiating substance may be endotoxin, yeast cell wall, bacterial capsule, or immunoglobulin A. Also called **properdin system.**

alternator, a device for generating an electric current that changes polarity a specified number of times per second.

alternobaric vertigo, a condition of dysequilibrium caused by unequalized pressure differences in the middle ear, as may be experienced by divers during ascent. The pressure difference exerts its effect on the oval window of the inner ear.

alt hor, (in prescriptions) abbreviation for the Latin phrase *alternis horis,* meaning 'every other hour.'

altitude /al′tityŏŏd/ [L, *altitudo,* height], level of elevation of any location on earth with reference to a fixed surface point, which is usually sea level. Several types of health effects are associated with altitude extremes, including a greater intensity of ultraviolet radiation that results from a thinner atmosphere. There are fewer molecules per liter of atmosphere and lower oxygen partial pressure. At an altitude of 5500 m, inspired oxygen pressure is only 50% of that at sea level, although demands of physical effort and cellular respiration are the same at both altitudes. High-altitude intolerance is usually associated with a blood or pulmonary disorder. See also **altitude sickness.**

altitude anoxia [L, *altus,* high; Gk, *a,* without, *oxys,* sharp, *genein,* to produce], oxygen deprivation in a high-altitude atmosphere.

altitude sickness, a syndrome associated with the relatively low partial pressure (reduced barometric pressure) of oxygen in the atmosphere at altitudes encountered during mountain climbing or travel in unpressurized aircraft. The acute symptoms may include dizziness, headache, irritability, breathlessness, and euphoria. Older people and those affected by pulmonary or cardiac disorders may suffer pulmonary edema, heart failure, or prostration, requiring emergency treatment and removal to lower altitudes. A chronic form of altitude sickness is characterized by an increased production of red blood cells, resulting in blood that is thick and difficult to move through the circulatory system. Also called **acute mountain sickness, Monge's disease, "the bends."** See also **polycythemia.**

altretamine, an antineoplastic agent.

■ INDICATIONS: It is used for palliative treatment of recurrent, persistent ovarian cancer following a first-line treatment with cisplatin or an alkylating agent-based combination.

■ CONTRAINDICATIONS: Known hypersensitivity to this drug, severe bone marrow depression, severe neurologic toxicity, and pregnancy prohibits its use.

■ ADVERSE EFFECTS: Among the more serious adverse reactions are hepatic toxicity, leukopenia, thrombocytopenia, and anemia.

altruism /al′trōō·iz′əm/, a sense of unconditional concern for the welfare of others. It may be expressed at the level of the individual, group, or the larger social system.

alum /al′əm/ [L, *alumen*], a topical astringent, used primarily in lotions and douches.

alum bath, a bath taken in water containing the mineral salt alum, used primarily for skin disorders.

alumina /ah-loo′mĭ-nah/, **1.** aluminum oxide. **2.** (in pharmaceuticals) aluminum hydroxide.

aluminum (Al) /əlōō′minəm/ [L, *alumen* alum], a widely used metallic element and the third most abundant of all the elements. Its atomic number is 13; its atomic weight (mass) is 26.97. It occurs in the ores feldspar, mica, and kaolin but most abundantly in bauxite. Aluminum is commonly obtained by purifying bauxite to produce alumina, which is reduced to aluminum. It is light and durable and used extensively in the manufacture of aircraft components, prosthetic devices, and dental appliances. Its compounds are components of many antacids, antiseptics, and astringents. Aluminum salts, such as aluminum hydroxychloride, can cause allergic reactions in susceptible individuals. Aluminum hydroxychloride is the most commonly used agent in antiperspirants and is also effective as a deodorant.

aluminum acetate solution.   See **Burow's solution.**

aluminum attenuator,   an aluminum filter used to control the hardness of an x-ray beam. The attenuator removes low-energy x-ray photons before they can reach the patient and be absorbed.

aluminum hydroxide [L, *alumen,* alum; Gk, *hydor,* water, *oxys,* sharp; L, *gelare,* to congeal],   an antacid that works by chemical neutralization and also by adsorption of hydrochloric acid, gases, and toxins.

aluminum oxide, Al_2O_3, occurring naturally as various minerals; used in the production of abrasives, refractories, ceramics, catalysts, and used in chromatography and to strengthen dental ceramics.

Alupent,   trademark for a beta-adrenergic bronchodilator (metaproterenol sulfate).

Alu sequences,   a family of repeated sequences found in large numbers in the human genome.

alve-, alveolo-,   prefix meaning 'trough, channel, cavity': *alveolate, alveolus.*

alveobronchitis [L, *alveolus,* little hollow; Gk, *brongchos,* windpipe, *itis,* inflammation],   inflammation of the alveoli and bronchioles. Also called alveobronchiolitis. See also **bronchopneumonia.**

alveolar /alvē′ələr/ [L, *alveolus,* little hollow],   pertaining to an alveolus.

alveolar adenocarcinoma [L, *alveolus,* little hollow],   a neoplasm in which the tumor cells form alveoli.

alveolar air,   the respiratory gases in an alveolus of the lung. Alveolar air can be analyzed for its content of oxygen, carbon dioxide, or other gases by collecting the last portion of air expelled by maximum exhalation. Also called **alveolar gas.**

alveolar air equation,   a mathematical expression relating the approximate alveolar oxygen tension to the arterial partial pressure of carbon dioxide, the fractional inspired oxygen, and the ratio of carbon dioxide production to oxygen consumption.

alveolar-arterial end-capillary gas pressure difference, the gas pressure difference between the partial pressure of a gas, such as CO_2, in alveolar air and that in pulmonary capillary blood as the blood leaves the alveoli. It is measured in torr or mm Hg.

alveolar-arterial gas pressure difference,   the difference between the partial pressure of a gas, such as CO_2, in the alveoli and that in systemic arterial blood. The difference may indicate ventilation-perfusion mismatching. A negative difference indicates that the partial pressure of the gas is higher in systemic arterial blood than it is in alveolar air. It is measured in torr or mm Hg.

alveolar bone.   See **alveolar process.**

alveolar canal,   any of the canals of the maxilla through which the posterior superior alveolar blood vessels and the nerves to the upper teeth pass. Also called **dental canal.**

alveolar-capillary membrane,   a lung tissue structure, varying in thickness from 0.4 to 2 μm, through which diffusion of oxygen and carbon dioxide molecules occurs during the respiration process. It consists of an alveolar cell separated from a capillary cell by an interstitial space and is essentially a fluid barrier.

Exchange of gases between an alveolus and a lung capillary

Alveolar-capillary membrane *(Chabner, 2001)*

alveolar carcinoma.   See **bronchioloalveolar carcinoma.**

alveolar cell carcinoma,   a malignant pulmonary neoplasm that arises in a bronchiole and spreads along alveolar surfaces. The tumor consists of cuboidal or nonciliated columnar epithelial cells with abundant eosinophilic cytoplasm that may contain droplets of mucus. This form of lung cancer is often characterized by a severe cough and copious sputum. Also called **bronchiolar carcinoma, bronchioloalveolar carcinoma.**

alveolar cleft,   a break in the continuity of the alveolar process, usually congenital. It typically occurs with a cleft lip and/or a cleft palate. See also **cleft lip, cleft palate.**

alveolar cyst,   an air-filled cavity in a lung or visceral tissues caused by rupture of an alveolus.

alveolar dead space.   See **dead space.**

alveolar distending pressure,   the pressure difference between the alveoli and the intrapleural space.

alveolar duct,   any of the air passages in the lung that branch out from the respiratory bronchioles. From the ducts arise the alveolar sacs.

alveolar edema,   an accumulation of fluid within the alveoli. The cause is usually the movement of blood components through the pulmonary capillary walls as a result of a change in osmotic pressure, an increased permeability of the walls, or related factors.

alveolar fiber,   any of the many white, collagenous fibers of the periodontal ligament that extend from the alveolar process to the intermediate plexus, where their terminations mix with those of the cemental fibers. Alveolar fibers surround the tooth and assist in resisting horizontal movements.

alveolar fistula.   See **dental fistula.**

alveolar gas.   See **alveolar air.**

alveolar gas volume,   the aggregate volume of gas in the alveoli of the lungs. It is indicated by the symbol V_A.

alveolar gingiva.   See **attached gingiva.**

alveolar macrophage,   a cell of the reticuloendothelial system in the lungs that engulfs and digests foreign substances inhaled into the alveoli.

alveolar microlithiasis,   a disease characterized by the presence of calcium phosphate deposits in the alveoli and other parts of the bronchopulmonary system. The fine, sand-like deposits may cause the entire lung to appear radiopaque. The disease is familial in about half of cases.

alveolar period,   the period or phase in lung development beginning in utero after the terminal saccular period (about 32 to 36 weeks) and lasting until about 8 years of age. The terminal alveolar saccules subdivide several more times and mature alveoli form. Also called *alveolar phase.*

alveolar periosteum [L, *alveolus,* little hollow; Gk, *peri,* near, *osteon,* bone], a dense layer of connective tissue that lines the alveolar cavities of the upper and lower jaws, joining the bones to the horizontal fibers on the cementum of the teeth. See also **periosteum.**

alveolar pressure (P_A), the pressure in the alveoli of the lungs.

alveolar process, the portion of the maxilla or the mandible that forms the dental arch and serves as a bony investment for the teeth. Its cortical covering is continuous with the compact bone of the body of the maxilla or the mandible and with the spongy bone of the body of the jaws. Also called **alveolar bone.** See also **alveolar ridge.**

alveolar proteinosis, a disorder marked by the accumulation of plasma proteins, lipoproteins, and other blood components in the alveoli of the lungs. The disease tends to affect previously healthy young adults, with a higher incidence among males than females. The cause is unknown, and clinical signs vary, although only the lungs are affected. Some patients are asymptomatic, whereas others experience dyspnea and an unproductive cough. The condition may be treated with bronchopulmonary lavage. There is a risk of secondary infections.

alveolar ridge, the bony ridge of the maxilla or the mandible that contains the alveoli of the teeth. See also **alveolar process.**

alveolar sac [L, *alveolus,* little hollow; Gk, *sakkos*], an air sac at one of the terminal cavities of lung tissue.

alveolar septum, interalveolar septum.

alveolar sinus. See **dental fistula.**

alveolar socket [L, *alveolus,* little hollow; OFr, *soket*], a cavity in the alveolar process of the maxilla and mandible that accommodates a tooth.

alveolar soft part sarcoma, a tumor in subcutaneous or fibromuscular tissue, consisting of numerous large round or polygonal cells in a netlike matrix of connective tissue.

alveolar ventilation, the volume of air that ventilates all the perfused alveoli, equal to total ventilation minus dead space ventilation. The normal average is between 4 and 5 liters per minute.

alveolectomy /al′vē·əlek′təmē/ [L, *alveolus* + Gk, *ektomē,* excision], the excision of a portion of the alveolar process performed to aid the extraction of a tooth or teeth, modify the alveolar contour after tooth extraction, or prepare the mouth for dentures.

alveoli /al·vē′ō·lī/, See **alveolus.**

alveolitis /al′vē·əlī′tis/, inflammation of the alveoli caused by the inhalation of an allergen. It is characterized by acute episodes of dyspnea, cough, sweating, fever, weakness, and pain in the joints and muscles lasting from 12 to 18 hours. Recurrent episodes may lead to chronic obstructive pulmonary disease with weight loss, increasing exertional dyspnea, and interstitial fibrosis. X-ray films of the lungs may show cellular thickening of alveolar septa and ill-defined generalized infiltrates. Kinds of alveolitis include **bagassosis, farmer's lung,** and **pigeon breeder's lung.**

alveoloplasty /alvē′əlōplas′tē/, reconstruction by plastic surgery of a dental alveolus.

alveolotomy /al′vē·əlot′əmē/, incision of a dental alveolus performed to drain pus from a dental infection.

alveolus *pl.* alveoli /alvē′ələs/ [L, little hollow], **1.** a small outpouching of walls of alveolar space through which gas

exchange between alveolar air and pulmonary capillary blood takes place. The term is often used interchangeably with acinus. See also **alveolar sac, dental alveolus, pulmonary alveolus. —alveolar,** *adj.* **2.** a tooth socket.

Alveoli *(Thibodeau and Patton, 2003)*

alvine constipation. See **obstructive constipation.**

alymphocytosis /alim′fōsītō′sis/ [Gk, *a,* not; L, *lympha,* water; Gk, *kytos,* cell, *osis,* condition], a severe reduction in the total number of circulating lymphocytes in the blood. Compare **aplastic anemia, lymphocytopenia.** See also **leukocyte, lymphocyte.**

Alzheimer's disease (AD) /ôl′zīmərz/, [Alois Alzheimer, German neurologist, 1864–1915], progressive mental deterioration characterized by confusion, memory failure, disorientation, restlessness, agnosia, speech disturbances, inability to carry out purposeful movement, and hallucinosis. The patient may become hypomanic, refuse food, and lose sphincter control without focal impairment. The disease sometimes begins in middle life with slight defects in memory and behavior, but the symptoms worsen dramatically after the age of 70. Although it occurs with equal frequency in men and women, the familial risk is four times that of the general population. Typical pathologic features are miliary amyloid plaques in the cortex and fibrillary degeneration (tangles) in layers containing pyramidal ganglion cells. The cerebral cortex atrophies with widening of the cerebral sulci, especially in the frontal and temporal regions. Diagnostic criteria consist of a failure in at least three cognitive functions, including memory, use of language, visuospatial skills, personality, and calculating skills. The symptoms frequently begin with an inability to incorporate new knowledge despite the retention of old information, an inability to recall words, and an inability to orient to one's surroundings. Only palliative treatment is available.

■ NURSING CONSIDERATIONS: Nursing care is concerned primarily with promoting activity and sleep and preventing agitation, violence, and injury. Death usually occurs 8 to 12 years after the first symptoms appear. Also called **senile dementia-Alzheimer type (SDAT).**

Alzheimer's sclerosis [Alois Alzheimer; Gk, *sklerosis,* hardening], the degeneration of small cerebral blood vessels resulting in mental changes.

Am, symbol for the element **americium.**

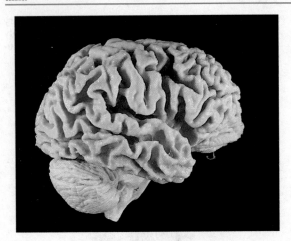

**Alzheimer's disease: narrowing
of cerebral cortical gyri**
(Kumar, Cotran, and Robbins, 1997)

Alzhemer's disease: senile plaque
*(Kumar, Cotran, and Robbins, 1997/courtesy Eileen Bigio, MD,
Department of Pathology, University of Texas
Southwestern Medical Center)*

ama, abbreviation for **against medical advice.**

AMA, 1. abbreviation for **American Medical Association. 2.** abbreviation for **antimitochondrial antibody. 3.** abbreviation for **active matrix array.**

amalgam /əmal′gəm/ [Gk, *malagma,* soft mass], **1.** a mixture or combination. **2.** an alloy of mercury, silver, and other metals commonly used as a dental filling. **3.** an alloy, usually made with mercury and another metal, in which the proportions of the metal components may be varied according to the desired hardness of the amalgam. Hardness can vary from that of a hard metal to that of a pliable plastic.

amalgam carrier, (in dentistry) an instrument used to pick up a quantity of amalgam and transfer it into a prepared tooth cavity (cavity prep) or mold.

amalgam carver, a dental instrument for shaping soft amalgam used in some tooth cavity fillings or restorations.

amalgam condenser, (in dentistry) an instrument used for compacting soft amalgam in filling teeth.

amalgam core, a rigid base for retaining a cast crown restoration, used in the replacement of a damaged tooth crown. The core may be held in place by undercuts, slots, pins, or the pulp chamber of an endodontically treated tooth. Compare **cast core, composite core.** See also **core.**

amalgam tattoo, a discoloration of the gingiva or buccal membrane caused by particles of silver that migrate from an amalgam filling and become embedded under the tissue surface. The condition causes no symptoms and is left untreated.

Amalgam tattoo *(Regezi, Sciubba, and Jordan, 2003)*

Amanita [Gk, *amanitai,* fungus], a genus of mushrooms. Some species, such as *Amanita phalloides,* are poisonous, causing hallucinations, GI upset, and pain that may be followed by liver, kidney, and central nervous system damage.

amantadine hydrochloride /əman′tədēn/, an antiviral and antiparkinsonian agent.

■ INDICATIONS: It is prescribed in the prophylaxis and early treatment of influenza virus A and in the treatment of parkinsonian symptoms and drug-induced extrapyramidal reactions.

■ CONTRAINDICATIONS: It is used with caution in patients with congestive heart failure and during pregnancy and lactation. Known hypersensitivity to this drug prohibits its use.

■ ADVERSE EFFECTS: Among the most serious adverse reactions are central nervous system effects and livedo reticularis. Nausea, dizziness, insomnia, nervousness, blurred vision, and slurred speech also may occur.

amastia /əmas′tē-ə/ [Gk, *a, mastos,* not breast], absence of the breasts in women caused by a congenital defect, an endocrine disorder resulting in faulty development, lack of development of secondary sex characteristics, or a bilateral mastectomy. Also called **amazia.**

amaurosis /am′ôrō′sis/ [Gk, *amauroein,* to darken], blindness, especially lack of vision resulting from a systemic cause such as disease of the optic nerve or brain, diabetes, renal disease, after acute gastritis or systemic poisoning produced by excessive use of alcohol or tobacco, rather than from damage to the eye itself. Unilateral or, more rarely, bilateral amaurosis may follow an emotional shock and may continue for days or months. One kind of congenital amaurosis is transmitted as an autosomal recessive trait. —**amaurotic**, *adj.*

amaurosis fugax /foo′gaks/, transient episodic blindness caused by decreased blood flow to the retina. Compare **amaurosis.**

amaurosis partialis fugax, transitory partial blindness, usually caused by vascular insufficiency of the retina or optic nerve as a result of carotid artery disease. Other related symptoms include dizziness, nausea, and vomiting.

amaurotic. See **amaurosis.**

amaurotic familial idiocy. See **Tay-Sachs disease.**

amazia. See **amastia.**

amb-. See **ambi-.**

amber [Ar, *anbar*], a hard fossilized resin derived from pine trees. An oil of amber, *Oleum succini,* has been used in some pharmaceutical preparations.

amber mutation [Ar, *anbar,* ambergris], a genetic alteration that causes the synthesis of a polypeptide chain to terminate prematurely because the triplet of nucleotides that normally codes for the next amino acid in the chain becomes uracil-adenine-guanine, the sequence that signals the end of the chain. One of three possible **nonsense mutations.** Also called **ochre mutation** and **opal mutation.**

ambi-, ambo-, amb-, prefix meaning "on both sides" or 'both': *ambidexterity, ambomalleal.*

ambidextrous /am′bēdek′strəs/ [L, *ambo,* both, *dexter,* right], able to use either the left or right hand to perform a task.

ambient /am′bē·ənt/ [L, *ambire,* on both sides], pertaining to the surrounding area or atmosphere, usually a defined area such as a room or other large enclosed space.

ambient air standard, the maximum tolerable concentration of any air pollutant, such as lead, nitrogen dioxide, particules, or sulfur dioxide. Research and medical evidence show the strong correlation between many diseases and toxic chemicals, but little is known about the precise effects and movement of airborne pollutants.

ambient noise [L, *ambiens,* around; ME, clamor], the total noise in a given environment.

ambient pressure, the atmospheric pressure, or pressure in the environment or surrounding area. It is given a reference value of zero (0) cm H_2O.

ambient temperature [L, *ambi,* around, *temperatura*], the temperature of the environment.

ambiguous /ambig′yoo·əs/ [L, *ambiguus,* to wander], having more than one direction, development, or interpretation or meaning.

ambiguous genitalia [L, *ambigere,* to go around], external genitalia that are not normal and morphologically typical of either sex, as occurs in pseudohermaphroditism.

ambilateral. See **ambi-.**

ambiopia. See **diplopia.**

ambivalence /ambiv′ələns/ [L, *ambo,* both, *valentia,* strength], **1.** a state in which a person concomitantly experiences conflicting feelings, attitudes, drives, desires, or emotions, such as love and hate, tenderness and cruelty, pleasure and pain toward the same person, place, object, or situation. To some degree, ambivalence is normal. Treatment in severe, debilitating cases consists of psychotherapy appropriate to the underlying cause. **2.** uncertainty and fluctuation caused by an inability to make a choice between opposites. **3.** a continuous oscillation or fluctuation. —**ambivalent,** *adj.*

ambivalent [L, *ambo,* both, *valentia,* strength], **1.** having equal power on both sides. **2.** (in psychology) having equally strong but opposing emotions, as love and hate for the same person.

Ambiguous genitalia *(Zitelli and Davis, 1997)*

ambivert /am′bivurt′/ [L, *ambo,* both, *vertere,* to turn], a person who possesses characteristics of both introversion and extroversion.

amblyopia /am′blē·ō′pē·ə/ [Gk, *amblys,* dull, *ops,* eye], reduced vision in an eye not correctable by a manifest refraction and with no obvious pathologic or structural cause. Typically, the vision in an amblyopic eye is 2 lines or more worse than in the fellow eye. See also **toxic amblyopia.**

amblyopia cruciata. See **crossed amblyopia.**

ambo-. See **ambi-.**

ambon [Gk, raised stage], a fibrocartilaginous ring that surrounds the cavity of a long bone socket.

Ambu bag, trademark for a resuscitator bag used to assist respiratory ventilation. See also **bag-valve-mask resuscitator.**

ambulance /am′byələns/, a vehicle designed to transport patients who are not able to be transported in a normal manner. It may be used under emergency or nonemergency conditions and is equipped with supplies and personnel to provide patient care en route.

ambulation: walking, a nursing outcome from the Nursing Outcomes Classification (NOC) defined as ability to walk from place to place. See also **Nursing Outcomes Classification.**

ambulation: wheelchair, a nursing outcome from the Nursing Outcomes Classification (NOC) defined as ability to move from place to place in a wheelchair. See also **Nursing Outcomes Classification.**

ambulatory /am′byələtôr′ē/ [L, *ambulare,* to walk about], able to walk, hence describing a patient who is not confined to bed or designating a health service for people who are not hospitalized.

ambulatory anesthesia, anesthesia done on an outpatient basis for ambulatory surgery.

ambulatory automatism, aimless wandering or moving about or performance of mechanical acts without conscious awareness of the behavior. See also **fugue, poriomania.**

ambulatory blood pressure monitoring (ABPM), the recording a patient's blood pressure at regular intervals under normal living and working conditions.

ambulatory care, health services provided on an outpatient basis to those who visit a hospital or other health care facility and depart after treatment on the same day.

ambulatory electrocardiograph. See **Holter monitor.**

ambulatory schizophrenia, a mild form of psychosis, characterized mainly by a tendency to respond to questions with vague and irrelevant answers. The person also may seem somewhat eccentric and wander aimlessly.

ambulatory splint. See **functional splint.**

ambulatory surgery center, a medical facility designed and equipped to handle surgery cases, such as cataracts, herniorrhaphy, and meniscectomy, that do not require overnight hospitalization. Most patients who are in relatively good health may receive treatment at ambulatory surgery centers. The centers may be part of a community general hospital, a specialty hospital, or an independent medical facility with prearranged hospital support. The centers are staffed with health professionals as in conventional surgery departments.

Ambu simulator, trademark for a manikin used in teaching cardiopulmonary resuscitation.

AM care /ā·em′/, routine hygienic care that is given patients before breakfast or early in the morning.

amcinonide /amsin′ōnīd/, a topical corticosteroid.

■ INDICATION: It is used to treat inflammatory skin conditions.

■ CONTRAINDICATIONS: Circulation impairment or known hypersensitivity to steroids prohibits its use.

■ ADVERSE EFFECTS: Among the most common adverse reactions are itching, stinging, burning, and less frequently, various skin eruptions. Systemic side effects may result from prolonged or excessive application.

amdinocillin pivoxil, an ester of amdinocillin, administered orally in the treatment of urinary tract infections; the form used can be the ester or the hydrochloride salt of the ester.

ameba /əmē′bə/ [Gk, *amoibe,* change], a microscopic, single-celled, parasitic organism. Several species may be parasitic in humans, including *Entamoeba coli* and *E. histolytica.* Also spelled **amoeba.** See also **amebiasis. —amebic,** *adj.*

-ameba, -amoeba, suffix meaning a '(specified) protozoan': *caudameba, Entamoeba.*

amebiasis /am′ēbī′əsis/, an infection of the intestine or liver by species of pathogenic amebas, particularly *Entamoeba histolytica,* acquired by ingesting fecally contaminated food or water. Infected carriers can be asymptomatic (luminal ambiasis); they may develop invasive intestinal disease with dysentery, colitis, or appendicitis or invasive extraintestinal disease with peritonitis and liver or lung abscess. Infection is most serious in infants, the elderly, and debilitated people. Amebiasis may require treatment with luminal amebicides (iodoquinole, paromycin) to eradicate cysts and/or systemic treatment with metronidazole. Also spelled **amoebiasis.** See also **ameba, amebic abscess, amebic dysentery, hepatic amebiasis.**

amebic. See **ameba.**

amebic abscess /əmē′bik/, a collection of pus formed by disintegrated tissue in a cavity, usually in the liver, caused by the protozoan parasite *Entamoeba histolytica.* Cysts of the organism, ingested in fecally contaminated food or water, pass into the intestine, where active trophozoites of the parasite are released. The trophozoites enter the intestinal mucosa, causing ulceration, nausea, vomiting, abdominal pain, and severe diarrhea, and they may invade the

Amebiasis of the colon *(Kumar, Cotran, and Robbins, 2003)*

liver and produce an abscess. Oral metronidazole and chloroquine hydrochloride administered orally or intramuscularly are used in treating hepatic amebic abscesses. See also **amebiasis.**

Aspirate of hepatic amebic abscess
(Silverberg, DeLellis, and Frable, 1997)

amebic carrier state, a condition in which a patient may be a carrier of amebic organisms without showing signs or symptoms of an amebic infection. A **precocious carrier** may appear healthy but may subsequently develop the amebic infection.

amebic dysentery, an inflammation of the intestine caused by infestation with *Entamoeba histolytica.* It is characterized by frequent, loose stools flecked with blood and mucus. Intestinal amebiasis may be accompanied by symptoms of liver involvement. Also called **intestinal amebiasis.** See also **amebiasis, hepatic amebiasis.**

amebic hepatitis, an inflammation of the liver caused by an amebic infection, usually after an attack of amebic dysentery.

amebicide /əmē′bəsīd/, a drug or other agent that is destructive to amebae.

amebic liver abscess, the abscess formed in hepatic amebiasis, resulting from liquefaction necrosis caused by entrance of *Entamoeba histolytica* into the portal circulation.

ameboid movement /əmē′boid/ [Gk, *amoibe,* ameba, *eidos,* form; L, *movere,* to move], the ameba-like movement of certain types of body cells that can migrate through tissues, such as white blood cells. The movement generally consists of extension of a portion of the cell membrane probably caused by internal rearrangement/movement of the cytoskeleton. See also **diapedesis.**

amelanotic /am'ilənot'ik/ [Gk, *a, melas,* not black], pertaining to tissue that is unpigmented because it lacks melanin.

amelanotic melanoma, a melanoma that lacks melanin. See also **melanoma.**

Ameloblastoma *(Regezi, Sciubba, and Jordan, 2003)*

Amelanotic malignant melanoma *(du Vivier, 1993)*

amelia /əmē'lyə/ [Gk, *a, melos,* not limb], **1.** a birth defect, marked by the absence of one or more limbs. The term may be modified to indicate the number of legs or arms missing at birth, such as tetramelia for the absence of all four limbs. **2.** a psychologic trait of apathy or indifference associated with certain forms of psychosis.

amelification /əmel'ifikā'shən/ [OFr, *amel,* enamel; L, *facere,* to make], the differentiation of ameloblasts, or enamel cells, into the enamel of the teeth.

amelioration [L, *ad,* to, *melior,* better], an improvement in conditions.

ameloblast /am'ilōblast'/ [OFr, *amel* + Gk, *blastos,* germ], an epithelial cell from which tooth enamel is formed. **—ameloblastic,** *adj.*

ameloblastic fibroma, an odontogenic neoplasm in which simultaneous proliferation of mesenchymal and epithelial tissues occurs without the formation of dentin or enamel.

ameloblastic hemangioma, a highly vascular tumor of cells covering the dental papilla. See also **hemangioma.**

ameloblastic odontoma, a malignant tumor of the jaw that forms cementum, dentin, enamel, and pulp tissue. See also **composite odontoma.**

ameloblastic sarcoma, a malignant odontogenic tumor, characterized by the proliferation of epithelial and mesenchymal tissue without the formation of dentin or enamel.

ameloblastoma /am'əlōblastō'mə/ [OFr, *amel* + Gk, *blastos,* germ, *oma*], a rare, highly destructive, benign, rapidly growing tumor of the jaw. Also called **adamantinoma, adamantoblastoma, epithelioma adamantinum.**

amelodentinal /am'əlōden'tinəl/ [OFr, *amel* + L, *dens,* tooth], pertaining to both the enamel and the dentin of the teeth.

amelogenesis /am'əlōjen'əsis/ [OFr, *amel* + Gk, *genein,* to produce], the formation of the enamel of the teeth. **—amelogenic,** *adj.*

amelogenesis imperfecta, a condition characterized by a brown coloration of the teeth and resulting from either severe hypocalcification or hypoplasia of the enamel. The condition, which is inherited as an autosomal dominant trait, is classified according to severity: in agenesis, there is a complete lack of enamel; in enamel hypoplasia, defective matrix formation causes the enamel to be normal in hardness but deficient in quantity; and in enamel hypocalcification, defective maturation of ameloblasts results in enamel that is normal in quantity but soft and undercalcified. Also called **hereditary brown enamel, hereditary enamel hypoplasia.** Compare **dentinogenesis imperfecta.** See also **enamel hypocalcification, enamel hypoplasia.**

amenorrhea /ā'menərē'ə/ [Gk, *a, men,* not month, *rhoia,* to flow], the absence of menstruation. Amenorrhea is normal before sexual maturity, during pregnancy, after menopause, and during the intermenstrual phase of the monthly hormonal cycle; it is otherwise caused by dysfunction of the hypothalamus, pituitary gland, ovary, or uterus, by the congenital absence or surgical removal of both ovaries or the uterus, or by medication. **Primary amenorrhea** is the failure of menstrual cycles to begin. **Secondary amenorrhea** is the cessation of menstrual cycles once established. Also spelled **amenorrhoea.** See also **dietary amenorrhea, hypothalamic amenorrhea, postpill amenorrhea. —amenorrheic.** *adj.*

amentia /āmen'shə/ [Gk, *a,* not; L, *mens,* mind], **1.** former term for mental retardation. **2.** dementia.

American Academy of Allergy and Immunology (AAAI), a national organization of physicians specializing in the diagnosis and treatment of allergies and immune system disorders.

American Academy of Audiology, a professional association for audiologists.

American Academy of Nursing (AAN), the honorary organization of the American Nurses Association, created to recognize superior achievement in nursing in order to promote advances and excellence in nursing practice, education, and research. A person elected to membership is given the title of Fellow of the American Academy of Nursing and may use the abbreviation FAAN as an honorific.

American Academy of Physical Medicine and Rehabilitation (AAPMR), a national association of professional health care workers concerned with the diagnosis of physical impairment and the development of therapies and devices to improve physical function.

American Academy of Physicians Assistants (AAPA), a national organization of physicians' assistants or associates.

American Association for Respiratory Therapy (AART), a national organization of respiratory therapists and other health workers involved in improving the ventilatory function of the respiratory tract.

American Association of Colleges of Nursing (AACN), a national organization of baccalaureate and higher degree programs in nursing that was established to address issues in nursing education.

American Association of Critical Care Nurses (AACN), a national organization of nurses working in critical care units.

American Association of Industrial Nurses (AAIN), a national professional association of nurses working in industry and concerned with issues in occupational health.

American Association of Medical Colleges (AAMC), a national organization of faculty members and deans of medical schools and colleges that was established to address issues in medical education.

American Association of Neurological Nurses (AANN), a national organization of nurses working in the field of neurology.

American Association of Neuroscience Nurses (AANN), a national organization of nurses working with neurologically impaired patients. The organization is affiliated with the American Association of Neurological Surgeons.

American Association of Nurse Anesthetists (AANA), a professional association of certified registered nurse anesthetists. See also **nurse anesthetist.**

American Association of Pathologists and Bacteriologists (AAPB), a national professional organization of specialists in pathology and bacteriology.

American Association of Retired Persons (AARP), a voluntary U.S. organization of older persons, who may or may not be retired, with the goal of improving the welfare of persons over 50 years of age. The AARP advises members of Congress and state legislatures about legislation affecting older individuals.

American Association of University Professors (AAUP), a national organization of faculty members of institutions of higher learning. The AAUP represents faculty in matters of academic freedom, appointment policies, and procedures and serves as the bargaining agent for the faculties of some universities.

American College of Emergency Physicians (ACEP), a national professional organization of physicians specializing in emergency medicine.

American College of Obstetricians and Gynecologists (ACOG), the national organization of obstetricians and gynecologists. It is concerned with the education of physicians in the specialty standards of practice, the continued education and well-being of its members, and the board certification of eligible members as fellows of the organization.

American College of Physicians (ACP), a national professional organization of physicians.

American College of Prosthodontists, an organization of dentists who specialize in the restoration of dental or oral prostheses, such as dentures, artificial crowns, and bridges, and in the diagnosis and treatment of temporomandibular joint and maxillofacial disorders.

American College of Radiology (ACR), a national professional organization of physicians who specialize in radiology.

American College of Surgeons (ACS), a national professional organization of physicians who specialize in surgery.

American Dental Hygienists' Association (ADHA), the largest organization of dental hygienists in the United States. Its mission is to advance the art and science of dental

hygiene by increasing the awareness of and ensuring access to quality oral health care; by promoting the highest standards of dental hygiene education, licensure, practice, and research; and by representing the interests of dental hygienists. The ADHA is structured on local, state, and national levels and has its national headquarters in Chicago.

American Hospital Association (AHA), a national organization of individuals, institutions, and organizations that works to improve health services for all people. The AHA publishes several journals and newsletters.

American Joint Committee on Cancer (AJCC), a nonprofit organization that creates and publishes systems of classification for cancer staging, such as the TNM staging system and Collaborative Stage Data collection systems.

American Journal of Nursing, the professional journal of the American Nurses Association (ANA). It contains articles of general and specialized clinical interest to nurses and is an important resource regarding the profession in the United States.

American leishmaniasis, a group of infections caused by various species of the parasitic protozoa *Leishmania* of Central and South America, characterized by cutaneous lesions at the site of the sandfly bite and transmitting infection and causing disfiguring ulcerative lesions of the nose, mouth, and throat or visceral disease. Illness may be prolonged, rendering patients susceptible to serious secondary infections. Kinds of American leishmaniasis are **chiclero ulcer, espundia, forest yaws,** and **uta.** Also called **mucocutaneous leishmaniasis, New World leishmaniasis.** See also **leishmaniasis.**

American Medical Association (AMA), a professional association whose membership is made up of approximately half of the total licensed physicians in the United States, including practitioners in all recognized medical specialties, as well as general primary care physicians. The AMA is governed by a board of trustees and house of delegates who represent various state and local medical associations and U.S. government agencies such as the Public Health Service and medical departments of the army, navy, and air force. The AMA maintains directories of all qualified physicians (including nonmembers) in the United States, including graduates of foreign medical colleges; researches prescription and nonprescription drugs; advises congressional and state legislators regarding proposed health care laws; and publishes a variety of journals that report on scientific and socioeconomic developments in the field of medicine. See also **British Medical Association, Canadian Medical Association.**

American mountain fever. See **Colorado tick fever.**

American National Standards Institute (ANSI), a private nonprofit organization that coordinates voluntary developments of standards for medical and other devices in the United States and represents the United States in matters related to international standardization.

American Nephrology Nurses' Association (ANNA), an organization of nurses and technicians working in the fields of dialysis and renal diseases.

American Nurses Association (ANA), the national professional association of registered nurses in the United States. It was founded in 1896 to improve standards of health and the availability of health care given in order to foster high standards for nursing, to promote the professional development of nurses, to advance the economic and general welfare of nurses, and to project a positive and realistic view of nursing. The ANA is made up of 54 constituent associations, from the 50 states, the District of Columbia, Guam, and the Virgin Islands, and the Federal Nurses Association

(FedNA), representing more than 900 district associations. National conventions are held biennially in even-numbered years. Members may join one or more of the five divisions on nursing practice: Community Health, Gerontological, Maternal and Child Health, Medical-Surgical, and Psychiatric and Mental Health Nursing. These divisions are coordinated by the Congress for Nursing Practice. The Congress evaluates changes in the scope of practice, monitors scientific and educational developments, encourages research, and develops statements that describe ANA policies regarding legislation affecting nursing practice. In addition, the ANA is politically active on the federal level in all issues relevant to nursing and the public. Statistical services enable the association to fulfill its role as the most authoritative source of data on nursing in the United States. ANA publications include *American Nurse, Publications List,* and *The American Journal of Nursing.*

American Nurses Association—Political Action Committee (ANA-PAC), an organization that raises funds for political contributions to candidates for public office at the state and national levels. Formerly called **Nurses' Coalition for Action in Politics (N-CAP).**

American Occupational Therapy Association. See **AOTA.**

American Psychiatric Association (APA), a national professional association for physicians who specialize in psychiatry. It is concerned with the development of standards for psychiatric facilities, the formulation of mental health programs, the dissemination of data, and the promotion of psychiatric education and research. It publishes the *Diagnostic and Statistical Manual of Mental Disorders (DSM).*

American Red Cross, one of more than 120 national organizations that seek to reduce human suffering through various health, safety, and disaster relief programs in affiliation with the International Committee of the Red Cross. The committee and all Red Cross organizations evolved from the Geneva Convention of 1864, following the example and urging of Swiss humanitarian Jean Henri Dunant, who aided wounded French and Austrian soldiers at the Battle of Solferino in 1859. The American Red Cross has more than 1.3 million members in about 1300 chapters throughout the United States. Some 97% of Red Cross staff is volunteer. Chapters maintain small paid staffs and employ some professionals but depend largely on the volunteers. The American Red Cross blood program collects and distributes more blood than any other single U.S. agency and coordinates distribution of blood and blood products to the U.S. Defense Department on request or during national emergencies. The organization annually collects about 4 million blood donations and gives blood to more than 4000 hospitals. American Red Cross nursing and health programs include courses in the home on parenthood, prenatal and postnatal care, hygiene, and venereal disease. Nursing students may enroll for service in American Red Cross community programs and during disasters. Four area offices at Alexandria, Virginia; Atlanta, Georgia; St. Louis, Missouri; and San Francisco, California, supervise and assist 70 divisions of the American Red Cross and direct field staff members assigned to military installations. National headquarters of the organization is at 17th and D Streets, NW, Washington, DC 20006. The President of the United States is honorary chairman of the organization, for which a 50-member board of governors, all volunteers, develops policy. The symbol of the American Red Cross, like that of most other Red Cross societies throughout the world, is a red cross on a field of white; in Switzerland it is a white cross on a red field, in Muslim countries a red crescent, and in Israel a red star of David.

American Registry of Radiologic Technologists (ARRT), a national certifying body for radiologic technologists in the disciplines of radiography, nuclear medicine, radiation therapy, mammography, computed tomography, magnetic resonance imaging, quality management and cardiovascular-interventional technology. Certification is awarded following passage of an examination in each of these areas.

American Sign Language (Ameslan, ASL), a method of manual communication used by some deaf persons. Messages are conveyed by manipulation of the hands and fingers. ASL is a distinct language, with its own grammar and syntax. See also **sign language.**

American Society of Parenteral and Enteral Nutrition (ASPEN), an organization that provides education, support, and accreditation to persons who specialize in nutrition that is provided through IV, enteral, or related types of feeding.

American Speech, Language, and Hearing Association (ASHA), a professional association that certifies audiologists and speech-language pathologists.

American Standard Safety System, a system of specifications for threaded high-pressure connections between compressed gas cylinders and their attachments.

Americans With Disabilities Act, legislation approved by the U.S. Congress in July 1990, that would bar discrimination against persons with physical or mental disabilities. The Act defines disability as a condition that "substantially limits" such activities as walking or seeing, and it applies to persons with acquired immunodeficiency syndrome (AIDS), as well as to diabetes, cancer, alcoholics and substance abusers undergoing treatment. The law requires employers to make "reasonable accommodations" for workers who are otherwise qualified to carry out their job duties.

American Type Culture Collection (ATCC), a U.S. nonprofit, nongovernmental organization that is concerned with the preservation of specimens of cellular and microbiologic cultures and with the distribution of the cultures to research centers and laboratories in the academic, scientific, and medical communities.

americium (Am) /am′ərish′ē·əm/, a synthetic radioactive element of the actinide group. Its atomic number is 95; its atomic mass is 243.

Ameslan /am′islan/, abbreviation for **American Sign Language.**

Ames test /āmz/, a method of testing substances for possible carcinogenicity by exposing a strain of *Salmonella* bacteria to a sample of the substance. The rate of mutations observed is interpreted as an indication of the carcinogenic potential of the substance tested. Also called **mutagenicity test.**

amethopterin. See **methotrexate.**

ametropia /am′itrō′pē·ə/ [Gk, *ametros,* irregular, *opsis,* sight], a condition characterized by an optic defect involving an error of refraction, such as astigmatism, hyperopia, or myopia. **—ametropic,** *adj.*

AMI, abbreviation for **acute myocardial infarction.**

Amicar, trademark for a hemostatic (aminocaproic acid).

amicrobic /am′īkrob′ik/, not caused by or related to microbes.

amidase /am′i·dās/, **1.** an enzyme that catalyzes the formation of a monocarboxylic acid and ammonia by hydrolytic cleavage of the C—N bond of a monocarboxylic acid amide. **2.** more generally, a term used in the recommended and trivial names of some hydrolases acting on amides, particularly those acting on linear amides.

amide, **1.** a chemical compound formed from an organic acid by the substitution of an amino (NH_2, NHR, or NR_2) group for the hydroxyl of a carboxyl (COOH) group. **2.** a chemical compound formed by the deprotonation of ammonia, NH_3, or a primary (RNH_2) or secondary (R_2Nh) amine.

amide local anesthetic, any of more than two dozen compounds containing an amide chemical group that are safe, versatile, and effective local anesthetics. If hypersensitivity to a drug in this group precludes its use, one of the ester-compound local anesthetics may provide analgesia without adverse effect. Examples of amide local anesthetics are **bupivacaine, lidocaine, mepivacaine,** and **prilocaine.**

amido-, prefix meaning 'the presence of the radical NH_2 along with the radical CO': *amidoacetal, amidobenzene.*

amifostine, a cytoprotective agent for cisplatin.

■ INDICATIONS: This drug is used to reduce renal toxicity when cisplatin is given to treat ovarian cancer. It also reduces xerostomia in radiation therapy for head and neck cancer.

■ CONTRAINDICATIONS: Known hypersensitivity to mannitol or aminothiol, hypotension, dehydration, and lactation prohibit the use of this drug.

■ ADVERSE EFFECTS: Dizziness, somnolence, sneezing, flushing, hiccups, hypocalcemia, rash, and chills are among this drug's side effects. Common side effects include hypotension, nausea, and vomiting.

Amigo, trademark for a battery-operated scooterlike vehicle that gives mobility to some patients who cannot walk.

amikacin sulfate /am′ikā′sin/, an aminoglycoside antibiotic.

■ INDICATIONS: It is prescribed in the treatment of various severe infections caused by susceptible strains of gram-negative bacteria.

■ CONTRAINDICATIONS: Concurrent use of certain diuretics or known hypersensitivity to this or other aminoglycosides prohibits its use. The drug is used with caution in patients who have impaired renal function or myasthenia gravis and those under the influence of neuromuscular blockers or other nephrotoxins.

■ ADVERSE EFFECTS: Among the most serious adverse reactions are nephrotoxicity, auditory and vestibular ototoxicity, and neuromuscular blockade. GI disturbances, pain at the site of injection, and hypersensitivity reactions may occur.

Amikin, trademark for an aminoglycoside antibiotic (amikacin sulfate).

amiloride hydrochloride /am′ilôr′id/, a potassium-sparing diuretic with antihypertensive activity.

■ INDICATIONS: It is prescribed as adjunctive therapy in the treatment of congestive heart failure or hypertension. It is often given with a thiazide medication.

■ CONTRAINDICATIONS: Concurrent use of potassium-conserving agents, hyperkalemia, impaired renal function, or known hypersensitivity to this drug prohibits its use.

■ ADVERSE EFFECTS: Among the most serious adverse reactions are headache, diarrhea, nausea and vomiting, anorexia, hyperkalemia, dizziness, encephalopathy, impotence, muscle cramps, photosensitivity, irregular heart rhythm, mental confusion, and paresthesia.

amiloxate /am′il-ok′sāt/, an absorber of ultraviolet B radiation, used topically as a sunscreen.

amine /am′in, əmēn′/ [L, *ammonia*], (in chemistry) an organic derivative of ammonia in which one or more hydrogen atoms are replaced by alkyl or aryl groups.

amine pump, *informal.* an active transport system in the presynaptic nerve endings that takes up released amine neurotransmitters. Adverse reactions to some drugs, notably tricyclic antidepressants, block this function, resulting in a high concentration of norepinephrine in cardiac tissue and resultant tachycardia and arrhythmia. See also **monoamine oxidase inhibitor.**

amino-, prefix for a chemical name indicated by the monovalent radical NH_2.

aminoacetic acid. See **glycine.**

amino acid /əmē′nō/, an organic chemical compound composed of one or more basic amino groups and one or more acidic carboxyl groups. Twenty of the more than 100 amino acids that occur in nature are the building blocks of proteins. Peptide linkages between them form polypeptides or proteins (for example the structural components of muscle). The eight **essential amino acids** are isoleucine (Ile), leucine (Leu), lysine (Lys), methionine (Met), phenylalanine (Phe), threonine (Thr), tryptophan (Trp), and valine (Val). Arginine (Arg) and histidine (His) are essential in infants. Cysteine (Cys) and tyrosine (Tyr) are semiessential because they may be synthesized from methionine (Met) and phenylalanine (Phe), respectively. The main nonessential amino acids are alanine (Ala), asparagine (Asn), aspartic acid (Asp), glutamine (Glm), glutamic acid (Glu), glycine (Gly), proline (Pro), and serine (Ser). From their structures, the amino acids can be classified as basic (arginine, histidine, lysine), acidic (aspartic acid, glumatic acid), or neutral (the remainder); each group is transported across cell membranes by different carrier methods.

Basic chemical structure of an amino acid

amino acid group, a category of organic chemicals containing the monovalent amine radical NH_2, an acid or COOH, and a group idiosyncratic to that particular amino acid group. Proteins are composed of various proportions of about 20 common amino acids.

aminoacidopathy /ə·mē′nō·as′id·op′ə·thē/, any of various disorders caused by a defect in an enzymatic step in the metabolic pathway of one or more amino acids or in a protein mediator necessary for transport of an amino acid into or out of a cell.

amino acid residue, an amino acid molecule that has lost a water molecule by becoming joined to a molecule of another amino acid.

aminoaciduria /amē′nō·as′ido�ardr′ē·ə/, the abnormal presence of amino acids in the urine that usually indicates an inborn metabolic defect, as in cystinuria. Also called **acidaminuria.**

aminobenzene. See **aniline.**

aminobenzoate /ah-me′no-ben′zo-āt/, *p*-aminobenzoate, any salt or ester of *p*-aminobenzoic acid; the potassium salt is administered orally as an antifibrotic in some dermatologic disorders; various substituted esters, such as padimate O, are used as topical sunscreens.

aminobenzoic acid /-benzō′ik/, a metabolic product of the catabolism of the amino acid tryptophan. Also called **anthranilic acid.** See also **paraaminobenzoic acid (PABA).**

aminocaproic acid /əmē′nōkəprō′ik, am′inō-/, a hemostatic.

■ INDICATION: It is prescribed to stop excessive bleeding that results from hyperfibrinolysis.

■ CONTRAINDICATION: Active intravascular coagulation prohibits its use.

■ ADVERSE EFFECTS: Among the most serious adverse reactions are thrombosis and hypotension. Inhibition of ejaculation, nasal congestion, diarrhea, and allergic reactions also may occur.

aminoglycoside antibiotic. See **antibiotic.**

aminohydrolase. See **deaminase.**

aminolevulinic acid (ALA)[1] /am′inōlev′ōōlin′ik/, the aliphatic precursor of heme. It is formed in the body from the condensation of glycine and succinyl coenzyme A and undergoes further condensation to form porpholbilinogen. Aminolevulinic acid may be detected in the urine of some patients with porphyria, liver disease, and lead poisoning.

aminolevulinic acid[2], a photochemotherapeutic agent.

■ INDICATIONS: It is used to treat nonhyperkeratotic actinic keratoses of the face and scalp.

■ CONTRAINDICATIONS: Known hypersensitivity to porphyrins contraindicates this drug's use.

■ ADVERSE EFFECTS: Side effects include crusting, hypopigmentation or hyperpigmentation, ulceration, pain, itching, bleeding, and pustules at the site of application.

aminolevulinic acid hydrochloride, the hydrochloride salt of aminolevulinic acid, applied topically in the treatment of nonhyperkeratotic actinic keratoses of the face and scalp. It is metabolized to protoporphyrin IX, a photosensitizer, which accumulates in the skin at the sites of application; on exposure of the sites to light of appropriate energy and wavelength together with oxygen, a photodynamic reaction occurs with cytotoxic effects.

aminophylline /am′ənōfil′in, əmē′nō-/, a bronchodilator.

■ INDICATIONS: It is prescribed in the treatment of bronchospasm associated with asthma, emphysema, and bronchitis.

■ CONTRAINDICATIONS: Known hypersensitivity to this drug or other xanthine medication prohibits its use. It is used with caution in patients who have peptic ulcer and those in whom cardiac stimulation would be harmful.

■ ADVERSE EFFECTS: Among the more serious adverse reactions are GI disturbances, central nervous system stimulation, palpitations, tachycardia, nervousness, and seizures.

aminophylline poisoning, an adverse reaction to an excessive intake of a methylxanthine drug such as caffeine or theophylline. The patient appears alternately restless, excited, and lethargic. Symptoms may include nausea, diarrhea, vomiting, abdominal pain, and GI bleeding; headache, tinnitus, thirst, delirium, and seizures; tachycardia, cardiac arrhythmias, and blood pressure changes.

aminopyrine /-pī′rin/, a white chemical compound with analgesic and antipyretic effects. Its continued or excessive use may lead to agranulocytosis.

aminosalicylic acid. See **paraaminosalicylic acid (PAS, PASA).**

5-aminosalicylic acid /ah-me′no-sal′ĭ-sil′ik/, mesalamine.

aminosuccinic acid. See **aspartic acid.**

aminotransferase /-trans′fərās/, enzymes that catalyze the transfer of an amino group from an amino acid to an alpha-keto acid, with pyridoxal phosphate and pyridoxamine phosphate acting as coenzymes. Aspartate amino transferase (AST), normally present in serum and various tissues, especially in the heart and liver, is released by damaged cells, and, as a result, a high serum level of AST may be diagnostic in myocardial infarction or hepatic disease. Alanine aminotransferase (ALT), a normal constituent of serum and especially in the liver, is released by injured tissue and may be present in high concentrations in the sera of patients with acute liver disease. Also called **transaminase** /transam′inās/.

amiodarone hydrochloride, an oral antiarrhythmic drug.

■ INDICATIONS: It is prescribed for the treatment of life-threatening recurrent ventricular fibrillation and recurrent, hemodynamically unstable ventricular tachycardia refractory to other drugs; not considered first-line therapy due to toxicities.

■ CONTRAINDICATIONS: This drug should not be given to patients with severe sinus-node dysfunction or second- and third-degree atrioventricular block or when episodes of bradycardia have resulted in syncope, except when used in conjunction with a pacemaker. It also should not be used during pregnancy or in combination with certain other drugs such as ritonavir or certain quionolone antibiotics (e.g., sparfloxacin, moxifloxacin, gatifloxacin).

■ ADVERSE EFFECTS: Among the most serious adverse effects are pulmonary toxicity, liver dysfunction, nausea, vomiting, constipation, anorexia, malaise, fatigue, tremor, involuntary movements, visual disorders, bradycardia, cyanosis, and congestive heart failure.

Amipaque, trademark for an intrathecal and intravascular diagnostic drug (metrizamide).

amitosis /am′ətō′sis/ [Gr, *a, mitos,* not thread], cell division in which there is simple fission of the nucleus and cytoplasm (as in bacteria) without the complex stages of chromosome separation that occur in mitosis. —**amitotic,** *adj.*

amitriptyline /am′itrip′tilin/, a tricyclic antidepressant.

■ INDICATION: It is prescribed in the treatment of depression, has unlabeled uses for treating neuropathic pain and headaches.

■ CONTRAINDICATIONS: Concomitant administration of monoamine oxidase inhibitors, recent myocardial infarction, or known hypersensitivity to this drug or to other tricyclic medication prohibits its use. It is used with caution in patients having a seizure disorder, cardiovascular disease, or at risk for suicide.

■ ADVERSE EFFECTS: Among the more common adverse reactions are sedation and anticholinergic effects. A variety of cardiovascular and central nervous system effects may occur. This agent interacts with many other drugs.

AML, abbreviation for **acute myelocytic leukemia.**

amlexanox /am-lek′sah-noks/, a topical antiulcerative agent used in treatment of recurrent aphthous stomatitis.

amlodipine /am-lo′dĭ-pēn/, a calcium channel blocking agent administered orally in the form of the besylate salt in treatment of hypertension and chronic stable and vasospastic angina.

ammoni-, ammono-, prefix meaning 'ammonium': *ammoniemia, ammonolysis.*

ammonia (NH_3) /amō′nē·a/ [Gk, *ammoniakos,* salt of Ammon, Egyptian god], a colorless pungent gas produced by the decomposition of nitrogenous organic matter. Some of its many uses are as a fertilizer, an aromatic stimulant, a detergent, and an emulsifier.

ammoniacal fermentation /am′ənī′əkəl/, the production of ammonia and carbon dioxide from urea by the enzyme urease.

ammonia exposure, an adverse reaction to ammonia, which is formed as a product of amino acid and nucleic acid catabolism. Ammonia is converted to urea in the liver and excreted by the kidneys. In liver diseases such as cirrhosis, ammonia may accumulate in the blood, resulting in neurologic damage. Preventive measures include administering antibiotics that restrict the growth of ammonia-producing bacteria and limiting the amount of protein in the diet.

ammonia level test, a blood test used to help diagnose severe liver diseases such as fulminant hepatitis, cirrhosis, and hepatic encephalopathy.

ammonium (NH_4^+), an NH_4^+ ion formed by the reaction of ammonia (NH_3) with a hydrogen ion (H^+). The ammonium ion is highly soluble in water but does not pass easily through cell membranes, as does the ammonia molecule, and its rate of excretion is influenced in part by the acidity of urine. The lower the pH, the greater the proportion of ammonium ions present, assuming a constant level of ammonia production from amino acid metabolism.

Ammon's horn. See **hippocampus.**

ammonuria /am′ōnŏŏr′ē-ə/, urine that contains an excessive amount of ammonia.

amnesia /amnē′zhə/ [Gk, *a, mnasthai,* to forget], a loss of memory caused by brain damage or by severe emotional trauma. Kinds of amnesia include **anterograde amnesia, posttraumatic amnesia,** and **retrograde amnesia.**

amnesiac /amnē′sē-ak/, a person with a loss of memory caused by brain damage or severe emotional trauma.

amnesic /amnē′sik/ [Gk, *a, mnasthai,* to forget], in a state of forgetfulness or showing signs of memory loss or impairment.

amnesic aphasia [Gk, *a, mnasthai + a, phasis,* without speech], an inability to remember spoken words or to use words for names of objects, circumstances, or characteristics.

amnestic apraxia /amnes′tik/, the inability to carry out a movement in response to a request because of a lack of ability to remember the request. See also **apraxia.**

amnio-, prefix meaning 'amnion': *amniogenesis, amniorrhexis.*

amniocentesis /am′nē-ōsentē′sis/ [Gk, *amnos,* lamb's caul, *kentesis,* pricking], an obstetric procedure in which a small amount of amniotic fluid is removed for laboratory analysis. It is usually performed between the sixteenth and twentieth weeks of gestation to aid in the diagnosis of fetal abnormalities.

■ METHOD: With the use of ultrasound scanning techniques the position of the fetus and the location of the placenta are determined. The skin on the mother's abdomen is aseptically prepared, and a local anesthetic is usually injected. A needle attached to a syringe is introduced into a part of the uterus where there is the least chance of perforating the placenta or scratching the fetus. Between 20 and 25 ml of amniotic fluid is aspirated. Amniocentesis is performed to diagnose various genetic defects, including chromosomal abnormalities, neural tube defects, and Tay-Sachs disease. It is also performed to discover the sex of the fetus if certain sex-linked genetic defects are suspected. Later in pregnancy, amniocentesis may be performed to assess fetal lung maturity by testing the lecithin-sphingomyelin (L/S) ratio and the presence of phosphatidyl-glycerol (PG) in the laboratory before elective delivery. The fluid may be tested for the concentration of creatinine, another indicator of fetal maturity. When postmaturity is suspected, amniocentesis is performed to examine the amniotic fluid for meconium.

■ NURSING CONSIDERATIONS: Proof of informed consent must

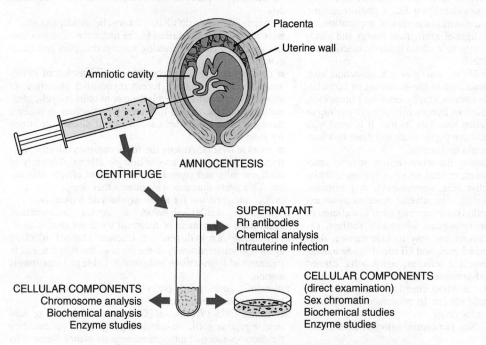

Amniocentesis: laboratory use of fluid aspirant
(Lowdermilk and Perry, 2004)

be signed by the woman before amniocentesis. Specifically stated in the consent form are the reasons for performing the procedure and the facts that fluid is to be removed after needle puncture of the uterus, that ultrasound imaging techniques are usual adjuncts, that the procedure may fail to give the results intended, and that spontaneous abortion, nausea, abdominal pain, or fetal injury may occur. The woman is reassured that complications and failure are rare; she is given emotional support before, during, and after the procedure. In testing for genetic abnormalities 10 days to 2 weeks is usually necessary for tissue culture before a diagnosis may be made; this waiting period may be extremely stressful for the mother. The woman is warned to report any signs of infection or of the onset of labor. Rh immune globulin should be given to pregnant women who are Rh negative.
■ OUTCOME CRITERIA: Spontaneous abortion occurs in approximately 1% of women undergoing amniocentesis. Perforation of the placenta or a blood vessel in the umbilical cord or placenta may cause hemorrhage or isoimmunization and hemolytic disease of the fetus, possibly leading to fetal death. Maternal and fetal infection with attendant morbidity or mortality may occur, but it is rare. Premature rupture of the membranes, premature labor, or trauma to the fetus or umbilical cord may occur. Compare **chorionic villus sampling.**

Amniocentesis: placement of needle *(Chabner, 2004)*

amniography /am′nē·og′rəfē/, a procedure used to detect placement of the placenta by x-ray examination with injection of a radiopaque contrast medium into the amniotic fluid. It is seldom used, having been largely supplanted by ultrasonography.

amnioinfusion, a nursing intervention from the Nursing Interventions Classification (NIC) defined as infusion of fluid into the uterus during labor to relieve umbilical cord compression or to dilute meconium-stained fluid. See also **Nursing Interventions Classification.**

amnion /am′nē·on/ [Gk, *amnos,* lamb's caul], a membrane, continuous with and covering the fetal side of the placenta, that forms the outer surface of the umbilical cord. Compare **chorion.**

amnionitis /am′nē·ōnī′tis/, an inflammation of the amnion. The condition may develop after early rupture of the fetal membranes.

amnioscopy /am′nē·os′kəpē/, direct visual examination of

the fetus and amniotic fluid with an endoscope that is inserted into the amniotic cavity through the uterine cervix or an incision in the abdominal wall.

amniotic /am′nē·ot′ik/, pertaining to the amnion.

amniotic band disruption sequence syndrome, an abnormal condition of fetal development characterized by the development of fibrous bands within the uterus that entangle the fetus, leading to deformities in structure and function. The syndrome is associated with a variety of congenital defects, including clubbed feet, missing limbs, simian creases, and skull and visceral defects. It can be detected in the womb. Interventions are specific to the varied symptoms, and genetic counseling is applied.

Amniotic bands *(Zitelli and Davis, 1997)*

amniotic cavity [Gk, *amnion,* fetal membrane; L, *cavum*], the fluid-filled cavity of the amniotic sac surrounding the fetus.

amniotic fluid, a liquid produced by the fetal membranes and the fetus. It surrounds the fetus throughout pregnancy, protecting it from trauma and temperature variations, providing freedom of fetal movements, and helping to maintain the fetal oxygen supply. The volume totals about 1000 ml at term. In addition to providing the fetus with physical protection, the amniotic fluid is a medium of active chemical exchange. It is secreted and resorbed by cells lining the amniotic sac at a rate of 500 ml/hr at term and is swallowed, metabolized, and excreted as fetal urine at a rate of 50 ml/hr. Its chemical constituents are those of maternal and fetal plasma in different concentrations. Its pH is close to neutral. Amniotic fluid itself is clear, though desquamated fetal cells and lipids give it a cloudy appearance.

amniotic fluid embolism [Gk, *amnion;* L, *fluere,* to flow; Gk, *embolos,* plug], a quantity of amniotic fluid that enters the maternal blood system during labor and/or delivery and becomes lodged in a vessel. It is usually fatal to the mother if it is a pulmonary embolism.

amniotic fold, an embryonic growth feature observed in many vertebrates, particularly birds and reptiles. It consists of flaps of ectoderm and mesoderm that grow over the back of an embryo to form the amnion.

amniotic sac, a thin-walled bag that contains the fetus and amniotic fluid during pregnancy. It has a capacity of 4 to 5 L at term. The wall of the sac extends from the margin of the placenta. The amnion, chorion, and decidua that make up the wall are each a few cell layers thick. They are closely applied—though not fused—to each other and to the wall of the uterus. The intact sac and its fluid provide for the equilibration of hydrostatic pressure within the uterus. During labor, the sac effects the uniform transmission of the force of uterine contractions to the cervix for dilation. See also **amnion, chorion, decidua.**

amniotomy /am′nē·ot′əmē/, the artificial rupture of the fetal membranes (ARM). It is usually performed to stimulate or accelerate the onset of labor. The procedure is painless.

amobarbital /am′ōbär′bətal/, a barbiturate sedative-hypnotic.

■ INDICATIONS: It is prescribed as an anticonvulsant and a pre-anesthetic and for short-term treatment of insomnia.

■ CONTRAINDICATIONS: Porphyria or known hypersensitivity to barbiturates prohibits its use. It is also contraindicated in patients with marked liver impairment or respiratory disease.

■ ADVERSE EFFECTS: Among the most serious adverse reactions are respiratory and circulatory depression, drug hangover, and various allergic reactions. It also interacts with many other drugs.

A-mode, amplitude modulation in diagnostic ultrasonography. It represents the time required for the ultrasound beam to strike a tissue interface and return its signal to the transducer. The greater the reflection at the interface, the larger the signal amplitude on the A-mode screen. See also **B-mode, M-mode.**

A-mode ultrasound [L, *ultra,* beyond, *sonus,* sound], a display of ultrasonic echoes in which the horizontal axis of the cathode ray tube display represents the time required for the return of the echo and the vertical axis represents the strength of the echo. The mode is used in echoencephalography. See also **A-mode.**

amoeba. See **ameba.**

amoebiasis. See **amebiasis.**

amoebic dysentery. See **amebic dysentery.**

amok [Malay, *amoq,* furious], a psychotic frenzy with a desire to kill anybody encountered. The murderous episodes may follow periods of severe depression.

amoric /ah-mo′rik/, without particles.

amorph /ā′môrf, əmôrf′/ [Gk, *a, morphef,* not shape], **1.** a mutant allele that has little or no effect on the expression of a trait. Compare **antimorph, hypermorph, hypomorph.** —**amorphic,** *adj.* **2.** abbreviation for *amorphous,* as in amorph IZS (amorphous insulin zinc suspension).

amorphic, (in genetics) pertaining to a gene that is inactive or nearly inactive so that it has no determinable effect.

amorphous /əmôr′fəs/ [Gk, *a,* not, *morphe,* form], **1.** describing an object that lacks definite visible shape or form. **2.** (in chemistry) a substance that is not crystalline.

amorphous crystals, shapeless, ill-defined crystals, usually phosphates.

amoxapine /əmok′sepin/, a tricyclic antidepressant (secondary amine subclass).

■ INDICATION: It is prescribed in the treatment of mental depression.

■ CONTRAINDICATIONS: It is used with caution in conditions in which anticholinergics are contraindicated, in seizure disorders, and in cardiovascular disorders. Concomitant administration of monoamine oxidase inhibitors, recent myocardial infarction, or known hypersensitivity to this drug prohibits its use.

■ ADVERSE EFFECTS: Among the most serious adverse reactions are sedation and anticholinergic side effects. A variety of GI, cardiovascular, and neurologic reactions may also occur. It is involved in many drug interactions.

amoxicillin /əmok′səsil′in/, a beta-lactam semisynthetic oral penicillin antibiotic.

■ INDICATIONS: It is prescribed in the treatment of infections caused by a susceptible gram-negative or gram-positive bacteria.

■ CONTRAINDICATION: Known hypersensitivity to any penicillin prohibits its use.

■ ADVERSE EFFECTS: Among the most serious adverse reactions are anaphylaxis, nausea, and diarrhea. Allergic reactions and rashes are common.

Amoxil, trademark for a beta-lactam antibiotic (amoxicillin).

AMP, abbreviation for **adenosine monophosphate.**

ampere (A) /am′pēr/ [André M. Ampere, French physicist, 1775–1836], a unit of measurement of the amount of electric current. An ampere, according to the meter-kilogramsecond (MKS) system, is the amount of current passed through a resistance of 1 ohm by an electric potential of 1 volt; in the International System (SI), an ampere is a unit of electric current that carries a charge of 1 coulomb through a conductor in 1 second. The standard international ampere is the amount of current that deposits 0.001118 g of silver per second when passed, according to certain specifications, through a silver nitrate solution. See also **ohm, volt, watt.**

amperometry /am′parom′ətrē/, the measurement of current at a single applied potential.

amph-. See **amphi-.**

amphetamine poisoning, toxic effects of overdosage of amphetamines. Symptoms usually include excitement, tremors, tachycardia, hallucinations, delirium, convulsions, and circulatory collapse.

amphetamines /amfet′əmēnz/, a group of nervous system stimulants, including amphetamine and its chemical congeners dextroamphetamine and methamphetamine, that are subject to abuse because of their ability to produce wakefulness, euphoria, and weight loss. Abuse leads to compulsive behavior, paranoia, hallucinations, and suicidal tendencies. Amphetamines have many street names, such as **black beauties, lid poppers, pep pills, speed** (an injectable form), and **ice** (a crystalline form of methamphetamine that is smoked). See also **crack, dextroamphetamine sulfate, methamphetamine hydrochloride.**

amphetamine sulfate, a colorless water-soluble salt of amphetamine that stimulates the central nervous system. It has been used to treat certain respiratory complaints, fatigue, narcolepsy, and effect weight loss. It formerly was used to treat obesity.

amphi-, amph-, ampho-, prefix meaning 'on both sides, around, double': *amphiarthrosis, amphodiplopia.*

amphiarthrosis. See **cartilaginous joint.**

amphidiarthrodial joint /am′fēdī′ärthrō′dē·əl/ [Gk, *amphi,* both kinds], a type of joint that combines amphiarthrosis with diarthrosis, permitting movement in more than one direction, such as that of the lower jaw.

amphigenesis. See **amphigony.**

amphigenetic /am′fijənet′ik/ [Gk, *amphi,* both sides, *genein,* to produce], **1.** produced by the union of gametes from both sexes. **2.** bisexual; having both testicular and ovarian tissue. Compare **hermaphroditism, pseudohermaphroditism.**

amphigenous inheritance /amfij′ənəs/, the acquisition of genetic traits and conditions from both parents. Also called **biparental inheritance, duplex inheritance.**

amphigonadism /am′figō′nədiz′əm/, true hermaphroditism; the presence of both testicular and ovarian tissue. —**amphigonadic,** *adj.*

amphigony /amfig′ənē/ [Gk, *amphi + gonos,* generation], sexual reproduction. Also called **amphigenesis.** —**amphigonic** /am'figon'ik/, *adj.*

amphikaryon /am'fiker'ē·on/ [Gk, *amphi* + *karyon,* nucleus], a nucleus containing the diploid number of chromosomes. —**amphikaryotic,** *adj.*

amphimixis /am'fimik'sis/ [Gk, *amphi* + *mixis,* mingling], **1.** the union of germ cells in reproduction so that both maternal and paternal hereditary characteristics are derived; interbreeding. **2.** the union and integration of oral, anal, and genital libidinal impulses in the development of heterosexuality.

amphipathic /-path'ik/ [Gk, *amphi* both + *pathos* suffering], pertaining to a molecule having two sides with characteristically different properties, such as a detergent, which has both a polar (hydrophilic) end and a nonpolar (hydrophobic) end but is long enough so that each end demonstrates its own solubility characteristics.

ampho-. See **amphi-.**

Amphojel, trademark for aluminum hydroxide gel.

amphoric breath sound /amfôr'ik/ [Gk, *amphoreus,* jug], an abnormal, resonant, hollow, blowing sound heard with a stethoscope over the thorax. It indicates a cavity opening into a bronchus or a pneumothorax.

amphoteric /am'fōter'ik/ [Gk, *amphoteros,* pertaining to both], a substance that can act as an acid or base, depending on conditions.

amphotericin B /am'fəter'əsin/, an antifungal medication.
■ INDICATIONS: It is prescribed for topical or systemic use in the treatment of fungal infections.
■ CONTRAINDICATION: Known hypersensitivity to this drug prohibits its use.
■ ADVERSE EFFECTS: When it is used systemically, among the most serious adverse reactions are anaphylaxis, thrombophlebitis, blood dyscrasias, nephrotoxicity, nausea, and fever; chills and shaking may occur on administration. With topical use, local hypersensitivity reactions are the most common adverse reactions.

amphotericin B cholesteryl complex, amphotericin B complexed with cholesteryl sulfate in a 1:1 ratio; administered by IV infusion in the treatment of disseminated aspergillosis in patients refractory to or intolerant of conventional amphotericin B therapy.

amphotericin B lipid complex, amphotericin B complexed with two phospholipids in a 1:1 drug-to-lipid ratio; administered by IV infusion in the treatment of invasive fungal infections in patients who are refractory to or intolerant of conventional amphotericin B therapy.

amphotericin B liposomal complex, amphotericin B intercalated into a single bilayer liposome; administered by IV infusion in the treatment of severe systemic fungal infections and visceral leishmaniasis in patients refractory to or intolerant of conventional amphotericin B therapy.

amphoterism /-ter'izəm/ [Gk, *amphoteros,* pertaining to both], a quality of a chemical compound that permits it to act as an acid or a base.

ampicillin /am'pəsil'in/, a semisynthetic aminopenicillin.
■ INDICATIONS: It is prescribed in the treatment of infections caused by a broad spectrum of sensitive gram-negative and gram-positive organisms.
■ CONTRAINDICATION: Known hypersensitivity to any penicillin prohibits its use.
■ ADVERSE EFFECTS: Among the most serious adverse reactions are anaphylaxis, nausea, and diarrhea. Fever, rashes, allergic reactions, and suprainfection also may occur.

ampicillin sodium, the sodium salt of ampicillin, prescribed as an antibiotic to treat gram-positive organisms and some gram-negative organisms.

amplification /am'plifikā'shən/ [L, *amplificare,* to make wider], **1.** a genetic engineering process in which the amount of plasmid DNA increases in proportion to the amount of bacterial DNA by treatment with certain substances, including chloramphenicol. **2.** the replication in bulk of an entire gene library. See also **polymerase chain reaction.** —**amplify,** *v.*

amplifier, a device that controls power from a mechanical, electrical, hydraulic, or other source so that the output is greater than the input.

amplifier T lymphocytes, a T lymphocyte of the CD8 cell type that modifies a developing immune response by releasing nonspecific signals to which other T lymphocytes (either effector or suppressor cells) respond.

amplitude /am'plityōōd/ [L, *amplus,* wide], width or breadth of range or extent, such as amplitude of accommodation or amplitude of convergence.

amplitude of accommodation (AA), the total accommodative power of the eye, determined by the difference between the refractive power for farthest vision and that for nearest vision.

amplitude of convergence, the difference in the power needed to turn the eyes from their far point to their near point of convergence. Also called **fusional amplitude, vergence ability.**

amprenavir, an antiviral (protease inhibitor).
■ INDICATIONS: It is used to treat HIV in combination with other antiretroviral agents.
■ CONTRAINDICATIONS: Known hypersensitivity to this drug prohibits its use.
■ ADVERSE EFFECTS: Life-threatening side effects include Stevens-Johnson syndrome and acute hemolytic anemia. Other serious adverse effects include new-onset diabetes, hyperglycemia, and exacerbation of preexisting diabetes mellitus. Common side effects include diarrhea, abdominal pain, nausea, paresthesia, and rash.

ampule /am'pyōōl/ [Fr, *ampoule,* phial], a small, sterile glass or plastic container that usually contains a single dose of a solution. Also spelled ampoule.

Ampule *(Potter and Perry, 2005)*

ampulla /ampōōl'ə/ [L, flasklike bottle], a rounded, saclike dilation of a duct, canal, or any tubular structure, such as the lacrimal duct, semicircular canal, uterine tube, rectum, or vas deferens.

ampulla of the bile duct. See **hepatopancreatic ampulla.**

ampulla of the rectum, a flask-shaped dilation near the end of the rectum.

ampulla of Vater. See **hepatopancreatic ampulla.**

ampullar crest, the most prominent part of a localized thickening of the membrane that lines the ampullae of the semicircular ducts, covered with neuroepithelium containing endings of the vestibular nerve.

ampullary aneurysm. See **saccular aneurysm.**

ampullary tubal pregnancy /ampōō'lərē, am'pəler'ē/, a kind of tubal pregnancy in which implantation occurs in the ampulla of one of the fallopian tubes. See also **tubal pregnancy.**

ampullula /ampōōl'yələ/, a spherical dilation of a minute lymph or blood vessel or duct. Compare **ampulla.**

amputation /am'pyōōtā'shən/ [L, *amputare*, to excise], the surgical removal of a part of the body or a limb or part of a limb to treat recurrent infections or gangrene in peripheral vascular disease, to remove malignant tumors, and to treat severe trauma. The part is removed and a shaped flap is cut from muscular and cutaneous tissue to cover the end of the bone. A section may be left open for drainage if infection is present. After surgery a lower leg amputation is elevated on a pillow for no more than 24 to 48 hours, and, if necessary, protected with plastic from urinary and fecal contamination. Vital signs are monitored carefully. If a soft dressing is used, it is watched for excessive bleeding. The stump is moved frequently to prevent circulatory complications, contractures, and tissue necrosis. If the dressing is rigid (a cast), it must remain in place for 8 to 14 days. Should the cast come off accidentally, the stump must be wrapped tightly at once with an elastic compression bandage and plans must be made to replace the cast. The patient is fit for a prosthesis, either delayed or immediately. Medication may relieve incisional and phantom limb pain. Kinds of amputation include **closed amputation, congenital amputation, open amputation, primary amputation,** and **secondary amputation.**

amputation care, a nursing intervention from the Nursing Interventions Classification (NIC) defined as promotion of physical and psychological healing after amputation of a body part. See also **Nursing Interventions Classification.**

amputation flap, a flap of skin used to cover the end of an amputation stump.

amputation neuroma, a form of traumatic neuroma that may develop near the stump after the amputation of an extremity.

amputation-stump bandage, an elastic figure-eight bandage applied to cover the stump after an amputation. It helps control edema and shape the remaining portion of the limb.

amputee /am'pyətē'/, a person who has had one or more extremities traumatically or surgically removed. See also **congenital amputation.**

AMRA, abbreviation for *American Medical Records Association.*

amrinone lactate /am'rinōn/, previous name for inamrinone lactate.

Amsler grid [Marc Amsler, Swiss ophthalmologist, 1891–1968], a checkerboard grid of intersecting dark horizontal and vertical lines with one dark spot in the middle. To discover a visual field defect, the person simply covers or closes one eye and looks at the spot with the other. A visual field

Flap amputation

Secured flap amputation

Amputation flaps *(Beare and Myers, 1998)*

Start of second bandage

Amputation-stump bandaging for above-the-knee stump
(Lewis, Heitkemper, and Dirksen, 2004)

defect is perceived as a defect, distortion, blank, or other fault in the grid. The person may record the defects directly on a paper copy of the grid that may be kept as a permanent record. Used in testing for macular degeneration.

AMT, abbreviation for *American Medical Technologists.*

amu, abbreviation for **atomic mass unit.**

amusia /ə·myōō'zē·ə/ [Gk, *amousia,* want of harmony], inability to recognize the significance of sounds manifest as loss of the ability to recognize or produce music.

amyelia /am'ī·ēl'yə/ [Gk, *myelos,* marrow], the absence of a spinal cord.

amyelinic neuroma /amī'əlin'ik/ [Gk, *a, myelos,* without marrow, *neuron,* nerve, *oma*], a tumor that contains only nonmyelinated nerve fibers.

amygdala /amig'dələ/ [Gk, *amygdale,* almond], an almond-shaped mass of gray matter in the front portion of the temporal lobe of the brain that may play a major role in memory processing and "learned fear."

amygdalin /əmig′dəlin/ [Gk, *amygdale*, almond], a naturally occurring cyanogenic glycoside obtained from bitter almonds and apricot pits. It has been promoted as a potential cancer remedy under the trademark of Laetrile. Also called **vitamin B$_{17}$.**

amygdaloid /-dəloid/, resembling a tonsil.

amygdaloid fossa [Gk, *amylon, eidos,* starchlike; L, *fossa,* ditch], a space in the wall of the oropharynx, between the pillars of the fauces, that is occupied by the palatine tonsil. Also called **tonsillar fossa.**

amygdaloid nucleus [Gk, *amygdale,* almond, *eidos,* form; L, *nucleus,* nut], one of the basal nuclei, found near the inferior horn of the lateral ventricle. Also called amygdale.

amyl-. See **amylo-.**

amyl alcohol /am′il/ [Gk, *amylon,* starch], a colorless, oily liquid with the formula $C_5H_{11}OH$, that is only slightly soluble in water but can be mixed with ethyl alcohol, chloroform, or ether.

amyl alcohol, tertiary. See **amylene hydrate.**

amylase /am′ilās/ [Gk, *amylon,* starch], an enzyme that catalyzes the hydrolysis of starch into smaller carbohydrate molecules. Alpha-amylase, found in saliva, pancreatic juice, malt, certain bacteria, and molds, catalyzes the hydrolysis of starches to dextrins, maltose, and maltotriose. Beta-amylase, found in grains, vegetables, malt, and bacteria, is involved in the hydrolysis of starch to maltose. Normal blood findings are 56 to 190 IU/L. See also **enzyme.**

amylase test, an easily and rapidly performed blood or urine test that is most specific for pancreatitis and other pancreatic disorders. Elevated amylase levels may also indicate nonpancreatic disorders such as bowel perforation, penetrating peptic ulcer, duodenal obstruction, and others.

amylene hydrate /am′əlēn/, a clear, colorless liquid, $(CH_3)_2C(OH)CH_2CH_3$ with a camphorlike odor, miscible with alcohol, chloroform, ether, or glycerin and used as a solvent and a hypnotic.

amylic fermentation /əmil′ik/, the formation of amyl alcohol from sugar.

amyl nitrite, a vasodilator.

■ INDICATION: It is prescribed to relieve the vasospasm of angina pectoris and as an adjunct in the treatment of cyanide poisoning.

■ CONTRAINDICATION: Known hypersensitivity to this drug or to other nitrites prohibits its use as does head trauma and narrow-angle glaucoma.

■ ADVERSE EFFECTS: Among the serious adverse reactions are hypotension, allergic reactions, nausea, headache, and dizziness.

amylo-, amyl-, combining form meaning 'starch': *amylodextrin, amylase.*

amylobarbitone. See **amobarbital.**

amyloid /am′iloid/ [Gk, *amylon,* starch, *eidos,* form], **1.** pertaining to or resembling starch. **2.** a starchlike protein-carbohydrate complex that is deposited abnormally in some tissues during certain chronic disease states, such as amyloidosis, rheumatoid arthritis, tuberculosis, and Alzheimer's disease.

amyloid degeneration, degeneration with deposition of amyloid in the tissue.

amyloid disease. See **amyloidosis.**

amyloid liver [Gk, *amylon,* starch, *eidos,* form; AS, *lifer*], liver in which the cells have been infiltrated with amyloid deposits. Also called **albuminous liver.**

amyloidosis /am′iloidō′sis/ [Gk, *amylon + eidos,* form, *osis,* condition], a disease in which a waxy, starchlike glycoprotein (amyloid) accumulates in tissues and organs, impairing their function. There are two major forms of the condition.

Primary amyloidosis usually occurs with multiple myeloma. Patients with **secondary amyloidosis** usually suffer from another chronic infectious or inflammatory disease, such as tuberculosis, osteomyelitis, rheumatoid arthritis, or Crohn's disease. The cause of both types of amyloidosis is unknown. Almost all organs are affected, most often the heart, lungs, tongue, and intestines in primary amyloidosis, and the kidneys, liver, and spleen in the secondary type. Elderly patients tend to experience cardiac effects of the disease. Diagnosis is made through biopsy of the suspected organ. There is no known cure for amyloidosis, and treatment in the secondary type is aimed at alleviating the underlying chronic disease. Patients with renal amyloidosis are frequently candidates for kidney dialysis and transplantation.

Amyloidosis of the kidney *(Kumar, Cotran, and Robbins, 2003)*

amyloid osteopathy, local osteoarticular lytic lesions often found in patients with hemodialysis-associated amyloidosis.

amyloid precursor protein (APP), a large transmembrane glycoprotein expressed on the cell surface and of uncertain function; it may be cleaved on the cell surface to a soluble form. Alternatively, cleavage may follow endocytosis, and in some cases then yields abnormal 40 to 43 amino acid peptides, which aggregate to form Ab amyloid, associated with Alzheimer's disease.

amylolysis /am′ēlol′isis/ [Gk, *amylon,* starch, *lysis,* loosening], the digestive process whereby starch is converted into sugars and dextrins by hydrolysis or by enzymatic activity.

amylopectinosis. See **Andersen's disease.**

amylophagia /am′ĭ-lo-fa′jah/, the habit of eating starch, such as laundry starch, a form of pica.

amylopsin, pancreatic amylase.

amylose /am′ə·lōs/ [Gk, *amylon,* starch + *-ose,* carbohydrate suffix], a lesser constituent of starch consisting of a chain of glucose residues; it stains blue with iodine.

amyoplasia congenita. See **arthrogryposis multiplex congenita.**

amyotonia /ā′mī·ōtō′nē·ə/ [Gk, *a, mys,* not muscle, *tonos,* tone], an abnormal condition of skeletal muscle, characterized by a lack of tone, weakness, and wasting, usually the result of motor neuron disease. See also **myotonia. —amyotonic,** *adj.*

amyotrophic lateral sclerosis (ALS) /ā′mī-ōtrof′ik/ [Gk, *a, mys + trophe,* nourishment], a degenerative disease of the motor neurons, characterized by weakness and atrophy of the muscles of the hands, forearms, and legs, spreading to involve most of the body and face. It results from degeneration of the motor neurons of the anterior horns and corticospinal tracts, beginning in middle age and progressing rapidly, causing death within 2 to 5 years. There is no known treatment. Also called **Lou Gehrig's disease, wasting palsy.** See also **Aran-Duchenne muscular atrophy.**

Amytal Sodium, trademark for a barbiturate (sodium amobarbital).

an-, ana-, prefix meaning 'not, without': *anoxia, analgesia.*

-an, -ian, suffix meaning 'belonging to, characteristic of, similar to': *protozoan, salpingian.*

ANA, 1. abbreviation for **American Nurses Association.** 2. abbreviation for **antinuclear antibody.**

ana (āa, āā, AA). See **āa, āā, AA.**

anabolic steroid /an'əbol'ik/ [Gk, *anaballein,* to build up], any one of several compounds derived from testosterone or prepared synthetically to promote general body growth, to oppose the effects of endogenous estrogen, or to promote masculinizing effects. All such compounds cause a mixed androgenic-anabolic effect.

■ INDICATIONS: Anabolic steroids are prescribed in the treatment of aplastic anemia, red-cell aplasia, and hemolytic anemia and in anemias associated with renal failure, myeloid metaplasia, and leukemia.

■ CONTRAINDICATIONS: They are contraindicated in palliation of carcinoma of the breast; in pregnancy and serious cardiac, renal, and hepatic diseases; and with known hypersensitivity.

■ ADVERSE EFFECTS: Among the most serious adverse effects are acne, growth of facial hair, and hoarsening or deepening of the voice; other masculinizing features are common. Continued use of these compounds in women may also produce prominent musculature, excessive body hair, and hypertrophy of the clitoris.

anabolism /ənab'əliz'əm/ [Gk, *anaballein,* to build up], constructive metabolism characterized by the conversion of simple substances into the more complex compounds of living matter. Compare **catabolism. —anabolic** /an'əbol'ik/, *adj.*

anabolite /ənab'ōlīt/ [Gk, *anaballein,* to build up], a product of the process of anabolism.

anacatadidymus /an'əkat'ədid'iməs/ [Gk, *ana,* up, *kata,* down, *didymos,* twin], conjoined twins that are fused in the middle but separated above and below.

anaclisis /an'əklī'sis/ [Gk, *ana + klisis,* leaning], 1. a condition, normal in childhood but pathologic in adulthood, in which a person is emotionally dependent on other people. 2. a condition in which a person consciously or unconsciously chooses a love object because of a resemblance to the mother, father, or other person who was an important source of comfort and protection in infancy. **—anaclitic** /an'əklit'ik/, *adj.*

anaclitic depression /an'əklit'ik/, a syndrome occurring in infants, usually after sudden separation from the mothering person. Symptoms include apprehension, withdrawal, detachment, incessant crying, refusal to eat, sleep disturbances, and, eventually, stupor leading to severe impairment of the infant's physical, social, and intellectual development. If the mothering figure or a substitute is made available within 1 to 3 months, the infant recovers quickly with no long-term effects. See also **hospitalism.**

anacrotic /an'əkrot'ik/, pertaining to anacrotism, or a pulse with more than one expansion of the artery and observed as a double heartbeat.

anacrotic pulse [Gk, *ana + krotos,* stroke], a pulse characterized by a transient drop in amplitude of the primary elevation on a sphygmographic tracing. It is seen in valvular aortic stenosis.

anacrotism /ənak'rətiz'əm/ [Gk, *ana, krotos,* stroke], a condition characterized by two arterial expansions per heartbeat and observed as a notch on the ascending limb of an arterial pulse pressure tracing. **—anacrotic,** *adj.*

anacusis /an'əkoo'sis/ [Gk, *a, akouein,* not to hear], a total loss of hearing.

anadicrotic pulse /an'ədīkrot'ik/ [Gk, *ana + dis,* twice, *krotos,* stroke], (on a sphygmographic tracing) a pulse characterized by two transient drops in amplitude on the curve of primary elevation.

anadidymus /an'ədid'iməs/ [Gk, *ana + didymos,* twin], conjoined twins that are united at the pelvis and lower extremities but are separated in the upper half. Also called **duplicatus anterior.**

anadipsia /an'ədip'sē·ə/ [Gk, *ana + dipsa,* thirst], extreme thirst, often occurring in the manic phase of bipolar mood disorder. The condition is the result of dehydration caused by the excessive perspiration, electrolyte imbalance, continuous urination, and relentless physical activity produced by the intense excitement characteristic of the manic phase. See also **polydipsia.**

Anadrol-50, trademark for an androgen (oxymetholone).

anaemia. See **anemia.**

anaerobe /aner'ōb/ [Gk, *a + aer,* not air, *bios,* life], a microorganism that grows and lives in the complete or almost complete absence of oxygen. An example is *Clostridium botulinum.* Anaerobes are widely distributed in nature and in the body. Types include the **facultative anaerobe** and the **obligate anaerobe.** Compare **aerobe, microaerophile.** See also **anaerobic infection.**

anaerobic /an'ərō'bik/, 1. pertaining to the absence of air or oxygen. 2. able to grow and function without air or oxygen.

anaerobic catabolism, the breakdown of complex chemical substances into simpler compounds, with the release of energy, in the absence of oxygen.

anaerobic exercise, any short-duration exercise that is powered primarily by metabolic pathways that do not use oxygen. Such pathways produce lactic acid, resulting in metabolic acidosis. Examples of anaerobic exercise include sprinting and weight lifting. Compare **aerobic exercise.** See also **active exercise, passive exercise.**

anaerobic glycolysis. See **glycolysis.**

anaerobic infection, an infection caused by an anaerobic organism, usually occurring in deep puncture wounds that exclude air or in tissue that has diminished oxygen-reduction potential as a result of trauma, necrosis, or overgrowth of bacteria. Examples of anaerobic infection are **gangrene** and **tetanus.** See also *Clostridium.*

anaerobic myositis. See **gas gangrene.**

anaesthesia. See **anesthesia.**

anaesthetic. See **anesthetic.**

anaesthetist. See **anesthetist.**

anagen, the first phase of the hair cycle, during which synthesis of the hair takes place.

anagrelide, an antiplatelet agent.

■ INDICATIONS: This drug is prescribed for essential thrombocythemia.

■ CONTRAINDICATIONS: Known hypersensitivity to this drug and hypotension prohibit its use.

■ ADVERSE EFFECTS: Life-threatening effects include congestive heart failure, myocardial infarction, cardiomyopathy, cardiomegaly, complete heart block, atrial fibrillation, anemia, thrombocytopenia, ecchymosis, and lymphadenoma. Other serious effects include tachycardia, palpitations, arrhythmia, and seizures. Common side effects include postural hypotension and rash.

anakinra, an antirheumatic agent and immunomodulator used to reduce the signs and symptoms of moderate to severe active rheumatoid arthritis in adult patients.

Ana-Kit, trademark for an insect sting treatment emergency kit containing chlorpheniramine epinephrine in a sterile 1-ml syringe.

anal /ā′nəl/ [L, *anus*], pertaining to the anus.

anal agenesis. See **imperforate anus.**

anal canal, the final portion of the alimentary tract, about 4 cm long, between the rectum and the anus.

anal character, (in psychoanalysis) type of personality exhibiting patterns of behavior originating in the anal phase of childhood. It is characterized by extreme orderliness, obstinacy, perfectionism, cleanliness, punctuality, and miserliness, or their extreme opposites. Also called **anal personality.** See also **anal stage, psychosexual development.**

anal column, the highly vascular longitudinal folds of the anal canal, in which are found the hemorrhoidal blood vessels.

anal crypt, the depression between rectal columns that encloses networks of veins that, when inflamed and swollen, are called hemorrhoids.

anal cryptitis, inflammation of the mucous membrane of the anal crypts.

analeptic. See **central nervous system stimulant.**

anal eroticism, (in psychoanalysis) libidinal fixation at or regression to the anal stage of psychosexual development, often reflected in such personality traits as miserliness, stubbornness, and overscrupulousness. Also called **anal erotism.** Compare **oral eroticism.** See also **anal character.**

anal fissure, a painful linear ulceration or laceration of the skin at the margin of the anus. Also called **fissure-in-ano.**

anal fistula, an abnormal opening on the cutaneous surface near the anus, usually resulting from a local crypt abscess and also common in Crohn's disease. A perianal fistula may or may not communicate with the rectum. Also called **fistula-in-ano.**

anal folds, slight elevations flanking the anal membrane and derived from the cloacal folds; they form the margin of the anus.

analgesia /an′əljē′zē-ə/ [Gk, *a, algos,* without pain], a decreased or absent sensation of pain.

analgesic /an′əljē′zik/, **1.** relieving pain. **2.** a drug that relieves pain. The opioid analgesics act on the central nervous system and alter the patient's perception; they are more often used for severe pain. The nonopioid analgesics act primarily at the periphery, do not produce tolerance or dependence, and do not alter the patient's perception; they are used for mild to moderate pain. See also **pain intervention.**

analgesic administration, a nursing intervention from the Nursing Interventions Classification (NIC) defined as use of pharmacologic agents to reduce or eliminate pain. See also **Nursing Interventions Classification.**

analgesic administration: intraspinal, a nursing intervention from the Nursing Interventions Classification (NIC) defined as administration of pharmacologic agents into the epidural or intrathecal space to reduce or eliminate pain. See also **Nursing Interventions Classification.**

analgesic nephropathy [Gk, *a, algos,* without pain, *nephros,* kidney, *pathos,* disease], kidney damage resulting from the consumption of excessive amounts of nonsteroidal antiinflammatory drugs (NSAIDs) or similar analgesic medications.

analgia [Gk, *ana,* without, *algos,* pain], an absence of pain.

anal incontinence [L, *anus, incontinentia,* an inability to retain], the lack of voluntary control over fecal discharge.

anal membrane. See **cloacal membrane.**

Analgesic nephropathy *(Kumar, Abbas, and Fausto, 2005)*

anal membrane atresia. See **imperforate anus.**

analog /an′əlog/ [Gk, *analogos,* proportionate], **1.** a substance, tissue, or organ that is similar in appearance or function to another but differs in origin or development, such as the eye of a fly and the eye of a human. **2.** a drug or other chemical compound that resembles another in structure or constituents but has different effects. Also spelled **analogue.** Compare **homolog.**

analog computer, a computer that processes information as a physical quantity, such as voltage, amperage, weight, or length and presents results of calculations that can be continuously varied and measured. Compare **hybrid computer.**

analogous /ənal′əgəs/ [Gk, *analogos,* proportionate], similar in function but different in origin or structure, such as wings of birds and flies.

analog signal, a continuous electrical signal representing a specific condition, such as temperature, electrocardiogram waveforms, telephones, or computer modems.

analog-to-digital converter, a device for converting analog information, such as temperature or electrocardiographic waveforms, into digital form for processing by a digital computer. Also called **A/D converter.**

analogue. See **analog.**

analogy /ənal′əjē/ [Gk, *analogos*], similar to a degree in function or form but different in structure or origin.

anal orifice [L, *orificium,* an opening], **1.** the external opening at the end of the anal canal. **2.** the anus, surrounded by the anal sphincter muscle.

anal pecten, the corrugated epithelium within the anal transitional zone between the pectinate line and the anocutaneous line.

anal personality. See **anal character.**

anal phase. See **anal stage.**

anal plug, a mass of epithelial cells that temporarily occludes the anal canal in the embryo.

anal reflex, a superficial neurologic reflex obtained by stroking the skin or mucosa of the region around the anus, which normally results in a contraction of the external anal sphincter. This reflex may be lost in disease of the pyramidal tract above the upper lumbar spine level (S3-S4). See also **superficial reflex.**

anal region, the part of the perineal region that surrounds the anus.

anal sadism, (in psychoanalysis) a sadistic form of anal eroticism, manifested by such behavior as aggressiveness and selfishness. Compare **oral sadism.**

anal sphincter, either of two sphincters (the *internal* and *external anal sphincters*) that open and close to control evacuation of feces from the anus.

anal stage, (in psychoanalysis) the pregenital period in psychosexual development, occurring between 1 and 3 years of age, when preoccupation with the function of the bowel and the sensations associated with the anus are the predominant source of pleasurable stimulation. It is regarded as an important determinant of ultimate personality type. Adult patterns of behavior associated with fixation on this stage include extreme neatness, orderliness, cleanliness, perfectionism, and punctuality or their extreme opposites. Also called **anal phase.** See also **anal character, psychosexual development.**

anal stenosis. See **imperforate anus.**

anal verge [L, *anus* + *vergere,* to bend], the area between the anal canal and the perianal skin.

analysand /ənal'isand'/, a person undergoing psychoanalysis.

analysis /ənal'əsis/ [Gk, *ana* + *lyein,* to loosen], **1.** the separation of substances into their constituent parts and the determination of the nature, properties, and composition of compounds. In chemistry, **qualitative analysis** is the determination of the elements present in a substance; **quantitative analysis** is the determination of how much of each element is present in a substance. **2.** an informal term for **psychoanalysis. —analytic,** *adj.* **analyze,** *v.*

analysis of variance (ANOVA), a series of statistical procedures for comparing differences among three or more groups to determine if differences are due to chance. It is accomplished by examining the differences within the groups as well.

analyst /an'əlist/, **1.** a psychoanalyst. **2.** a person who analyzes the chemical, physical, or other properties of a substance or product.

analyte /an'əlīt/, any substance that is measured. The term is usually applied to a component of blood or other body fluid.

analytic. See **analysis.**

analytic chemistry, a branch of chemistry that deals with identification (qualitative) and measurement (quantitative) of the components of chemical compounds or mixtures of compounds.

analytic psychology /an'əlit'ik/, **1.** the system in which phenomena such as sensations and feelings are analyzed and classified by introspective rather than by experimental methods. Compare **experimental psychology. 2.** also called **Jungian psychology,** a system of analyzing the psyche according to the concepts developed by Carl Gustav Jung. It differs from the psychoanalysis of Sigmund Freud in stressing a "collective unconscious" and a mystic, religious factor in the development of the personal unconscious while minimizing the role of sexual influence on early emotional and psychologic development.

analyze. See **analysis.**

analyzing /an'əlī'zing/, (in five-step nursing process) a category of nursing behavior in which the health care needs of the client are identified and the goals of care are defined. The nurse interprets data; identifies problems (nursing diagnoses) involving the patient, the patient's family, and significant others; defines goals and establishes priorities; integrates the information; and projects the expected outcomes of nursing activities. Although analyzing follows assessing and precedes planning in the five steps of the nursing process, in practice, analyzing is integral to effective nursing practice at all steps of the process. See also **assessing, evaluating, implementing, nursing process, planning.**

anamnesis /an'amnē'sis/ [Gk, *anamimneskein,* to recall], **1.** remembrance of the past. **2.** the accumulated data concerning a medical or psychiatric patient and the patient's background, including family, previous environment, experiences, and, particularly, recollections, for use in analyzing his or her condition. Compare **catamnesis.**

anamnestic /an'amnes'tik/, **1.** pertaining to amnesia or memory. **2.** pertaining to the immunologic memory and the immune response to an antigen to which immunocompetent cells have been exposed.

ANA-PAC, abbreviation for **American Nurses Association-Political Action Committee.**

anaphase /an'əfāz/ [Gk, *ana* + *phainein,* to appear], the third of four stages of nuclear division in mitosis and in each of the two divisions of meiosis. In anaphase of mitosis and of the second meiotic division, the centromeres divide, and the two chromatids, which are arranged along the equatorial plane of the spindle, separate and move to the opposite poles of the cell, forming daughter chromosomes. In anaphase of the first meiotic division, the pairs of homologous chromosomes separate from each other and move intact to the opposite poles of the cell. See also **cytokinesis, interphase, meiosis, metaphase, mitosis, prophase, telophase.**

Anaphase (© Ed Reschke/used with permission)

anaphia /ənā'fē·ə/, an inability to perceive tactile stimuli.

anaphoresis, (in electrophoresis) the movement of anions in a solution or suspension toward the anode.

anaphylactic /an'əfilak'tik/ [Gk, *ana,* up, *phylaxis,* protection], pertaining to anaphylaxis.

anaphylactic hypersensitivity, an immediate, systemic hypersensitivity response to an exogenous antigen medicated by immunoglobulin E or G. It can be triggered by many substances, including drugs, especially penicillin and other antibiotics; foreign proteins used as therapeutic agents, such as insulin, vaccines, allergen extracts, and muscle relaxants; insect venom, especially from bees, wasps, hornets, and fire ants; and certain foods such as shellfish, berries, chocolate, eggs, and nuts. Also called **type I hypersensitivity.** Compare **cell-mediated immune response, cytotoxic anaphylaxis,** immune complex hypersensitivity. See also **anaphylactic shock, immunoglobulin.**

anaphylactic reactions [Gk, *ana, phylaxis,* protection; L, *re, agere,* to act], acute allergic responses involving IgE-mediated antigen-stimulated mast cell activation resulting in histamine release. Exposure to the antigen may result in dyspnea, airway obstruction, shock, urticaria, and, in some cases, death. Anaphylactic reactions may be caused by Hymenoptera (bee) stings, foods, allergen extract; medications, or exercise. Rapid administration of subcutaneous epinephrine is the treatment of choice for severe reactions.

anaphylactic shock, a severe and sometimes fatal systemic allergic reaction to a sensitizing substance, such as a

drug, vaccine, specific food, serum, allergen extract, insect venom, or chemical. This condition may occur within seconds to minutes from the time of exposure to the sensitizing factor (allergen) and is commonly marked by respiratory distress and vascular collapse. The quicker the systemic atopic reaction occurs in the individual after exposure, the more severe the associated shock is likely to be.
■ OBSERVATIONS: The first symptoms are intense anxiety, weakness, and a feeling of impending doom. Sweating and shortness of breath may occur. These are often followed, often quickly, by pruritus and urticaria. Other symptoms include hypotension, shock, arrhythmia, respiratory congestion, laryngeal edema, nausea, and diarrhea.
■ INTERVENTIONS: Treatment requires the immediate injection of intramuscular or subcutaneous epinephrine with vigorous massage of the injection site to ensure faster distribution of the drug. The airway is maintained, and the patient is carefully monitored for signs of laryngeal edema, which may require the insertion of an endotracheal tube or a cricothyrotomy and oxygen therapy. The signs of laryngeal edema include stridor, hoarseness, and dyspnea. Cardiopulmonary resuscitation may be required for cardiac arrest.
■ NURSING CONSIDERATIONS: Nursing care of patients experiencing anaphylactic shock requires appropriate emergency treatment and the close monitoring of the patient for respiratory distress, hypotension and decreased circulatory volume. Patients with a history of severe allergic reactions are instructed to avoid offending allergens; some patients must carry emergency anaphylaxis kits. Such kits contain injectable epinephrine, such as an Epi-Pen Auto-Injector.

anaphylactoid purpura. See **Henoch-Schönlein purpura.**

anaphylatoxin /an′əfī′lətok′sin/, a polypeptide derived from complement. Along with other mechanisms, it mediates changes in mast cells leading to the release of histamine and other immunoreactive or inflammatory reactive substances.

anaphylaxis /an′əfilak′sis/ [Gk, *ana* + *phylaxis,* protection], an exaggerated, life-threatening hypersensitivity reaction to a previously encountered antigen. It is mediated by antibodies of the E or G class of immunoglobulins and results in the release of chemical mediators from mast cells. The reaction may consist of a localized wheal and flare of generalized itching, hyperemia, angioedema, and in severe cases vascular collapse, bronchospasm, and shock. The severity of symptoms depends on the original sensitizing dose of the antigen, the number and distribution of antibodies, and the route of entry and dose of subsequently encountered antigen. Penicillin injection is the most common cause of anaphylactic shock. Insect stings, radiopaque contrast media containing iodide, aspirin, antitoxins prepared with animal serum, and allergens used in testing and desensitizing patients who are hypersensitive also produce anaphylaxis in some individuals. Kinds of anaphylaxis are **aggregate anaphylaxis, antiserum anaphylaxis, cutaneous anaphylaxis, cytotoxic anaphylaxis, indirect anaphylaxis,** and **inverse anaphylaxis. —anaphylactic,** *adj.*
■ OBSERVATIONS: Manifestations can range from mild to severe. Mild symptoms include queasiness, anxiety, hives, itching, flushing, sneezing, nasal congestion, runny nose, cough, conjunctivitis, abdominal cramps, and tachycardia. Moderate reactions include a range of symptoms, including malaise; urticaria; pulmonary congestion, dyspnea, wheezing, and bronchospasm; hoarseness; edema of the periorbital tissue and/or tongue, larynx, and pharynx; dysphagia; nausea; vomiting; diarrhea; hypotension; syncope and confusion. Severe anaphylaxis presents with pallor and cyanosis;

stridor, airway occlusion, and hypoxia. If not treated immediately, respiratory arrest, cardiac arrhythmia, circulatory collapse, seizures, coma, and death rapidly ensue.
■ INTERVENTIONS: Treatment centers on immediate and aggressive management of emerging symptoms. Maintaining the airway and blood pressure is critical. Epinephrine and other drugs are used to counteract effects of mediator release and to block further mediator release. Vasopressors are used to maintain blood pressure. Intubation or tracheostomy may be necessary to maintain an airway.
■ NURSING CONSIDERATIONS: The patient suffering an allergic reaction needs careful monitoring for signs of respiratory distress, hypotension, and decreased circulatory volume. Nursing interventions for anaphylactic shock center on promotion of adequate ventilation and tissue perfusion. Airway needs are maintained, vital signs monitored for hypotension, blood gases monitored for acidosis; ECG monitored for dysrhythmias; fluid volume replaced with IV solutions. Education about prevention of future attacks should include instruction in prophylaxis, such as avoidance of known allergens, wearing a medical alert identification bracelet or necklace that identifies allergies, and ensuring that all medical records have allergies highlighted in a prominent place. Those with severe allergic reactions should consider carrying an anaphylaxis kit with preloaded epinephrine syringes.

anaphylaxis management, a nursing intervention from the Nursing Interventions Classification (NIC) defined as promotion of adequate ventilation and tissue perfusion for a patient with a severe allergic (antigen-antibody) reaction. See also **Nursing Interventions Classification.**

anaplasia /an′əplā′zhə/ [Gk, *ana* + *plassein,* to shape], a change in the structure and orientation of cells, characterized by a loss of differentiation and reversion to a more primitive form. Anaplasia is characteristic of malignancy. Compare **aplasia. —anaplastic** /an′əplas′tik/, *adj.*

anaplastic [Gk, *ana,* backward, *plassein,* to mold], pertaining to anaplasia.

anaplastic astrocytoma. See **glioblastoma multiforme.**

anapnea /anap′nē·ə/ [Gk, *ana, pnoia,* breath], respiration or restoration of breathing after a period of halted respiration.

anapophysis /an′ə·pof′i·sis/ [Gk, *an-,* not, without + *apophysis,* a growing away], an accessory vertebral process, especially one on a thoracic or lumbar vertebra.

Anaprox, trademark for a nonsteroidal antiinflammatory drug (naproxen sodium).

anarthria /anär′thrē·ə/ [Gk, *a, arthron,* not joint], a loss of control of the muscles of speech, resulting in the inability to articulate words. The condition is usually caused by damage to a central or peripheral motor nerve.

anasarca /an′əsär′kə/ [Gk, *ana* + *sarx,* flesh], severe generalized, massive edema. Anasarca often occurs in severe cardiovascular renal disease. See also **edema. —anasarcous,** *adj.*

anastomose /ənas′təmōs/ [Gk, *anastomoien,* to provide a mouth], to open a channel or passage between two vessels or cavities that are normally separate.

anastomosis *pl.* **anastomoses** /ənas′tōmō′sis/ [Gk, *anastomoien,* to provide a mouth], **1.** a connection between two vessels. **2.** a surgical joining of two ducts, blood vessels, or bowel segments to allow flow from one to the other. A vascular anastomosis may be performed to bypass an aneurysm or a vascular or arterial occlusion. With the patient under anesthesia, a section of the saphenous vein or a synthetic prosthesis is grafted to the prepared vessels. Postoperative nursing care includes preventing tissue injury and wound infection. Lack of blood flow may allow the graft to close. Pulses distal to the anastomosis are evaluated and often. Capillary filling time and the color and temperature of the skin are checked. Prophylactic antibiotic therapy may be started within hours. Urinary output is monitored. Kinds of anastomoses are **end-to-end anastomosis, side-to-side anastomosis.** See also **aneurysm, bypass.**

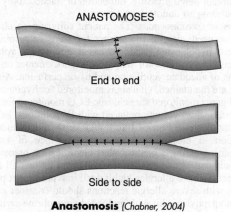

ANASTOMOSES

End to end

Side to side

Anastomosis *(Chabner, 2004)*

anastomosis at elbow joint, a convergence of blood vessels at the elbow joint, consisting of various veins and portions of the brachial and deep brachial arteries and their branches.

anastomotic /ənas′təmot′ik/, pertaining to or resembling an anastomosis.

anastrozole, a nonsteroidal aromatase inhibitor.

■ INDICATIONS: It is prescribed in the treatment of advanced breast cancer for postmenopausal women whose disease has not responded to treatment with tamoxifen.

■ CONTRAINDICATIONS: The drug is usually effective only in patients with estrogen-dependent tumors.

■ ADVERSE EFFECTS: The side effects most often reported include diarrhea, fatigue, nausea, headache, hot flashes, and back pain.

anatomic [Gk, *ana* + *temnein,* to cut], pertaining to the structure of the body.

anatomic age, the estimated age of an individual based on the stage of development or deterioration of the body as compared to that of other persons of the same chronologic age.

anatomic crown, the portion of the dentin of a tooth that is covered by enamel. See also **artificial crown, clinical crown, partial crown.**

anatomic curve, the curvature of the different segments of the vertebral column. In the lateral contour of the back, the cervical and lumbar curves appear concave, the thoracic and sacral curves appear convex.

anatomic dead space. See **dead space.**

anatomic height of contour, an imaginary line that encircles a tooth at the level of greatest circumference. Also called **surveyed height of contour.** See also **height of contour.**

anatomic impotence. See **impotence.**

anatomic incontinence, urinary incontinence associated with instability or excessive mobility of the bladder neck and adjacent urethra.

anatomic neck of the humerus [Gk, *ana,* up, *temnein,* to cut; AS, *hnecca;* L, *humerus,* shoulder], the portion of the humerus where there is a slight constriction adjoining the head.

anatomic pathology [Gk, *ana,* up, *temnein,* to cut, *pathos,* disease, *logos,* science], the study of the effects of disease on the structure of the body.

anatomic position, a standard position of the body: standing erect, facing directly forward, feet pointed forward and slightly apart, and arms hanging down at the sides with palms facing forward. This position is used as a reference to describe sites or motions of various parts of the body.

Face forward

Arms at sides

Palms directed forward

Standing erect

Toes directed forward

Anatomic position *(Applegate, 2000)*

anatomic snuffbox, a small, cuplike depression on the back of the hand near the wrist formed by the tendons reaching toward the thumb and index finger as the thumb is abducted, the wrist flexed, and the digits extended.

anatomic topography [Gk, *ana* + *temnein,* to cut, *topos,* place, *graphein,* to write], a system of identification of a body part in terms of the region in which it is located and its nearby structures.

anatomic zero joint position, the beginning point of a joint range of motion.

anatomy /ənat′əmē/ [Gk, *ana* + *temnein,* to cut], **1.** the study, classification, and description of structures and organs of the body. **2.** the structure of an organism. See also **applied anatomy, comparative anatomy, gross anatomy, microscopic anatomy, surface anatomy.** Compare **physiology.**

anatripsis /an′ətrip′sis/, a therapy that involves rubbing or friction with or without a simultaneous application of a medicine.

ANC, abbreviation for **absolute neutrophil count,** calculated by adding the number of segmented neutrophils and the number of basal neutrophis and multiplying the sum by the total white blood cell count. The formula is ANC = Total WBC count × (% neutrophils + % bands)/100.

A.N.C., abbreviation for **Army Nurse Corps.**

-ance. See **-ency.**

Ancef, trademark for a semisynthetic cephalosporin antibiotic (cefazolin sodium).

ancestor [L, *antecessorem*], one from whom a person is descended, through the mother or the father. The term assumes a direct line of descent, excluding collateral family members of previous generations.

anchorage [Gk, *agkyra,* anchor], surgical fixation of a movable body part.

ancillary /an′sələr′ē/ [L, *ancillaris,* handmaid], pertaining to something that is subordinate, auxiliary, or supplementary.

Ancobon, trademark for an antifungal (flucytosine).

anconeus /angkō′nē·əs/ [Gk, *agkon,* elbow], one of seven superficial muscles of the posterior forearm. A small triangular muscle, it originates on the dorsal surface of the lateral condyle of the humerus and inserts in the olecranon process of the ulna. It functions to extend the forearm and abduct the ulna in pronation.

ancrod /ang′krod/, the venom of the Malayan pit viper, used to remove fibrinogen from the circulation, to prevent clotting of the blood.

-ancy. See **-ency.**

ancylo-, ancyl, anchyl-, anchylo-, ankylo-, ankyl-, combining form meaning 'bent or crooked, curved, stiff, fixed': *ancylostoma, ankylosis.*

Ancylostoma /ang′kilos′təmə/ [Gk, *agkylos,* crooked, *stoma,* mouth], a genus of nematode that is an intestinal parasite and causes hookworm disease. See also **Necator.**

ancylostomiasis /an′səlos′təmī′əsis/, hookworm disease, more specifically that caused by *Ancylostoma duodenale, A. braziliense,* or *A. caninum.* Infection by *A. duodenale* is generally more harmful and less responsive to treatment than that by *Necator americanus,* which is the hookworm most often found in the southern United States. Larvae enter the host via the skin; the adult worm lives in the intestine. The adult worms abrade the intestinal wall eventually causing severe anemia and debilitation. Clinical manifestations and treatment are similar for all types of hookworms. Infection may be prevented by eliminating fecal pollution of soil and by wearing shoes. See also **hookworm.**

Andersen's disease [Dorothy H. Andersen, American pathologist, 1901–1963], a rare glycogen storage disease characterized by a genetic deficiency of branching enzyme (alpha-1:4, alpha 1:6 transglucosidase), causing the deposition in tissues of abnormal glycogen with long inner and outer chains. Infants with the disease are normal at birth but fail to thrive and soon show hepatomegaly, splenomegaly, and hypotonia of muscle associated with the progressive development of liver cirrhosis or heart failure of unknown mechanisms. Diagnosis is by enzyme assays of white blood cells and fibroblasts. There is no specific therapy for the disease, which is usually fatal in the first few years of life. Also called **amylopectinosis, brancher glycogen storage disease, glycogen storage disease type IV.**

Andersen's syndrome /an′der-senz/, bronchiectasis, cystic fibrosis, and vitamin A deficiency. Also called *Andersen's triad.*

Anderson-Hynes pyeloplasty, dismembered pyeloplasty.

-andr-, combining form designating an androgen (steroid hormone).

andreioma, androblastoma. See **arrhenoblastoma.**

andro-, andr-, prefix meaning 'man or male': *androcyte, androgen.*

androgamone /an′drōgam′ōn/ [Gk, *andros,* man, *gamos,* marriage], a chemical secreted by male gametes that is believed to attract female gametes.

androgen /an′drəjin/ [Gk, *andros + genein,* to produce], any steroid hormone that increases male characteristics. Natural hormones, such as testosterone and its esters and analogs, are primarily used as substitutional therapy during the male climacteric. —**androgenic** /an′drōjen′ik/, *adj.*

androgenetic alopecia, a progressive, diffuse, symmetric loss of scalp hair. In men it begins in the 20s or early 30s with hair loss from the crown and the frontal and temple regions, ultimately leaving only a sparse peripheral rim of scalp hair (*male pattern alopecia* or *male pattern baldness*). In females it begins later, with less severe hair loss in the front area of the scalp. In affected areas, the follicles produce finer and lighter terminal hairs until terminal hair production ceases, with lengthening of the anagen phase and shortening of the telogen phase of hair growth. The cause is unknown, but is believed to be a combination of genetic factors and increased response of hair follicles to androgens.

androgenic [Gk, *andros,* man, *genein,* to produce], pertaining to the production or development of masculine characteristics.

androgynous /androj′inəs/, **1.** (of a man or woman) having some characteristics of both sexes. Social role, behavior, personality, and appearance are reflections of individuality and are not determined by gender. **2.** hermaphroditic. Compare **gynandrous.** —**androgyny** /-droj′ənē/, *n.*

android [Gk, *andros + eidos,* form], pertaining to something that is typically masculine, or manlike, such as an android pelvis.

android obesity, obesity in which fat is localized around the waist and in the upper body, most frequently seen in men and having a poorer prognosis for morbidity and mortality than the gynoid type.

android pelvis, a type of pelvis with a structure characteristic of the male. It is not uncommon in women. The bones are thick and heavy, and the inlet is heart-shaped. The sacrum inclines anteriorly, the side walls are convergent, and the pubic arch is small. The diameters of the midplane and the outlet are smaller than in the normal gynecoid pelvis. Vaginal delivery is likely to be difficult unless the overall pelvis is large and the fetus small. See also **pelvis.**

andrology /androl′əjē/ [Gk, *andros,* man, *logos,* science], the study of the health of males.

androma. See **arrhenoblastoma.**

andropause /an′drəpôs/, a change of life for males that may be expressed in terms of a career change, divorce, or reordering of life. It is associated with a decline in androgen levels that occurs in men during their late forties or early fifties. See also **menopause.**

androstenedione test, a blood test used to identify the presence of androstenedioine, a precursor of testosterone. May be used orally by some athletes to enhance performance or increase body bulk.

androsterone /andros′tərōn/ [Gk, *andros + stereos,* solid], originally believed to be the principal male sex hormone, it is used less frequently in therapy since the discovery of testosterone. The greater potency of several other male sex hormones has relegated androsterone largely to historic biochemical interest. See also **anabolic steroid, testosterone.**

-ane, suffix designating a saturated hydrocarbon of the methane series: *butane, propane.*

anecdotal /an′əkdot′əl/ [Gk, *anekdotos,* unpublished], pertaining to knowledge based on isolated observations and not yet verified by controlled scientific studies.

anecdotal records, medical findings usually based on one or a few observed episodes of patient care, as distinguished from results compiled in a large-scale scientific or systematic study.

anechoic /an′ekō′ik/, (in ultrasonography) free of echoes.

Anectine, trademark for a depolarizing neuromuscular blocker (succinylcholine chloride), used as an adjunct to anesthesia.

anejaculation, failure of ejaculation of semen from the urinary meatus in sexual intercourse.

anemia /ənē′mē·ə/ [Gk, *a + haima,* without blood], a decrease in hemoglobin in the blood to levels below the normal range of 12-16 g/dL for women and 13.5-18 g/dL for men. Anemia may be caused by a decrease in red cell production, an increase in red cell destruction, or a loss of blood. A morphologic classification system describes anemia by the hemoglobin content of the red cells (normochromic or hypochromic) and by differences in red cell size (macrocytic, normocytic, or microcytic). Also spelled **anaemia.** See also **hemolytic anemia, hypoplastic anemia, iron deficiency anemia, iron metabolism.**

■ OBSERVATIONS: Depending on severity, anemia may be accompanied by clinical findings that stem from the diminished oxygen-carrying capacity of the blood. Signs and symptoms include fatigue, exertional dyspnea, dizziness, headache, insomnia, and pallor. Signs may also include confusion or disorientation. Anorexia, dyspepsia, palpitations, tachycardia, cardiac dilation, and systolic murmurs also may occur. Iron deficiency is the most common causative factor. Additional laboratory studies may be required to establish the less common forms of anemia.

■ INTERVENTIONS: The therapeutic response to anemia is variable and depends on the causative factors. Moderate to severe anemia, with hemoglobin levels that are below 7 to 8 g/dL, may require transfusion of one or more units of blood (packed red blood cells), especially if the condition is acute and specific clinical signs are present. Depending on the kind of anemia, treatment includes providing supplements of the deficient component, eliminating the cause of the blood loss, or alleviating the hemolytic component. The latter may involve administration of adrenal corticosteroids or splenectomy. Appropriate laboratory tests are repeated at intervals to monitor the response and need for continued therapy. Erythropoietin injections may be used to stimulate red cell production when anemia is secondary to chronic renal failure, the anemia of chronic disease, or in chemotherapy.

-anemia, -anaemia, -nemia   suffix meaning (condition of) red blood cell deficiency: *achylanemia, melanemia, sulfanemia.*

anemia of chronic disease,   a decrease in the number of circulating erythrocytes as a result of a chronic inflammatory state.

anemia of pregnancy,   a condition of pregnancy characterized by a reduction in the concentration of hemoglobin in the blood. It may be physiologic or pathologic. In physiologic anemia of pregnancy, the reduction in concentration results from dilution because the plasma volume expands more than the red blood cell volume. The hematocrit in pregnancy normally drops several points below its pregnancy level. In pathologic anemia of pregnancy, the oxygen-carrying capacity of the blood is deficient because of disordered erythrocyte production or excessive loss of erythrocytes through destruction or bleeding. Pathologic anemia is a common complication of pregnancy occurring in approximately half of all pregnancies. Disordered production of erythrocytes may result from nutritional deficiency of iron, folic acid, or vitamin B_{12}, or from sickle cell or other chronic disease, malignancy, chronic malnutrition, or exposure to toxins. Destruction of erythrocytes may result from inflammation, chronic infection, sepsis, autoimmune disorders, microangiopathy, or a hematologic disease in which the red cells are abnormal. Excessive loss of erythrocytes through bleeding may result from abortion, bleeding hemorrhoids, intestinal parasites such as hookworm, placental abnormalities such as placenta previa and premature separation, or postpartum uterine atony.

anemic /ənē′mik/ [Gk, *a,* without, *haima,* blood],   pertaining to anemia. See also **Cabot rings.**

anemic anoxia,   a condition characterized by an oxygen deficiency in body tissues, resulting from a decrease in the number of erythrocytes or in the amount of hemoglobin in the blood.

anemic infarct.   See **pale infarct.**

anemo-,   prefix meaning 'wind': *anemophobia.*

anencephalus /an′ən·sef′ə·ləs/,   an infant with anencephaly.

anencephaly /an′ensef′əlē/ [Gk, *a + encephalos,* without brain],   congenital absence of major portions of the brain and malformation of the brainstem. The cranium does not close and the vertebral canal remains a groove. Transmitted genetically, anencephaly is not compatible with life. It can be detected early in gestation by amniocentesis and analysis or by ultrasonography. See also **neural tube defect. —anencephalous,** *adj.*

Anencephaly *(Kumar, Cotran, and Robbins, 2003)*

anephric /ā·nef′rik/ [Gk, *a, nephros* without kidney],   without kidneys.

anephrogenesis /anef′rōjen′əsis/ [Gk, *a,* without, *nephros,* kidney, *genein,* to produce],   the condition of being born without kidneys.

anergia /ənur′jə/,   **1.** a condition of lethargy or lack of physical activity. **2.** a diminished or absent sensitivity to commonly used test antigens.

anergic /ənur′jik/,   pertaining to a lack of energy or activity.

anergic stupor,   a kind of dementia characterized by quietness, listlessness, and nonresistance.

anergy /an′ərjē/ [Gk, *a, ergon,* not work],   **1.** lack of activity, lack of energy leading to inactivity. **2.** an immunodeficient condition characterized by a lack of or diminished reaction to an antigen or group of antigens. This state may be seen in advanced tuberculosis and other serious infections, acquired immunodeficiency syndrome, and some malignancies. **—anergic,** *adj.*

aneroid /an′əroid/,   not containing a liquid; used especially to describe a device in contrast to one that performs a similar function that does contain liquid, such as an aneroid sphygmomanometer, which does not contain a column of liquid mercury.

aneroid barometer,   a device consisting of a flexible spring in a sealed, evacuated metal box that is used to measure atmospheric pressure. It is less accurate than a mercury barometer and is generally used for nonscientific work.

Anestacon,   trademark for a local anesthetic jelly (2% lidocaine hydrochloride) used for endourethral and endotracheal procedures.

anesthesia /an′esthē′zhə/ [Gk, *anaisthesia,* lack of feeling],   the absence of all sensation, especially sensitivity to pain, as induced by an anesthetic substance or by hypnosis or as occurs with traumatic or pathophysiologic damage to nerve tissue. Anesthesia induced for medical or surgical purposes may be topical, local, regional, or general and is named for the anesthetic agent used, the method or procedure followed, or the area or organ anesthetized. Also spelled **anaesthesia.** See also **general anesthesia, local anesthesia, regional anesthesia, topical anesthesia,** and specific anesthetic agents.

Comparison of types of anesthesia

Type	Expected result	Method of administration	Risks
General	Reversible unconsciousness Analgesia Anesthesia Amnesia Muscle relaxation (immobility) Depression of reflexes	Inhalation Intravenous injection	Oral or dental injury Cardiac or respiratory arrest Residual muscle paralysis Hyptertension Hypotension Hypothermia Hyperthermia Renal dysfunction Neurologic dysfunction
Regional			
Spinal	Analgesia Anesthesia Muscle relaxation	Anesthetic agent injected into the cerebrospinal fluid (CSF) in the subarachnoid space	Hypotension Total spinal anesthesia (inadvertent high level of spinal anesthesia, causing respiratory arrest and complete paralysis) Neurologic complications (tinnitis, arachnoiditis, meningitis, paresthesias, bowel/bladder dysfunction, paralysis) Headache Infection
Epidural	Analgesia Anesthesia Muscle relaxation	Anesthetic agent injected into epidural space and CSF	Dural puncture Intravascular injection with possible convulsions, hypotension, cardiac arrest Hypotension Total spinal anesthesia Neurologic complications Hematoma Infection
Nerve block	Anesthesia of selected nerve	Local anesthetic injected around peripheral nerve	Inadvertent intravascular injection Nerve damage Infection
Intravenous (Bier block)	Anesthesia of extremity (usually used on upper extremity)	Anesthetic agent injected into veins of arm or leg while using a pneumatic tourniquet	Pain from tourniquet Overdose or toxicity of anesthetic agent Infection
Monitored anesthesia care	Analgesia Anesthesia Amnesia Decreased level of consciousness with ability for purposeful responses to verbal and tactile stimuli Ability to independently maintain airway Safe monitoring of patient Anxiety relief	Anesthesia provider present to monitor patient May supplement local or regional anesthetic with analgesics, sedatives, or amnestics	Same as for local or regional Respiratory depression with use of adjuvant drugs
Sedation and analgesia (conscious sedation)	Ability to maintain independent cardiorespiratory function Decreased level of consciousness with ability for purposeful responses to verbal and tactile stimuli Sedation Analgesia Amnesia Anxiety relief Rapid safe return to activities of daily living	Intravenous injection May or may not have anesthesia provider in attendance; RN may have responsibility for patient monitoring	Oversedation Respiratory depression, apnea Airway obstruction Hypotension Aspiration
Local	Depresses peripheral nerves and blocks conduction of pain impulses	Administration of anesthetic agent by surgeon to a specific area of the body by topical application or local infiltration	Allergic reaction Toxicity Cardiac or respiratory arrest Anxiety due to "awake" state of patient Infection

From Phipps WJ et al: *Medical-surgical nursing: health and illness perspectives,* ed 7, St Louis, 2003, Mosby.

anesthesia administration, a nursing intervention from the Nursing Interventions Classification (NIC) defined as preparation for and administration of anesthetic agents and monitoring of patient responsiveness during administration. See also **Nursing Interventions Classification.**

Common postanesthesia problems

Apnea, hypoventilation, and hypoxia
Contributing factors
  Airway obstruction
  Respiratory depressant drugs
  Residual effects of muscle relaxants
  Pain
  Constrictive abdominal or thoracic dressings
Treatment
  Airway maintenance
  Oxygen administration
  Reversal of anesthetic agents by narcotic antagonists and
    anticholinesterases
  Respiratory stimulants
  Wake-up regimen
  Pain relief
Hypotension
Contributing factors
  Hypovolemia (blood loss; fluid deficit)
  Cutaneous vasodilation with rewarming
  Loss of sympathetic tone
  Myocardial dysfunction
  Drugs
  Technical problems
Treatment
  Determine cause
  Replace volume deficits
  Place patient in Trendelenburg position
  Administer vasopressors
Hypertension
Contributing factors
  Pain
  Delirium and agitation
  Hypoxia
  Hypercarbia
  Excess fluid administration
  Moderate hypothermia
  Gastric or bladder distension
  Preoperative hypertension
Treatment
  Determine cause
  Drug therapy (analgesics; sedation)

From Beare PG, Myers JL: *Principles and practice of adult health nursing,* ed 3, St Louis, 1998, Mosby.

anesthesia machine, an apparatus for administering inhalation anesthetic gases and vapors that is capable of controlling ventilation. Although there are many different models, all have the following features: a delivery system for gas; a flowmeter to measure gas flow; vaporizers for volatilizing and combining the anesthetic agents with oxygen and carrier gases; a circuit for delivering the gas to the patient; monitoring equipment or gauges; and a ventilator and a scavenging system to contain and discharge excess gas.

anesthesia patients, classification of, the system by which the American Society of Anesthesiologists classifies patients in five categories by physical status. Class I includes patients who are healthy and who are without organic, phys-

iologic, biochemical, or psychiatric problems. Class II includes patients who have mild to moderate systemic disease, whether involving or extraneous to the condition requiring anesthesia, such as anemia, mild diabetes, moderate hypertension, obesity, or chronic bronchitis. Class III includes patients who have severe systemic disturbances or disease, whether or not related to the procedure requiring surgical anesthesia. Class IV includes patients who have severe systemic disease that is a constant threat to life that may or may not be related to the intended surgical procedure. Class V includes the moribund patient who is not expected to survive more than 24 hours with or without surgical intervention, such as a person in shock with a ruptured abdominal aneurysm or a massive pulmonary embolus. The letter *E* is added to the Roman numeral to indicate an emergency procedure, as when the condition of a patient scheduled for an elective herniorrhaphy requires emergency treatment when the hernia strangulates.

anesthesia screen, a metal, inverted U-shaped frame that attaches to the sides of an operating table, 12 to 18 inches above a patient's upper chest. It is covered with a sheet to prevent contamination of an operative site on the chest or abdomen by airborne infection from the patient and the anesthetist and to provide a wide sterile field for the surgeon.

anesthesiologist /an′əsthē′zē·ol′əjist/, a physician who completes an accredited of residency in anesthesia. Although anesthesiologists do administer anesthesia directly, they more often supervise nurse anesthetists in the delivery of anesthesia, act as consultants, head anesthesia departments or divisions, or direct intensive care units or pain management clinics. Compare **nurse anesthetist.**

anesthesiologist assistant (AA), an allied health professional who, under the supervision of a licensed anesthesiologist, assists in developing and implementing the anesthesia care plan. Duties may include collecting preoperative data, such as taking an accurate health history and performing an appropriate physical examination; performing various preoperative tasks, such as the insertion of IV and arterial lines, central venous pressure monitors, and special catheters; managing the airway and administering drugs for induction and maintenance of anesthesia; administering supportive therapy, such as IV fluids and vasodilators; providing recovery room care and performing other functions and tasks relating to care in an intensive care unit or pain clinic; providing anesthesia monitoring services; and performing administrative and educational functions and tasks.

anesthesiologist's assistant (AA), an allied health professional who assists the anesthesiologist in collecting preoperative data, such as taking the health history and performing an appropriate physical examination; in performing various preoperative tasks, such as the insertion of IV and arterial lines, central venous pressure monitors, and special catheters; in managing the airway and administering medications for induction and maintenance of anesthesia; in administering supportive therapy, such as IV fluids and vasodilators; in providing postanesthesia care unit (PACU) care under the care of a registered nurse with expertise in preanesthesia care and in performing other functions and tasks relating to care in an intensive care unit or pain clinic; in providing anesthesia monitoring services; and in performing administrative functions and tasks, such as staff education.

anesthesiology /-ol′əjē/, the branch of medicine that is concerned with the relief of pain and with the administration of medication to relax muscles and obliterate consciousness during surgery. It is a specialty requiring competency in general medicine, a broad understanding of surgical procedures, and a comprehensive knowledge of clinical obstetrics, chest medicine, neurology, pediatrics, pharmacology, biochemistry, cardiology, and cardiac and respiratory physiology. See also **anesthesiologist, nurse anesthetist.**

anesthetic /an′esthet′ik/, a drug or agent that is capable of producing a complete or partial loss of feeling (anesthesia). Also spelled **anaesthetic.**

anesthetist /ənes′thətist/, a person who administers anesthesia. Also spelled **anaesthetist.** See also **nurse anesthetist.** Also called anesthesia technician.

anesthetize /ənes′thətīz/ [Gk, *anaisthesia,* lack of feeling], to induce a state of anesthesia.

anetoderma /an′ətōdur′mə/ [Gk, *anetos,* relaxed, *derma,* skin], an idiopathic clinical change produced by focal damage to elastin fibers that results in looseness of skin. There is no known effective treatment.

Anetoderma *(Goldman et al, 2004)*

aneuploid /an′yŏŏploid/ [Gk, *a, eu,* not good, *ploos,* fold, *eidos,* form], **1.** an individual, organism, strain, or cell that has a chromosome number that is not an exact multiple of the haploid number characteristic of the species. **2.** pertaining to such an individual, organism, strain, or cell. Also called **aneuploidic** /-ploi′dik/. Compare **euploid.** See also **monosomy, trisomy.**

aneuploidy /an′yŏŏploi′dē/, any variation in chromosome number that involves individual chromosomes rather than entire sets of chromosomes. There may be fewer chromosomes, as in Turner's syndrome (one X chromosome in females), or more chromosomes, as in Down syndrome (three copies of chromosome 21). Such individuals have various abnormal physiologic and morphologic traits. See also **chromosomal aberration.** Compare **euploidy.** See also **monosomy, trisomy.**

aneurysm /an′yŏŏriz′əm/ [Gk, *aneurysma,* widening], a localized dilation of the wall of a blood vessel. It may be caused by atherosclerosis and hypertension, or, less frequently, by trauma, infection, or a congenital weakness in the vessel wall. Aneurysms are common in the aorta but also occur in peripheral vessels, especially in the popliteal arteries of older people. A sign of large arterial aneurysm is a

pulsating swelling that produces a blowing murmur on auscultation. Small aneurysms may produce no sound at all. An aneurysm may rupture, causing hemorrhage, or thrombi may form in the dilation and give rise to emboli that may obstruct smaller vessels. Also called **vascular tumor.** Kinds of aneurysms include **aortic, bacterial, berry, cerebral, compound, dissecting, fusiform, mycotic, racemose, Rasmussen's, saccular, varicose,** and **ventricular aneurysm.** —**aneurysmal** /an′yooriz′məl/, *adj.*

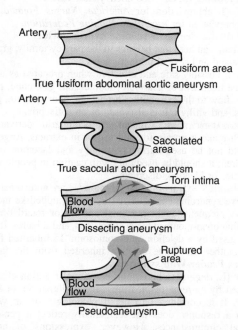

Aneurysms *(Lewis, Heitkemper, and Dirksen, 2004)*

aneurysmal bone cyst, a cystic lesion that tends to develop in the metaphyseal region of long bones but may occur in any bone, including the vertebrae. It may produce pain and swelling and generally increases in size gradually. It is usually removed surgically, but radiation may be used in cases when the tumor is not readily accessible.

Aneurysmal bone cyst *(Silverberg, DeLellis, and Frable, 1997)*

aneurysmal thrill, a vibration that can be felt over an aneurysm. In arterial aneurysms, the vibration is felt only in systole, but in arteriovenous aneurysms it is felt during both systole and diastole.

aneurysmal varix [Gk, *aneurysma,* a widening; L, *varix,* a dilated vein], a varicose vein in which the enlargement is due to an acquired communication with an adjacent artery. Also called **aneurysmoid varix.**

aneurysmectomy, surgical removal of an aneurysm.

aneurysm needle, a needle equipped with a handle, used to ligate aneurysms.

aneurysmoid varix. See **aneurysmal varix.**

ANF, **1.** abbreviation for *American Nurses Foundation.* **2.** abbreviation for *Australian Nursing Federation.*

angel dust. See **phencyclidine hydrochloride.**

angelica, an herb that belongs to the parsley family, grown in Iceland and several northern areas.

■ USES: Possibly safe and effective when prepared as a tea for the treatment of heartburn, indigestion, gas, colic, poor blood flow to the extremities, bronchitis, poor appetite, psoriasis, and vitiligo. It is also used as an antiseptic.

■ CONTRAINDICATIONS: Contains furocoumarin derivatives which make it unsafe for oral use or in extracts. Angelica should not be used during pregnancy and lactation or in children; it should be used only with caution in people with diabetes or bleeding disorders.

Angelman's syndrome /ān′jəl·mənz/, an autosomal recessive syndrome characterized by jerky puppetlike movements, frequent laughter, mental and motor retardation, a peculiar open-mouthed facial expression, and seizures. It can be caused by a deletion on chromosome 15 inherited from the mother; the same deletion inherited from the father causes **Prader-Willi syndrome.**

anger [L, *angere,* to hurt], an emotional reaction characterized by extreme displeasure, rage, indignation, or hostility. It is considered to be of pathologic origin when such a response does not realistically reflect a person's actual circumstances. However, expressions of anger vary widely in different individuals and cultures and may be considered functional under certain controlled circumstances.

anger control assistance, a nursing intervention from the Nursing Interventions Classification (NIC) defined as facilitation of the expression of anger in an adaptive nonviolent manner. See also **Nursing Interventions Classification.**

angi-. See **angio-.**

angiitis /anjē·ī′tis/ [Gk, *angeion,* vessel, *itis*], inflammation of a vessel, chiefly a blood or lymph vessel. See also **vasculitis.**

angina /anjī′nə, an′jinə/ [L, *angor,* quinsy (strangling)], **1.** a spasmodic, cramplike choking feeling. **2. angina pectoris. 3.** characterized by a feeling of choking, suffocation, or crushing pressure and pain. Kinds of angina are **decubitus, intestinal, Ludwig's, stable, preinfarction, Prinzmetal's, streptococcal** and **unstable. —anginal,** *adj.*

-angina, suffix meaning 'severe ulceration, usually of the mouth or throat.'

anginal /anji′nal/, pertaining to angina.

angina pectoris, a paroxysmal thoracic pain caused most often by myocardial anoxia as a result of atherosclerosis or spasm of the coronary arteries. The pain usually radiates along the neck, jaw, and shoulder and down the inner aspect of the left arm. It is frequently accompanied by a feeling of suffocation and impending death. Attacks of angina pectoris are often related to exertion, emotional stress, eating, and exposure to intense cold. The pain may be relieved by rest and vasodilation of the coronary arteries by medication, such as nitroglycerin. Also called **cardiac pain.**

■ OBSERVATIONS: The chief symptom of stable angina is a highly variable, transient, substernal pain that typically starts with physical or emotional exertion and subsides with rest. It may range from a vague ache to an intense crushing sensation. Radiation to the left shoulder, arm, or jaw or to the back is common but does not occur in all cases. Attacks are exacerbated by cold. The most severe class of angina is a constant pain present even at rest. Symptom patterns tend to be consistent and stable for a given individual. Any change in symptom patterns, such as an increase in attack frequency or intensity should be viewed as serious. Such changes are known as unstable angina and are associated with the deterioration of atherosclerotic plaque. The pain in unstable angina is frequently not fully relieved by rest. Unstable angina is often a precursor to myocardial infarction. Tests include a treadmill test to deliberately induce an angina attack and check for ECG changes. A test dose of nitroglycerin is given to evaluate degree of pain relief. Serum lipids and cardiac enzymes are run to screen for cardiac risk factors. Nuclear imaging, angiography, and PET may be indicated to check myocardial perfusion and determine presence of underlying coronary artery disease (CAD).

■ INTERVENTIONS: The first line of treatment is aggressive modification of risk factors, such as smoking, obesity, physical inactivity, elevated lipids, and elevated blood pressure. Drug therapy focuses on prevention of myocardial insufficiency and pain relief and include nitrates, beta-blockers, and calcium channel blockers. Prophylactic aspirin and statins are given for individuals with known CAD, and aspirin and heparin are used to treat intracoronary clotting in unstable angina and prevent progression to myocardial infarction. Coronary artery bypass is used for selected individuals who present with severe angina, localized CAD, no history of MI, and good ventricular function. Percutaneous coronary intervention may be performed to compress plaque and stent placement may be done to keep the coronary artery open. Angioplasty may be used to remove obstructive atherosclerotic lesions. Unstable angina necessitates immediate hospitalization, bed rest, and ECG monitoring for possible MI.

■ NURSING CONSIDERATIONS: Nursing plays a large role in reducing risk behaviors through smoking cessation protocols, dietary modification (low fat and low sodium diet with complex carbohydrates and fruits), consistent aerobic exercise routines (three to four times weekly), and stress reduction activities. Patient education is tailored to the individual's symptom set and includes identification of precipitating factors and education to prevent or control those factors. Education about medication effects and side effects is essential. The individual should be able to recognize and report unstable angina symptoms. Nursing intervention during an acute attack is aimed at maintaining adequate tissue perfusion and relieving pain. This includes assessment and monitoring of vital signs and ECG patterns and auscultation of heart and lung sounds; administration of oxygen; prompt administration of nitrates and narcotic analgesics as needed. Rest and cessation of all activity should occur until pain subsides. The nurse should provide comfortable positioning, and supportive calm reassurance to reduce anxiety.

angina sine dolore /sē′nə dolôr′ə, sī′nē/, a painless episode of coronary insufficiency. See also **silent ischemia.**

angina trachealis. See **croup.**

angio-, angei-, angi-, combining form meaning 'a vessel, usually a blood vessel': *angioblastic, angiitis.*

angioblast /an′jēō·blast′/ [Gk, *angeion,* vessel + *blastos,* germ], **1.** the mesenchymal tissue of the embryo from which the blood cells and blood vessels differentiate. **2.** an individual vessel-forming cell.

angioblastic cords, cordlike masses of splanchnic mesenchymal cells ventral to the primordial coelom; they arrange themselves side by side to form the primordia of the endocardial heart tubes. Also called **angiogenic cell clusters.**

angioblastic meningioma /an′jē-ōblas′tik/, a tumor of the blood vessels of the meninges covering the spinal cord or the brain.

angioblastoma *pl.* **angioblastomas, angioblastomata** /an′jē-ōblastō′mə/ [Gk, *angeion,* vessel, *blastos,* germ, *oma*], a tumor of blood vessels in the brain. Kinds of angioblastomas are **angioblastic meningioma** and **cerebellar angioblastoma.**

angiocardiogram /an′jē-ōkär′dē-ōgram′/, a series of radiographic images produced by angiocardiography.

angiocardiography /-kär′dē-og′rəfē/ [Gk, *angeion* + *kardia,* heart, *graphein,* to record], the process of producing a radiograph of the heart and its great vessels. A radiopaque contrast medium is injected directly into the heart by a catheter introduced through the antecubital or femoral vein. X-ray films are taken as the contrast medium passes through the heart and great vessels. Also called **cardiac angiography.** See also **angiography.**

angiocardiopathy /-kär′dē-op′əthē/ [Gk, *angeion,* vessel, *kardia,* heart, *pathos,* disease], a disease of the blood vessels of the heart.

angiocarditis /-kärdī′tis/, inflammation of the heart and large blood vessels.

angiocatheter /an′jē-ōkath′ətər/, a hollow, flexible tube inserted into a blood vessel to withdraw or instill fluids.

angiochondroma *pl.* **angiochondromas, angiochondromata** /an′jē-ōkondrō′mə/ [Gk, *angeion* + *chondros,* cartilage, *oma*], a cartilaginous tumor characterized by an excessive formation of blood vessels.

angioedema /an′jē-ō′idē′mə/, a dermal, subcutaneous, or submucosal swelling that is acute, painless, and of short duration. It may involve the face, neck, lips, larynx, hands, feet, genitalia, or viscera. Angioedema may be hereditary or the result of food or drug allergy, infection, emotional stress, or a reaction to blood products. Treatment depends on the cause. Severe angioedema may require subcutaneous injections of epinephrine, intubation, or tracheotomy to prevent respiratory obstruction. Prevention depends on the identification and avoidance of causative factors. Also called **angioneurotic edema.** See also **anaphylaxis, serum sickness, urticaria.**

angioendothelioma. See **hemangioendothelioma.**

angiofibroma *pl.* **angiofibromas, angiofibromata** /an′jē-ōfībrō′mə/ [Gk, *angeion* + L, *fibra,* fiber; Gk, *oma*], an angioma containing fibrous tissue. Also called **fibroangioma, telangiectatic fibroma.**

angiogenesis /an′jē-ōjen′əsis/ [Gk, *angeion* + *genesis,* origin], the ability to evoke blood vessel formation, a common property of malignant tissue. The presence of angiogenesis in breast tissue is regarded as a precursor of histologic evidence of breast cancer.

angiogenesis inhibitor, a group of drugs that prevent growth of new blood vessels into a solid tumor.

angiogenic cell clusters, angioblastic cords.

angiogenin /an′jē-ōjen′in/, a protein that mediates the formation of blood vessels. A single-chain basic protein cloned from molecules of the tumor angiogenesis factor (TAF) in human colon cancer cells. Angiogenin is used experimentally to stimulate the development of new blood vessels in

Angioedema *(Callen et al, 2000)*

wound healing, stroke, or coronary heart disease. See also **tumor angiogenesis factor.**

angioglioma *pl.* **angiogliomas, angiogliomata** /an′jē-ōglē-ō′mə/ [Gk, *angeion* + *glia,* glue, *oma*], highly vascular tumor composed of neuroglia.

angiogram /an′jē-əgram/ [Gk, *angeion,* vessel, *gramma,* writing], a radiographic image of a blood vessel following injection of a radiopaque contrast medium. Also called **arteriogram.**

angiograph /an′jē-əgraf/ [Gk, *angeion,* vessel, *graphein,* to record], an instrument that records the patterns of pulse waves. See also **sphygmograph.**

angiography /an′jē-og′rəfē/ [Gk, *angeion* + *graphein,* to record], the x-ray visualization of the internal anatomy of the heart and blood vessels after the intravascular introduction of radiopaque contrast medium. The procedure is used as a diagnostic aid in myocardial infarction, vascular occlusion, calcified atherosclerotic plaques, cerebrovascular accident, portal hypertension, renal neoplasms, renal artery stenosis as a causative factor in hypertension, pulmonary emboli, and congenital and acquired lesions of pulmonary vessels. The contrast medium may be injected into an artery or vein or introduced into a catheter inserted in a peripheral artery and threaded through the vessel to a visceral site. Because the iodine in the contrast medium may cause a marked allergic reaction in some patients and may lead to death in severe cases, testing for hypersensitivity is indicated before the radiopaque substance is used. After the procedure the patient is monitored for signs of bleeding at the puncture site, and bed rest for a number of hours is indicated. —**angiographic,** *adj.*

angiohemophilia. See **von Willebrand's disease.**

angioimmunoblastic lymphadenopathy with dysproteinemia (AILD), a systemic disorder resembling lymphoma, characterized by fever, night sweats, weight loss, and generalized lymphadenopathy; there is a cellular infiltrate of lymphocytes, immunoblasts, and plasma cells, change or effacement of lymph node architecture, hepatosplenomegaly, maculopapular rash, polyclonal hypergammaglobulinemia, and Coombs-positive hemolytic anemia. It is considered to be a nonmalignant hyperimmune reaction to chronic antigenic stimulation; there is proliferation of B cells and profound deficiency of T cells. The disease follows a progressive but variable course; some patients have long survival without chemotherapy, whereas others have a rapid course with death from overwhelming infection.

Angiography (Brunwald, 2001)

angiokeratoma *pl.* **angiokeratomas, angiokeratomata** /an'jē·ōker'ətō'mə/ [Gk, *angeion* + *keras,* horn, *oma*], a vascular, horny neoplasm on the skin, characterized by clumps of dilated blood vessels, clusters of warts, and thickening of the epidermis, especially the scrotum and the dorsal aspect of the fingers and toes.

angiokeratoma circumscriptum, a rare skin disorder characterized by discrete papules and nodules in small patches on the legs or on the trunk.

angiokeratoma corporis diffusum, an uncommon familial disease in which glycolipids are stored in many parts of the body, especially in the venal and cardiovascular systems, causing vasomotor, urinary, and cutaneous disorders and, in some cases, muscular abnormalities. Characteristic signs of the disease are dilation of blood vessels in the "bathing suit areas," edema, hypertension, and cardiomegaly, especially enlargement of the left ventricle; diffuse nodularity of the skin; albumin, erythrocytes, leukocytes, and casts in the urine; and vacuoles in muscle bundles. Also called **Fabry's disease, diffuse angiokeratoma, glycolipidosis.**

Angiokeratoma corporis diffusum (Callen et al, 2000)

angiokeratomata. See **angiokeratoma.**

angiolipoma *pl.* **angiolipomas, angiolipomata** /an'jē·ōlipō'mə/ [Gk, *angeion* + *lipos,* fat, *oma*], a benign neoplasm containing blood vessels and tissue. Also called **lipoma cavernosum, telangiectatic lipoma.**

angioma *pl.* **angiomas, angiomata** /an'jē·ō'mə/ [Gk, *angeion,* vessel, *oma* tumor], any benign tumor with blood vessels (hemangioma) or lymph vessels (lymphangioma). Most angiomas are congenital; some, such as cavernous hemangiomas, may disappear spontaneously.

-angioma, suffix meaning a 'tumor composed chiefly of blood and lymph vessels': *fibroangioma, glomangioma.*

angioma arteriale racemosum /ärtir'ē·ā'lē ras'əmō'səm/ [Gk, *angeion* + *oma* + L, *arteria,* airpipe, *racemus,* grape], a vascular neoplasm characterized by the intertwining of many small, newly formed dilated blood vessels. Normal blood vessels become affected.

angioma cavernosum. See **cavernous hemangioma.**

angioma cutis, a nevus composed of a network of dilated blood vessels.

angioma lymphaticum. See **lymphangioma.**

angioma serpiginosum /sərpij'inō'səm/ [Gk, *angeion* + *oma* + L, *serpere,* to creep], a cutaneous disease characterized by rings of tiny vascular points appearing as red dots.

angiomatosis /an'jē·ōmətō'sis/, a condition characterized by numerous vascular tumors.

angiomyoma *pl.* **angiomyomas, angiomyomata** /-mī·ō'mə/ [Gk, *angeion* + *mys,* muscle, *oma*], a tumor composed of vascular and muscular tissue elements.

angiomyoneuroma. See **glomangioma.**

angiomyosarcoma *pl.* **angiomyosarcomas, angiomyosarcomata** /-mī'ōsärkō'mə/ [Gk, *angeion* + *mys* muscle, *sarx,* flesh, *oma*], a tumor containing vascular, muscular, and connective tissue elements.

angioneuroma. See **glomangioma.**

angioneurotic anuria /-nŏŏrot'ik ənyŏŏr'ē·ə/ [Gk, *angeion* + *neuron,* nerve, *a* + *ouron,* not urine], an abnormal condition characterized by an almost complete absence of urination caused by destruction of tissue in the renal cortex.

angioneurotic edema. See **angioedema.**

angioneurotic gangrene [Gk, *angeion* + *neuron,* nerve, *gaggraina*], the death and putrefaction of tissue caused by an interruption of the blood supply resulting from thrombotic arteries or veins.

angiopathy /an'jē·op'əthē/ [Gk, *angeion,* vessel, *pathos,* disease], a disease of the blood vessels.

angioplasty /an'jēōplas'tē/ [Gk, *angeion,* vessel, *plassein,* to mold], the reconstruction of blood vessels damaged by disease or injury.

angiopoiesis /-poi·ē'sis/ [Gk, *angeion,* vessel, *poien,* to make], the process of blood vessel formation.

angiorrhaphy /an'jē·ôr'əfē/ [Gk, *angeion,* vessel, *rhaphe,* suture], the repair by suture of any blood vessel.

angiosarcoma /-särkō'mə/, a rare, malignant tumor consisting of endothelial and fibroblastic tissue that proliferates and eventually surrounds vascular channels. The condition usually occurs in older persons. Angiosarcoma has been associated with exposure to vinyl chloride and arsenic. Also called **hemangiosarcoma, malignant hemangioendothelioma.** Compare **angioma.**

angiosclerosis /-sklerō'sis/ [Gk, *angeion,* vessel, *skleros,* hard, *osis,* condition], a thickening and hardening of the walls of the blood vessels. See also **atherosclerosis.**

angioscope /an'jē·əskōp'/, a type of microscope that permits inspection of the capillary vessels.

angiospasm /an'jē·ōspaz'əm/, a sudden, transient constric-

Angiosarcoma *(Callen et al, 2000)*

tion of a blood vessel. Also called **vasomotor spasm, vasospasm.** See also **vasoconstriction.**

angiostrongyliasis /an′jē·ō·stron′ji·lī′ə·sis/, infection by a species of *Angiostrongylus,* usually *A. cantonensis* in humans; infection comes after eating contaminated raw hosts such as snails, slugs, prawns, or crabs. The larval worms migrate to the central nervous system and cause eosinophilic meningitis.

Angiostrongylus [Gk, *angeion,* vessel + *strongylos,* round], a genus of parasitic nematodes; species *A. cantonensis* and *A. costaricensis* normally infect other animals but can cause angiostrongyliasis in humans.

angiotensin /-ten′sin/ [Gk, *angeion* + L, *tendere,* to stretch], a polypeptide in the blood that causes vasoconstriction, increased blood pressure, and the release of aldosterone from the adrenal cortex. Angiotensin is formed by the action of renin on angiotensinogen, an alpha-2-glycoprotein that is produced in the liver and constantly circulates in the blood. Renin, stimulated by juxtaglomerular cells in the kidney in response to decreased blood volume and serum sodium, acts as an enzyme in the conversion of angiotensinogen to angiotensin I, which is rapidly hydrolyzed to form the active compound, angiotensin II. The vasoconstrictive action of angiotensin II decreases the glomerular filtration rate, and the concomitant action of aldosterone promotes sodium retention, with the result that blood volume and sodium reabsorption increase. Plasma angiotensin II increases during the luteal phase of the menstrual cycle and is probably responsible for an elevated level of aldosterone during that period. Angiotensin is inactivated by peptidases, called angiotensinases, in plasma and tissues.

angiotensin-converting enzyme (ACE), a glycoprotein (dipeptidyl carboxypeptidase) that catalyzes the conversion of angiotensin I to angiotensin II by splitting two terminal amino acids. ACE-inhibiting agents are used in hypertension control and for protection of the kidneys in diabetes mellitus.

angiotensin-converting enzyme (ACE) inhibitor, a protease inhibitor found in serum that promotes vasodilation by blocking the formation of angiotensin II and slowing the degradation of bradykinin and other kinins. It decreases sodium retention, water retention, blood pressure, and heart size and increase cardiac output.

angiotensin-converting enzyme (ACE) test, a blood test used to detect angiotensin.

angiotensinogen /-tensin′əjən/, a serum glycoprotein produced in the liver that is the precursor of angiotensin.

angiotensin sensitivity test (AST), a test for sensitivity to angiotensin II by infusion of angiotensin II amide into the right cubital vein. Angiotensin is metered in doses that increase by 1 ng/kg/min at 5-minute intervals. A positive AST result is an effective pressor dose, or one that causes a 20 mm Hg rise in diastolic blood pressure at an infusion rate of less than 10 ng/kg/min.

angle /ang′gəl/ [L, *angulus*], **1.** the space or the shape formed at the intersection of two lines, planes, or borders. The divergence of the lines, planes, or borders may be measured in degrees of a circle. **2.** (in anatomy and physiology) the geometric relationships between the surfaces of body structures and the positions affected by movement.

angle board, a device used in denistry to establish reproducible angular relationships between a patient's head, the x-ray beam, and the x-ray film during radiography.

angle-closure glaucoma. See **glaucoma.**

angle former, a hoe-shaped, paired dental instrument whose cutting edges are at an oblique angle to the axis of the blade. It is used to accent angles in class III dental caries. Also called **bayonet angle former.**

angle of convergence, an angle formed between the visual axis of an eye focused on an object and a median line.

angle of incidence, the angle at which an ultrasound beam hits the interface between two different types of tissues, such as the facing surfaces of bone and muscle. The angle is also affected by the difference in acoustic impedance of the different tissues.

angle of iris, the angle formed between the cornea and the iris at the periphery of the anterior chamber of the eye. The aqueous fluid normally drains through this angle, which may be blocked in glaucoma. Also called **filtration angle.**

angle of Louis [Pierre C. A. Louis, French physician, 1787–1872], the sternal angle between the manubrium and the body of the sternum.

angle of mandible, the measure in degrees of the relationship between the body and the ramus of the mandible. It is used in cephalometric measurements of skull radiographs. Also called **gonial angle.**

angle of refraction [L, *angulus* + *refringere,* to break apart], the angle that a refracted ray of light makes with a line perpendicular to the refracting surface at the point of refraction. Also called **refracting angle.**

angle of Treitz /trīts/ [Wenzel Treitz, Czech physician, 1819–1872], a sharp curve or flexure at the junction of the duodenum and jejunum.

Angle's Classification of Malocclusion (modified) [Edward Hartley Angle, American orthodontist, 1855–1930], a classification of the various types of malocclusion, or abnormal contact between the teeth of the maxilla and those of the mandible. The classification is based on where the buccal groove of the mandibular first molar contacts the mesiobuccal cusp of the maxillary first molar: on the cusp (Class I, neutroclusion, or normal occlusion); distal to the cusp by at least the width of a premolar (Class II, distocclusion); or mesial to the cusp (Class III, mesiocclusion). Each class contains two or more types or divisions. See also **classification of malocclusion.**

angor /ang′gôr/, a condition of extreme distress, usually occurring in abdominal or pectoral angina or during a sudden attack of blindness.

angstrom (Å) /ang′strəm/ [Anders J. Angström, Swedish physicist, 1814–1874], a unit of measure of length equal to 0.1 nanometer (1/10,000,000,000 meter), or 10^{-10} meter. Also called **angstrom unit.**

angular artery /ang′gu·lər är′tə·re/, a branch of the facial artery that supplies the lacrimal sac, lower eyelid, and nose.

**Angle's classification of malocclusion:
Class I malocclusion**
(Seidel et al, 2003/courtesy Drs. Abelson and Cameron)

**Angle's classification of malocclusion:
Class III malocclusion**
(Seidel et al, 2003/courtesy Drs. Abelson and Cameron)

angular cheilitis, single or multiple fissures and cracks at the corner of the mouth on one side or both sides, which in advanced stages may spread to the lips and cheeks. Causes include primary or superimposed infection with microorganisms, such as *Candida albicans,* staphylococci, or streptococci; poor hygiene; drooling of saliva; overclosure of the jaws in patients without teeth or with ill-fitting dentures; riboflavin deficiency; or other causes. Also called perlèche.

angular gyrus /ang′gyələr/ [L, *angulus* + Gk, *gyros*], a folded convolution in the inferior parietal lobe where it unites with the temporal lobe of the cerebral cortex.

angular movement [L, *angularis,* sharply bent], one of the four basic movements allowed by the various joints of the skeleton. It is a movement in which the angle between two adjoining bones is decreased, as in flexion, or increased, as in extension. Compare **circumduction, gliding, rotation.**

angular spinal curvature [L, *angulus* + *spina,* backbone, *curvatura,* bend], a sharp bending or sloping of the vertebral column. See also **gibbus.**

angular stomatitis, inflammation at the corner of the mouth.

angular vein, one of a pair of veins of the face, formed by the junction of the frontal and the supraorbital veins. At the root of the nose each angular vein receives the flow of venous blood from the infraorbital, the superior palpebral, the inferior palpebral, and the external nasal veins, becoming the first part of one of the two facial veins.

angulated fracture /ang′gyəlā′tid/, a fracture in which the fragments of bone are at angles to one another.

angulation [L, *angulatus,* bent], **1.** an angular shape or formation. **2.** the discipline of precisely measuring angles, as in mechanical drafting and surveying. **3.** (in radiography) the direction of the primary beam of radiation in relation to the object being radiographed and the film used to record its image. See also **horizontal angulation, vertical angulation.**

anhedonia /an′hēdō′nē·ə/ [Gk, *a* + *hedone,* not pleasure], the inability to feel pleasure or happiness in response to experiences that are ordinarily pleasurable. It is often a characteristic of major depression and schizophrenia. —**anhedonic,** *adj.*

anhidrosis /an′hidrō′sis, an′hī-/ [Gk, *a* + *hidros,* without sweat], an abnormal condition characterized by inadequate perspiration.

anhidrotic /an′hidrot′ik, an′hī-/, **1.** pertaining to anhidrosis. **2.** an agent that reduces or suppresses sweating.

anhidrotic ectodermal dysplasia, a congenital X-linked disorder fully expressed in males, or rarely an autosomal recessive trait with full expression in both sexes, characterized by ectodermal dysplasia associated with aplasia or hypoplasia of the sweat glands, hypothermia, alopecia, anodontia, conical teeth, and typical facies with frontal bossing, midfacial hypoplasia, saddle nose, large chin, and thick lips. Also called **Christ-Siemens-Touraine syndrome, congenital ectodermal defect, hypohidrotic ectodermal dysplasia.**

Anhidrotic ectodermal dysplasia
(Hordinsky, Sawaya, and Scher, 2000)

anhydrase /anhī′drās/ [Gk, *a,* not, *hydor,* water], an enzyme that catalyzes the elimination of water molecules from certain compounds, as carbonic anhydrase dehydrates carbonic acid, thereby controlling the amount of carbon dioxide in the blood and lungs.

anhydration. See **dehydration.**

anhydride /anhī′drīd/ [Gk, *a* + *hydor,* without water], a chemical compound derived by the removal of water from one or more substances, especially an acid.

anhydrous /anhī′drəs/ [Gk, *a,* without, *hydor,* water], an absence of water.

anicteric /an′ikter′ik/ [Gk, *a* + *icterus,* not jaundice], pertaining to the absence of jaundice.

anicteric hepatitis, a mild form of hepatitis in which there is no jaundice (icterus). Symptoms include anorexia, GI disturbances, and slight fever. Aspartate aminotransferase and alanine aminotransferase are elevated. The infection may be mistaken for influenza or be undetected. Compare **hepatitis.** See also **acute anicteric hepatitis, jaundice.**

anidean /anid'ē·ən/ [Gk, *a* + *eidos,* not form], formless; shapeless; denoting an undifferentiated mass, such as an anideus. Also **anidian, anidous** /an'idəs/.

anideus /anid'ē·əs/, an anomalous, rudimentary embryo consisting of a simple rounded mass with little indication of the body parts. A kind of anideus is **embryonic anideus.** Also called **fetus anideus.**

anidian, anidous. See **anidean.**

anileridine hydrochloride, the hydrochloride salt of anileridine; administered orally in the treatment of moderate to severe pain.

aniline ($C_6H_5NH_2$) /an'ilēn/, [Ar, *alnil,* indigo], an oily, colorless poisonous liquid with a strong odor and burning taste, formerly extracted from the indigo plant and now made synthetically from nitrobenzene and used in the manufacture of aniline dyes. Industrial workers exposed to aniline are at risk of developing methemoglobinemia and bone marrow depression. Also called **amidobenzene, benzenamine.**

aniline dye, one containing aniline; such dyes are an important cause of poisoning in the workplace.

anilingus /ā'niling'gəs/, sexual stimulation of the anus by the tongue or lips.

anilism [Ar, *alnil,* indigo; Gk, *ismos,* state], a condition of poisoning resulting from exposure to aniline compounds. Symptoms generally include cyanosis, weakness, cold sweats, irregular pulse, breathing difficulty, coma, convulsions, and possible sudden heart failure. Also called **anilinism.** See also **aniline.**

anima /an'imə/ [L, soul], **1.** the soul or life. **2.** the active ingredient in a drug. **3.** (in Jungian psychology) a person's true inner unconscious being or personality, as distinguished from overt personality, or persona. **4.** (in analytic psychology) the female component of the male personality. Compare **animus.**

animal, a multicellular organism that subsists on the breakdown of organic substances taken into the body, usually by ingestion. Most animals are capable of movement as a result of the actions of nervous tissue and muscle tissue, which are unique to animals.

animal-assisted therapy, a nursing intervention from the Nursing Interventions Classification (NIC) defined as purposeful use of animals to provide affection, attention, diversion, and relaxation. See also **Nursing Interventions Classification.**

animal pole [L, *anima*], the active, formative part of an ovum. It contains the nucleus and the bulk of the cytoplasm and is the site where the polar bodies form. In mammals, the animal pole is also the site where the inner cell mass develops and gives rise to germ layers, such as the ectoderm. Also called **germinal pole.** Compare **vegetal pole.**

animal starch. See **glycogen.**

animation, **1.** the state of being alive. **2.** an ability to put into action a vivid appearance of life.

animus /an'iməs/ [L, spirit], **1.** the active or rational soul; the animating principle of life. **2.** (in analytic psychology) the male component of the female personality. **3.** (in psychiatry) a deep-seated antagonism that is usually controlled but may erupt with virulence under stress. Compare **anima.**

anion /an'ī·ən/ [Gk, *ana* + *ion,* backward going], a negatively charged ion that is attracted to the positive electrode (anode) in electrolysis. Compare **cation.**

anion-exchange resin, any one of the simple organic polymers with high molecular weights that exchange the resin anions with other anions in solution. Compare **cation-exchange resin.**

anion gap, the difference between the concentrations of serum cations and anions, determined by measuring the concentrations of sodium cations and chloride and bicarbonate anions. It is helpful in the diagnosis and treatment of acidosis, and it is estimated by subtracting the sum of chloride and bicarbonate concentrations in the plasma from that of sodium. It is normally about 8 to 14 mEq/L and represents the negative charges contributed to plasma by unmeasured ions or ions other than those of chloride and bicarbonate, mainly phosphate, sulfate, organic acids, and plasma proteins. Anions other than chloride and bicarbonate normally constitute about 12 mEq/L of the total anion concentration in plasma. Acidosis can develop with or without an associated anion increase. An increase in the anion gap often suggests diabetic ketoacidosis, drug poisoning, renal failure, or lactic acidosis and usually warrants further laboratory tests.

anion gap test, a calculation used to help identify the causes of metabolic acidosis, most of which are associated with an increased anion gap. It is a calculation derived from blood electrolyte values. Used to measure the difference between cations (NA^+) and (K^+) and anions (Cl^-) and bearbonalt (HCO_3).

anionic /an'ī·on'ik/ [Gk, *ana,* not, *ion,* going], pertaining to an anion.

aniridia /an'i·rid'ē·ə/ [Gk, *a,* without + *iris*], absence of the iris, a usually bilateral, hereditary anomaly; often a rudimentary stump is visible through a gonioscope.

anisakiasis /an'i·sə·kī'ə·sis/, infection of humans or other animals with a nematode of the family Anisakidae, usually *Anisakis marina.* Human infection is usually caused by third-stage larvae eaten in undercooked infected marine fish such as herring; the larvae then burrow into the stomach wall, producing an eosinophilic granulomatous mass. Also called **eosinophilic granuloma.**

Anisakis /an'i·sa'kis/ [Gk, *an-,* not, without + Gk, *isos,* equal + Gk, *akis,* point], a genus of nematodes of the family Anisakidae; species *A. marina* is the usual cause of human anisakiasis.

anise /an'is/, the fruit of the *Pimpinella anisum* plant. Extract of anise is used in the preparation of carminatives and expectorants.

aniseikonia /an'īsīkō'nē·ə/ [Gk, *anisos,* unequal, *eikon,* image], an abnormal ocular condition in which each eye perceives the same image as being of a different form and size.

anismus /ānis'məs/, extreme contraction of the external sphincter of the anus.

aniso-, anis- /anī'sō-/, prefix meaning 'unequal, asymmetric, or dissimilar': *aniseikonia, anisognathous.*

anisocoria /-kôr'ē·ə/ [Gk, *anisos,* unequal, *kore,* pupil], an inequality of the diameter of the pupils of the two eyes.

Anisocoria *(Lemmi and Lemmi, 2000)*

Unequal pupils of anisocoria *(Phipps et al, 2003)*

Ankle clonus *(Elkin, Perry, and Potter, 2004)*

anisocytosis /anī′sōsītō′sis/ [Gk, *anisos* + *kytos,* cell], an abnormal condition of the blood characterized by excessive red blood cells of variable and abnormal size. Compare **poikilocytosis.** See also **macrocytosis, microcytosis.**

anisogamete /-gam′ēt/ [Gk, *anisos* + *gamos,* marriage], a gamete that differs considerably in size and structure from the one with which it unites, as the macrogamete and microgamete of certain sporozoa. Compare **heterogamete, isogamete. —anisogametic,** *adj.*

anisogamy /an′īsog′əmē/, sexual conjugation of gametes that are of unequal size and structure, as in certain thallophytes and sporozoa. Compare **heterogamy, isogamy. —anisogamous,** *adj.*

anisognathy /an′īsōnath′ik/ [Gk, *anisos* + *gnathos,* jaw], an abnormal condition in which the maxillary and mandibular arches or jaws are of significantly different sizes. **—anisognathic,** *adj.*

anisokaryosis /anī′sōker′ē·ō′sis/, a significant variation in nuclear size among cells of the same general type. **—anisokaryotic,** *adj.*

anisomastia /anī′sōmas′tē·ə/, a condition in which one female breast is much larger than the other.

anisometropia /anī′sōmetrō′pē·ə/ [Gk, *anisos* + *metron,* measure, *ops,* eye], an abnormal ocular condition characterized by a difference in the refractive powers of the eyes.

anisopia /an′īsō′pē·ə/, a condition in which the visual power of one eye is greater than that of the other.

anisopiesis /an′īsōpī·ē′sis/ [Gk, *anisos,* unequal, *piesis,* pressure], a condition of unequal arterial blood pressure on the left and right sides of the body.

ankh /ängk/, an ancient Egyptian symbol of life. It resembles a cross with a loop instead of the top beam.

ankle [AS, *ancleow*], **1.** the joint of the tibia and fibula of the leg with the talus of the foot. **2.** the part of the leg where this joint is located.

ankle-arm index (AAI). See **ankle-brachial index.**

ankle bandage, a figure-eight bandage looped under the sole of the foot and around the ankle. The heel may be covered or left exposed, although covering is preferable because it prevents "window edema."

ankle bone. See **talus.**

ankle-brachial index (ABI), the ratio of ankle systolic blood pressure to arm systolic blood pressure. It is calculated by dividing the higher of the left and right ankle pressures by the higher of the two brachial artery pressures. Also called **ankle-arm index (AAI).**

ankle clonus, an involuntary tendon reflex that causes repeated flexion and extension of the foot. It may be caused by pressure on the foot or corticospinal disease.

ankle-foot orthosis (AFO), any of a variety of protective external devices that can be applied to the ankle area to prevent injury in a high-risk athletic activity, to protect a previous injury such as a sprain, or to assist patients with chronic joint instability with walking. An AFO is often used by patients who are unable to dorsiflex the ankle during gait. It may be used to maintain anatomic position in a person that has a footdrop.

Ankle-foot orthosis *(Modified from Sorrentino, 2000)*

ankle joint [AS, *ancleow* + L, *jungere,* to join], a synovial hinge joint between the leg and the foot. The rounded malleolar prominences on each side of the joint form a mortise for the upper surface of the talus.

ankle reflex. See **Achilles tendon reflex.**

ankylo-. See **ancylo-.**

ankyloblepharon /ang′kə·lō·blef′ə·ron/ [Gk, *agkylos,* crooked + *blepharon,* eyelid], the adhesion of the ciliary edges of the eyelid to each other.

ankyloblepharon-ectodermal dysplasia-clefting syndrome. See **Hay-Wells syndrome.**

ankyloglossia /ang′kilōglos′ē·ə/ [Gk, *agkylos,* crooked, *glossa* tongue], a severe restriction of tongue movement as a result of fusion or adherence of the tongue to the floor of the mouth. Partial ankyloglossia (also called **tongue-tie**) is caused by a lingual frenum that is abnormally short or is attached too close to the tip of the tongue; this condition may

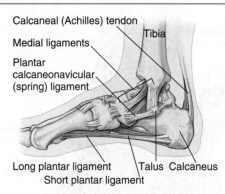

Calcaneal (Achilles) tendon
Tibia
Medial ligaments
Plantar calcaneonavicular (spring) ligament
Long plantar ligament
Short plantar ligament
Talus Calcaneus

Ankle joint of the right foot: medial view

be surgically corrected by a simple excision. Complete ankyloglossia requires extensive surgical reconstruction of the tongue and the floor of the mouth.

Ankyloglossia *(Zitelli and Davis, 1997)*

ankylosed /ang′kilōst/, pertaining to the immobility of a joint resulting from pathologic changes in it or in adjacent tissues.

ankylosing spondylitis /ang′kilō′sing/, a chronic inflammatory disease of unknown origin, first affecting the spine and adjacent structures and commonly progressing to eventual fusion (ankylosis) of the involved joints. In extreme cases a forward flexion of the spine, called a "poker spine" or "bamboo spine," develops. The disease primarily affects males under 30 years of age and generally follows a course of 20 years. There is a strong hereditary tendency. In addition to the spine, the joints of the hip, shoulder, neck, ribs, and jaw are often involved. When the costovertebral joints are involved, the patient may have difficulty in expanding the rib cage while breathing. Ankylosing spondylitis is a systemic disease, often affecting the eyes and heart. Many patients also have inflammatory bowel disease. The aim of treatment is to reduce pain and inflammation in the involved joints, usually with nonsteroidal antiinflammatory drugs. Physical therapy helps keep the spine as erect as possible to prevent flexion contractures. In advanced cases, surgery may

be performed to straighten a badly deformed spine. Compare **rheumatoid arthritis.** See also **ankylosis.** Also called

Ankylosing spondylitis *(Goldman et al, 2004)*

Marie-Strümpell disease.

ankylosis /ang′kilō′sis/ [Gk, *ankylosis,* bent condition], **1.** fixation of a joint, often in an abnormal position, usually resulting from destruction of articular cartilage and subchondral bone, as occurs in rheumatoid arthritis. It may also occur in immobilized patients when active or passive range of motion is not provided. Also called **true ankylosis. 2.** Surgically induced fixation of a joint to relieve pain or provide support. Also called **arthrodesis, fusion.**

anlage /on′lägə/ [Ger, *Anlage,* disposition, aptitude], (in embryology) the undifferentiated layer of cells from which a particular organ, tissue, or structure develops; primordium rudiment. See also **blastema.**

ANLL, abbreviation for **acute nonlymphocytic leukemia.** See **acute myelocytic leukemia.**

ANNA, abbreviation for **American Nephrology Nurses' Association.**

anneal [AS, *aelan,* to burn], **1.** a method of tempering metals, glass, or other materials by controlled heating and cooling to make them more malleable and ductile. **2.** a process whereby two separate strands of nucleic acid interact to form a duplex molecule, often by using a related technique of controlled heating and cooling.

annexa. See **adnexa.**

annihilation /əni′ələ′shən/, the total transformation of matter into energy, as when an antimatter positron collides with an electron. Two photons are created, each with an energy equaling the mass of the individual particles at rest.

annular. See **anular.**

annular ligament. See **anular ligament.**

annulus /an′yələs/ [L, a ring], any ring-shaped structure, such as the outer edge of an intervertebral disk.

annulus conjunctivae. See **conjunctival ring.**

anodal [Gk, *ana* + *hodas,* way], relating to an anode.

anode, the electrode at which oxidation occurs.

anodic stripping voltammetry /əno'dik, anod'ik/,　a process of electroanalytic chemistry used to detect trace metals. It involves the use of a metal-exchange reagent that releases lead or other metals from macromolecular binding sites.

anodontia /an'odon'te·ə/ [Gk, *a*, not, *odous*, tooth],　a congenital defect in which some or all of the teeth are missing. The term is generally applied to cases in which most teeth are missing and no tooth follicles are present.

anodyne /an'ədīn/ [Gk *a* + *odyne*, not pain],　a drug that relieves or lessens pain. Compare **analgesic.**

anomalo-, anomal-,　combining form meaning 'uneven, deviation from normal, or irregular': *anomalopia, anomalous.*

anomalous　/ə·nom'ə·ləs/ [Gr. *anomalos*],　irregular; marked by deviation from the natural order. Applied particularly to congenital and hereditary defects.

anomalous trichromacy,　anomalous trichromatic vision.

anomalous trichromatism,　anomalous trichromatic vision.

anomaly /ənom'əle/ [Gk, *anomalos*, irregular],　**1.** deviation from what is regarded as normal. **2.** congenital malformation, such as the absence of a limb or the presence of an extra finger. **—anomalous,** *adj.*

anomia /əno'me·ə/ [Gk, *a* + *onoma*, without name],　a form of aphasia characterized by the inability to name objects. Comprehension and repetition are unaffected.

anomie /an'əme/,　a state of apathy, alienation, anxiety, personal disorientation, and distress, resulting from the loss of social norms and goals previously valued. Also spelled **anomy.**

anonychia /an'o·nik'e·ə/ [Gk, *a*, *onyx* without nail],　absence of the nail(s).

anoopsia /an'o·op'se·ə/ [Gk, *ana*, up, *ops*, eye],　a strabismus in which one or both eyes are deviated upward. Also called **hypertropia.**

Anopheles /ənof'əlez/ [Gk, *anopheles*, harmful],　a genus of mosquito, many species of which transmit malaria-causing parasites to humans. See also **malaria, Plasmodium.**

anopia /ano'pe·ə/ [Gk, *a* + *ops*, not eye],　blindness resulting from a defect in or the absence of one or both eyes.

-anopia, -anopsia, 1. suffix meaning '(condition involving) nonuse or arrested development of the eye': *hemianopia, quadrantanopsia.* **2.** suffix meaning '(condition of) defective color vision': *cyanopia, tritanopia.*

anoplasty /an'oplas'te/ [L, *anus* + Gk, *plassein*, to shape],　a restorative operation on the anus.

-anopsia.　See **-anopia.**

anorchia /anôr'ke·ə/ [Gk, *a* + *orchis*, not testis],　congenital absence of one or both testes. Also called **anorchism.**

anorchidism,　congenital absence of one or both testicles. See **anorchia.**

anorectal /ān'orek'təl, a'no-/ [L, *anus* + *rectus*, straight],　pertaining to the anal and rectal portions of the large intestine.

anorectal abscess [L, *anus* + *rectus*, straight, *abscedere*, to go away],　an abscess in the area of the anus and rectum. See also **abscess.**

anorectal stricture [L, *anus* + *rectus*, straight, *strictura*, compression],　a narrowing of the anorectal canal. It is sometimes congenital but also may result from surgery to correct a fissure or to remove hemorrhoids.

anorectic /an'orek'tik/,　**1.** pertaining to anorexia. **2.** lacking appetite. **3.** causing a loss of appetite, as an anorexiant drug. Also called **anorectous, anorexiant, anorexic.**

anorectoperineal muscles,　bands of smooth muscle fibers extending from the perineal flexure of the rectum to the membranous urethra in the male.

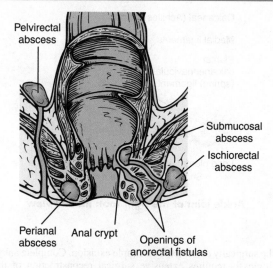

Pelvirectal abscess

Submucosal abscess

Ischiorectal abscess

Perianal abscess　　　Anal crypt

Openings of anorectal fistulas

Common sites of anorectal abscess
(Lewis, Heitkemper, and Dirksen, 2004)

anorexia /an'orek'se·ə/ [Gk, *a* + *orexis*, not appetite],　lack or loss of appetite, resulting in the inability to eat. The condition may result from poorly prepared or unattractive food or surroundings, unfavorable company, or various physical and psychologic causes. Compare **pseudoanorexia.** See also **anorexia nervosa.**

anorexia nervosa,　a disorder characterized by a prolonged refusal to eat, resulting in emaciation, amenorrhea, emotional disturbance concerning body image, and fear of becoming obese. The condition is seen primarily in adolescents, predominantly in girls, and is usually associated with emotional stress or conflict, such as anxiety, irritation, anger, and fear, which may accompany a major change in the person's life. Treatment consists of measures to improve nourishment, followed by therapy to overcome the underlying emotional conflicts.

anorexiant /an'orek'se·ənt/,　a drug or other agent that suppresses the appetite, such as amphetamine. See also **anorectic.**

anorexic.　See **anorectic.**

anorgasmy /an'ôrgaz'me/,　failure to achieve orgasm. Inability to experience orgasm during sexual intercourse or masturbation.

anorthopia /an'ôrtho'pe·ə/,　a visual disorder in which straight lines appear to be curved or angular. The person also may have a diminished perception of symmetry.

anosigmoidoscopy /an'osig'moidos'kəpe/,　a procedure in which an endoscope is used for direct examination of the lining of the anus, rectum, and sigmoid colon.

anosmia /anoz'me·ə/ [Gk, *a* + *osme*, without smell],　loss or impairment of the sense of smell. It usually occurs as a temporary condition resulting from a head cold or respiratory infection or when intranasal swelling or other obstruction prevents odors from reaching the olfactory region. It becomes a permanent condition when the olfactory neuroepithelium or any part of the olfactory nerve is destroyed as a result of intracranial trauma, neoplasms, or disease, such as atrophic rhinitis or the chronic rhinitis associated with the granulomatous diseases. In some instances, the condition may be caused by psychologic factors, such as a phobia or fear associated with a particular smell. Kinds of anosmia include **anosmia gustatoria** and **preferential anosmia.** Also called **anosphresia, olfactory anesthesia. —anosmatic, anosmic,** *adj.*

anosmia gustatoria, the inability to smell foods.

anosmic [Gk, *a* + *osme,* without smell], pertaining to a loss of the sense of smell.

anosognosia /an′əsog·nō′zhə/, [Gk, *a* + *nosos,* not disease, *gnosis,* knowing], lack of awareness or denial of a neurologic defect, or illness in general especially paralysis, on one side of the body. It may be attributable to a lesion in the right parietal lobe of the brain.

anosphresia. See **anosmia.**

anotia /anō′tē·ə/ [Gk, *a,* without, *ous,* ear], a congenital absence of one or both ears.

ANOVA, abbreviation for **analysis of variance.**

anovaginal /ā′nōvaj′inəl/ [L, *anus* + *vagina,* sheath], pertaining to the perineal region of the anus and vagina.

anovarianism. See **anovarism.**

anovarism /an·ō′vər·iz·əm/ [Gk, *a,* without; L, *ovum,* egg], absence of the ovaries. Also called **anovarianism.**

anovesical /-ves′ikəl/ [L, *anus* + *vesicula,* small bladder], pertaining to the anus and bladder.

anovular /anov′yələr/ [Gk, *a,* not, *ovulum*], pertaining to menstrual discharge not associated with the production or release of an ovum.

anovular menstruation [Gk, *a* + *ovulum,* not egg], menstrual bleeding that occurs although ovulation has not taken place. The ovum either remains within the follicle and undergoes degeneration or in rare cases becomes impregnated, resulting in an ovarian pregnancy.

anovulation /an′ovyəlā′shən/, failure of the ovaries to produce, mature, or release eggs. The condition may be a result of ovarian immaturity or postmaturity; of altered ovarian function, as in pregnancy and lactation; of primary ovarian dysfunction, as in ovarian dysgenesis; or of disturbance of the interaction of the hypothalamus, pituitary gland, and ovary, caused by stress or disease. Hormonal contraceptives prevent conception by suppressing ovulation. Anovulation may be an adverse side effect of medications prescribed in the treatment of other disorders. —**anovulatory** /anov′yələtôr′ē/, *adj.*

anoxemia /an′oksē′mē·ə/, a deficiency of oxygen in the blood. Also spelled **anoxaemia.** See also **hypoxia.**

anoxia /anok′sē·ə/ [Gk, *a* + *oxys,* not sharp], an abnormal condition characterized by a local or systemic lack of oxygen in body tissues. It may result from an inadequate supply of oxygen to the respiratory system, an inability of the blood to carry oxygen to the tissues, or a failure of the tissues to absorb the oxygen from the blood. Kinds of anoxia include **anemic anoxia** and **stagnant anoxia.** See also **hypoxemia, hypoxia. —anoxic,** *adj.*

-ans, suffix meaning '-ing': *penetrans, proliferans.*

ansa *pl.* **ansae** /an′sə/ [L, handle], (in anatomy) a looplike structure resembling a curved handle of a vase.

ansa cervicalis, one of three loops of nerves in the cervical plexus, branches of which innervate the infrahyoid muscles. Also called **ansa hypoglossi.**

-anserin, suffix designating a serotonin antagonist.

ANSER system, a pattern of questionnaires for studying developmental defects in children.

ANSI, abbreviation for **American National Standards Institute.**

ant-. See **anti-.**

Antabuse, trademark for a blocker of alcohol oxidation (disulfiram).

antacid /antas′id/ [Gk, *anti,* against, *acidus,* sour], **1.** opposing acidity. **2.** a drug or dietary substance that buffers, neutralizes, or absorbs hydrochloric acid in the stomach. Nonsystemic antacids containing aluminum and calcium are constipating; those containing magnesium have a laxative effect. Systemic antacids such as sodium bicarbonate are rarely used.

antagonism /antag′əniz′əm/ [Gk, *antagonisma,* struggle], **1.** an inhibiting action between physiologic processes, such as muscle actions. An example is the opposition between the biceps and the triceps of the arm. The biceps flexes the arm while the triceps extends it. **2.** opposing actions of drugs.

antagonist /antagə′nist/ [Gk, *antagonisma,* struggle], **1.** one who contends with or is opposed to another. **2.** (in physiology) any agent, such as a drug or muscle, that exerts an opposite action to that of another or competes for the same receptor sites. Kinds of antagonists include the **antimetabolite, associated antagonist, direct antagonist,** and **narcotic antagonist.** Compare **agonist. 3.** (in dentistry) a tooth in the upper jaw that articulates during mastication or occlusion with a tooth in the lower jaw. —**antagonistic,** *adj.,* **antagonize,** *v.*

antagonistic reflexes [Gk, *antagonisma* + L, *reflectere,* to bend back], two or more reflexes initiated at the same time that produce opposite effects. The most adaptive or persistent response occurs.

antagonize. See **antagonist.**

antazoline /an-taz′o-lēn/, a derivative of ethylenediamine, used as an antihistamine; the phosphate salt is applied topically to the eyes in treatment of allergic conjunctivitis.

ante-, prefix meaning 'before in time or in place': *anteflexion, antepartal.*

antebrachial region /an′tə·brā′kē·əl/ [L. *ante,* before + *brachium,* arm], an anatomical term denoting the forearm, divided into the anterior or palmar antebrachial region and the posterior or dorsal antebrachial region.

antebrachium. See **forearm.**

antecardium. See **epigastric region.**

antecedent /an′ti·sē′dənt/ [L, *antecedentem*], a thing or period that precedes others in time or order.

antecubital /-kyoo͞o′bitəl/ [L, *ante,* before, *cubitum,* elbow], in front of the elbow; at the bend of the elbow.

antecubital fossa [L, *ante,* before, *cubitum,* elbow, *fossa,* ditch], a depression at the bend of the elbow.

antecurvature /-kur′vəchər/, a slight degree of anteflexion or forward curvature.

antefebrile. See **antipyretic.**

anteflexion /-flek′shən/ [L, *ante* + *flectare,* bend], an abnormal position in which an organ is tilted acutely forward, folded over on itself.

Anteflexion of the uterus *(Beare and Myers, 1998)*

antegonial notch /-gō′nē·əl/ [L, *ante* + *gonia,* angle], a depression or concavity commonly present on the lower edge of the mandible on each side, immediately in front of the angle, or corner of the jaw.

antegrade /an′təgrād/ [L, *ante,* before, *gredi,* to go], moving forward, or proceeding toward the front. Also called **anterograde.**

antegrade colonic enema, creation of a continent stoma in the right colon through which an irrigation fluid may be infused; used in the management of chronic evacuation disorders. Also called *antegrade colonic irrigation.*

-antel, combining form designating an anthelmintic.

ante mortem [L, *ante,* before, *mors,* death], before death.

antenatal. See **prenatal.**

antenatal care. See **antepartal care.**

antenatal diagnosis. See **prenatal diagnosis.**

antepartal /an′təpär′təl/ [L, *ante* + *parturire,* to have labor pains], pertaining to the period spanning conception and labor.

antepartal care, care of a pregnant woman during the time in the maternity cycle that begins with conception and ends with the onset of labor. A medical, surgical, gynecologic, obstetric, social, and family history is taken, with particular emphasis on the discovery of familial or transmissible diseases. A physical examination is performed, including observation and evaluation of all body systems and pelvic organs. The vaginal part of the pelvic examination may include estimation of the size of the pelvis; a Papanicolaou (Pap) smear; and tests for *Neisseria gonorrhoeae, Candida albicans, Chlamydia* spp., *Trichomonas vaginalis,* syphilis, genital herpes, and other viral infections. Blood pressure, weight, urinalysis primarily for glucose and protein, measurement of the height of the fundus, and auscultation of the fetal heart are routinely performed at monthly intervals or even more frequently in the second and third trimesters. Laboratory tests are performed to determine blood type and Rh factor, rubella antibody titers, hematocrit, and hemoglobin or complete blood count. Ultrasound and/or amniocentesis may be performed if certain fetal abnormalities are suspected. Also called **antenatal care, prenatal care.** See also **intrapartal care, postpartal care.**

antepartum hemorrhage [Gk, *ante,* before; L, *parturire,* to have labor pains; Gk, *haima,* blood, *rhegnynai,* to burst forth], bleeding from the uterus during a pregnancy in which the placenta appears to be normally situated, particularly after the 28th week.

antepyretic /-pīret′ik/ [L, *ante,* before; Gk, *pyretos,* fever], before the onset of fever. Also called **antefebrile.**

anterior (A) /antir′ē·ər/ [L, *ante* + *prior,* foremost], **1.** the front of a structure. **2.** pertaining to a surface or part situated toward the front or facing forward. Compare **posterior.** See also **ventral.**

anterior Achilles bursitis. See **Albert's disease.**

anterior asynclitism. See **asynclitism.**

anterior atlantoaxial ligament /atlan′tō·ak′sē·əl/, one of five ligaments connecting the atlas to the axis. It is fixed to the inferior border of the anterior arch of the atlas and to the ventral surface of the body of the axis. Compare **posterior atlantoaxial ligament.**

anterior atlantooccipital membrane, one of two broad, densely woven fibrous sheets that form part of the atlantooccipital joint between the atlas and the occipital bone. Also called **anterior atlantooccipital ligament.** Compare **posterior atlantooccipital membrane.**

anterior axillary line (AAL), an imaginary vertical line on the body wall continuing the line of the anterior axillary fold with the upper arm.

anterior cardiac vein, one of several small vessels that return deoxygenated blood from the ventral portion of the myocardium of the right ventricle to the right atrium. See also **coronary sinus.**

anterior central gyrus. See **precentral gyrus.**

anterior cerebral commissure [L, *ante* + *prior,* foremost, *cerebrum,* brain, *commissura,* ajoining], a bundle of fibers in the anterior wall of the forebrain connecting the olfactory bulb and cortex on one side with the similar structures on the other side.

anterior chamber [L, *ante* + *prior,* foremost; Gk, *kamara,* an arched cover], the part of the anterior cavity of the eye in front of the iris. It contains the aqueous humor.

anterior column. See **anterior horn.**

anterior common ligament. See **anterior longitudinal ligament.**

anterior corticospinal tract, a group of nerve fibers in the anterior funiculus of the spinal cord, originating in the cerebral cortex.

anterior cruciate ligament, a strong band that arises from the posterior middle part of the lateral condyle of the femur, passes anteriorly and inferiorly between the condyles, and is attached to the depression in front of the intercondylar eminence of the tibia.

anterior crural nerve. See **femoral nerve.**

anterior cutaneous nerve, one of a pair of cutaneous branches of the cervical plexus. It arises from the second and the third cervical nerves and divides into the ascending and the descending branches. The ascending branches are distributed to the cranial, the ventral, and the lateral parts of the neck. The descending branches are distributed to the skin of the ventral and lateral parts of the neck as far down as the sternum.

anterior determinants of cusp, the characteristics of the anterior teeth that determine the cusp elevations and the fossa depressions in restoration of the postcanine teeth. Such determinants include occlusion, alignment overlaps, and the capacity to disocclude conjointly with condylar trajectories.

anterior drawer sign or test, a test for rupture of the anterior cruciate ligament. The result is positive if there is increased anterior glide of the tibia when the knee is flexed at a 90-degree angle. See also **drawer sign.**

anterior elastic lamina. See **Bowman's lamina.**

anterior fontanel, a diamond-shaped unossified area between the frontal and two parietal bones just above an infant's forehead at the junction of the coronal and sagittal sutures. Also called soft spot *(informal).* See also **fontanel.**

anterior guide, the portion of a dental articulator that is contacted by the incisal guide pin to maintain the selected separation of the upper and lower members of the articulator. The anterior guide influences the changing relationships of mounted casts in eccentric movements. Also called **incisal guide.** Compare **condylar guide.**

anterior horn [L, *ante* + *prior,* foremost, *cornu,* horn, *spina,* spine; Gk, *chorde,* string], one of the hornlike projections of gray matter into the white matter of the spinal cord. The anterior, or ventral, horn contains efferent fibers innervating skeletal muscle tissue. Also called **anterior column.**

anterior horn cell, a large nerve cell, the body of a motor neuron, in the anterior column of the spinal cord.

anterior longitudinal ligament, the broad, strong ligament attached to the ventral surfaces of the vertebral bodies. It extends from the occipital bone and the anterior tubercle of the atlas to the sacrum. Also called **anterior common ligament.** Compare **posterior longitudinal ligament.**

anterior mediastinal node, a node in one of the three

groups of thoracic visceral nodes of the lymphatic system that drains lymph from the nodes of the thymus, the pericardium, and the sternum. The nodes are located ventral to the brachiocephalic veins and to the arterial trunks from the aortic arch. Compare **posterior mediastinal node.** See also **lymph, lymphatic system, lymph node.**

anterior mediastinum, a caudal portion of the mediastinum in the middle of the thorax, bounded ventrally by the body of the sternum and parts of the fourth through the seventh ribs and dorsally by the parietal pericardium, extending downward as far as the diaphragm. Compare **middle mediastinum, posterior mediastinum, superior mediastinum.**

anterior nares, the ends of the nostrils that open anteriorly into the nasal cavity and allow the inhalation and the exhalation of air. Each is an oval opening that measures about 1.5 cm anteroposteriorly and about 1 cm in diameter. The anterior nares connect with the nasal fossae. Also called **nostrils.** Compare **posterior nares.**

anterior nasal spine, the sharp anterosuperior projection at the anterior extremity of the line of union of the two maxillae.

anterior neuropore, the opening of the embryonic neural tube in the anterior portion of the forebrain. Compare **posterior neuropore.** See also **horizon.**

anterior pituitary. See **adenohypophysis.**

anterior rhizotomy [L, *anterior,* foremost; Gk, *rhiza,* root, *temnein,* to cut], the surgical cutting of the ventral root of a spinal nerve, usually to relieve persistent spasm, involuntary movement, or intractable pain.

anterior temporal artery, anterior temporal branch of middle cerebral artery: *origin,* middle cerebral artery; *branches,* none; *distribution,* cortex of anterior temporal lobe.

anterior tibial artery, one of the two divisions of the popliteal artery, arising in back of the knee, dividing into six branches, and supplying various muscles of the leg and foot. Compare **posterior tibial artery.**

anterior tibial node, one of the small lymph glands of the lower limb, lying on the interosseous membrane near the proximal portion of the anterior tibial vessels. Compare **inguinal node, popliteal node.**

anterior tooth, any of the incisors or canines. Compare **posterior tooth.**

anterior triangle of the neck, a triangular area bounded by the median line of the neck in front, the lower border of the mandible, and a line extending back to the sternocleidomastoid muscle.

antero-, anter- /an′tərō-/, prefix denoting front: *anterolateral.*

anterocclusion /an′tərōkloo͞′shən/ [L, *ante* + *occludere,* to shut], a malocclusion in which the mandibular teeth are anterior to their normal position relative to the maxillary teeth. Compare **anteversion.**

anteroexternal. See **anterolateral.**

anterograde. See **antegrade.**

anterograde amnesia [L, *ante* + *prior,* foremost, *gredi,* to go], **1.** the inability to recall events that occur after the onset of amnesia. **2.** the inability to form new memories. Compare **anterograde memory, retrograde amnesia.**

anterograde memory, the ability to recall past events but not recent occurrences. Compare **anterograde amnesia.**

anteroinferior /an′tərō-infir′ē·ər/, situated in front of but at a lower level, such as the anteroinferior spine of the ilium.

anterointernal. See **anteromedial.**

anterolateral /-lat′ərəl/, in front and on each side of another structure or object.

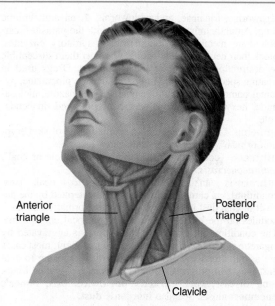

Anterior triangle of the neck *(Seidel et al, 2003)*

anterolateral thoracotomy, a surgical technique in which entry to the chest is made with an incision below the breast but above the costal margins. The incision involves the pectoralis, serratus anterior, and intercostal muscles. Compare **median sternotomy, posterolateral thoracotomy.** See also **thoracotomy.**

anteromedial /an′tər·ō·mē′dē·əl/, located anteriorly and to the medial side; also called **anterointernal.**

anteromedial central arteries of anterior communicating artery, branches of the anterior communicating artery that supply the corpus callosum, septum pellucidum, lentiform nucleus, and caudate nucleus.

anteroposterior (AP) /an′tərōpostir′ē·ər/ [L, *ante* + *prior,* foremost, *posterus,* coming after], from the front to the back of the body.

anteroposterior diameter of the pelvic outlet, the distance between the middle of the symphysis pubis and the upper border of the third sacral vertebra.

anteroposterior vaginal repair, a surgical procedure in which the upper and lower walls of the vagina are reconstructed to correct relaxed tissue. Relaxed vaginal tissue may result from aging changes, childbirth, or surgical trauma or may be inherited.

anterosuperior, situated in front of but at a higher level, such as the anterosuperior spine of the ilium.

anteversion /-vur′shən/ [L, *ante* + *versio,* turning], **1.** an abnormal position of an organ in which it is tilted or bent forward on its axis, away from the midline. **2.** (in dentistry) the tipping or the tilting of teeth or other mandibular structures more anteriorly than normal. Compare **anterocclusion. 3.** the angulation created in the transverse plane between the neck and shaft of the femur. The normal angle is between 15 and 20 degrees.

anteverted /an′tivur′tid/, inclined or turned forward, as for example a uterus.

anthelmintic /ant′helmin′tik/ [Gk, *anti* + *helmins,* against worms], **1.** pertaining to a substance that destroys or prevents the development of parasitic worms, such as filariae, flukes, hookworms, pinworms, roundworms, schistosomes, tapeworms, trichinae, and whipworms. **2.** an anthelmintic drug. An anthelmintic may interfere with the parasites' carbohydrate metabolism, inhibit their respiratory enzymes, block their neuromuscular action, or render them susceptible to destruction by the host's macrophages. Drugs used in treating specific helmintic infections include piperazine, pyrantel pamoate, pyrvinium pamoate, mebendazole, niclosamide, hexylresorcinol, diethylcarbamazine, and thiabendazole.

-anthema, suffix meaning a '(specified) type of skin eruption or rash': *enanthema, exanthema.*

anthraco-, combining form meaning 'carbuncle or coal': *anthraconecrosis, anthracosis.*

anthracosis /an'thrəkō'sis/ [Gk, *anthrax,* coal, *osis,* condition], a chronic lung disease characterized by the deposit of coal dust in the lungs and by the formation of black nodules on the bronchioles, resulting in focal emphysema. The condition occurs in coal miners and is aggravated by cigarette smoking. There is no specific treatment; most cases are asymptomatic, and preventing further exposure to coal dust may halt progress of the condition. Also called **black lung disease, coal worker's pneumoconiosis, miner's pneumoconiosis.** See also **inorganic dust.**

anthralin /an'thrəlin/, a topical antipsoriatic.

■ INDICATIONS: It is prescribed in the treatment of psoriasis and chronic dermatitis.

■ CONTRAINDICATIONS: Known hypersensitivity to this drug prohibits its use. It is not applied to acute psoriatic eruptions or near the eyes.

anthranilic acid. See **aminobenzoic acid.**

anthrax /an'thraks/ [Gk, *anthrax,* coal, carbuncle], an acute infectious disease caused by spore-forming bacteria and occurring most frequently in herbivores (cattle, goats, sheep). It is caused by the bacterium *Bacillus anthracis.* Humans can become infected through skin contact, ingestion, or inhalation of spores from infected animals or animal products. Person-to-person transmission of inhalational disease does not occur. Anthrax in animals is usually fatal. Inhalation causes the most serious form of anthrax in humans, but it is most often acquired when a break in the skin has direct contact with infected animals and their hides. The cutaneous form begins with a reddish brown lesion that ulcerates and then forms a dark scab surrounded by brawny edema. The signs and symptoms that follow include internal hemorrhage, muscle pain, headache, fever, nausea, and vomiting. The pulmonary form, called woolsorter's disease, is often fatal unless treated early. Treatment for both forms is ciprofloxacin or erythromycin. Contaminated surfaces should be cleaned with a 5% hypochlorite solution. A vaccine is available for veterinarians and for others for whom anthrax is an occupational hazard. The incubation period for anthrax is 2 to 60 days. Anthrax is an important potential bioterrorism agent. Also called **malignant pustule.**

anthrax vaccine, a cell-free protein extract of cultures of *Bacillus anthracis,* used for immunization against anthrax.

anthropo-, prefix meaning 'man or human': *anthropocentric, anthropoid.*

anthropoid /an'thrəpoid/ [Gk, *anthropos,* human, *eidos,* form], a noun or adjective generally applied to humanlike apes or other primates; also used to describe a certain kind of pelvis in gynecology and obstetrics.

anthropoid pelvis [Gk, *anthropos,* human, *eidos,* form], a type of pelvis in which the inlet is oval; the anteroposterior diameter is much greater than the transverse. The posterior portion of the space in the true pelvis is much greater than the anterior portion. If the pelvis is large, vaginal delivery is not compromised, but the occiput posterior position of the

Anthrax *(Swartz, 2002)*

fetus is favored. This type of pelvis is present in 40% of women who are not Caucasian and in more than 25% of Caucasian women. See also **pelvis.**

anthropology [Gk, *anthropos,* human, *logos,* science], the science of human beings, from animal-like characteristics to social and environmental aspects.

anthropometry /an'thrəpom'ətrē/ [Gk, *anthropos + metron,* measure], the science of measuring the human body as to height, weight, and size of component parts, including skinfolds, to study and compare the relative proportions under normal and abnormal conditions. Also called **anthropometric measurement. —anthropometric,** *adj.*

Anthropometric measurements

Test	Gender	Normal values	Values showing malnutrition
Triceps skinfold (TSF)	Male	11-12.5 mm	7.5-11 mm
	Female	15-16.5 mm	10-15 mm
Mid upper arm circumference (MUAC)	Male	26-29 cm	20-26 cm
	Female	26-28.5 cm	20-26 cm
Arm muscle circumference (AMC)	Male	23-25 cm	16-23 cm
	Female	20-23 cm	14-20 cm
AMC = MUAC − 0.314 = TSF			

anthropomorphism /an'thrəpōmôr'fizəm/ [Gk, *anthropos,* human, *morphe,* form], the assignment of human shapes and qualities to other animals.

anti-, ant-, prefix meaning 'against or over against': *anti-alexin, antacid.*

antiadrenergic /an'ti·ad'rənur'jik, an'tī-/ [Gk, *anti* + L, *ad* + *ren,* to kidney], **1.** pertaining to the blocking of the effects of impulses transmitted by the adrenergic postganglionic fibers of the sympathetic nervous system. **2.** an anti-adrenergic agent. Drugs that block the response to norepinephrine bound to alpha-adrenergic receptors reduce the tone of smooth muscle in peripheral blood vessels, causing increased peripheral circulation and decreased blood pressure. Alpha$_1$-blocking agents include ergotamine derivatives, used in treating migraine; phenoxybenzamine and phentolamine, administered for Raynaud's disease, pheochromocytoma, and diabetic gangrene; and tolazoline hydrochloride, administered for spastic vascular disease. Agents that block beta$_1$-adrenergic receptors decrease the rate and force of heart contractions among other effects. Propranolol and its congeners are beta-blocking agents and are administered for hypertension, angina, and arrhythmias. Also called **sympatholytic.** Compare **adrenergic.**

antiagglutinin /-əglōō'tinin/ [Gk, *anti*, against; L, *agglutinare*, to glue], a specific antibody that counteracts the effects of an agglutinin.

antiamebic /an'ti·ə·mē'bik/, pertaining to a medication that treats amebic infections.

antianabolic /-an'əbol'ik/, pertaining to drugs or other agents that inhibit or retard anabolic processes, such as cell division and the creation of new tissue by protein synthesis.

antianaphylaxis /-an'əfilak'sis/ [Gk, *anti*, against, *ana*, back, *phylaxis*, protection], a procedure to prevent anaphylactic reactions by injecting a patient with small desensitizing doses of the antigen. Also called allergy immunotherapy.

antianemic /-ənē'mik/ [Gk, *anti* + *a* + *haima*, without blood], **1.** pertaining to a substance or procedure that counteracts or prevents a deficiency of erythrocytes. **2.** an agent used to treat or to prevent anemia. Whole blood is transfused in the treatment of anemia resulting from acute blood loss, and packed red cells are usually administered when the deficiency is caused by chronic blood loss. Transfusions of blood components are used in the treatment of aplastic anemia. Iron deficiency anemia, the most common form of anemia, is usually treated with oral preparations of ferrous sulfate, fumarate, or gluconate, but a parenteral preparation is indicated for people who are unable to absorb iron from the GI tract or for those who respond with nausea and diarrhea to oral administration of iron. Cyanocobalamin is administered parenterally in the treatment of pernicious anemia. Folic acid is prescribed to correct a deficiency of that vitamin in the anemias accompanying general malnutrition or alcoholic cirrhosis and to treat the common anemia of infants who are on an exclusive milk diet. A combination of folic acid and vitamin B_{12} is prescribed for people who are anemic as a result of an inadequate dietary intake of both vitamins.

antianginal drug /-anji'nəl/, any medication that reduces myocardial oxygen consumption or increases oxygen supply to the myocardium to prevent symptoms of angina pectoris.

antiantibody /an'ti·an'tibod'ē/ [Gk, *anti* + *anti* + AS, *bodig*], an immunoglobulin formed as the result of the administration of an antibody that acts as an immunogen. The antiantibody then interacts with the antibody. See also **antibody, immune gamma globulin.**

antiantitoxin /-tok'sin/ [Gk, *anti* + *anti* + *toxikon*, poison], an antiantibody that may form in the body during immunization, inhibiting or counteracting the effect of the antitoxin administered. See also **antiantibody.**

antianxiety agent, a drug that reduces anxiety. The group includes the benzodiazepine derivatives (diazepam and drugs related to it) and a few less widely used non-benzodiazepines such as meprobamate and hydroxyzine. Prolonged high dosage of benzodiazepine agents leads to tolerance and physical dependence, and sudden discontinuation of them may cause withdrawal symptoms. Also called **anxiolytic.**

antiarrhythmic /-ərith'mik/ [Gk, *anti* + *rhythmos*, rhythm], **1.** pertaining to a procedure or substance that prevents, alleviates, or corrects an abnormal cardiac rhythm. **2.** an agent used to treat a cardiac arrhythmia. A defibrillator that delivers a precordial electric shock is often used to restore a normal rhythm to rapid, irregular atrial or ventricular contractions. A pacemaker may be implanted in a patient with an extremely slow heart rate or other arrhythmia. The electrode catheter of an external pacemaker may be threaded through a vein to the heart in cases of ventricular standstill or complete heart block. Two of the major antiarrhythmic drugs are lidocaine, which increases the threshold of electrical stimulation in the ventricles during diastole, and a combination of disopyramide, procainamide, and quinidine, which decreases the excitability of the myocardium and prolongs the refractory period. The beta-adrenergic blocking agent propranolol may be used in treating arrhythmias. Isoproterenol is indicated for complete heart block and ventricular arrhythmias requiring an increased force of cardiac contractions to establish a normal rhythm. Atropine may be used in the treatment of bradycardia, a sedative in the treatment of tachycardia, and digitalis in the treatment of atrial fibrillation. Calcium blockers control arrhythmias by inhibiting calcium ion influx across the cell membrane of cardiac muscle, thus slowing atrioventricular (AV) conduction and prolonging the effective refractory period within the AV node. See also **arrhythmia.**

antiarthritic /-ärthrit'ik/ [Gk, *anti*, against, *arthron*, joint, *itis*, inflammation], pertaining to a therapy that relieves symptoms of arthritis.

antibacterial /-baktir'ē·əl/ [Gk, *anti* + *bakterion*, small staff], **1.** pertaining to a substance that kills bacteria or inhibits their growth or replication. **2.** an antibacterial agent. Antibiotics synthesized chemically or derived from various microorganisms exert their bactericidal or bacteriostatic effect by interfering with the production of the bacterial cell wall; by interfering with protein synthesis, nucleic acid synthesis, or cell membrane integrity; or by inhibiting critical biosynthetic pathways in the bacteria.

antiberiberi factor. See **thiamine.**

antibiotic /-bī·ot'ik/ [Gk, *anti* + *bios*, life], **1.** pertaining to the ability to destroy or interfere with the development of a living organism. **2.** an antimicrobial agent, derived from cultures of a microorganism or produced semisynthetically, used to treat infections. The penicillins, derived from species of the fungus *Penicillium* or manufactured semisynthetically, consist of a thiazolidine ring fused to a beta-lactam ring connected to side chains; these agents exert their action by inhibiting mucopeptide synthesis in bacterial cell walls during multiplication of the organisms. Penicillin G and V are widely used in treating many gram-positive coccal infections but are inactivated by the enzyme penicillinase produced by strains of staphylococci; cloxacillin, dicloxacillin, methicillin, nafcillin, and oxacillin are penicillinase-resistant penicillins. Broad-spectrum penicillins effective against gram-negative organisms are ampicillin and carbenicillin. Hypersensitivity reactions, such as rash, fever, bronchospasm, vasculitis, and anaphylaxis, are relatively common side effects of penicillin therapy. Aminoglycoside antibiotics, composed of amino sugars in glycoside linkage, interfere with the synthesis of bacterial proteins and are used primarily for treating infections caused by gram-negative organisms. The aminoglycosides include gentamicin derived from *Micromonospora*, semisynthetic amikacin, kanamycin, neomycin, streptomycin, and tobramycin. These agents commonly cause nephrotoxic and ototoxic reactions as well as GI disturbances. Macrolide antibiotics, consisting of a large lactone ring and deoxamino sugar, interfere in protein synthesis of susceptible bacteria during multiplication without affecting nucleic acid synthesis. Oleandomycin, which is added to feed to improve the growth of poultry and swine, and broad-spectrum erythromycin, used to treat various gram-positive and gram-negative infections and intestinal amebiasis, are macrolides derived from species of *Streptomyces*. Erythromycin may cause mild allergic reactions and GI discomfort, but nausea, vomiting, and diarrhea occur infrequently with the usual oral dose. Polypeptide antibiotics derived from species of *Streptomyces* or certain soil bacilli vary in their spectra; most agents are nephrotoxic and otdtoxic. Bacitracin and vancomycin are polypeptides used to treat severe staphylococcal infections; capreomycin and vancomycin are antituberculosis agents; and gramicidin is included in ointments for topical infections. Among polypeptide antibiotics effective against gram-negative organisms, colistin and neomycin are administered for diarrhea caused by enteropathogenic *Escherichia coli.* The tetracyclines, including the prototype derived from *Streptomyces,* chlortetracycline, demeclocycline, doxycycline, minocycline, and oxytetracycline, are active against a wide range of grampositive and gram-negative organisms and some rickettsiae. Antibiotics in this group are primarily bacteriostatic and are thought to exert their effect by inhibiting protein synthesis in the organisms. Tetracycline therapy may cause GI irritation, photosensitivity, renal toxicity, and hepatic toxicity. Administering a drug of this group in patients during the last half of pregnancy or before 8 years of age may result in permanent discoloration of the teeth. The cephalosporins, derived from the soil fungus *Cephalosporium* or produced semisynthetically, inhibit bacterial cell wall synthesis and resist the action of penicillinase. They are used in treating infections of the respiratory tract, urinary tract, middle ear, and bones, as well as septicemia caused by a wide range of grampositive and gram-negative organisms. The group includes cefadroxil, cefamandole, cefazolin, cephalexin, cephaloglycin, cephaloridine, cephalothin, cephapirin, and cephradine. Treatment with a cephalosporin may cause nausea, vomiting, diarrhea, enterocolitis, or an allergic reaction, such as a rash, angioneurotic edema, or exfoliative dermatitis; use of antibiotics in this group is contraindicated in patients who have shown hypersensitivity to a penicillin. Chloramphenicol, a broad-spectrum antibiotic initially derived from *Streptomyces venezuelae,* inhibits protein synthesis in bacteria. Because the drug may cause life-threatening blood dyscrasias, its use is reserved for the treatment of acute typhoid fever, serious gram-negative infections (including *Haemophilus influenzae* meningitis), and rickettsial diseases.

antibiotic anticancer agents, drugs that block mammalian cell proliferation in addition to microbial proliferation, making them too dangerous for treating bacterial infections but useful for treating cancer. Examples include bleomycin, dactinomycin, daunorubicin, and mitomycin.

antibiotic resistant, pertaining to strains of microorganisms that either developed a resistance to antibiotic medications or were never sensitive to the drug.

antibiotic sensitivity test, a laboratory method for determining the susceptibility of organisms to therapy with antibiotics. After the infecting organism has been recovered from a clinical specimen, it is cultured and tested against several antibiotic drugs, often in two groups, gram-positive and gram-negative. If the growth of the organism is inhibited by the action of the drug, it is reported as sensitive to that antibiotic. If the organism is not susceptible to the antibiotic, it is reported as resistant to that drug. See also **Gram's stain, sensitivity test.**

antibody (Ab) /an'tibod'ē/ [Gk, *anti* + AS, *bodig*], an immunoglobulin produced by lymphocytes in response to bacteria, viruses, or other antigenic substances. An antibody is specific to an antigen. Each class of antibody is named for its action. Antibodies include agglutinins, bacteriolysins, opsonins, and precipitin. Also called **immune body.** See also **antiantibody, antigen determinant, plasma protein, T cell.**

antibody absorption, the process of removing or tying up

undesired antibodies in an antiserum reagent by allowing them to react with undesired antigens.

antibody-instructive model, a hypothetical explanation for antibody formation. It postulates that each antigenic contact in the life of an individual causes a new antibody to develop, as when a B cell comes in contact with an antigen and subsequently produces plasma cells and memory cells. The model maintains that the random contact of B cells with antigens induces the reticuloendothelial system to instruct memory cells to produce antibodies against antigens at any time. This model is not supported by experimental evidence in favor of the **antibody-specific model.**

antibody-specific model, a proposed explanation for antibody formation which states that precommitted clones of lymphoid cells that are produced in the fetus are capable of interacting with a limited number of antigenic determinants with which they may have contact. Any such cells that encounter their specific antigenic determinant in utero are destroyed or suppressed. This action removes cells programmed to produce endogenous autoantibodies and prevents the development of autoimmune diseases, leaving intact those cells capable of reacting with exogenous antigens. The model holds that the body contains an enormous number of diverse clones of cells, each genetically programmed to synthesize a different antibody. Any antigen entering the body selects the specific clone programmed to synthesize the antibody for that antigen and stimulates the cells of the clone to proliferate and produce more of the same antibody. Also called **clonal selection model.** Compare **antibody-instructive model.** See also **autoimmunity.**

antibody therapy, the administration of parenteral immunoglobulins as a treatment for patients with immunodeficiency diseases.

antibody titer, the concentration of antibodies circulating in the bloodstream of an individual. A rising titer usually indicates the body's response to antigens associated with a developing infection.

antibromic. See **deodorant.**

anticancer diet /-kan'sər/, a diet, based on recommendations of the American Cancer Society (ACS), National Cancer Institute (NCI), and National Academy of Sciences, to reduce cancer risk factors associated with eating habits.

anticarcinogenic /-kär'sinəjen'ik/ [Gk, *anti,* against, *karkinos,* crab, *oma,* tumor, *genein,* to produce], pertaining to a substance or device that neutralizes the effects of a cancer-causing substance.

anticholinergic /-kō'lənur'jik/ [Gk, *anti* + *chole,* bile, *ergein,* to work], **1.** pertaining to a blockade of acetyl-choline receptors that results in the inhibition of the transmission of parasympathetic nerve impulses. **2.** an anticholinergic agent that functions by competing with the neurotransmitter acetylcholine for its receptor sites at synaptic junctions. Anticholinergic drugs are used to treat spastic disorders of the GI tract, to reduce salivary and bronchial secretions before surgery, or to dilate the pupil. Some anticholinergic agents reduce parkinsonian symptoms but are never considered primary agents for therapy. Atropine in large doses stimulates the central nervous system and in small doses acts as a depressant. Among numerous cholinergic blocking agents are atropine, belladonna, glycopyrrolate, hyoscyamine sulfate, methixene hydrochloride, trihexyphenidyl, and scopolamine. Also called **cholinergic-blocking, parasympatholytic.**

anticholinergic agent. See **anticholinergic.**

anticholinergic poisoning, poisoning caused by overdosage with an anticholinergic agent or by ingestion of plants such as jimsonweed that contain belladonna alkaloids. It is characterized by dry mouth, hot, dry, flushed skin, fixed and dilated pupils, sinus tachycardia, urinary retention, disorientation, agitation, impairment of short-term memory, slurred speech, hallucinations, respiratory depression, seizures, and coma; in rare cases death may occur. Treatment is by induced emesis and administration of activated charcoal; physostigmine may be used in severe cases to reverse the anticholinergic effects.

anticholinesterase /an'tikol'ənes'tərās/, a drug that inhibits or inactivates the action of acetylcholinesterase. Drugs of this class cause acetylcholine to accumulate at the junctions of various cholinergic nerve fibers and their effector sites or organs, allowing potentially continuous stimulation of cholinergic fibers throughout the central and peripheral nervous systems. Anticholinesterase drugs include physostigmine, neostigmine, edrophonium, and pyridostigmine. Neostigmine and pyridostigmine are prescribed in the treatment of myasthenia gravis; edrophonium in the diagnosis of myasthenia gravis and the treatment of overdosage of curariform drugs. Many agricultural insecticides have been developed from anticholinesterases; these are the highly toxic chemicals called organophosphates. Nerve gases developed as potential chemical warfare agents contain potent, irreversible forms of anticholinesterase.

anticipation /antis'ipā'shən/, an appearance before the expected time of a periodic sign or symptom, as a malarial paroxysm or a hereditary disorder.

anticipatory adaptation /antis'əpətôr'ē/ [L, *anticipare,* to receive before], the act of adapting to a potentially distressing situation before actually confronting the problem, as when a person tries to relax before learning the results of a medical examination.

anticipatory grief, feelings of grief that develop before, rather than after, a loss.

anticipatory guidance[1], the psychologic preparation of a person to help relieve fear and anxiety of an event expected to be stressful. An example is the preparation of a child for surgery by explaining what will happen and what it will feel like and showing equipment or the area of the hospital where the child will be. It is also used to prepare parents for normal growth and development.

anticipatory guidance[2], a nursing intervention from the Nursing Interventions Classification (NIC) defined as preparation of patient for an anticipated developmental and/or situational crisis. See also **Nursing Interventions Classification.**

anticipatory vomiting, vomiting occurring in anticipation of a second episode of something that triggered it previously, such as a migraine or chemotherapy.

anticoagulant /-kō·ag'yələnt/ [Gk, *anti* + *coagulare,* curdle], 1. pertaining to a substance that prevents or delays coagulation of the blood. 2. an anticoagulant drug. Heparin is a potent anticoagulant that interferes with the formation of thromboplastin, with the conversion of prothrombin to thrombin, and with the formation of fibrin from fibrinogen. Phenindione derivatives administered orally or by injection are vitamin K antagonists that prevent coagulation by inhibiting the formation of vitamin K–dependent clotting factors. See also **antithrombotic.**

anticoagulant citrate phosphate dextrose adenine solution, citrate phosphate dextrose adenine.

anticoagulant citrate phosphate dextrose solution, citrate phosphate dextrose.

anticoagulant therapy [Gk, *anti* + L, *coagulare,* to curdle; Gk, *therapeia*], the therapeutic use of anticoagulants to discourage formation of blood clots within a blood vessel. Its main purpose is preventive; however, thrombolytic action of an anticoagulant can destroy a clot and thereby improve the condition of the ischemic tissue supplied by the affected vessel. Conditions in which this therapy is used include occlusive vascular disease, such as coronary occlusion, cerebrovascular and venous thrombosis, and pulmonary embolism. It is administered prophylactically when major surgery is planned for a patient with a history of arterial stasis and for patients who must be immobilized for a prolonged period of time.

anticodon /an'tikō'don/ [Gk, *anti* + *caudex,* book], a sequence of three nucleotides found in transfer RNA. Each anticodon pairs complementarily with a specific codon of messenger RNA during protein synthesis and specifies a particular amino acid in the protein. See also **genetic code, transcription, translation.**

anticomplement, a substance other than an antigen-antibody complex that activates serum complement, resulting in complement fixation.

anticonvulsant /-kənvul'sənt/ [Gk, *anti* + L, *convellere,* to shake], 1. pertaining to a substance or procedure that prevents or reduces the severity of epileptic or other convulsive seizures. 2. an anticonvulsant drug. Hydantoin derivatives, especially phenytoin, apparently exert their anticonvulsant effect by stabilizing the cell membrane and decreasing intracellular sodium, with the result that the excitability of the epileptogenic focus is reduced. Phenytoin prevents the spread of excessive discharges in cerebral motor areas and suppresses arrhythmias originating in the thalamus, frontal lobes, and other brain areas. Succinic acid derivatives, valproic acid, and various barbiturates are among the drugs prescribed to limit or prevent absence seizures. Some benzodiazepines also have been shown to be useful as anticonvulsants. Many of these agents have a potential for producing fetal malformations when administered to pregnant women.

antideformity positioning and splinting /-dəfōr'mitē/, the use of splints, braces, or similar devices to prevent or control contractures or other musculoskeletal deformities that may result from disuse, burns, or other injuries. Examples include the application of an axillary or airplane splint to prevent adduction contracture of the shoulder and a neck conformer splint to prevent flexion contractures of the neck.

antidepressant /-dəpres'ənt/, pertaining to a substance or a measure that prevents or relieves depression.

antidiabetic /-dī'əbet'ik/, pertaining to an agent that prevents or relieves symptoms of diabetes.

antidiarrheal /-dī'ərē'əl/, a drug or bulk-forming agent that relieves the symptoms of diarrhea. The most effective antidiarrheal drugs are opioid derivatives, which slow intestinal motility to permit greater time for the absorption of water and electrolytes. Bulk-forming agents improve stool consistency, but may not decrease fluid and electrolyte loss. Infectious diarrhea (e.g., traveler's diarrhea) may require antibiotics if severe.

antidiuretic /-dī'əret'ik/ [Gk, *anti* + *dia,* through, *ourein,* to urinate], 1. of or pertaining to the suppression of urine formation. 2. an antidiuretic hormone (vasopressin), produced in hypothalamic nuclei and stored in the posterior lobe of the pituitary gland, that suppresses urine formation by permitting the resorption of water collecting ducts in the kidneys. **—antidiuresis,** *n.*

antidiuretic hormone (ADH), a hormone that decreases the production of urine by increasing the reabsorption of water by the renal tubules. ADH is secreted by cells of the hypothalamus and stored in the posterior lobe of the pituitary gland. ADH released in response to a decrease in blood volume or an increased concentration of sodium or other substances in plasma, or by pain, stress, or the action of certain drugs. ADH causes contraction of smooth muscle in the digestive tract and blood vessels, especially capillaries, arterioles, and venules. Acetylcholine, methacholine, nicotine, large doses of barbiturates, anesthetics, epinephrine, and norepinephrine stimulate ADH release; ethanol and phenytoin inhibit production of the hormone. Increased intracranial pressure promotes inappropriate increases and decreases in ADH. Synthetic ADH is used in the treatment of diabetes insipidus (caused by decreased ADH levels). Normal values are 1 to 5 pg/ml or less than 1.5 ng/L. Also called **vasopressin.**

antidiuretic hormone (ADH) test, a blood test that may be used to diagnose diabetes insipidus (both the neurogenic and nephrogenic forms) and the syndrome of inappropriate ADH secretion (SIADH), which is associated with tumors, pulmonary diseases, infection, trauma, Addison's disease, and myxedema.

anti-DNA antibody test, a blood test that is useful for the diagnosis and follow-up of systemic lupus erythematosus (SLE). High titers characterize SLE, while low to moderate levels may indicate other rheumatic diseases as well as chronic hepatitis, infectious mononucleosis, and biliary cirrhosis.

antidotal /-dō'təl/ [Gk, *anti,* against, *dotos,* that which is given], a substance that renders a poison or drug ineffective. See also **antidote.**

antidote /an'tidōt/ [Gk, *anti + dotos,* that which is given], a drug or other substance that opposes the action of a poison. An antidote may be mechanical, such as activated charcoal which absorbs poisons in the GI tract and prevents their absorption; chemical, acting to neutralize the toxin; or physiologic, acting to oppose the action of the poison, as when a sedative is given to a person who has ingested a large amount of a stimulant, or when a receptor blocker is administered to a person who has taken a large dose of the receptor agonist.

antidromic conduction /an'tidrom'ik/ [Gk, *anti + dromos,* course], the conduction of a neural impulse backward from a receptor in the midportion of an axon. It is an unnatural phenomenon and may be produced experimentally. Because synaptic junctions allow conduction in one direction only, any backward, antidromic impulses that occur fail to pass the synapse, dying at that point. Compare **orthodromic conduction.**

antidyskinetic /an'te-, an'ti-dis'kĭ-net'ik/, 1. relieving or preventing dyskinesia. 2. an agent that relieves or prevents dyskinesia.

antiembolism hose /-em'bəliz'əm/ [Gk, *anti + embolos,* plug], elasticized stockings worn to prevent the formation of emboli and thrombi, especially in patients who have had surgery or who have been restricted to bed. Return flow of the venous circulation is promoted, preventing venous stasis and dilation of the veins, conditions that predispose individuals to varicosities and thromboembolic disorders. Abbreviated **AE hose** or **TED (thromboembolic disorder) hose.**

antiemetic /-imet'ik/ [Gk, *anti + emesis,* vomiting], 1. pertaining to a substance or procedure that prevents or alleviates nausea and vomiting. 2. an antiemetic drug or agent. Chlorpromazine and other phenothiazines are sometimes effective antiemetic agents. In motion sickness, scopolamine and antihistamines provide relief. SHT_3-receptor antagonists such as dolasteron and the corticosteroid dexamethasone may relieve chemotherapy-induced nausea. Cannabis derivatives such as dronabinol may also alleviate the nausea induced by certain antineoplastic drugs in cancer patients.

Antiembolism hose *(Elkin, Perry, and Potter, 2004)*

antiepileptic. See **anticonvulsant.**

antiestrogen drug /-es'trəjən/, any of a group of hormone-based products used predominantly in cancer chemotherapy. The group includes tamoxifen. They are used mainly in treating estrogen-dependent tumors, such as breast cancer.

antifebrile. See **antipyretic.**

antifibrillatory /-fibril'ətôr'ē/, a medication or other agent that suppresses either atrial or ventricular fibrillation.

antifilarial, 1. destructive to filariae. 2. an agent having this effect.

antiflux /an'ti·fluks/ [Gk, *anti,* against + L, *fluere,* to flow], a substance that prevents the attachment of solder.

antifungal /-fung'gəl/, 1. pertaining to a substance that kills fungi or inhibits their growth or reproduction. 2. an antifungal, antibiotic drug. Amphotericin B and ketoconazole, both effective against a broad spectrum of fungi, probably act by binding to sterols in the fungal cell membrane and changing the membrane's permeability. Griseofulvin, another broad-spectrum antifungal agent, binds to the host's new keratin and renders it resistant to further fungal invasion. Miconazole inhibits the growth of common dermatophytes, including yeastlike *Candida albicans;* nystatin is effective against yeast and yeastlike fungi. Also called **antimycotic.**

antigalactic /-gəlak'tik/, pertaining to a drug or other agent that prevents or reduces milk secretion in some mothers of newborns.

anti-GBM disease, a kidney disorder in which the glomerular basement membrane is damaged by an antigenantibody reaction. The kidney itself may serve as the antigenic target in the reaction.

antigen /an'tijən/ [Gk, *anti + genein,* to produce], a substance, usually a protein, that the body recognizes as foreign and that can evoke an immune response.

antigen-antibody reaction, a process of the immune system in which immunoglobulin-coated B cells recognize a specific antigen and stimulate antibody production. T cells also play an essential role in the reaction. An antigen-antibody reaction begins with the binding of antigens to antibodies to form antigen-antibody complexes. These complexes may render toxic antigens harmless, agglutinize antigens on the surface of microorganisms, or activate the complement system by exposing the complement-binding sites on antibodies. Certain complement proteins immediately bind to these sites and trigger the activity of the other complement proteins, which cause antigen-bearing cells to lyse. Antigen-antibody reactions may start immediately with antigen contact or as much as 48 hours later. They normally produce immunity but may also be responsible for allergy, autoimmunity, and fetomaternal hematologic incompatibility. In the immediate allergic response, the antigen-antibody reaction activates certain enzymes and causes an imbalance between those enzymes and their inhibitors. Simultaneously released into the circulation are several pharmacologically active substances, including acetylcholine, bradykinin, histamine, immunoglobulin G, and leukotaxine. See also **allergen, allergic reaction, humoral immunity, serum sickness.**

antigen determinant, a short sequence of amino acids in an antigen molecule that assume a particular shape and bind to a corresponding site of an antibody molecule or T cell receptor. Also called **epitope.** See also **antibody.**

antigenic /-jen'ik/, provoking an immune response or reacting with antibodies. Also called **immunogenic.**

antigenic drift [Gk, *anti,* against, *genein,* to produce; AS, *drifan,* drift], the tendency of a virus or other microorganism to gradually alter its genetic makeup, periodically producing a mutant antigen requiring new antibodies and vaccines to combat its effects. See also **influenza.**

antigenicity /an'tijənis'ətē/, the ability to cause the production of antibodies. The degree of antigenicity of a substance depends on the kind and amount of that substance and on the degree to which the host is sensitive to it and able to produce antibodies. See also **antigen-antibody reaction.**

antigenic shift, a sudden, major change in the antigenicity of a virus, seen especially in influenza viruses, resulting from the recombination of the genomes of two different strains; it is associated with pandemics, because hosts do not have immunity to the new strain. See also **antigenic drift**.

antigen presentation, presentation of ingested antigens on the surface of macrophages near histocompatibility antigens.

antigen-presenting cell, a cell that can break down protein antigens into peptides and present the peptides, in conjunction with major histocompatibility complex class II molecules, on the cell surface, where they can interact with T cell receptors. Macrophages are one type of antigen-presenting cell.

antigen processing, the steps that occur in an immune response after a protein is recognized as a foreign.

antigen unit, the smallest amount of antigen required to fix one unit of complement.

antigenuria /an'tĭ-jĕ-nu're-ah/, the presence of a specific antigen in the urine.

antigerminal pole. See **vegetal pole.**

antiglaucoma /an'te-glaw-ko'mah, -glou-ko'mah/, preventing or alleviating glaucoma.

antiglobulin /an'tiglob'yōōlin/ [Gk, *anti* + L, *globulus,* small globe], an antibody that occurs naturally or is prepared in laboratory animals to be used against human globulin. Specific antiglobulins are used in the detection of specific antibodies, as in blood typing. See also **antiglobulin test, Coombs' test, precipitin.**

antiglobulin test, a test for the presence of antibodies that coat and damage red blood cells as a result of any of several diseases or conditions. The test can detect Rh antibodies in maternal blood and is used to anticipate hemolytic disease of the newborn. It is also used to diagnose and screen for autoimmune hemolytic anemias and to determine the compatibility of blood types. When exposed to a sample of the patient's serum, the antiglobulin serum causes agglutination if human globulin antibody or its complement is present. Also called **Coombs' test.** See also **autoimmune disease, erythroblastosis fetalis.**

antigravity muscles /-grav'itē/, the muscle groups involved in stabilization of joints or other body parts by op-

posing the effects of gravity. Examples include the muscles of the jaw that automatically keep the mandible raised and the mouth closed.

anti-G suit. See **military antishock trousers.**

antihemophilic C factor. See **factor XI.**

antihemophilic factor (AHF) /-hē'mōfil'ik/, blood factor VIII, a systemic hemostatic.

■ INDICATION: It is prescribed in the treatment of hemophilia A, a deficiency of factor VIII.

■ CONTRAINDICATION: There are no known contraindications.

■ ADVERSE EFFECTS: The most serious adverse reaction is hepatitis, which occurs because the factor is obtained from pools of human plasma. Allergic reactions may also occur.

antihemophilic factor plasma [Gk, *anti,* against, *haima,* blood, *philein,* to love; L, *facere,* to make; Gk, *plassein,* to mold], blood plasma that contains the antihemophilic factor VIII.

antihemophilic factor (recombinant), a sterile, purified, concentrate produced by recombinant technology using cultured hamster cell lines that have been transfected with a gene for human coagulation factor VIII and having biological activity comparable with that of plasma-derived coagulation factor VIII; used to prevent or arrest hemorrhage during surgery or other procedures in patients with hemophilia A, administered intravenously.

antihemorrhagic /-hē'môraj'ik/, any drug or agent used to prevent or control bleeding, such as thromboplastin or thrombin, either of which mediates the blood clotting process.

antihidrotic /-hidrot'ik/ [Gk, *anti,* + *hidros,* sweat], an agent that inhibits or prevents the production of sweat, and antiperspirant.

antihistamine /-his'təmin/ [Gk, *anti* + *histos,* tissue, amine (ammonia compound)], any substance capable of reducing the physiologic and pharmacologic effects of histamine, including a wide variety of drugs that block histamine receptors. Many such drugs are readily available as nonprescription medicines for the management of allergies. Toxicity resulting from the overuse of antihistamines and their accidental ingestion by children is common and sometimes fatal. These substances do not completely stop the release of histamine, and the ways in which they act on the central nervous system are not completely understood. The antihistamines are divided into histamine H_1 and H_2 blockers, depending on the responses to histamine they prevent. The H_1 blocking drugs, such as the alkylamines, ethanolamines, ethylenediamines, and piperazines, are effective in the symptomatic treatment of acute allergies. Second-generation H_1 blockers, such as cetirizine (Zyrtec), fexofenadine (Allegra), and loratadine (Claritin), cause less sedation. The H_2 blocking drugs are effective in the control of gastric secretions and are often used in the treatment of gastroesophageal reflux disease. Antihistamines can both stimulate and depress the central nervous system.

antihistamine poisoning, an adverse reaction to an excessive intake of antihistamine medication. Symptoms include fatigue, lethargy, delirium, hallucinations, loss of voluntary muscle control, hyperreflexia, tachycardia, dilated pupils, and in severe cases coma.

antihistaminic [Gk, *anti* + *histos,* tissue, amine], pertaining to a substance that counteracts the effects of histamine.

anti-Hu antibody, any of the polyclonal IgG autoantibodies directed against the proteins of the Hu antigen family; they are associated with paraneoplastic sensory neuronopathy and encephalomyelitis in small cell lung carcinoma and, more rarely, sarcoma and neuroblastoma. Also called *type 1 antineuronal antibody (ANNA-1).*

antihypercholesterolemic /-hī′pərkō′les′tərōlē′mik/, a drug that prevents or controls an increase of cholesterol in the blood. See also **antilipidemic.**

antihyperglycemic /an′te-, an′ti-hi′per-gli-se′mik/, **1.** counteracting high levels of glucose in the blood. **2.** antihyperglycemic agent.

antihyperglycemic agent, an agent that counteracts high levels of glucose in the blood. See also **hypoglycemic agent**.

antihyperkalemic /an′te-, an′ti-hi′per-kah-le′mik/, **1.** effective in decreasing or preventing hyperkalemia. **2.** an agent with this effect.

antihyperlipidemic /an′te-, an′ti-hi′per-lip′ĭde′mik/, **1.** promoting a reduction of lipid levels in the blood. **2.** an agent that promotes a reduction of lipid levels in the blood.

antihypertensive /-hī·pərten′siv/, **1.** pertaining to a substance or procedure that reduces high blood pressure. **2.** an antihypertensive agent. Various drugs achieve their antihypertensive effect by depleting tissue stores of catecholamines in peripheral sites, by stimulating pressor receptors in the carotid sinus and heart, by blocking autonomic nerve impulses that constrict blood vessels, by stimulating central inhibitory alpha$_2$ receptors, or by direct vasodilation. Thiazides and other diuretic agents reduce blood pressure by decreasing blood volume. Among the numerous drugs used to treat hypertension are adrenergic blockers (alpha$_1$ and nonselective beta blockers), angiotensin-converting enzyme inhibitors, nonnitrate vasodilators (such as hydrazine and nesiritide), beta blockers, calcium channel blockers, angiotensin receptor blockers, and thiazide diuretics.

antihypertensive agent, an agent that reduces high blood pressure; there are many different types of drugs that do this. Diuretics inhibit the reabsorption of sodium in the renal tubules, causing an increase in urinary excretion of sodium and a decrease in the plasma volume and extracellular fluid volume. Drugs that act on adrenergic control of blood pressure include beta-adrenergic blocking agents, such as propranolol, which act at beta-adrenergic receptors in the heart and kidneys to reduce cardiac output and renin secretion; and others, such as methyldopa, that act on alpha-adrenergic mechanisms in the central or sympathetic nervous system to reduce peripheral vascular resistance. Vasodilatators act directly on the arterioles to produce the same effect. Almost every case of hypertension can be controlled by one of these drugs or a combination of them. The proper combination is determined by the response of the individual patient. In some cases several drugs must be tried before the right combination is found.

antihypoglycemic /an′te-, an′ti-hi′po-gli-se′mik/, **1.** counteracting hypoglycemia. **2.** an agent that counteracts hypoglycemia.

antihypotensive /-hī′pōten′siv/, pertaining to any medication or other agent that tends to increase blood pressure. Compare **antihypertensive.**

antiimmune /an′ti-imyo͞on′/ [Gk, anti + L, immunis, free from], pertaining to the prevention or inhibition of immunity. See also **immune response.**

antiinfection vitamin. See **vitamin A.**

antiinfective /-infek′shəs/ [Gk, anti + L, inficere, to stain], pertaining to an agent that prevents or treats infection.

antiinflammatory /-inflam′ətor′ē/ [Gk, anti + L, inflammare, to set afire], pertaining to a substance or procedure that counteracts or reduces inflammation.

antiinhibitor coagulant complex (AICC), a concentrated fraction from pooled human plasma, which includes vitamin K-dependent coagulation factors (factors II, VII, IX, and X), factors of the kinin-generating system, and factor VIII coagulant antigen. It is administered intravenously as an antihemorrhagic in hemophilic patients with factor VIII inhibitors. Its mechanism of action has not been elucidated but may be due at least in part to its factor Xa content.

antiinitiator /-inish′ē·ātər/, a substance that is a potential cocarcinogen but that may protect cells against cancer development if given before exposure to an initiator. An example is the food additive butylated hydroxytoluene (BHT). An antiinitiator given after exposure to an initiator may also act as a promoter and encourage rather than block cancer development.

antileprotic /-leprot′ik/, a drug or other agent that is effective in treating leprosy.

antilipidemic /an′tilip′ĭde′mik/ [Gk, anti + lipos, fat, haima, blood], **1.** pertaining to a regimen, diet, or agent that reduces the amount of lipids in the serum. Antilipidemic diets and drugs are prescribed to reduce the risk of atherosclerotic cardiovascular disease for two reasons: atheromatous plaques contain free cholesterol, and lower serum cholesterol levels and lower incidence of coronary heart disease are found in populations consuming a low-fat diet than in those on a high-fat diet. **2.** a drug used to reduce the amount of lipids in the serum. A number of pharmacologic agents are used to reduce serum lipids. Among drugs used to reduce serum lipids are bile acid sequestrants and statins. Cholestyramine and colestipol exert their antilipemic action by combining with bile acids in the intestine to form an insoluble complex that is excreted in the feces; they may reduce serum cholesterol but prevent the absorption of essential fat-soluble vitamins and may be associated with several serious side effects. Colestipol also binds and removes bile acids from the intestine. A newer class of statins interfere with the biosynthesis of cholesterol. See also **hyperlipidemia.**

Antilirium, trademark for an acetylcholinesterase drug inhibitor (physostigmine salicylate).

antimalarial /-məler′ē·əl/, **1.** pertaining to a substance that destroys or suppresses the development of malaria plasmodia or to a procedure that exterminates the mosquito vectors of the disease, such as spraying insecticides or draining swamps. **2.** an antimalarial drug that destroys or prevents the development of plasmodia in human hosts. Chloroquine hydrochloride and hydroxychloroquine sulfate are effective against *Plasmodium vivax, P. malariae,* and certain strains of *P. falciparum.* Patients with drug-resistant *P. falciparum* are often treated with a combination of quinine, pyrimethamine, and sulfadoxine. See also **malaria.**

antimalarial agent, an antiprotozoal agent particularly effective against the malaria parasite.

antimessage, a strand of viral RNA that cannot act as messenger RNA because of its negative coding sequence. It must be converted to a positive-strand sequence by a viral transcriptase before its message can be translated in a host cell.

antimetabolite /-mətab′əlīt/ [Gk, anti + metabole, change], a drug or other substance that is an antagonist to or resembles a normal human metabolite and interferes with its function in the body, usually by competing for its receptors or enzymes. Among the antimetabolites used as antineoplastic agents are the folic acid analog methotrexate and the pyrimidine analog fluorouracil. Antineoplastic mercaptopurine, an analog of the nucleotide adenine and the purine base hypoxanthine, is a metabolic antagonist of both compounds. Thioguanine, another member of a large series of purine analogs, interferes with nucleic acid synthesis. Cytarabine, used in the treatment of acute myelocytic leukemia, is a synthetic nucleoside that resembles cytidine and kills cells that actively synthesize deoxyribonucleic acid (DNA), apparently by inhibiting the enzyme DNA polymerase.

antimicrobial /-mīkrō'bē·əl/ [Gk, *anti* + *mikros*, small, *bios*, life], **1.** pertaining to a substance that kills microorganisms or inhibits their growth or replication. **2.** an agent that kills or inhibits the growth or replication of microorganisms. See also **antibiotic.**

antimicrobial drugs [Gk, *anti* + *mikros*, small *bios*, life, Fr, + *drogue*], drugs that destroy or inhibit the growth of microorganisms.

antimicrobic /-mīkrob'ik/, any agent that prevents or destroys microorganisms or inhibits their growth.

Antiminth, trademark for an anthelmintic (pyrantel pamoate).

antimitochondrial antibody (AMA) /-mī'tōkon'drē·əl/, an antibody that acts specifically against mitochondria. These antibodies are not normally present in the blood of healthy people. A laboratory test for the presence of antibodies in the blood is a valuable diagnostic aid in liver disease. Low titers may occur in chronic hepatitis, drug-induced hepatotoxicity, and various other diseases. High titers are virtually diagnostic of primary biliary cirrhosis.

antimitochondrial antibody (AMA) test, a blood test that is used primarily to help diagnose primary biliary cirrhosis. Patients with chronic active hepatitis, drug-induced cholestasis, autoimmune hepatitis, extrahepatic obstruction, or acute infection may also test positive for AMA.

antimitotic /-mītot'ik/, inhibiting cell division.

antimony (Sb) /an'təmō'nē/ [L *antimonium*], a bluish, crystalline metallic element occurring in nature. Various antimony compounds are used in the treatment of filariasis, leishmaniasis, lymphogranuloma, schistosomiasis, and trypanosomiasis and as emetics.

antimony poisoning, toxic effect caused by the ingestion or inhalation of antimony or antimony compounds, characterized by vomiting, sweating, diarrhea, and a metallic taste in the mouth. Irritation of the skin or mucous membrane may result from external exposure. Severe poisoning resembles arsenic poisoning. Antimony and antimony compounds are common ingredients of many substances used in medicine and industry.

antimorph /an'təmôrf/ [Gk, *anti* + *morphe*, form], a mutant allele that inhibits or antagonizes the influence of the normal allele in the expression of a trait. Compare **amorph, hypermorph, hypomorph.**

antimuscarinic /-mus'kərin'ik/ [Gk, *anti* + L, *musca*, fly], effective against the poisonous activity of muscarine. See also **muscarinic.**

antimutagen /-myoo'təjən/ [Gk, *anti* + L, *mutare*, to change; Gk, *genein*, to produce], **1.** any substance that reduces the rate of spontaneous mutations or counteracts or reverses the action of a mutagen. **2.** any technique that protects cells against the effects of mutagens. —**antimutagenic,** *adj.*

antimyasthenic /an'te-, an'ti-mi'as-then'ik/, **1.** counteracting or relieving muscular weakness in myasthenia gravis. **2.** an agent that counteracts or relieves muscular weakness in myasthenia gravis.

antimycotic. See **antifungal.**

antimyocardial antibody (AMA) test, a blood test used to detect an autoimmune source of myocardial injury and disease, such as rheumatic heart disease, cardiomyopathy, postthoracotomy syndrome, and postmyocardial infarction. This test may also be used to monitor these conditions' response to treatment.

antineoplastic /-nē'ōplas'tik/ [Gk, *anti* + *neos*, new, *plasma*, something formed], **1.** pertaining to a substance, procedure, or measure that prevents the proliferation of cells, **2.** a chemotherapeutic agent that controls or kills cancer cells.

Drugs used in the treatment of cancer are cytotoxic but are generally more damaging to dividing cells than to resting cells. Cycle-specific antineoplastic agents are more effective in killing proliferating cells than in killing resting cells, and phase-specific agents are most active during a specific phase of the cell cycle. Most anticancer drugs prevent the proliferation of cells by inhibiting the synthesis of deoxyribonucleic acid (DNA) by various mechanisms. Alkylating agents, such as nitrogen mustard derivatives, ethylenimine derivatives, and alkyl sulfonates, interfere with DNA replication by causing cross-linking of DNA strands and abnormal pairing of nucleotides. Antimetabolites exert their action by interfering with the formation of compounds required for cell division. The folic acid analog methotrexate and 5-fluorouracil, a pyrimidine analog, inhibit enzymes required for the formation of the essential DNA constituent thymidine. Hypoxanthine analog 6-mercaptopurine and 6-thioguanine, an analog of guanine, interfere with the biosynthesis of purines. Vinblastine and vincristine, alkaloids derived from the periwinkle plant, disrupt cell division by interfering with the formation of the mitotic spindle. Antineoplastic antibiotics, such as doxorubicin, daunomycin, and mitomycin, block or inhibit DNA synthesis; dactinomycin and mithramycin interfere with ribonucleic acid synthesis. Cytotoxic chemotherapeutic agents may be administered orally, intravenously, or by infusion. All have untoward and unpleasant side effects and are potentially immunosuppressive and dangerous. Estrogens and androgens, although not considered antineoplastic agents, frequently cause tumor regression when administered in high doses to patients with hormone-dependent cancers. See also **alkylating agent, antimetabolite.**

antineoplastic antibiotic, a chemical substance derived from a microorganism or a synthetic analog of the substance, used in cancer chemotherapy. Dactinomycin, used in the treatment of Wilms' tumor, testicular carcinoma, choriocarcinoma, rhabdomyosarcoma, and some other sarcomas, exerts its antineoplastic effect by interfering with ribonucleic acid (RNA) synthesis. Mithramycin, with a similar mechanism of action, is also administered for testicular cancer and for trophoblastic neoplasms. Doxorubicin, a broad-spectrum agent that is especially useful in treating breast carcinoma, lymphomas, sarcomas, and acute leukemia, and closely related daunomycin, which is also effective in acute leukemias, block the biosynthesis of RNA. Mitomycin C, prescribed for gastric, breast, cervical, and head and neck carcinomas, cross-links strands of deoxyribonucleic acid (DNA). Bleomycin, used in the treatment of squamous cell carcinomas of the head and neck, testicular carcinoma, and lymphomas, damages DNA and prevents its repair. Antineoplastic antibiotics depress bone marrow and usually cause nausea and vomiting; several cause alopecia.

antineoplastic hormone, a chemically synthesized or a synthetic analog of the naturally occurring compound used to control certain disseminated cancers. Hormonal therapy is designed to counteract the effect of an endogenous hormone required for tumor growth. The estrogens diethylstilbestrol (DES) and ethinyl estradiol may be used in palliative treatment of a prostatic carcinoma that is nonresectable or unresponsive to radiotherapy. An androgen, such as testosterone propionate, testolactone, or fluoxymesterone, may be administered postoperatively to control disseminated breast cancer in women whose tumor is estrogen-dependent. The antiestrogen tamoxifen produces responses in many patients with advanced estrogen-dependent breast cancer. Paradoxically, large doses of estrogen, frequently used to control disseminated breast cancer in postmenopausal women, apparently check the growth of tumors by inhibiting the secretion of estrogen by the adrenal gland. Some progestins produce a favorable response in women with disseminated endometrial carcinoma and, occasionally, in patients with prostatic or renal cancers. These progestins include megestrol acetate, medroxyprogesterone acetate, and 17-alphahydroxyprogesterone caproate.

antineoplaston, a naturally occurring peptide, amino acid derivative, or carboxylic acid proposed to control neoplastic cell growth using the patient's own biochemical defense system, which works jointly with the immune system.

antineuritic vitamin. See **thiamine.**

antineutrophil cytoplasmic antibody test, a blood test used to diagnose Wegener's granulomatosis (WG). It is also used to follow the course of the disease, monitor its response to therapy, and detect early relapse.

antinuclear antibody (ANA) /-noo'klē-ər/, an autoantibody that reacts with nuclear material. Antinuclear antibodies are found in the blood serum of patients with rheumatoid arthritis, systemic lupus erythematosus, Sjögren's syndrome, polymyositis, and a number of nonrheumatic disorders ranging from lymphomas and leukemias to adverse drug reactions. The antibodies are often detected with an immunofluorescent assay technique.

antinuclear antibody (ANA) test, a blood test used primarily to help diagnose systemic lupus erythematosus (SLE), although a positive result may also indicate other autoimmune diseases such as Sjögren's syndrome, scleroderma, Raynaud's disease, mixed connective tissue disease, rheumatoid arthritis, primary biliary cirrhosis, thyroiditis, and chronic active hepatitis.

antiodontalgia /an'ti-ō'dontal'jə/, a toothache remedy.

antioncogene /an'ti-on'kəjēn/, a tumor-suppressing gene. It may act by controlling cellular growth. When an antioncogene is inactivated, tumor cellular proliferation begins and tumor activity accelerates.

antioxidant /-ok'sidənt/, a chemical or other agent that inhibits or retards oxidation of a substance to which it is added. Examples include butylated hydroxyanisole (BHA) and butylated hydroxytoluene (BHT). These substances are added to foods or the packaging of foods containing fats or oils to prevent oxygen from combining with the fatty molecules, thereby causing them to become rancid.

antioxidation /-ok'sidā'shən/, the prevention of oxidation.

antiparallel /-per'ələl/ [Gk, *anti + parallelos,* side-by-side], pertaining to molecules, such as strands of DNA, that are parallel but are oriented in opposite directions.

antiparasitic /-per'əsit'ik/ [Gk, *anti + parasitos,* guest], **1.** pertaining to a substance or procedure that kills parasites or inhibits their growth or reproduction. **2.** an antiparasitic drug such as an amebicide, an anthelmintic, an antimalarial, a schistosomicide, a trichomonacide, or a trypanosomicide.

antiparkinsonian /-pär'kənsəniz'əm/, pertaining to a substance or procedure used to treat parkinsonism. Drugs for this neurologic disorder are of two kinds: those that compensate for the lack of dopamine in the corpus striatum of parkinsonism patients, and anticholinergic agents that counteract the activity of the abundant acetylcholine in the striatum. Synthetic levodopa, a dopamine precursor that crosses the blood-brain barrier, is administered to patients to reduce the rigidity, sluggishness, dysphagia, drooling, and instability characteristic of the disease, but the drug does not alter the relentless course of the disorder. Centrally active cholinergic blockers, notably benztropine, biperiden, procyclidine, and trihexyphenidyl, may relieve tremors and rigidity and improve mobility. The antiviral agent amantadine is often effective in the treatment of parkinsonism; its mecha-

nism of action is not established, but it apparently increases release of dopamine in the brain. Therapeutic approaches to the relief of the symptoms of parkinsonism include alcohol injection, cautery, cryosurgery, and surgical excision performed to destroy the globus pallidus (reducing rigidity) and parts of the thalamus (reducing tremor). Extrapyramidal symptoms similar to those of idiopathic parkinsonism are frequently induced by antipsychotic drugs. See also **tardive dyskinesia.**

antipathic /-path'ik/, pertaining to a strong or excessive aversion or dislike.

antipathy /antip'əthē/ [Gk, *anti + pathos,* suffering], a strong feeling of aversion or antagonism to particular objects, situations, or individuals.

antiperistalsis /-per'əstal'sis/, a wave of contractions in the digestive tract that moves toward the oral end of the tract. In the duodenum, stomach, or esophagus it results in regurgitation. Also called **reverse peristalsis.**

antiperistaltic /-per'əstal'tik/ [Gk, *anti + peristellein,* to wrap around], **1.** pertaining to a substance that inhibits or diminishes peristalsis. **2.** an antiperistaltic agent. Opioids, such as paregoric, diphenoxylate, and loperamide hydrochloride, are antiperistaltic agents used to provide symptomatic relief in diarrhea. Anticholinergic (parasympatholytic) drugs reduce spasms of intestinal smooth muscle and are frequently prescribed to decrease excessive GI motility.

antipernicious anemia factor. See **cyanocobalamin.**

antiplatelet /-plat'lit/, any agent that destroys platelets or inhibits their function.

antipode /an'tipōd/, something that is diametrically opposite.

antipraxia /prak'sē·ə/, a condition in which functions or symptoms appear to oppose each other.

antiprogestin /-prōjes'tin/, a substance that interferes with the production, uptake, or effects of progesterone. The most common example is mifepristone.

antiprotease, a substance that is capable of preventing the digestion of proteins.

antiprothrombin /prōthrom'bin/, a substance that inhibits the conversion of prothrombin to thrombin.

antiprotoplasmatic /-prō'təplasmat'ik/, pertaining to agents that damage the protoplasm of cells.

antiprotozoal /an'te-, an'ti-pro-to-zo'al/, **1.** destroying protozoa or checking their growth or reproduction. **2.** antiprotozoal agent.

antiprotozoal agent, an agent that destroys protozoa or checks their growth or reproduction. Antimalarial agents are one type.

antipruritic /-prŏŏrit'ik/ [Gk, *anti + L, prurire,* to itch], **1.** pertaining to a substance or procedure that tends to relieve or prevent itching. **2.** an antipruritic drug. Topical anesthetics, corticosteroids, and antihistamines are used as antipruritic agents.

antipsoriatic /an'tisôr'ē·at'ik/ [Gk, *anti + psora,* itch], pertaining to an agent that relieves the symptoms of psoriasis.

antipsychotic /-sīkot'ik/ [Gk, *anti + psyche,* mind, *osis,* condition], **1.** pertaining to a substance or procedure that counteracts or diminishes symptoms of a psychosis. **2.** an antipsychotic drug. Phenothiazine derivatives are the oldest antipsychotics for use in the treatment of schizophrenia and other major affective disorders. They apparently act by enhancing the filtering mechanisms of the reticular formation in the brainstem and by blocking central dopamine receptors. See also **neuroleptic, tranquilizer.**

antipsychotic agent, any drug that favorably modifies psychotic symptoms; categories include the phenothiazines, butyrophenones, thioxanthenes, dibenzodiazepines, diphenylbutylpiperidines, dihydroindolones, and dibenzoxazepines. They are chemically diverse but pharmacologically similar. Formerly called *major tranquilizer.*

antipyresis /-pīrē'sis/ [Gk, *anti* + *pyretos,* fever], treatment to reduce and ameliorate fever.

antipyretic /-pīret'ik/ [Gk, *anti* + *pyretos,* fever], **1.** pertaining to a substance or procedure that reduces fever. **2.** an antipyretic agent. Such drugs usually lower the thermodetection set point of the hypothalamic heat regulatory center, with resulting vasodilation and sweating. Widely used antipyretic agents are acetaminophen, aspirin, and NSAIDs. Also called **antifebrile, antithermic.**

antipyretic bath, a bath in which tepid water is used to reduce body temperature.

antipyrotic /-pīrot'ik/ [Gk, *anti* + *pyr,* fire], pertaining to the treatment of burns or scalds.

antirabies serum, antiserum obtained from the blood serum or plasma of animals immunized with rabies vaccine; used for postexposure prophylaxis against rabies if rabies immune globulin is unavailable.

antirachitic /-rəkit'ik/, pertaining to an agent used to treat rickets.

antiretroviral /an'te-, an'ti-ret'ro-vi'ral/, **1.** effective against retroviruses. **2.** an agent with this quality.

anti-Rh agglutinin, an antibody to the Rh antigen present on Rh+ red blood cells that causes these cells to clump (agglutinate). This antibody is produced by Rh– persons after exposure to Rh+ red blood cells, as when an Rh– mother is pregnant with an Rh+ fetus.

antirheumatic /-rōōmat'ik/ [Gk, *anti* + *rheumatismos,* that which flows], pertaining to the relief of symptoms of any painful or immobilizing disorder of the musculoskeletal system.

anti-Ri antibody, an autoantibody having neuronal binding characteristics similar to those of anti-Hu antibody but directed against a different RNA-binding site; it is associated with paraneoplastic opsoclonus-myoclonus in small cell lung carcinoma cancer of the breast and fallopian tube. Also called *type 2 antineuronal antibody (ANNA-2).*

antiscorbutic vitamin. See **ascorbic acid.**

antiseborrheic /-seb'ərē'ik/, pertaining to a drug or agent that is applied to the skin to control seborrhea or seborrheic dermatitis.

antisense /an'tēsens/, pertaining to an RNA molecule that is complementary to the messenger RNA (mRNA) produced by transcription of a given gene. Antisense RNA synthesized in the laboratory will hybridize with the complementary mRNA molecules, thereby blocking the synthesis of specific proteins.

antisense strand, the strand of a double-stranded nucleic acid that is complementary to the sense strand, in DNA being thus the template strand on which the mRNA is synthesized. Compare **sense strand.**

antisepsis /-sep'sis/ [Gk, *anti* + *sepein,* putrefaction], destruction of microorganisms to prevent infection.

antiseptic /-sep'tik/, **1.** tending to inhibit the growth and reproduction of microorganisms. **2.** a substance that tends to inhibit the growth and reproduction of microorganisms when applied to living tissue. See also **disinfectant.**

antiseptic dressing, a fabric or pad treated with a solution and applied to a wound or an incision to prevent or treat infection. The solution may be an antiseptic, germicidal, or bacteriostatic.

antiseptic gauze, a dressing permeated with a solution to prevent infection.

antiserum *pl.* **antisera, antiserums** /an'tisir'əm/ [Gk, *anti* + L, whey], serum of an animal or human containing antibodies against a specific disease, used to confer passive immunity to that disease. Antisera do not provoke the production of antibodies. There are two types of antiserum: antitoxin is an antiserum that neutralizes the toxin produced by specific bacteria, but it does not kill the bacteria; antimicrobial serum acts to destroy bacteria by making them more susceptible to the leukocytic action. Polyvalent antiserum acts on more than one epitope; monovalent antiserum acts on only one. Antibiotic drugs have largely replaced antimicrobial antisera. Caution is always to be used in administration of antiserum of any kind, since hepatitis or hypersensitivity reactions can result. Also called **immune serum.** Compare **vaccine.**

antiserum anaphylaxis, an exaggerated hypersensitivity in a normal person after the injection of serum from a sensitized individual. Also called **passive anaphylaxis.** Compare **active anaphylaxis.**

antishock garment, trousers designed to apply pressure on circulation in the lower part of the body, thereby increasing the amount of blood in the upper part.

antisialogog /-sī·al'əgōg'/ [Gk, *anti* + *sialon,* saliva, *agogos,* leading], a drug that reduces saliva secretion.

antismooth muscle antibody test, a blood test used primarily to help diagnose autoimmune chronic active hepatitis, although a low-level positive result may also be associated with viral infections, malignancy, multiple sclerosis, primary biliary cirrhosis, and *Mycoplasma* infections.

antisocial personality /-sō'shəl/ [Gk, *anti* + L, *socius,* companion], a person who exhibits attitudes and overt behavior contrary to the customs, standards, and moral principles accepted by society. Also called **psychopathic personality, sociopathic personality.** See also **antisocial personality disorder.**

antisocial personality disorder, a condition characterized by repetitive behavioral patterns that are contrary to usual moral and ethical standards and cause a person to experience continuous conflict with society. Symptoms include aggressiveness, callousness, impulsiveness, irresponsibility, hostility, a low frustration level, a marked emotional immaturity, and poor judgment. A person who has this disorder overlooks the rights of others, is incapable of loyalty to others or to social values, is unable to experience guilt or to learn from past behaviors, is impervious to punishment, and tends to rationalize his or her behavior or to blame it on others. Also called **antisocial reaction.**

antispasmodic /-spazmod'ik/, a drug or other agent that prevents smooth muscle spasms, as in the uterus, digestive system, or urinary tract. Belladonna and dicyclomine hydrochloride are among drugs used in antispasmodic preparations. See also **anticholinergic, cholinergic blocking agent.**

antispastic /an'te-, an'ti-spas'tik/, antispasmodic with specific reference to skeletal muscle.

antisperm antibody (ASA), any of various surface-bound antibodies found on sperm after infection, trauma to the testes, or vasectomy; they interfere with the fertilization process or result in nonviable zygotes.

antispermatozoal antibody test, a fluid analysis or blood test used as an infertility screening test. The test may be done on both men and women to detect the presence of sperm antibodies that may diminish fertility.

antistreptolysin-O test (ASOT, ASO, ASLT) /an'tistrep'təlī'sinō'/, a streptococcal antibody test for finding and measuring serum antibodies to streptolysin-O, an exotoxin produced by most group A and some group C and G streptococci. The test is often used as an aid in the diagnosis of rheumatic fever and glomerulonephritis. A low titer of antistreptolysin-O antibody is present in most people, since streptococcal infection is common. Elevated or increasing titers indicate a recent infection. The normal findings for adults are equal to or less than 160 Todd units/ml. See also **Lancefield's classification.**

antithermic. See **antipyretic.**

antithrombin /-throm'bin/, a substance that inhibits the action of thrombin.

antithrombotic /-thrombot'ik/, preventing or interfering with the formation of a thrombus or blood coagulation.

antithymocyte globulin (ATG) /an'tithi'məsīt/, the gamma globulin fraction of antiserum derived from animals that have been immunized against human thymocytes; an immunosuppressive agent that causes specific destruction of T lymphocytes, used in treatment of allograft rejection. The term is sometimes used interchangeably with *antilymphocyte globulin.*

antithymocyte globulin (rabbit), a purified gamma globulin obtained from rabbits immunized with human thymocytes; administered intravenously in the treatment of acute rejection occurring after renal transplantation and experimentally in the treatment of rejection occurring after various other transplant procedures.

antithyroglobulin antibody test, a blood test used primarily in the differential diagnosis of thyroid diseases such as Hashimoto's thyroiditis or chronic lymphocytic thyroiditis in children. This test is usually performed in conjunction with the antithyroid microsomal antibody test.

antithyroid drug /-thī'roid/, a preparation that inhibits the synthesis of thyroid hormones and is commonly used in the treatment of hyperthyroidism. The major antithyroid drugs are thioamides, such as propylthiouracil, and methimazole. In the body such substances interfere with the incorporation of iodine into the tyrosyl residues of thyroglobulin required for the production of the hormones thyroxine and triiodothyronine. These drugs are often used to control hyperthyroidism during an anticipated remission and before a thyroidectomy.

antithyroid microsomal antibody test, a blood test used primarily in the differential diagnosis of thyroid diseases such as Hashimoto's thyroiditis or chronic lymphocytic thyroiditis in children. This test is usually performed in conjunction with the antithyroglobulin antibody test.

antitoxin /-tok'sin/ [Gk, *anti* + *toxikon,* poison], a subgroup of antisera usually prepared from the serum of horses immunized against a particular toxin-producing organism, such as botulism antitoxin given therapeutically in botulism and tetanus and diphtheria antitoxins given prophylactically to prevent those infections.

antitrismus /-tris'məs/, a tonic muscular spasm that forces the mouth to open.

antitrust /-trust'/, (in law) against the operation, establishment, or maintenance of a monopoly in the manufacture, production, or sale of a commodity, provision of a service, or practice of a profession.

antitrypsin /-trip'sin/, a protein, produced in the liver, that blocks the action of trypsin and other proteolytic enzymes. A deficiency of antitrypsin is associated with emphysema, in which the basic lesion is believed to result from effects of proteolytic enzymes on the walls of the alveoli. Also called **alpha-antitrypsin.**

antitubercular /-tŏŏbur'kyələr/, any agent or group of drugs used to treat tuberculosis. At least two drugs, and usually three, are required in various combinations in pulmonary tuberculosis therapy. These include isoniazid (INH), ethambutol (EMB), streptomycin (SM), and rifampin (RMP). Supplements of pyridoxine (vitamin B_6) also may be needed to relieve the symptoms of peripheral neuritis that can occur as an INH side effect.

antitumor antibodies, natural products that interfere with deoxyribonucleic acid (DNA) in such a way as to prevent its further replication and the transcription of ribonucleic acid.

antitussive /an'titus'iv/ [Gk, *anti* + L, *tussive,* cough], **1.** against a cough. **2.** any of a large group of opioid and nonopioid drugs that act on the central and peripheral nervous systems to suppress the cough reflex. Because the cough reflex is necessary for clearing the upper respiratory tract of obstructive secretions, antitussives should not be used with a productive cough. Codeine and hydrocodone are potent opioid antitussives. Dextromethorphan is an effective antitussive with no dependence liability. Antitussives are administered orally, usually in a syrup with a mucolytic or expectorant and alcohol, or, sometimes, in a capsule with an antihistaminic and a mild analgesic.

antiurolithic /an'te-u'ro-lith'ik/, **1.** preventing formation of urinary calculi. **2.** an agent that so acts.

antivenin /an'tiven'in/ [Gk, *anti* + L, *venenum,* poison], a suspension of venom-neutralizing antibodies prepared from the serum of immunized horses. Antivenin confers passive immunity and is given as a part of emergency first aid for various snake and insect bites. Also called **antivenom.**

Antivert, trademark for an antihistaminic antivertigo agent (meclizine hydrochloride).

antiviral, destructive to viruses.

antivirus software, a software program written so that on execution (this is usually automatic on boot up) it scans the hard drive and related processors to identify, isolate and eradicate the virus. Modern antivirus software requests updates automatically on a schedule set either by default or by the user.

antivitamin factor [Gk, *anti* + L, *vita,* life, amine], a substance that inactivates a vitamin.

antixerophthalmic vitamin. See **vitamin A.**

anti-Yo antibody, polyclonal IgG autoantibody directed against Purkinje cells and associated with paraneoplastic cerebellar degeneration in small cell lung carcinoma and cancer of the breast or ovary. Also called *anti-Purkinje cell antibody (APCA).*

Anton's syndrome [Gabriel Anton, German neuropsychiatrist, 1858–1933], a form of anosognosia in which a person with partial or total blindness denies being visually impaired, despite medical evidence to the contrary. The patient typically contrives excuses for the inability to see, such as suggesting that the light is inadequate.

Antopol-Goldman lesion, subepithelial hematoma of renal pelvis.

antr-. See **antro-.**

antra. See **antrum.**

antral gastritis [Gk, *antron,* cave], an abnormal narrowing of the antrum, or distal portion of the stomach. The narrowing is not a true gastritis, but a radiographic finding that may represent gastric ulcer or tumor.

antrectomy /antrek'təmē/, the surgical excision of the pyloric part of the stomach.

antro-, antr-, prefix meaning 'antrum or sinus': *antrocele, antrodynia.*

antrum, *pl.* **antra** [Gk, *antron,* cave], a cavity or chamber that is nearly closed and usually surrounded by bone. The cardiac antrum is a dilation of the esophagus. The fluid-filled cavity in a mature graafian follicle is also termed an antrum.

antrum cardiacum /an'trəm/, a constricted passage from the esophagus to the stomach, lying just inside the opening formed by the cardiac sphincter.

antrum of Highmore. See **maxillary sinus.**

Anturane, trademark for a uricosuric (sulfinpyrazone).

ANUG, abbreviation for **acute necrotizing ulcerative gingivitis.**

anular /an'yələr/ [L, *annulus,* ring], describing a ring-shaped lesion surrounding a clear, normal, unaffected disk of skin.

Anular psoriasis *(du Vivier, 1993)*

anular ligament, a ligament that encircles the head of the radius and holds it in the radial notch of the ulna. Distal to the notch, the anular ligament forms a complete fibrous ring.

anulus /an'yələs/, a ring of circular tissue, such as the whitish tympanic anulus around the perimeter of the tympanic membrane.

anuresis. See **anuria.**

anuria /ənoor'ē-ə/ [Gk, *a, ouron,* not urine], the absence of urine production or a urinary output of less than 100 ml per day. Anuria may be caused by kidney failure or dysfunction, a decline in blood pressure below that required to maintain filtration pressure in the kidney, or an obstruction in the urinary passages. A rapid decline in urinary output, leading ultimately to anuria and uremia, occurs in acute renal failure. Kinds of anuria include **angioneurotic anuria, obstructive anuria, postrenal anuria, prerenal anuria,** and **renal anuria.** Also called **anuresis** /an'yoore'sis/. —**anuric, anuretic,** *adj.* Compare **oliguria.**

anus /ā'nəs/, the outlet at the terminal end of the anal canal lying in the fold between the buttocks.

anxietas /angzī'ətas/ [L, anxiety], a state of anxiety, nervous restlessness, or apprehension, often accompanied by a feeling of oppression in the epigastrium. Kinds of anxietas are **anxietas presenilis** and **restless legs syndrome.**

anxietas presenilis [L, *anxietas + prae,* before, *senex,* aged], a state of extreme anxiety associated with the climacteric period of life.

anxietas tibiarum. See **restless legs syndrome.**

anxiety[1] /angzī'ətē/ [L *anxietas*], anticipation of impending danger and dread accompanied by restlessness, tension, tachycardia, and breathing difficulty not necessarily associated with an apparent stimulus. Kinds of anxiety include **castration anxiety, generalized** or **"free-floating" anxiety, separation anxiety, panic anxiety,** and **situational anxiety.**

anxiety[2], a nursing diagnosis accepted by the Fifth National Conference on the Classification of Nursing Diagnoses. Anxiety is defined as a vague, uneasy feeling, the source of which is often nonspecific or unknown to the individual.

■ DEFINING CHARACTERISTICS: The defining characteristics of anxiety may be subjective or objective. Subjective characteristics include increased tension, apprehension, persistent increased helplessness, and feelings of uncertainty, inadequacy, fear, overexcitability, distress, worry, and impending doom. Objective characteristics include increased heart rate, dilated pupils, restlessness, insomnia, glancing about, poor eye contact, trembling, facial tension, quivering voice, self-focus, increased perspiration, and expressed concern regarding life events.

■ RELATED FACTORS: Related factors include an unconscious conflict regarding essential values or goals of life; threat to self-concept; threat of death; threat to or of change in health status, the environment, or interaction patterns; situational or maturational crises; interpersonal transmission of contagion, and unmet needs.

anxiety attack, an acute, psychobiologic reaction manifested by intense anxiety and panic. Symptoms include palpitations, shortness of breath, dizziness, faintness, profuse sweating, pallor of the face and extremities, GI discomfort, and a vague feeling of imminent doom or death. Attacks usually occur suddenly, last from a few seconds to an hour or longer, and vary in frequency from several times a day to once a month. Treatment consists of reassurance, separation of the individual from anxiety-producing situations, administration of a sedative if necessary, and appropriate psychotherapy to identify the stresses perceived as threatening. See also **anxiety.**

anxiety complex. See **castration anxiety.**

anxiety control, a nursing outcome from the Nursing Outcomes Classification (NOC) defined as personal actions to eliminate or reduce feelings of apprehension and tension from an unidentifiable source. See also **Nursing Outcomes Classification.**

anxiety, death, a nursing diagnosis accepted by the Thirteenth National Conference on the Classification of Nursing Diagnoses. The condition is the apprehension, worry, or fear related to death or dying.

■ DEFINING CHARACTERISTICS: The condition is characterized by worrying about the impact of one's own death on significant others; feelings of powerlessness over issues related to dying; fear of loss of physical and/or mental abilities when dying; anticipated pain related to dying; deep sadness; fear of the process of dying; concerns of overworking the caregiver as terminal illness incapacitates self; concern about meeting one's creator or feeling doubtful about the existence of a higher being; total loss of control over any aspect of one's death; negative death images or unpleasant thoughts about any event related to death or dying; fear of delayed demise; fear of premature death because it prevents the accomplishment of important life goals; worry about being the cause of other's grief and suffering; fear of leaving family alone after death; fear of developing a terminal illness, and denial of one's own mortality or impending death.

■ RELATED FACTORS: Related factors are to be developed. See also **nursing diagnosis.**

anxiety disorder, a disorder in which anxiety is the most prominent feature. The symptoms range from mild, chronic tenseness, with feelings of timidity, fatigue, apprehension, and indecisiveness, to more intense states of restlessness and irritability that may lead to aggressive acts, persistent helplessness, or withdrawal. In extreme cases, the overwhelming emotional discomfort is accompanied by physical responses,

Physiological, behavioral, cognitive, and affective responses to anxiety

Physiological	Physiological—cont'd	Behavioral	Cognitive	Affective
Cardiovascular	*Neuromuscular*	Restlessness	Impaired attention	Edginess
Palpitations	Increased reflexes	Physical tension	Poor concentration	Impatience
Heart racing	Startle reaction	Tremors	Forgetfulness	Uneasiness
Increased blood pressure	Eyelid twitching	Startle reaction	Errors in judgment	Tension
Faintness*	Insomnia	Rapid speech	Preoccupation	Nervousness
Actual fainting*	Tremors	Lack of coordination	Blocking of thoughts	Fear
Decreased blood pressure*	Rigidity	Accident proneness	Decreased perceptual field	Fright
Decreased pulse rate*	Fidgeting	Interpersonal withdrawal	Reduced creativity	Alarm
	Pacing	Inhibition	Diminished productivity	Terror
Respiratory	Strained face	Flight	Confusion	Jitteriness
Rapid breathing	Generalized weakness	Avoidance	Hypervigilance	Jumpiness
Shortness of breath	Wobbly legs	Hyperventilation	Self-consciousness	
Pressure on chest	Clumsy movement		Loss of objectivity	
Shallow breathing			Fear of losing control	
Lump in throat	*Urinary Tract*		Frightening visual images	
Choking sensation	Pressure to urinate*		Fear of injury or death	
Gasping	Frequent urination*			
Gastrointestinal	*Skin*			
Loss of appetite	Face flushed			
Revulsion toward food	Localized sweating (palms)			
Abdominal discomfort	Itching			
Abdominal pain*	Hot and cold spells			
Nausea*	Face pale			
Heartburn*	Generalized sweating			
Diarrhea*				

From Stuart GW, Sundeen: *Principles and practice of psychiatric nursing,* ed 5, St Louis, 1995, Mosby.
*Parasympathetic response.

including tremor, sustained muscle tension, tachycardia, dyspnea, hypertension, increased respiration, and profuse perspiration. Other physical signs include changes in skin color, nausea, vomiting, diarrhea, restlessness, immobilization, insomnia, and changes in appetite, all occurring without identification of a known underlying organic cause. See also **anxiety, anxiety attack, anxiety reaction, anxiety state, obsessive-compulsive disorder, phobia.**

anxiety dream, a dream that is accompanied by restlessness and a gradual increase in pulse rate. Anxiety dreams tend to occur in children, who usually recall the content clearly.

anxiety level, a nursing outcome from the Nursing Outcomes Classification (NOC) defined as the severity of manifested apprehension, tension, or uneasiness arising from an unidentifiable source. See also **Nursing Outcomes Classification.**

anxiety reaction [L, *anxietas* + *re, agere,* to act], a clinical characteristic in which anxiety is the predominant feature or is experienced by a person facing a dreaded situation to the extent that his or her functioning is impaired. The reaction may be expressed as a panic disorder, a phobia, or a compulsion.

anxiety reduction, a nursing intervention from the Nursing Interventions Classification (NIC) defined as minimizing apprehension, dread, foreboding, or uneasiness related to an unidentified source of anticipated danger. See also **Nursing Interventions Classification.**

anxiety state [L, *anxietas* + *state*], a mental or emotional reaction characterized by apprehension, uncertainty, and irrational fear. Anxiety states may be accompanied by physiologic changes such as sweating, tremors, rapid heartbeat, dilated pupils, and dry mouth.

anxiolytic /angk′sē-ōlit′ik/, a drug used primarily to treat episodes of anxiety. Common kinds of anxiolytics include benzodiazepines, buspirone, and the barbiturates, which are important historically but are now used less often.

AOA, abbreviation for **Administration on Aging.**

AORN, abbreviation for **Association of Operating Room Nurses.**

aorta /ā·ôr′tə/ [Gk, *aerein,* to raise], the main trunk of the systemic arterial circulation, comprising four parts: the ascending aorta, the arch of the aorta, the thoracic portion of the descending aorta, and the abdominal portion of the descending aorta. It starts at the aortic opening of the left ventricle, rises a short distance, bends over the root of the left lung, descends within the thorax on the left side of the vertebral column, and passes through the aortic hiatus of the diaphragm into the abdominal cavity. It branches into the two common iliac arteries.

aortic /ā·ôr′tik/ [Gk, *aerein,* to raise], pertaining to the aorta.

aortic aneurysm, a localized dilation of the wall of the aorta caused by atherosclerosis, hypertension, or, less frequently, syphilis. The lesion may be a saccular distension, a fusiform or cylindrical swelling of a length of the vessel, or a longitudinal dissection between the outer and middle layers of the vessel wall. Syphilitic aneurysms almost always occur in the thoracic aorta and usually involve the aortic arch. The more common atherosclerotic aneurysms are usually in the abdominal aorta below the renal arteries and above the bifurcation of the aorta. These lesions often contain atheromatous ulcers covered by thrombi that may discharge emboli, causing obstruction of smaller vessels. See also **dissecting aneurysm.**

aortic angiogram. See **aortogram.**

aortic arch. See **arch of the aorta.**

aortic arch syndrome, any of a group of occlusive conditions of the aortic arch producing a variety of symptoms

Ruptured abdominal aortic aneurysm
(Kumar, Abbas, and Fausto, 2005)

Reduced cardiac output with angina and fatigue

Elevated left atrial pressure

Eventual pulmonary artery congestion and right ventricular failure may occur

Diastolic regurgitation through aortic valve

Left ventricular hypertrophy and dilatation and decreased cardiac output

Effects of aortic regurgitation *(Beare and Myers, 1998)*

related to obstruction of the large branch arteries, including the brachiocephalic, left common carotid, and left subclavian. It may be caused by atherosclerosis, Takayasu's arteritis, syphilis, and other conditions. Symptoms include syncope, temporary blindness, hemiplegia, aphasia, and memory loss.

aortic atresia [Gk, *aeirein* + *a, tresis,* a boring], a congenital anomaly in which the left side of the heart is defective and there is an imperforation of the aortic valve into the aorta.

aortic balloon pump. See **intraaortic balloon pump.**

aortic body, one of several small structures on the aortic arch that contain neural tissue sensitive to the chemical composition of arterial blood. The aortic bodies respond primarily to large reductions in blood oxygen content and trigger an increase in respiratory rate. See also **aortic-body reflex, carotid body.**

aortic-body reflex, a neural reflex in which a decrease in the oxygen content of arterial blood is sensed by the aortic bodies, which signal the medullary respiratory center to increase respiratory rate. See also **carotid-body reflex.**

aortic insufficiency, the flow of blood from the aorta back into the left ventricle during diastole, resulting from a failure of the aortic valve to close completely. Also called **aortic regurgitation.**

aortic notch [Gk, *aeirein,* to raise; OFr, *enochier*], the dicrotic notch on the descending limb of an arterial pulse sphygmogram. It marks the closure of the aortic valve.

aortic obstruction [L, *obstruere,* to build against], a blockage or impediment that interrupts the flow of blood in the aorta.

aorticopulmonary septum, a septum, formed by fusion of the bulbar ridges, that divides the bulbus cordis into aortic and pulmonary trunks.

aortic reconstruction, restoration of function to a damaged aorta as by bypass or aortoplasty.

aortic regurgitant murmur [Gk, *aeirein,* to raise; L, *re,* again, *gurgitare,* to flow, *murmur,* humming], a high-pitched, soft, blowing, decrescendo, early diastolic heart murmur that is a sign of aortic regurgitation.

aortic regurgitation, the flow of blood from the aorta back into the left ventricle during diastole, resulting from a failure of the aortic valve to close completely. Also called **aortic insufficiency.**

aortic sinus [Gk, *aeirein,* to raise; L, *sinus,* little hollow], any of three dilations, one anterior and two posterior, between the aortic wall and the semilunar cusps of the aortic valve. Also called **Petit's sinus, sinus of Morgagni, sinus of Valsalva.**

aortic stenosis (AS) [Gk, *aeirein* + *stenos,* narrow, *osis,* condition], a narrowing or stricture of the aortic valve secondary to congenital malformation or fusion of the cusps, as may result from rheumatic fever. Aortic stenosis obstructs the flow of blood from the left ventricle into the aorta, causing decreased cardiac output and pulmonary vascular congestion. It may lead to congestive heart failure. Clinical manifestations include faint peripheral pulses, exercise intolerance, angina-type pain, and a harsh midsystolic murmur often introduced by an ejection sound. Diagnosis is confirmed by cardiac catheterization or echocardiography. Surgical repair may be indicated. Surgery is followed by frequent examinations because recurrence of the stenosis and bacterial endocarditis are relatively common sequelae. Children with aortic stenosis are usually restricted from strenuous activities. See also **congenital cardiac anomaly, valvular heart disease.**

Aortic stenosis *(Damjanov and Linder, 2000)*

aortic thrill [Gk, *aeirein,* to raise; AS, *thyrlian*], a palpable chest vibration caused by aortic stenosis or an aortic aneurysm. It is usually felt in systole by placing the flat of the hand or the fingertips on the second intercostal space to the right of the sternum.

aortic valve, a valve in the heart between the left ventricle and the aorta. It is composed of three semilunar cusps that close in diastole to prevent blood from flowing back into the left ventricle from the aorta. The three cusps are separated by sinuses that resemble tiny buckets when they are filled with blood. These cup-shaped flaps grow from the lining of the aorta and, in systole, open to allow oxygenated blood to flow from the left ventricle into the aorta and on to the peripheral circulation. Compare **mitral valve, pulmonary valve, tricuspid valve.**

aortic valvular stenosis. See **subaortic stenosis.**

aortitis /ā′ôrtī′tis/, inflammation of the aorta. It occurs most frequently in tertiary syphilis and occasionally in rheumatic fever.

aortocoronary /ā·ôr′tōkôr′əner′ē/ [Gk, *aeirein* + L, *corona,* crown], pertaining to the aorta and coronary arteries.

aortocoronary bypass [AS, *bi,* alongside; Fr, *passer*], a surgical procedure, for treatment of angina pectoris or coronary vessel disease, in which a saphenous vein, mammary artery, or other blood vessel or a synthetic graft is used to build a shunt from the aorta to one of the coronary arteries in order to bypass a circulatory obstruction.

aortogram /ā·ôr′təgram/ [Gk, *aerein* + *gramma,* record], a radiographic image of the aorta made after the injection of a radiopaque contrast medium in the blood.

aortography /ā·ôrtog′rəfē/ [Gk, *aerein* + *graphein,* to record], a radiographic process in which the aorta and its branches are injected with any of various contrast media for visualization. **—aortographic,** *adj.*

aortopulmonary fenestration /ā·ôr′tōpul′məner′ē/ [Gk, *aerein* + L, *pulmoneus,* lung, *fenestra,* window], a congenital anomaly characterized by an abnormal fenestration in the ascending aorta and the pulmonary artery cephalad to the semilunar valve, allowing oxygenated and unoxygenated blood to mix, resulting in a decrease in the oxygen available in the peripheral circulation.

aosmic. See **anosmia.**

AOTA, abbreviation for *American Occupational Therapy Association.*

AOTF, abbreviation for *American Occupational Therapy Foundation.*

ap-, apo-, prefix meaning 'separation or derivation from; away from': *apeidosis, aponeurosis.*

AP, abbreviation for **anteroposterior.**

APA, **1.** abbreviation for *American Psychiatric Association.* **2.** abbreviation for *American Psychological Association.*

APACHE /əpach′ē/, abbreviation for *Acute Physiology and Chronic Health Evaluation,* a system of classifying severity of illnesses in intensive care patients.

apareunia /ā′pəroo′nē·ə/, an inability to perform sexual intercourse caused by a physical or psychologic sexual dysfunction.

apathetic. See **apathy.**

apathetic hyperthyroidism /ap′əthet′ik/, a form of thyrotoxicosis that tends to affect mainly older adults who have stereotyped "senile" physical features and whose behavior is apathetic and inactive rather than hyperkinetic. Medical treatment not only restores normal behavioral activity but also results in a loss of wrinkles and a more youthful physical appearance. Untreated, the pa-

tient is likely to succumb to the effects of stress or acute illness.

apathy /ap′əthē/ [Gk, *a, pathos,* not suffering], an absence or suppression of emotion, feeling, concern, or passion; an indifference to stimuli found generally to be exciting or moving. The condition is common in patients with neurasthenia, depressive disorders, and schizophrenia. **—apathetic,** *adj.*

apatite /ap′ətīt/ [Gk, *apate,* deceit], an inorganic mineral composed of calcium and phosphate that is found in the bones and teeth.

APC, **1.** abbreviation for *atrial premature contraction.* **2.** abbreviation for **adenomatous polyposis coli.**

APCC, **1.** abbreviation for *anti-inhibitor coagulant complex.* **2.** abbreviation for **activated prothrombin complex concentrate.**

APD, abbreviation for **adult polycystic disease.** See **polycystic kidney disease.**

apepsia /āpep′sē·ə/ [Gk, *a,* without, *pepsis,* digestion], a condition involving a failure of the digestive functions.

aperient /əpir′ē·ənt/ [L, *aperire,* to open], a mild laxative.

aperistalsis /āper′istal′sis/ [Gk, *a,* without, *peristellein,* to clasp], a failure of the normal waves of contraction and relaxation that move contents through the digestive tract.

aperitive /əper′itiv/ [L, *aperere,* to open], a stimulant of the appetite. Also called aperitif /əper′itif/.

Apert's syndrome /äperz′/ [Eugene Apert, French pediatrician, 1868–1940], a rare condition characterized by an abnormal craniofacial appearance in combination with partial or complete fusion of the fingers and toes. The specific cause of Apert's syndrome is unknown, but the condition appears to be the result of a primary germ plasm defect. A characteristic feature is the premature joining of cranial bones, with resultant growth disturbances. Signs of Apert's syndrome include a peaked and vertically elongated head, widespread and bulging eyes, and a high, arched posterior palate with bony defects of the maxilla and the mandible. The degree of fusion varies greatly and may be complete. Also called **acrocephalosyndactyly; acrocephalosyndactyly, type I.** See also **acrocephalosyndactyly.**

aperture /ap′ərchər/ [L, *apertura,* an opening], an opening or hole in an object or anatomic structure.

aperture of frontal sinus, an external opening of the frontal sinus into the nasal cavity.

aperture of glottis, an opening between the true vocal cords and the arytenoid cartilages.

aperture of larynx, an opening between the pharynx and larynx.

aperture of sphenoid sinus, a round opening between the sphenoid sinus and nasal cavity, situated just above the superior nasal concha.

apex *pl.* **apices** /ā′peks/ [L, tip], the top, the end, the summit, or the extremity of a structure, such as the apex of the heart or the apices of the teeth.

apex beat, a pulsation of the left ventricle of the heart, palpable and sometimes visible at the fifth intercostal space, approximately 9 cm to the left of the midline. Also called **apical beat.**

apexcardiogram (ACG) /-kär′dē·əgram′/, a graphic representation of the pulsations of the chest over the heart in the region of the cardiac apex. The purpose is to provide additional information regarding the diagnosis of ventricular abnormalities.

apexcardiography (ACG) /-kär′dē·og′rəfē/, the recording of heart pulsations obtained from the cardiac apex.

apex cordis [L, *apex* + *cordis,* of the heart], the pointed lower border of the heart. It is directed downward, forward, and to the left and is usually located at the level of the fifth intercostal space.

apexification /-if′ikā′shən/ [L, *apex* + *facere,* to make], a process of inducing tooth root development, usually by repeated treatments with calcium hydroxide, or of promoting apical closure of the root by the placement of hard material after an apicoectomy.

apexigraph /āpek′sigraf′/, a device used for determining the position of the apex of a tooth root.

apex murmur [L, *apex,* summit, *murmur,* humming], a heart sound heard best at the apex of the heart, which in most individuals is at the level of the fifth intercostal space. Also called **apical murmur.**

apex of the lung, the highest point of the lung as it extends to the level of the first rib at the base of the neck.

apex of urinary bladder, the superior area of the urinary bladder, opposite to the fundus. It is at the junction of the superior and inferolateral surfaces of the bladder, and from it the middle umbilical ligament (urachus) extends to the umbilicus. Also called *vertex* or *summit of bladder* and *vertex* or *summit of urinary bladder.*

apex pneumonia [L, *apex,* summit; Gk, *pnemon,* lung], pneumonia in which consolidation is limited to the upper lobe of one lung. Also called **apical pneumonia.**

apex pulmonis /pəlmō′nis/ [L, *apex* + *pulmoneus,* lung], the rounded upper border of each lung, projecting above the clavicle.

APF, acidulated phosphate fluoride, a preparation of sodium fluoride acidulated with phosphoric acid for topical application to the teeth in the prevention of dental caries.

Apgar score /ap′gär/ [Virginia Apgar, American anesthesiologist, 1909–1974], the evaluation of an infant's physical condition, usually performed 1 minute and again 5 minutes after birth, based on a rating of five factors that reflect the infant's ability to adjust to extrauterine life. Virginia Apgar, M.D., developed the system for the rapid identification of infants requiring immediate intervention or transfer to an intensive care nursery.
■ METHOD: The infant's heart rate, respiratory effort, muscle tone, reflex irritability, and color are scored from a low value of 0 to a normal value of 2. The five scores are combined, and the totals at 1 minute and 5 minutes are noted; for example, Apgar 9/10 is a score of 9 at 1 minute and 10 at 5 minutes.
■ NURSING CONSIDERATIONS: A low 1-minute score requires immediate intervention, including administration of oxygen, clearing of the nasopharynx, and usually transfer to an intensive care nursery. A baby with a low score that persists at 5 minutes requires expert care, which may include assisted ventilation, umbilical catheterization, cardiac massage, blood gas evaluation, correction of acid-base deficit, or medication to reverse the effects of maternal medication.
■ OUTCOME CRITERIA: A score of 0 to 3 represents severe distress, a score of 4 to 7 indicates moderate distress, and a score of 7 to 10 indicates an absence of difficulty in adjusting to extrauterine life. The 5-minute total score is normally higher than the 1-minute score. Because a normal, vigorous, healthy newborn almost always has bluish hands and feet at 1 minute, the first score for color will include a 1 rather than a perfect 2; however, at 5 minutes the blueness may have passed, and a score of 2 may be given. A 5-minute overall score of 0 to 1 correlates with a 50% neonatal mortality rate; infants who survive exhibit three times as many neurologic abnormalities at 1 year of age as do children with a 5-minute score of 7 or more.

Infant evaluation at birth—Apgar scoring system

Sign	0	1	2
Heart rate	Absent	Slow, <100	>100
Respiratory effort	Absent	Irregular, slow, weak cry	Good, strong cry
Muscle tone	Limp	Some flexion of extremities	Well-flexed
Reflex irritability	No response	Grimace	Cry, sneeze
Color	Blue, pale	Body pink, extremities blue	Completely pink

From Hockenberry MJ, et al: *Wong's nursing care of infants and children,* ed 7, St Louis, 2003, Mosby.

APHA, abbreviation for *American Public Health Association.*

aphacia, aphacic. See **aphakia.**

aphagia /əfā′jē-ə/ [Gk, *a* + *phagein,* not to eat], a condition characterized by the loss of the ability to swallow as a result of organic or psychologic causes. A kind of aphagia is **aphagia algera.** See also **dysphagia.**

aphagia algera, a condition characterized by the refusal to eat or swallow because doing so causes pain.

aphakia /əfā′kē-ə/ [Gk, *a, phakos,* not lens], (in ophthalmology) a condition in which the crystalline lens of the eye is absent, usually because it has been surgically removed, as in the treatment of cataracts. Also called **aphacia** /əfā′shə/. —**aphakic, aphacic,** *adj.*

aphakic /əfākik/ [Gk, *a,* without, *phakos,* lens], pertaining to the absence of the lens of the eye as a result of a congenital or surgical cause.

aphasia /əfā′zhə/ [Gk, *a* + *phasis,* not speech], an abnormal neurologic condition in which language function is disordered or absent because of an injury to certain areas of the cerebral cortex. The deficiency may be sensory or receptive, in which language is not understood, or expressive or motor, in which words cannot be formed or expressed. Aphasia may be complete or partial, affecting specific language functions. Most commonly, the condition is a mixture of incomplete expressive and receptive aphasia. It may occur after severe head trauma, prolonged hypoxia, or cardiovascular accident. It is sometimes transient, as when the swelling in the brain that follows a stroke or injury subsides and language returns. See also **Broca's area, Wernicke's aphasia.** —**aphasic,** *adj.*

aphemia /əfē′mē-ə/, a loss of the ability to speak. The term is applied to emotional disorders as well as neurologic causes. A person may be **aphemic** because a fear of speaking or a refusal to participate in verbal communication.

apheresis /əfer′əsis, af′ərē′sis/ [Gk, *aphairesis,* removal], a procedure in which blood is temporarily withdrawn, one or more components are selectively removed, and the rest of the blood is reinfused into the donor. The process is used in treating various disease conditions in the donor and for obtaining blood elements for treatment of other patients or for research purposes. Also called **pheresis.** See also **leukapheresis, plasmapheresis, plateletpheresis.**

-aphia, -haphia, suffix meaning a 'condition of the sense of touch': *hyperaphia, paraphia.*

aphonia /āfō′nē-ə/ [Gk, *a, phone,* without voice], a condition characterized by loss of the ability to produce normal speech sounds that results from overuse of the vocal cords, organic disease, or psychologic causes, such as anxiety.

Kinds of aphonia include **aphonia clericorum, aphonia paralytica, aphonia paranoica,** and **spastic aphonia.** See also **speech dysfunction.** —**aphonic, aphonous,** *adj.*

aphonia paralytica /par′əlit′ikə/, a condition characterized by a loss of the voice caused by paralysis or disease of the laryngeal nerves.

aphonia paranoica, an inability to speak that lacks an organic basis and that is characteristic of some forms of mental illness.

aphonic. See **aphonia.**

aphonic pectoriloquy /āfon′ik/, the abnormal transmission of voice sounds through a cavity or a serous pleural effusion, detected during auscultation of a lung.

aphonous. See **aphonia.**

aphoria /əfôr′ē·ə/, a condition in which physical weakness is not lessened as a result of exercise.

aphoric speech, abnormal speech in which vocalizations are whispered.

aphrasia /əfrā′zhə/, a form of aphasia in which a person may be able to speak single words or understand single words but is not able to communicate with words that are arranged in meaningful phrases or sentences.

-aphrodisia, suffix meaning a '(specified) condition of sexual arousal': *anaphrodisia, hypaphrodisia.*

aphronia /əfrō′nē·ə/ [Gk, *a, phronein,* not to understand], (in psychiatry) a condition characterized by an impaired ability to make commonsense decisions. —**aphronic,** *adj.*

aphthae /af′thē/ [Gk, *aphtha,* eruption], a common condition of shallow, painful ulcerations that usually affect the oral mucosa, but not underlying bone. Aphthae occasionally may affect other body tissues, including those of the GI tract and the external genitalia. See also **aphthous stomatitis, foot-and-mouth disease.** —**aphthous,** *adj.*

Aphthae *(Callen et al, 2000)*

aphthous fever. See **foot-and-mouth disease.**

aphthous stomatitis /af′thəs/ [Gk, *aptha,* eruption; *stoma,* mouth, *itis* inflammation], a recurring condition characterized by the eruption of painful ulcers (commonly called canker sores) on the mucous membranes of the mouth. Evidence suggests that the condition is an immune reaction. Heredity, some foods, emotional stress, cancer, and fever are also possible causes. See also **canker sore.**

Aphthous stomatitis *(Feldman, Friedman, and Sleisenger, 2002)*

APIC, abbreviation for **Association for Professionals in Infection Control and Epidemiology.**

apical /ap′ikəl, ā′pi-/ [L, *apex,* tip], **1.** pertaining to the summit or apex. **2.** pertaining to the end of a tooth root or the lumenal surface of a cell.

apical beat. See **apex beat.**

apical curettage [L, *apex;* Fr, scraping], debridement of the apical surface of a tooth and removal of diseased soft tissues in the surrounding bony crypt. Compare **apicoectomy, root curettage, subgingival curettage.**

apical fiber, one of the many fibers of the periodontal ligament. These fibers radiate around the apex of the tooth at approximately right angles to their cementum attachment, extending into the bone at the bottom of the alveolus. Apical fibers resist forces that tend to lift the tooth from the socket and, with the other fibers of the periodontal ligament, stabilize the tooth against tilting movements.

apical impulse. See **precordial movement.**

apical lordotic view /lôrdot′ik/, a radiograph made with the patient leaning backward at an angle of approximately 45 degrees, allowing visualization of the apices of the lung under the clavicle.

apical membrane, the layer of plasma membrane on the apical side (the side towards the lumen) of the epithelial cells in a body tube or cavity, separated from the basolateral membrane by the zonula occludens.

apical murmur. See **apex murmur.**

apical odontoid ligament /ōdon′toid/, a ligament connecting the axis to the occipital bone. It extends from the process of the axis to the anterior margin of the foramen magnum and lies between the two alar ligaments, blending with the anterior atlantooccipital membrane.

apical perforation, root perforation.

apical periodontitis [L, *apex,* summit; Gk, *peri,* near, *odous,* tooth, *itis,* inflammation], an inflammation of the tissues around the apex of a tooth root.

apical pneumonia. See **apex pneumonia.**

apical pulse, the heartbeat as heard with a stethoscope placed on the chest wall adjacent to the cardiac apex.

apicectomy. See **apicoectomy.**

apices. See **apex.**

apicitis /ap′isī′tis/, an inflammation of the apex of a body structure, such as the apex of a lung or root of a tooth.

apicoectomy /ap′isek′təmē/ [L, *apex* + Gk, *ektomē* excision], the surgical removal of the apex or the apical portion of a tooth root, usually in conjunction with apical curettage or root canal therapy. Also called **apicectomy root amputation, root resection.**

Apical pulse *(Elkin, Perry, and Potter, 2004)*

apicotomy /ā′pikot′əmē/, a surgical incision into the apex of a body structure.

apituitarism /ā′pityoo′itəriz′əm/ [Gk, *a*, without; L, *pituita*, phlegm; Gk, *ismos*, a state], an absence or loss of function of the pituitary gland.

APKD, abbreviation for *adult polycystic kidney disease.* See also **polycystic kidney disease.**

aplasia /əplā′zhə/ [Gk, *a, plassein*, not to form], **1.** a developmental failure resulting in the absence of an organ or tissue. **2.** (in hematology) a failure of the normal process of cell generation and development. See also **aplastic anemia, hyperplasia.**

aplasia cutis congenita [Gk, *a, plassein*; L, *cutis*, skin, *congenitus* born with], the congenital absence of a localized area of skin. The defect occurs predominantly on the scalp, less frequently on the limbs and trunk. It is usually covered by a thin, translucent membrane or scar tissue, or it may be raw and ulcerated. The condition is genetically transmitted, although the mode of inheritance is not known.

Aplasia cutis congenita *(Callen et al, 2000)*

aplastic /āplas′tik/ [Gk, *a, plassein*, not to form], **1.** pertaining to the absence or defective development of a tissue or organ. **2.** failure of a tissue to produce normal daughter cells by mitosis. See also **aplastic anemia.**

aplastic anemia, a deficiency of all of the formed elements of blood (specifically red blood cells, white blood cells, and platelets), representing a failure of the cell-generating capacity of bone marrow. Neoplastic disease of bone marrow and destruction of bone marrow by exposure to toxic chemicals, ionizing radiation, or some antibiotics or other medications are common causes. Also spelled **anaemia.** Compare **alymphocytosis, hemolytic anemia, hypoplastic anemia.** See also **aleukia, leukopenia.**

Aplastic anemia: bone marrow smear
(Carr and Rodak, 1999)

Apley's scratch test, a method for assessing the range of motion of the shoulders. The patient is asked to scratch his or her back while reaching over the head with one hand and behind the back with the other hand. The test requires abduction and lateral rotation of one shoulder and adduction and medial rotation of the other shoulder.

Aplisol, trademark for a tuberculin purified protein derivative used for tuberculin skin tests.

APMA, abbreviation for *American Podiatric Medical Society.*

AP mobile projection. See **AP portable chest radiograph.**

APN, abbreviation for **advanced practice nurse.**

apnea /apnē′ə, ap′nē·ə/, [Gk, *a + pnein*, not to breath], an absence of spontaneous respiration. Types of apnea include **cardiac apnea, deglutition apnea, periodic apnea of the newborn, primary apnea, reflex apnea, secondary apnea,** and **sleep apnea.** Also spelled **apnoea. —apneic,** *adj.*

apnea monitor [Gk, *a + pnein,* not to breathe], a bed surface for infants, designed to sound an alarm if the child stops breathing for a given period of time. It may be a bed pad (alarm mattress) or a nasal flow sensor.

apnea monitoring, the act of closely observing the respiration of individuals, particularly infants. The procedure may involve the use of electronic devices that detect changes in thoracic or abdominal movements and in heart rate. Such devices may include an alarm that sounds if breathing stops. See also **apnea monitor.**

apneic. See **apnea.**

apneumia /ap·noo′mē·ə/ [Gk, *a, pneumon,* without lung], congenital absence of the lungs.

apneustic breathing /apnoo′stik/ [Gk, *a, pneusis,* not breathing], a pattern of breathing characterized by a prolonged inspiratory phase followed by expiration apnea. The rate of apneustic breathing is usually around 1.5 breaths per minute. This breathing pattern is often associated with head injury.

apneustic center, an area in the lower portion of the pons that controls the inspiratory phase of respiration. Disorders involving abnormal stimulation of the apneustic center can produce a gasping type of ventilation with maximum inspirations. Also called **pontine respiratory center.**

apnoea. See **apnea.**

apocrine /ap′əkrīn, -krin/ [Gk, *apo,* from, *krinein,* to separate], **1.** pertaining to a cell that loses part of its cytoplasm during secretion. **2.** pertaining to sweat glands, which are most numerous in the axilla and the groin.

apocrine gland. See **eccrine gland, exocrine gland.**

apocrine miliaria. See **Fox-Fordyce disease.**

apocrine secretion [Gk, *apo* + *krinein*; L, *secernere,* to separate], a mammary gland type of secretion in which the end of the secreting cell is broken off and its contents expelled. The secretion thus contains cellular granules in addition to fluid.

apocrine sweat gland [Gk, *apo,* from, *krinein,* to separate], one of the large dermal exocrine glands located in the axillary, anal, genital, and mammary areas of the body. The apocrine glands become functional only after puberty. They secrete sweat containing nutrients consumed by skin bacteria. Bacterial waste products produce a characteristic odor. Compare **eccrine gland.** See also **exocrine gland.**

Pinched off portions of cells releasing secretory product
Pinched off portions of cells

Apocrine sweat gland (Applegate, 2000)

apodal /ə·pō′dəl/ [Gk, *a, pous,* without foot], having no feet. See also **symmelia.**

apodial symmelia. See **sirenomelia.**

apoenzyme /ap′ō·en′zīm/ [Gk, *apo* + *en,* into, *zyme,* ferment], the protein part of a holoenzyme. The nonprotein part is the prosthetic group, which is usually permanently attached to the apoenzyme.

apogee /ap′əjē/ [Gk, *apo* + *ge,* earth], the climax of a disease or the period of greatest severity of signs and symptoms, usually followed by a crisis.

apolipoprotein /ap′ōlip′ōprō′tēn/ [Gk, *apo* + *lipos,* fat, *protos,* first], the protein component of lipoprotein complexes.

apolipoprotein A-I, a protein component of lipoprotein complexes found in high-density lipoprotein (HDL) and chylomicrons. It is an activator of lecithin-cholesterol acyltransferase (LCAT), which forms cholesteryl esters in HDL. All apoproteins of plasma lipoproteins bind and transport lipid in the blood. A deficiency of apolipoprotein A-I is associated with low HDL levels and Tangier disease. See also **Tangier disease.**

apolipoprotein A-II, a protein component of lipoprotein complexes found in high-density lipoprotein (HDL) and chlyomicrons, which activates hepatic lipase. See also **apolipoprotein A-I**

apolipoprotein A-III, one found in high-density lipoproteins. Also called **apolipoprotein D.**

apolipoprotein B, apoprotein B-48, a protein component of lipoprotein involved in transport from the GI tract to the bloodstream.

apolipoprotein B-100, a protein component of lipoprotein involved in hepatic transport of lipid as very-low-density lipoprotein (VLDL) and low-density lipoprotein (LDL). Apoprotein B-100 links to cellulose LDL receptors. It is elevated in the plasma of patients with familial hyperlipoproteinemia. See also **hyperlipoproteinemia.**

apolipoprotein C, a class of apolipoproteins, apo C-I, C-II, and C-III, that occur in very-low-density lipoprotein (VLDL), high-density lipoprotein (HDL), and chylomicrons. Apo C-II activates lipoprotein lipase, which hydrolyzes triglycerides for transfer from VLDL and chylomicrons to tissues.

apolipoprotein C-I, a protein component of lipid that activates lecithin-cholesterol acyltransferase (LCAT).

apolipoprotein C-II, a protein component of chylomicrons and very-low-density lipoprotein (VLDL) that activates lipoprotein lipase (LPL), an enzyme that hydrolyzes triglyceride to free fatty acids and monoglycerides.

apolipoprotein D. See **apolipoprotein A-III.**

apolipoprotein E, a protein component of lipoprotein complexes found in very-low-density lipoprotein (VLDL), high-density lipoprotein (HDL), chylomicrons, and chylomicron remnants. It facilitates hepatic uptake of chylomicron and VLDL remnants and is elevated in patients with type III hyperlipoproteinemia. See also **hyperlipoproteinemia.**

apolipoproteins test, a blood test used to evaluate the risks of atherogenic disease of the heart and peripheral arteries. Specific levels of certain apolipoproteins are also associated with conditions such as Alzheimer's disease, familial hypercholesterolemia, some types of renal failure, nephrotic syndrome, and estrogen depletion in women over the age of 50.

aponeurosis *pl.* **aponeuroses** /ap′ōnŏŏrō′sis/ [Gk, *apo* + *neuron,* nerve, sinew], a strong flat sheet of fibrous connective tissue that serves as a tendon to attach muscles to bone or as fascia to bind muscles together or to other tissues at their origin or insertion.

aponeurosis of the external abdominal oblique, the strong membrane that covers the entire ventral surface of the abdomen and lies superficial to the rectus abdominis. Fibers from both sides of the aponeurosis interlace in the midline to form the linea alba. The upper part of the aponeurosis serves as the inferior origin of the pectoralis major; the lower part ends in the inguinal ligament.

aponeurotic fascia /-nŏŏrot′ik/ [Gk, *apo,* from, *neuron,* tendon], a thickened layer of connective tissue that provides attachment to a muscle.

aponeurotic fibroma, a recurrent benign tumor seen mainly in persons under 20 years of age, most often on the hand, occurring as a firm, fixed nodule composed of fibroblastic tissue with finely stippled calcifications, not attached to the overlying skin and infiltrating into surrounding soft tissue. Also called *juvenile aponeurotic fibroma.*

Aponomma hydrosauri, a tick that infests reptiles. It is the arthropod reservoir for *Rickettsia honei* on Flinders Island, Australia, and transmits Flinders Island spotted fever.

apophyseal /ap′əfiz′ē·əl/, pertaining to an apophysis. Also **apophysial.**

apophyseal fracture, a fracture that separates a projection (apophysis) of a bone from the main osseous tissue at a point of strong tendinous attachment.

apophysial. See **apophyseal.**

apophysis /əpof′isis/ [Gk, a growing away], any small projection, process, or outgrowth, usually on a bone without an

Anterior superior iliac spine

External oblique

Aponeurosis of external oblique

Inguinal ligament

Lacunar ligament

Femoral artery and vein

Pubic tubercle

Aponeurosis *(Drake, Vogl, and Mitchell, 2005)*

independent center of ossification. Examples include the zygomatic apophysis of the temporal bone and the basilar apophysis of the occipital bone.

apophysitis /əpof′əsī′tis/, inflammation of an outgrowth, projection, or swelling, especially a bony outgrowth that is still attached to the rest of the bone. Apophysitis occurs most frequently as a disorder of the foot caused by disease of the epiphysis of the quadrangular bone at the back of the tarsus.

apoprotein /ap′ōprō′tēn/, a polypeptide chain not yet complexed to its specific prosthetic group.

apoptosis /ā′pōtō′sis, ā′poptō′sis/ [Gk, *apo,* away, *ptosis,* falling], necrosis of keratinocytes in which the nuclei of the necrotic cells dissolve and the cytoplasm shrinks, rounds up, and is subsequently phagocytized. The term generally refers to "programmed" cell death.

aposia /āpō′shə/ [Gk, *a,* not, *posis,* thirst], a complete lack of thirst.

apothecaries' measure /əpoth′əker′ēz/ [Gk, *apotheke,* store], a system of graduated liquid volumes originally based on the minim, formerly equal to one drop of water but now standardized to 0.06 ml; 60 minims equals 1 fluid dram, 8 fluid drams equals 1 fluid ounce, 16 fluid ounces equals 1 pint, 2 pints equals 1 quart, 4 quarts equals 1 gallon. See also **apothecaries' weight, metric system.**

apothecaries' weight, a system of graduated amounts arranged in order of heaviness and based on the grain, formerly equal to the weight of a plump grain of wheat but now standardized to 65 mg; 20 grains equals 1 scruple, 3 scruples equals 1 dram, 8 drams equals 1 ounce, 12 ounces equals 1 pound. Compare **avoirdupois weight.** See also **apothecaries' measure, metric system.**

apothecary /əpoth′əker′ē/, [Gk, *apotheke,* store], a pharmacist. See also **apothecaries' measure, apothecaries' weight.**

apparatus /ap′ərat′əs/ [L, *ad,* toward, *parare,* to make ready], a device or a system composed of different parts that act together to perform some special function.

apparent death. See **death.**

apparent leukonychia, white discoloration of the nail that fades when pressure is applied and with maintenance of transparency of the nail plate.

appendage. See **appendix** (def. 1).

appendectomy /ap′əndek′təmē/, [L, *appendere* + Gk, *ektomē,* excision], the surgical removal of the vermiform appendix. The operation is performed in acute appendicitis to remove an inflamed appendix before it ruptures. If the appendix has perforated and risk of peritonitis is high, a drain may be left in the incision and the wound is left open, dressing changes are more frequent, and appropriate antibiotics are prescribed; ileus may develop within days, and pain may be acute. This procedure can be performed via laparoscope or open laparotomy. See also **abdominal surgery, peritonitis.**

appendical. See **appendiceal.**

appendical reflex /əpen′dikəl/, extreme tenderness at McBurney's point on the abdomen, a diagnostic finding in appendicitis.

appendiceal /ap′endish′əl/, pertaining to the vermiform appendix. Also **appendicial, appendical** /əpen′dikəl/.

appendiceal abscess. See **appendicular abscess.**

appendicectomy /əpen′disek′təmē/, **1.** surgical removal of the vermiform appendix. **2.** surgical removal of an appendage.

appendices. See **appendix.**

appendices epiploicae. See **appendix epiploica.**

appendicial. See **appendiceal.**

appendicitis /əpen′disī′tis/ [L, *appendere* + Gk, *itis*], inflammation of the vermiform appendix, usually acute, that, if undiagnosed, leads rapidly to perforation and peritonitis. The inflammation is caused by an obstruction such as a hard mass of feces or a foreign body in the lumen of the appendix, fibrous disease of the bowel wall, an adhesion, or a parasitic infestation. Appendicitis is most likely to occur in teenagers and young adults and is more prevalent in male patients.

■ OBSERVATIONS: The most common symptom is constant pain in the right lower quadrant of the abdomen around McBurney's point, which the patient describes as having begun as intermittent pain in midabdomen. Rebound pain occurs at McBurney's point as well. Pain may also occur on the left side. Extreme tenderness occurs over the right rectus muscle. To decrease the pain, the patient keeps knees bent to prevent tension of abdominal muscles. Appendicitis is characterized by vomiting, a low-grade fever of 99° to 102° F, an elevated white blood count, rebound tenderness, a rigid abdomen, and decreased or absent bowel sounds.

■ INTERVENTIONS: Treatment is appendectomy within 24 to 48 hours of the first symptoms because delay usually results in rupture and peritonitis as fecal matter is released into the peritoneal cavity. The fever rises sharply once peritonitis begins. The patient may have sudden relief from pain immediately after rupture, followed by increased, diffuse pain. The nurse is alert to the other indications of peritonitis: increasing abdominal distension, acute abdomen, rigid boardlike abdomen, tachycardia, rapid shallow breathing, and restlessness. If peritonitis is suspected, IV antibiotic therapy, fluids, and electrolytes are given. Kinds of appendicitis include **chronic appendicitis.** See also **McBurney's point, peritonitis.**

Acute appendicitis *(Zitelli and Davis, 1997)*

appendicitis pain [L, *appendere,* to hang upon, *poena,* penalty], severe general abdominal pain that develops rapidly and usually becomes localized in the lower right quadrant. It is accompanied by extreme tenderness over the right rectus muscle with rebound pain at McBurney's point. Occasionally, the pain is on the left side.

appendicular /ap'əndik'yələr/, **1.** pertaining to the vermiform appendix. **2.** pertaining to the limbs of the skeleton.

appendicular abscess, 1. an abscess on a limb. **2.** an abscess of the vermiform appendix. Also called **appendiceal abscess.**

appendicular skeleton, the bones of the limbs and their girdles, attached to the axial skeleton. See also **axial skeleton.**

appendix *pl.* **appendixes, appendices,** /əpen'diks/, **1.** an accessory part attached to a main structure. Also called **appendage. 2.** See **vermiform appendix.**

appendix dyspepsia [L, *appendere* + Gk, *dys,* difficult, *peptein,* to digest], an abnormal condition characterized by impairment of the digestive function associated with chronic appendicitis. See also **dyspepsia.**

appendix epididymidis /ep'ididim'idis/, a cystic structure sometimes found on the head of the epididymis. It represents a remnant of the mesonephros.

appendix epiploica *pl.* **appendices epiploicae** /əp'iplô'ik ə/ [L, *appendere* + Gk, *epiploon,* caul], one of the fat pads, 2 to 10 cm long, scattered through the peritoneum along the colon and the upper part of the rectum, especially along the transverse and the sigmoid parts of the colon.

appendixes. See **appendix.**

appendix vermiformis. See **vermiform appendix.**

apperception /ap'ərsep'shən/ [L, *ad,* toward, *percipere,* to perceive], **1.** mental perception or recognition. **2.** (in psychology) a conscious process of understanding or perceiving in terms of a person's previous knowledge, experiences, emotions, and memories. —**apperceptive,** *adj.*

appestat /ap'əstat/, a center in the hypothalamus of the brain that controls the appetite.

appetite[1] /ap'ətīt/ [L, *appetere,* to long for], a natural or instinctive desire, such as for food.

appetite[2], a nursing outcome from the Nursing Outcomes Classification (NOC) defined as the desire to eat when ill or receiving treatment.

apple picker's disease, an allergic reaction with respiratory complaints, associated with the handling of apples that have been treated with a fungicide.

apple sorter's disease, a form of contact dermatitis caused by chemicals used in washing apples.

appliance /əplī'əns/ [L, *applicare,* to apply], a device or instrument used to perform a specific medical function or to have a specific therapeutic effect.

application /ap'likā'shən/, a computer program used to process a particular type of data, such as payroll, inventory, data about patients, scheduling of procedures and activities, pharmacy requisition and control, recording of nursing notes, care planning, word processing, and spreadsheets.

applicator /ap'likā'tər/, a rodlike instrument with a piece of cotton on the end, used for the local application of medication or probing of wound pockets/crevices. Also called **cotton swab.**

applied anatomy /əplīd'/, the study of the structure of the organs of the body as it relates to the diagnosis and treatment of disease. Also called **practical anatomy.** See also **comparative anatomy, pathologic anatomy, radiologic anatomy, surgical anatomy.**

applied chemistry, the application of the study of chemical elements and compounds to industry and the arts.

applied kinesiology, a form of treatment using nutrition, physical manipulation, vitamins, diet, and exercise for the purpose of restoring and energizing the body. Weak muscles are proposed to be a source of dysfunctional health.

applied psychology, 1. the interpretation of historical, literary, medical, or other data according to psychologic principles. **2.** any branch of psychology that emphasizes practical rather than theoretic approaches and objectives, such as clinical psychology, child psychology, industrial psychology, and educational psychology.

applied science. See **science.**

AP portable chest radiograph, a radiographic examination of the chest performed with a portable x-ray machine in the room of an immobilized patient. The film holder is placed behind the patient and the x-ray tube in front. The patient is positioned as upright as possible to allow for visualization of fluid levels in the lungs. Also called **AP mobile projection.**

apposition /ap'əsish'ən/ [L, *apponere,* to put to], the placing of objects in proximity, as in the layering of tissue cells or juxtapositioning of facing surfaces side-by-side.

appositional growth, an increase in size by the addition of new tissue or similar material at the periphery of a particular part or structure, as in the addition of new layers in bone and tooth formation. Compare **interstitial growth.**

apposition suture, a suture that holds the margins of an incision close together.

approach, the steps in a particular surgical procedure from division of the most superficial parts of the anatomy through exposure of the operation site.

approach-approach conflict [L, *ad* + *propiare,* to draw near], a conflict resulting from the simultaneous presence of two or more incompatible impulses, desires, or goals, each of which is desirable. Also called **double-approach conflict.** See also **conflict.**

approach-avoidance conflict, a conflict resulting from the presence of a single goal or desire that is both desirable and undesirable. See also **conflict.**

appropriate for gestational age (AGA) infant /əprō'prē·it/ [L, *ad,* toward, *proprius,* ownership], a newborn whose size, growth, and maturation are normal for gestational age, whether delivered prematurely, at term, or later than term. Such infants, if born at term, fall within the average range of size and weight on intrauterine growth curves, measuring from 48 to 53 cm in length and weighing between 2700 and 4000 g.

approximal /əprok'siməl/ [L, *approximare,* to approach], close, or very near.

approximate /əprok'simāt/, [L, *ad + proximare,* to come near], **1.** to draw two tissue surfaces close together as in the repair of a wound or to draw the bones of a joint together as in physical therapy. **2.** almost correct.

approximator /əprok'səmā'tər/, a medical instrument used to draw together the edges of divided tissues, as in closing a wound or in repairing a fractured rib.

apraxia /əprak'sē·ə/ [Gk, *a + pressein,* not to act], an impairment in the ability to perform purposeful acts or to manipulate objects in the absence or loss of motor power sensation or coordination. **Ideational apraxia** is characterized by impairment caused by a loss of the perception of the use of an object. **Motor apraxia** is characterized by an inability to use an object or perform a task although it is understood. **Amnestic apraxia** is characterized by an inability to perform the function because of an inability to remember the command to perform it. **Apraxia of speech** is an inability to program the position of speech muscles and the sequence of muscle movements necessary to produce understandable speech, although understanding of speech remains intact. —**apraxic,** *adj.*

aprepitant, an antiemetic agent used for prevention of nausea.

Apresoline, trademark for a nonnitrate arteriolar vasodilator antihypertensive (hydralazine hydrochloride).

aprosody /āpros'odē/ [Gk, *a + prosodia,* not modulated voice], a speech disorder characterized by the absence of the normal variations in pitch, loudness, intonation, and rhythm of word formation.

aprosopia /ā'prəsō'pē·ə/ [Gk, *aprosopos,* faceless], a congenital absence of part or all of the facial structures. The condition is usually associated with other malformations.

aprotinin /ap'ro-ti'nin/, an inhibitor of proteolytic enzymes, used as an antihemorrhagic to reduce perioperative blood loss in patients undergoing cardiopulmonary bypass during coronary artery bypass graft; administered intravenously.

APTA, abbreviation for *American Physical Therapy Association.*

aptitude /ap'tətyood/ [L, *aptitudo,* ability], a natural ability, tendency, talent, or capability to learn, understand, or acquire a particular skill; mental alertness.

aptitude test, any of a variety of standardized tests for measuring an individual's ability to learn certain skills. Compare **achievement test, intelligence test, personality test, psychologic test.**

apyretic /ā'pīret'ik/ [Gk, *a + pyretos,* without fever], an afebrile condition.

apyrexia /ā'pīrek'sē·ə/ [Gk, *a + pyrexis,* without fever], an absence or remission of fever.

aq. See **aqua.**

AQ, abbreviation for **achievement quotient.**

aqua (aq) /ā'kwə/, the Latin word for water.

aqua amnii. See **amniotic fluid.**

AquaMEPHYTON, trademark for a vitamin K compound (phytonadione).

aquaphobia /ā'kwəfō'bē·ə/ [L, *aqua,* water; Gk, *phobos,* fear], irrational fear of water.

aquaporin /ak'wah-po'rin/, any of a family of proteins found in cell membranes and forming a functional component of water channels.

aquapuncture /-pungk'chər/ [L, *aqua,* water, *punctura,* puncture], the injection of water under the skin or spraying of a fine jet of water onto the skin surface to relieve a mild irritation.

aquatherapy. See **underwater exercise.**

aquathermia pad /-thur'mē·ə/, a waterproof plastic or rubber pad that can be applied to areas of muscle sprain, edema, or mild inflammation. The pad contains channels through which heated or cooled water flows. The device is connected by hoses to a bedside control unit that contains a temperature regulator, a motor for circulating the water, and a reservoir of distilled water. Although generally safer than a conventional heating pad, the aquathermia pad should be checked periodically to avoid the risk of accidental burns. Also called **water flow pad.**

Aquathermia pad *(Potter and Perry, 2005)*

aquatic exercise. See **underwater exercise.**

aqueduct /-dukt/ [L, *aqua,* water, *ductus,* act of leading], any canal, channel, or passage through or between body parts, as the cerebral aqueduct in the brain.

aqueduct of Sylvius. See **cerebral aqueduct.**

aqueductus /ak'wəduk'təs/, the Latin word for canal.

aqueous /ā'kwē·əs, ak'wē·əs/, [L, *aqua*], **1.** watery or waterlike. **2.** a medication prepared with water. See also **aqueous humor. 3.** solution containing water.

aqueous chambers [L, *aqua,* water; Gk, *kamara,* something with an arched cover], the anterior and posterior chambers of the eye, containing the aqueous humor.

aqueous extract, a water-based preparation of plant or animal substance containing the biologically active portion without the cellular residue.

aqueous humor, the clear, watery fluid circulating in the anterior chamber of the eye. It is produced by the ciliary body and is reabsorbed into the venous system at the iridocorneal angle by means of the sinus venosus, or canal of Schlemm.

aqueous phase, a fluid stage of a substance that is based on water in a liquid state, such as a solution of a substance in water.

aqueous solution [L, *aqua,* water + *solutus,* dissolved], a homogenous liquid preparation of any substance dissolved in water.

Ar, symbol for the element **argon.** Also used as an abbreviation for an aromatic group such as phenyl (C_6H_5).

AR, abbreviation for *assisted respiration.*

arabinosylcytosine. See **cytarabine.**

arachidonic acid /ar'əkidon'ik/ [L, *arachos,* a legume], a long-chain fatty acid that is a component of lecithin and a basic material in the biosynthesis of some prostaglandins. In mammals, arachidonic acid is synthesized from linoleic acid, which is an essential fatty acid.

arachnid [Gk, *arachne,* spider], an animal in the phylum Arthropoda, class Arachnida, which includes spiders, scorpions, mites, and ticks.

Flow of aqueous humor (Herlihy and Maebius, 2003)

arachnidism. See **arachnoidism.**

arachnitis /ar'əknī'tis/, inflammation of the arachnoid membrane covering the brain. Also called **arachnoiditis.**

arachno-, arachn-, combining form meaning 'arachnoid membrane or spider': *arachnoidal, arachnoidea.*

arachnodactyly /ərak'nōdak'tilē/ [Gk, *arachne,* spider, *dactylos,* finger], a congenital condition of having long, thin, spiderlike fingers and toes. It is seen in Marfan's syndrome.

Arachnodactyly in Marfan's syndrome
(Zitelli and Davis, 1997)

arachnoid /ərak'noid/ [Gk, *arachne,* spider, *eidos,* form], resembling a cobweb or spiderweb, such as the arachnoid membrane. See also **arachnoid membrane. —arachnoidal,** *adj.*

arachnoid cyst, a fluid-filled cyst between the layers of the leptomeninges, lined with arachnoid membrane, most commonly occurring in the sylvian fissure. Also called **leptomeningeal cyst.**

arachnoidism /ərak'noidiz'əm/ [Gk, *arachne,* spider, *eidos,* form], the condition produced by the bite of a venomous spider. Also called **arachnidism** /ərak'nīdiz'əm/.

arachnoiditis. See **arachnitis.**

arachnoid membrane, a thin, delicate membrane enclosing the brain and the spinal cord, interposed between the pia mater and the dura mater. The subarachnoid space lies between the arachnoid membrane and the pia mater, and the subdural space lies between the arachnoid membrane and the dura mater. Also called **arachnoid sheath.**

arachnoid sheath. See **arachnoid membrane.**

arachnoid villi /vil'ī/ [Gk, *arachne,* spider, *villus,* shaggy hair], projections of fibrous tissue from the arachnoid membrane.

arachnophobia /ərak'nōfō'bē·ə/, a morbid fear of spiders.

Aramine, trademark for a mixed-adrenergic agonist (metaraminol bitartrate).

Aran-Duchenne muscular atrophy /aran'dooshen'/ [François A. Aran, French physician, 1817–1861; Guillaume B.A. Duchenne, French neurologist, 1806–1875], a form of amyotrophic lateral sclerosis affecting the hands, arms, shoulders, and legs at the onset before becoming more generalized. Also **progressive spinal muscular atrophy.**

arbitrary inference /är'bitrer'ē in'fərəns/, a form of cognitive distortion in which a judgment based on insufficient evidence leads to an erroneous conclusion.

arbitrator /är'bətrā'tər/ [L, *arbiter,* umpire], an impartial person appointed to resolve a dispute between parties. The arbitrator listens to the evidence presented by the parties in an informal hearing and attempts to arrive at a resolution acceptable to both parties. **—arbitration,** *n.*

arborization test. See **ferning test.**

arbovirus /är'bōvī'rəs/, any one of more than 300 insect-borne viruses that cause infections characterized by a combination of two or more of the following: fever, rash, encephalitis, and bleeding into the viscera or skin. Dengue, yellow fever, and equine encephalitis are three common arboviral infections. Treatment is symptomatic for all arbovirus infections. Vaccines have been developed to prevent infection from some arboviruses.

arbutamine /ahr-bu'tah-mēn'/, a synthetic catecholamine used as a diagnostic aid in cardiac stress testing in patients unable to exercise sufficiently for the test; administered as the hydrochloride salt.

arc [L, *arcus,* bow], a part of the circumference of a circle.

ARC. See **AIDS-wasting syndrome.**

arcade [L, *arcus,* bow], an arch or series of arches.

arch, any anatomic structure that is curved or has a bowlike appearance. Also called **arcus.**

arch-. See **archi-.**

arch bar, any one of various types of wires, bars, or splints that conform to the arch of the teeth and are used in the treatment of fractures of the jaws and in the stabilization of injured teeth.

arche-. See **archi-.**

-arche, suffix meaning 'beginning': *menarche.*

archentera, archenteric. See **archenteron.**

archenteric canal. See **neurenteric canal.**

archenteron *pl.* **archentera** /arken'təron/ [Gk, *arche,* beginning, *enteron,* intestine], the primitive digestive cavity formed by the invagination into the gastrula which is lined with entoderm during the embryonic development of many animals. It corresponds to the tubular cavity in the vertebrates that connects the amniotic cavity with the yolk sac. Also called **archigaster, coelenteron, gastrocoele, primitive gut.** See also **gastrula. —archenteric,** *adj.*

archeocortex. See **olfactory cortex.**

arches of the foot [L, *arcus,* bow; AS, *fot*], the bony curves of the instep, including the longitudinal (anteroposterior) and the transverse arches.

Medial longitudinal arch

Lateral longitudinal arch

Normal longitudinal arch

Tibia
Fibula
Cuboid
Talus
Tarsals
Navicular
Cuneiforms
Calcaneus
Metatarsals
Phalanges

Transverse arch

Arches of the foot *(Thibodeau and Patton, 2003)*

archetype /är′kətīp′/ [Gk, *arche* + *typos,* type], **1.** an original model or pattern from which a thing or group of things is made or evolves. **2.** (in analytic psychology) an inherited primordial idea or mode of thought derived from the experiences of the human race and present in the subconscious of the individual in the form of drives, moods, and concepts. See also **anima. —archetypal, archetypic, archetypical,** *adj.*

archi-, arch-, arche-, prefix meaning 'first, beginning, or original': *archiblastoma, archetype.*

archiblastoma *pl.* **archiblastomas, archiblastomata** /är′kiblastō′mə/ [Gk, *arche* + *blastos,* germ, *oma*], a tumor composed of cells derived from the layer of tissue surrounding the germinal vesicle.

archigaster. See **archenteron.**

archinephric canal, archinephric duct. See **pronephric duct.**

archinephron. See **pronephros.**

archistome. See **blastopore.**

architectural barriers /är′kətek′chərəl/, architectural features of homes and public buildings that limit access and mobility of disabled persons. Wheelchair access, for example, requires ramped entryways, a minimum of 32-inch-wide doorways, a space of at least 60 inches by 60 inches for wheelchair turns, and counters no more than 26.5 inches above floor level.

architecture /är′kitek′chər/ [Gk, *architekton,* master builder], the basic structure of a computer, including the memory, central processing unit, and input/output devices.

architis /ärkī′tis/ [Gk, *archos,* anus, *itis,* inflammation], an inflammation of the anus. Also called **proctitis.**

arch length /ärch/, the distance from the distal point of the most posterior tooth on one side of the upper or lower jaw to the same point on the other side, usually measured through the points of contact between adjoining teeth. See also **available arch length.**

arch length deficiency, the difference in any dental arch between the length required to accommodate all the natural teeth and the actual length.

arch of the aorta, the proximal one of the four portions of the aorta, giving rise to three arterial branches called the innominate (brachiocephalic), left common carotid, and left subclavian arteries. The arch rises at the level of the border of the second sternocostal articulation of the right side, passes to the left in front of the trachea, bends dorsally, and becomes the descending aorta. Also called **aortic arch.**

arch width, the distance between the left and right opposite in the upper or lower jaw. The intercanine, interpremolar, or intermolar distance may be cited as the arch width.

arch wire, an orthodontic wire fastened to two or more teeth through fixed attachments, used to cause or guide tooth movement. See also **full-arch wire, sectional arch wire.**

arcing spring contraceptive diaphragm /är′king/, a kind of contraceptive diaphragm in which the flexible metal spring that forms the rim is a combination of a flexible coil spring and a flat band spring made of stainless steel. The latex or silicone rubber dome is approximately 4 cm deep, and the diameter of the rubber-covered rim is between 55–100 mm. Seven sizes, in increments of 0.5 cm, allow the clinician to fit the diaphragm to a particular woman. The kind of spring and the size of the rim in millimeters are stamped on the rim, for example, 75 mm arcing spring. This kind of diaphragm is prescribed for a woman whose vaginal musculature is relaxed and does not afford strong support, as in first-degree cystocele, rectocele, or uterine prolapse. Compare **coil spring contraceptive diaphragm, flat spring contraceptive diaphragm.** See also **contraceptive diaphragm fitting.**

arctation. See **stenosis.**

arcuate /är′kyoo·at/ [L, *arcuatus,* bowed], an arch or bow shape.

arcuate scotoma [L, *arcuatus* bowed; Gk, *skotoma,* darkness], an arc-shaped blind area that may develop in the field of vision of a person with glaucoma. It is caused by damage to nerve fibers in the retina.

arcus. See **arch.**

arcus senilis /senē′lis/ [L, bow, aged], an opaque ring, gray to white in color, that surrounds the periphery of the cornea. It is caused by deposits of cholesterol in the cornea or hyaline degeneration and occurs primarily in older persons. Also called **gerontoxon.**

Arcus senilis *(Kanski and Nischal, 1999)*

ardeparin, an anticoagulant.

■ INDICATIONS: This drug is used to prevent deep vein thrombosis after knee replacement surgery.

■ CONTRAINDICATIONS: The following conditions prohibit the use of this drug: known hypersensitivity to this drug, pork products, heparin, or other anticoagulants; hemophilia; leukemia with bleeding; thrombocytopenic purpura; cerebrovascular hemorrhage; cerebral aneurysm; severe hypertension; and other severe cardiac disease.

■ ADVERSE EFFECTS: Life-threatening consequences include intracranial bleeding, hemorrhage, anaphylaxis, and thrombocytopenia. Other adverse effects include fever, hypersensitivity, anemia, pruritus, superficial wound infection, ecchymosis, and rash.

ARDS, abbreviation for **adult respiratory distress syndrome.**

area /er′ē·ə/ [L, space], (in anatomy) a limited anatomic space that contains a specific structure of the body or within which certain physiologic functions predominate, such as the aortic area and the association areas of the cerebral cortex.

area restriction, a nursing intervention from the Nursing Interventions Classification (NIC) defined as a limitation of patient mobility to a specified area for purposes of safety or behavior management. See also **Nursing Interventions Classification.**

areata /erē·ā′tə/, occurring in patches, such as hair loss in alopecia areata.

area under the concentration curve (AUC), a method of measurement of the bioavailability of a drug based on a plot of blood concentrations sampled at frequent intervals. It is directly proportional to the total amount of unaltered drug in the patient's blood.

areflexia /ā′rēflek′sē·ə/, the absence of the reflexes.

Arenavirus /er′inəvī′rəs/, a genus of viruses usually transmitted to humans by contact with or inhalation of aerosolized excreta of wild rodents. Individual arenaviruses are identified with specific geographic areas, such as **Bolivian hemorrhagic fever** in one river valley in Bolivia; **Lassa fever** in Nigeria, Liberia, and Sierra Leone; and **Argentine hemorrhagic fever** in two agricultural provinces in Argentina. Arenavirus infections are characterized by slow onset, fever, muscle pain, rash, petechiae, hemorrhage, delirium, hypotension, and ulcers of the mouth. Treatment is supportive; there is no specific antimicrobial agent or vaccine. Fluid and electrolyte balance, rest, and adequate nutrition are the goals of treatment.

areola *pl.* **areolae,** /erē′ōlə/, **1.** a small space or a cavity within a tissue. **2.** a circular area of a different color surrounding a central feature, such as the discoloration about a pustule or vesicle. **3.** the part of the iris around the pupil.

areola mammae /mam′ē/, the pigmented, circular area surrounding the nipple of each breast. Also called **areola papillaris.**

areolar /erē′ələr/ [L, *areola,* little space], pertaining to an areola.

areolar gland, one of the large modified sebaceous glands in the areolae encircling the nipples of the breasts of women. The areolar glands secrete a lipoid fluid that lubricates and protects the nipple during nursing and contain smooth muscle bundles that cause the nipples to become erect when stimulated. Also called **gland of Montgomery.**

areolar tissue, a kind of connective tissue having little tensile strength and consisting of loosely woven fibers and areolae. It occupies the interspaces of the body. Also called **fibroareolar tissue.** Compare **fibrous tissue.**

Nucleus   Collagen fiber   Elastic fiber

Areolar tissue (© *Ed Reschke; used with permission*)

areolitis /er′ē·əlī′tis/, an inflammation of the areolas of the breasts.

ARF, abbreviation for **acute respiratory failure.** Also, abbreviation for **acute renal failure.**

Arg, abbreviation for the amino acid **arginine.**

argatroban /ahr-gat′ro-ban′/, an anticoagulant that binds to the thrombin active site and inhibits various thrombin-catalyzed reactions. It is used in the prophylaxis and treatment of thrombocytopenia resulting from treatment with heparin; administered intravenously.

argentaffin cell /är′jentaf′in/ [L, *argentum,* gleaming, *affinitas,* affinity], a cell containing granules that stain readily with silver and chromium. Such cells occur in most regions of the GI tract and are especially abundant in the crypts of Lieberkühn. Also called **enterochromaffin cell, Kulchitsky's cell.** See also **carcinoid, carcinoid syndrome.**

argentaffinoma *pl.* **argentaffinomas, argentaffinomata,** /är′jentaf′inō′mə/, a carcinoid tumor arising most often from argentaffin cells in epithelium of the crypts of Lieberkühn in the digestive tract. The neoplasm, which occurs primarily in middle-aged or elderly persons, starts as a nodule or plaque and progresses to a growth encircling the bowel. Highly vascular tumors formed of silver-staining argentaffin cells may also develop in the bronchi.

argentaffinoma syndrome. See **carcinoid syndrome.**

argentaffinomata. See **argentaffinoma.**

Argentine hemorrhagic fever, an infectious disease caused by an arenavirus transmitted to humans by contact with or inhalation of aerosolized excreta of infected rodents. Initially, it is characterized by chills, fever, headache, myalgia, anorexia, nausea, vomiting, and a general feeling of malaise. As the disease progresses, the victim may develop a high fever, dehydration, hypotension, flushed skin, abnormally slow heartbeat, bleeding from the gums and internal tissues, hematuria, and hematemesis. There may be involvement of the central nervous system, shock, and pulmonary edema. There is no specific treatment for the disease other than hydration, rest, warmth, and adequate nutrition. Rarely, IV fluids and dialysis are necessary. Usually, the prognosis is complete recovery. See also *Arenavirus,* **Bolivian hemorrhagic fever, Lassa fever.**

arginase /är′jinās/, an enzyme that catalyzes the hydrolysis of arginine during the urea cycle, producing urea and ornithine. The enzyme is found primarily in the liver but also occurs in the mammary gland, testes, and kidney.

arginase deficiency, an autosomal recessive aminoacidopathy involving the biosynthesis of urea; arginine is elevated in blood and urine and may cause secondary cystinuria; orotic aciduria is common, but hyperammonemia is rare. Clinical signs include psychomotor retardation, hepatomegaly, and scalp discoloration. Also called **argininemia.**

arginine (Arg) /är′jinin/, an amino acid formed during the urea cycle by the transfer of a nitrogen atom from aspartate to citrulline. It can also be prepared synthetically. Certain compounds made from arginine, especially arginine glutamate and arginine hydrochloride, are used intravenously in the management of conditions in which there is an excess of ammonia in the blood caused by liver dysfunction. See also **urea cycle.**

Chemical structure of arginine

argininemia /är′jininē′mē·ə/, arginase deficiency.

arginine vasopressin, vasopressin containing arginine, as that from humans and most other mammals; for medicinal uses. Also called **argipressin.**

argininosuccinic acidemia /ärjin′inō′suksin′ik/, an inherited amino acid metabolism disorder in which the lack of an enzyme, argininosuccinase, results in an excess of argininosuccinic acid in the blood. The condition is characterized by seizures and mental retardation. Treatment mainly involves a low-protein diet containing essential amino acids or amino acid analogs.

argipressin /ahr′gĭ-pres′in/, arginine vasopressin.

argon (Ar) /är′gon/ [Gk, *argos,* inactive], a colorless, odorless, chemically inactive gas and one of the six rare gases in the atmosphere. Its atomic mass is 39.95; its atomic number is 18. It forms no known compounds.

Argyll Robertson pupil [Douglas M.C.L. Argyll Robertson, Scottish ophthalmologist, 1837–1909], a pupil that constricts on accommodation but not in response to light. It is most often seen with miosis and in advanced neurosyphilis.

argyria /ärji′rē·ə/ [Gk, *argyros,* silver], a dull blue or gray coloration of the skin, conjunctiva, and internal organs caused by prolonged exposure to silver salts.

argyrophil /ärji′rəfil/ [Gk, *argyros,* silver, *philein,* to love], a cell or other object that is easily stained or impregnated with silver.

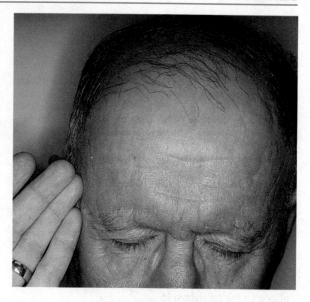

Argyria *(Callen et al, 2000)*

arhythmia. See **arrhythmia.**

ariboflavinosis /ärī′bōflā′vinō′sis/ [Gk, *a,* not, *ribose;* L, *flavus,* yellow; Gk, *osis*], a condition caused by deficiency of riboflavin (vitamin B_2) in the diet. It is characterized by bilateral lesions at the corners of the mouth, on the lips, and around the nose and eyes; by seborrheic dermatitis, and by various visual disorders. See also **riboflavin.**

Arica therapy, an alternative mental health treatment introduced by Oscar Ichazo that focuses on altered states of consciousness with a goal of increasing the powers of the mind. It requires a 40-day training program of physical exercise and meditation, climaxed by a mild form of sensory deprivation during which the patient practices self-observation.

Arimidex, trademark for an aromatase inhibitor (anastrozole) used for treating estrogen-receptor-positive breast cancer, primarily in postmenopausal women.

aripiprazole, an antipsychotic agent used to treat schizophrenia.

Aristocort, trademark for a glucocorticoid (triamcinolone).

-arit, combining form designating an antirheumatic drug.

arithmetic mean. See **mean.**

Arkansas stone /är′kənsô/, a fine-grained stone of novaculite used to sharpen surgical instruments.

Arlidin, trademark for a beta-adrenergic agonist peripheral vasodilator (nylidrin hydrochloride).

arm [L, *armus*], **1.** the portion of the upper limb of the body between the shoulder and the elbow. The bone of the arm is the humerus. The muscles of the arm are the coracobrachialis, the biceps brachii, the brachialis, and the triceps brachii. **2.** *nontechnical.* the arm and the forearm. See also **shoulder joint.**

ARM, abbreviation for *artificial rupture of (fetal) membranes.* See also **amniotomy.**

armamentarium /är′məmenter′ē·əm/ [L, *armamentum,* implement], the total therapeutic assets of a physician or medical facility, including medicines and equipment.

arm board, **1.** a board used to position the affected arm of a person with hemiplegia and of others with arm disabilities. It fastens to the arm rest of a wheelchair, supporting the flaccid arm in the correct position to prevent or decrease subluxation of the shoulder joint, and to prevent edema. **2.** a board used to keep the arm still to permit the drawing of blood or starting of an IV needle.

arm bone. See **humerus.**

arm cylinder cast, an orthopedic device of plaster of paris or fiberglass, used for immobilizing the upper limb from the wrist to the upper arm. It is most often applied to aid the healing of a dislocated elbow, for postoperative immobilization or positioning of the elbow, or in the correction of an elbow deformity.

armpit. See **axilla.**

Army Nurse Corps (ANC), a branch of the U.S. Army, founded February 2, 1901, with headquarters in Falls Church, Virginia.

Arneth's classification of neutrophils [Joseph Arneth, German physician, 1873–1953], a system expressed in chart form in which neutrophils are divided into five classes according to the number of segments of their nuclei and are further subdivided according to the shape of the nuclei. Immature neutrophils with a single lobed nucleus are placed on the far left side of the chart; those with multilobed nuclei are placed on the far right side.

Arnold-Chiari malformation /är′nəldkē·är′ē/ [Julius Arnold, German pathologist, 1835–1915; Hans Chiari, French pathologist, 1851–1916], a congenital herniation of the brainstem and lower cerebellum through the foramen magnum into the cervical vertebral canal. It is often associated with meningocele and spina bifida. See also **neural tube defect.**

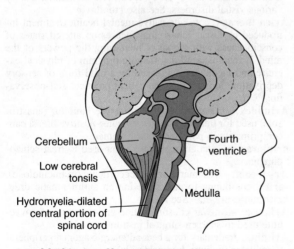

Arnold-Chiari malformation *(McCance and Huether, 2002)*

Arnold, Friedrich [German anatomist, 1803–1890], an investigator of structures and functions of the brain and nervous system, including the nerve center of the cough reflex.

-arol, combining form designating a dicoumarol-type anticoagulant.

AROM, 1. abbreviation for **active range of motion. 2.** abbreviation for *artificial rupture of (fetal) membranes.*

aroma [Gk, spice], any agreeable odor or pleasing fragrance, especially of food, drink, spices, or medication.

aromatase /ah-ro′mah-tās/, an enzyme activity occurring in the endoplasmic reticulum and catalyzing the conversion of testosterone to the aromatic compound estradiol.

aromatase inhibitors, a class of drugs that inhibit aromatase activity and thus block production of estrogens. It is used to treat breast cancer and endometriosis.

aromatherapy[1]**,** a form of herbal medicine that uses various oils from plants. The route of administration can be absorption through the skin or through inhalation. The action of antiviral and antibacterial agents is proposed to aid healing. The aromatic biochemical structures of certain herbs are thought to act in areas of the brain related to past experiences and emotions (e.g., limbic system).

aromatherapy[2]**,** a nursing intervention from the Nursing Interventions Classification (NIC) defined as the administration of essential oils through massage, topical ointments or lotions, baths, inhalation, douches, or compresses (hot or cold) to calm and soothe, provide pain relief, or enhance relaxation and comfort.

aromatic /er′ōmat′ik/, [Gk, *aroma,* spice], **1.** pertaining to a strong but agreeable odor such as a pleasant spicy odor. **2.** a stimulant or spicy medicine. **3.** pertaining to organic chemical structures including 6-carbon ring such as benzol.

aromatic alcohol, a fatty alcohol in which one or more of the hydrogen atoms of the hydrocarbon portion of the alcohol is replaced by an aromatic ring.

aromatic ammonia spirit [Gk, *aroma,* Ammon temple, ancient source of ammonium chloride salt, *spiritus,* breath], a strongly fragrant solution of ammonium carbonate in dilute liquid ammonia, oils, alcohol, and water. It is used as a reflex stimulus, antacid, and a carminative to relieve flatulence. Also called **aromatic spirit of ammonia.**

aromatic bath, a medicated bath in which aromatic substances or essential oils are added to the water.

aromatic compounds, organic compounds that contain a benzene, naphthalene, or analogous ring. Many of these compounds have agreeable odors, which accounts for the use of this term for such compounds.

aromatic elixir [Gk, *aroma* + Ar, *al-iksir,* philosophers' stone], a pleasant smelling flavoring agent added to some medications.

aromatic hydrocarbon [Gk, *aroma,* spice; *hydor,* water; L, *carbo,* coal], an organic compound that has a benzene or other aromatic ring, as distinguished from an open-chain aliphatic compound.

aromatic spirit of ammonia. See **aromatic ammonia spirit.**

arousal [OE, to rise], a state of responsiveness to sensory stimulation.

arousal level, the state of sensory stimulation needed to induce active wakefulness in a sleeping infant. Arousal levels range from deep sleep to drowsy state.

ARPKD, autosomal recessive polycystic kidney disease.

array [ME, *aray,* preparation], an arrangement or order of components or other objects, usually according to a predetermined system or plan.

arrector pili *pl.* **arrectores pilorum** /ä·rek′tor pī′lī/ [L, raisers of the hair], minute smooth muscles of the skin, attached to the connective tissue sheath of the hair follicles; when they contract they cause the hair to stand erect, producing the appearance called goose flesh.

arrest [L, *ad, restare,* to withstand], to inhibit, restrain, or stop, as to arrest the course of a disease. See also **cardiac arrest.**

arrested dental caries, tooth decay in which the area of decay has stopped progressing and infection is not present, but in which the demineralized area in the tooth remains as a cavity. Also called **eburnation of dentin.**

arrested development, the cessation of one or more phases of the developmental process in utero before normal completion, resulting in congenital anomalies. Also called **developmental arrest.**

arrested labor [L, *ad* + *restare,* to withstand, *labor,* work], an interruption in the labor process that may be caused by lack of uterine contractions.

arrheno-, prefix meaning 'male': *arrhenoblastoma, arrhenogenic.*

arrhenoblastoma /erē′nōblastō′mə/ [Gk, *arrhen,* male, *blastos,* germ, *oma,* tumor], an ovarian neoplasm whose cells mimic those in testicular tubules and secrete male sex hormone, causing virilization in females. Also called **andreioma, andreoblastoma, androma, arrhenoma, Sertoli-Leydig cell tumor.**

Arrhenoblastoma *(Fletcher, 2000)*

arrhenogenic /erē′nōjen′ik/, producing only male offspring.

arrhenokaryon /erē′nōker′ē·on/ [Gk, *arrhen,* male, *karyon,* nucleus], an organism that is produced from an egg that has only paternal chromosomes.

arrhenoma. See **arrhenoblastoma.**

arrhythmia /ərith′mē·ə, ərith′mē·ə/ [Gk, a + rhythmos, without rhythm], any deviation from the normal pattern of the heartbeat. Also spelled **arhythmia.** Compare **dysrhythmia. —arrhythmic, arrhythmical,** *adj.*

arrhythmic [Gk, *a, rhythmos,* without rhythm], pertaining to an absence or irregularity of normal rhythm in the heart's beating.

ARRT, abbreviation for **American Registry of Radiologic Technologists.**

arsenic (As) /är′sənik/ [Gk, *arsen,* strong], an element that occurs throughout the earth's crust in metal arsenides, arsenious sulfides, and arsenious oxides. Its atomic number is 33; its atomic mass is 74.92. The arsenic atom occurs in the elemental form and in trivalent and pentavalent oxidation states. This element has been used for centuries as a therapeutic agent and as a poison and continues to have limited use in some trypanosomicidal drugs such as melarsoprol and tryparsamide. The introduction of non-arsenic trypanosomicides with less dangerous side effects in the treatment of trypanosomiasis has greatly reduced its use. The average concentration in the human adult is about 20 mg, which is stored mainly in the liver, kidney, GI tract, and lungs. The mechanisms for the biotransformation of arsenics in humans are not well understood. Most arsenics are slowly excreted in the urine and feces, which accounts for the toxicity of the element. —**arsenic** /ärsen′ik/, *adj.*

arsenic poisoning, toxic effect caused by the ingestion or inhalation of arsenic or a substance containing arsenic, an ingredient in some pesticides, herbicides, dyes, and medicinal solutions. Small amounts absorbed over a period of time may result in chronic poisoning, producing nausea, headache, coloration and scaling of the skin, hyperkeratoses, anorexia, and white lines across the fingernails. Ingestion of large amounts of arsenic results in severe GI pain, diarrhea, vomiting, and swelling of the extremities. Renal failure and shock may occur, and death may result. Determination of the presence of arsenic in the urine, hair, or fingernails is diagnostic.

Arsenic keratoses *(Lawrence and Cox, 2002)*

arsenic stomatitis [Gk, *arsen,* strong; *stoma,* mouth, *itis,* inflammation], an abnormal oral condition associated with arsenic poisoning, characterized by dry, red, painful oral mucosa; ulceration; bleeding beneath the mucosa; and mobility of teeth. Compare **Atabrine stomatitis, bismuth stomatitis.** See also **arsenic poisoning.**

arsenic trihydride. See **arsine.**

arsenic trioxide, an oxidized form of arsenic, used in weed killers and rodenticides. It is also administered intravenously as an antineoplastic in the treatment of acute promyelocytic leukemia.

arsenism /ahr′sĕ-nizm/, chronic arsenic poisoning.

arsine /ahr′sēn/, any of several colorless, volatile arsenical bases that are highly toxic and carcinogenic; the most common one is AsH_3, arsenous trihydride. Some of these compounds have been used in warfare, and a major industrial use is in the production of microelectronic components. Inhalation leads to massive red blood cell hemolysis with secondary renal failure and jaundice. A garliclike odor may be noted with high concentrations.

ART, abbreviation for **active resistance training.**

Artane, trademark for an anticholinergic (trihexyphenidyl hydrochloride).

artefact. See **artifact.**

arterectomy /är′tərek′təmē/, the surgical removal of a segment of an artery.

arteri-. See **arterio-.**

arteria alveolaris inferior. See **inferior alveolar artery.**

arteriae corticales radiata, cortical radiate arteries. Arteries originating from the arcuate arteries of the kidney and distributed to the renal glomeruli. Also called *interlobular arteries of kidney* and *arteriae interlobulares renis.*

arteriae perforantes radiatae, perforating radiate arteries. Small arteries that are continuations of the cortical radiate arteries and perforate the renal capsule.

arterial /ärtir′ē·əl/ [Gk, *arteria,* airpipe], pertaining to an artery.

arterial bleeding. See **arterial hemorrhage.**

arterial blood gas (ABG), the oxygen and carbon dioxide content of arterial blood, measured by various methods to assess the adequacy of ventilation and oxygenation and the acid-base status of the body. Oxygen saturation of hemoglobin is normally 95% or higher. The partial pressure of arterial oxygen, normally 80 to 100 mm Hg, is increased in hyperventilation and decreased in cardiac decompensation, chronic obstructive pulmonary disease, and certain neuromuscular disorders. The partial pressure of carbon dioxide, normally 35 to 45 mm Hg, may be higher in emphysema, chronic obstructive pulmonary disease, and reduced respiratory center function; it may be lower in pregnancy and in the presence of pulmonary emboli and anxiety.

pressure, the resistance of the arterial walls, elasticity of vessels, the blood volume, and its viscosity.

arterial capillaries, microscopic blood vessels (capillaries) extending beyond the terminal ends of arterioles.

arterial catheter [Gk, *arteria,* airpipe, *katheter,* a thing lowered into], a tubular instrument that can be inserted into an artery either to draw blood or to measure blood pressure directly.

arterial circle of Willis. See **circle of Willis.**

arterial circulation [Gk, *arteria* + L, *circulare,* to go around], the movement of blood through the arteries directed away from the heart to the tissues, as opposed to venous circulation away from the tissues to the heart.

arterial hemorrhage, the loss of blood from an artery, often associated with vessel trauma or the removal of a large-bore arterial catheter. Also called **arterial bleeding.**

arterial insufficiency, inadequate blood flow in arteries. It may be caused by occlusive atherosclerotic plaques or emboli; damaged, diseased, or intrinsically weak vessels; arteriovenous fistulas; aneurysms; hypercoagulability states; or heavy use of tobacco. Signs of arterial insufficiency include pale, cyanotic, or mottled skin over the affected area, absent or decreased sensations, tingling, diminished sense of temperature, muscle pains, reduced or absent peripheral pulses, and, in advanced disease, arterial ulcers and atrophy of muscles in the involved extremity. Diagnosis includes checking and comparing peripheral pulses in contralateral extremities, angiography, ultrasound using a Doppler device, and skin temperature tests. Treatment may include a diet low in saturated fats, moderate exercise, sleeping on a firm mattress, use of a vasodilator, and, if indicated, surgical repair of an aneurysm or arteriovenous fistula. Use of tobacco products, prolonged standing, and sitting with the knees bent are discouraged.

Arterial blood gases

Parameter	Measurement	Value
Acid-base balance	pH: hydrogen ion concentration	Normal: 7.35-7.45 Alkalemia: ↑7.45 Acidemia: ↓7.35
Oxygenation	Pao₂: partial pressure of dissolved O₂ in blood	Normal: 80-100 mm Hg Hyperoxemia: ↑100 mm Hg Hypoxemia: ↓80 mm Hg 95%-98%
Ventilation	Sao₂: percentage of O₂ bound to hemoglobin Paco₂: partial pressure of CO₂ dissolved in blood	Normal: 35-45 mm Hg Hypercapnia: ↑45 mm Hg Hypocapnia: ↓35 mm Hg

From Phipps WJ et al: *Medical-surgical nursing: health and illness perspectives,* ed 7, St Louis, 2003, Mosby.

Arterial insufficiency *(Lemmi and Lemmi, 2000)*

arterial blood gases (ABG) test, a blood test used to provide information that helps assess and manage a patient's respiratory (ventilation) and metabolic (renal) acid/base and electrolyte homeostasis, and to assess adequacy of oxygenation.

arterial blood pressure (ABP), the pressure of the blood in the arterial system, which depends on the heart's pumping

arterial insufficiency of lower extremities, a condition characterized by hardening, thickening, and loss of elasticity of the walls of arteries in the legs. It causes decreased circulation, sensation, and function. Symptoms include sharp, cramping pain during exercise or rest at night; numbness; skin changes ranging from pallor to ulceration; thickened toenails; and loss of hair on the legs. Dorsalis pedis, posterior tibial, and popliteal pulses may be diminished or absent.

Laboratory studies usually show elevated plasma lipid levels. See also **claudication.**

arterialized flap, a flap whose blood supply in the new site is maintained by a vein that is grafted to an artery.

arterial line (A-line, Art-line), an arterial blood monitoring system consisting of a catheter inserted into an artery and connected to pressure tubing, a transducer, and a monitor. The device permits continuous direct blood pressure readings as well as access to the arterial blood supply when samples are needed for analysis.

arterial murmur, a sound produced by blood moving through a narrowed artery.

arterial nephrosclerosis [Gk, *arteria,* airpipe, *nephros,* kidney, *sklera,* hard, *osis,* condition], arteriosclerosis of the renal arteries, leading to deprivation of oxygenated blood to the kidney tissues and their destruction.

arterial network [L, *rete,* net: Gk, *arteria*], an anastomotic network of small arteries at a point before they branch into arterioles and capillaries. Also called **rete arteriosum.**

arterial palpitation [Gk, *arteria,* airpipe; L, *palpitare,* to flutter], a pulsation felt in an artery.

arterial pH, the hydrogen ion concentration of arterial blood. Normal range is 7.35 to 7.45.

arterial plethysmography, a manometric test that is usually performed to rule out occlusive disease of the lower extremities. It can also be used to identify arteriosclerotic disease in the upper extremity.

arterial port, the opening at the arterial end of a synthetic arteriovenous access device.

arterial pressure, the stress exerted by circulating blood on the artery walls. It is the product of the cardiac output and the systemic vascular resistance. A number of extrinsic and intrinsic factors regulate and maintain a reasonably constant arterial pressure. Extrinsic factors include neurologic stimulation and hormones such as catecholamines and prostaglandins. Intrinsic factors include chemoreceptors and pressure-sensitive receptors in the arterial walls that cause vasoconstriction or vasodilation. Arterial pressure is commonly measured with a sphygmomanometer and a stethoscope. Stress, hypervolemia, hypovolemia, and various drugs may alter the arterial pressure. Also called **arterial tension.** See also **blood pressure.**

arterial rete /rē′tē/ [Gk, *arteria,* airpipe; L, *rete,* net], a network of arteries and arterioles.

arterial sclerosis [Gk, *arteria,* airpipe, *sklerosis,* hardening], a thickening of the arteries. See also **arteriosclerosis, atherosclerosis.**

arterial tension. See **arterial pressure.**

arterial thrill, a vibration that can be felt over an artery. It is unusually associated with turbulent blood flow within the artery.

arterial wall, the fibrous and muscular wall of vessels that carry oxygenated blood from the heart to structures throughout the body, and of the pulmonary arteries that carry deoxygenated blood from the heart to the lungs. The wall of an artery has three layers: the **tunica intima,** the inner coat; the **tunica media,** the middle coat; and the **tunica adventitia,** the outer coat. Nerves from the sympathetic system constrict the vessel and thus control the flow of blood into the areas served by the artery. The middle layer in smaller arteries is almost entirely muscular and in larger arteries is more elastic. The thickness of the outer layer varies with the location of the artery. In protected areas, such as the abdominal and cranial cavities, the outer layer of associated arteries is very thin, but in more exposed locations, as in the limbs, it is much thicker.

arteria parietalis posterior, posterior parietal artery: or-

Tunica externa
(adventitia)
Connective tissue
Vasa vasorum

Tunica media
Smooth muscle

Tunica intima
Elastic fibers
Basement
membrane
Endothelium

Arterial wall *(Applegate, 2000)*

igin, terminal part of middle cerebral artery; *branches,* none; *distribution,* posterior parietal lobe.

arteria radicularis magna, artery of Adamkiewicz.

arteriectomy /ärtir′ē·ek′təmē/ [Gk, *arteria* + *ektomē,* excision], the surgical removal of a portion of an artery.

arteries. See **blood vessel.**

arterio-, arteri-, prefix meaning 'artery': *arteriosclerosis, arteritis.*

arteriocapillary /är·tēr′ē·ō·kap′i·lar′ē/ [Gk, *arteria* + L, *capillaris,* hairlike], pertaining to the arteries and the capillaries.

arteriofibrosis /ärtir′ē·ōfībrō′sis/, an inflammatory, fibrous thickening of the walls of the arteries and arterioles, resulting in a narrowing of the lumen of the vessels.

arteriogenic impotence, vasculogenic impotence caused by a disorder in the arteries supplying the penis, such as atherosclerosis or stenosis.

arteriogram /ärtir′ē·əgram′/, an x-ray film of an artery injected with a radiopaque medium. See also **arteriography.**

arteriography /ärtir′ē·og′rəfē/ [Gk, *arteria,* airpipe, *graphein,* to record], a method of radiologic visualization of arteries performed after a radiopaque contrast medium is introduced into the bloodstream or into a specific vessel by injection or through a catheter. See also **angiography. —arteriographic,** *adj.*

arteriole /ärtir′ē·ōl/ [L, *arteriola,* little artery], the smallest of the arteries. Blood flowing from the heart is pumped through the arteries, to the arterioles, to the capillaries, into the veins, and returned to the heart. The muscular walls of the arterioles constrict and dilate in response to both local factors and neurochemical stimuli; thus, arterioles play a significant role in peripheral vascular resistance and in regulation of blood pressure. Also called **arteriola.** See also **artery.**

arteriolosclerosis /ärtir′ē·ō′ləskləro′sis/, pathologic thickening, hardening, and loss of elasticity of arteriolar walls.

arteriopathy /ärtir′ē·op′əthē/ [Gk, *arteria* + *pathos,* suffering], a disease of an artery.

arterioplasty /ärtir′ē·əplas′tē/ [Gk, *arteria* + *plassein,* to mold], surgical repair or reconstruction of an artery. The procedure is often performed to correct an aneurysm.

arteriosclerosis /ärtir′ē·ō′sklərō′sis/ [Gk, *arteria* + *sklerosis,* hardening], a common disorder characterized by thickening, loss of elasticity, and calcification of arterial walls. It results in a decreased blood supply, especially to the cerebrum and lower extremities. The condition often develops with aging and in hypertension, nephrosclerosis, scleroderma, diabetes, and hyperlipidemia. Typical signs and symptoms include intermittent claudication, changes in skin temperature and color, altered peripheral pulses, bruits over an involved artery, headache, dizziness, and memory defects. Vasodilators and exercise may relieve symptoms, but there is no specific treatment. Preventive measures include therapy for predisposing diseases, adequate rest and exercise, avoidance of stress, and discontinuation of tobacco use. Kinds of arteriosclerosis include **atherosclerosis** and **Mönckeberg's arteriosclerosis**. Also called **arterial sclerosis, hardening of the arteries**. —**arteriosclerotic**, *adj*.

arteriosclerosis obliterans [Gk, *arteria* + *skleros* + L, *obliterare*, efface], a gradual narrowing of the arteries with thrombosis and degeneration of the intima. The condition may lead to complete occlusion of an artery and subsequent gangrene.

arteriosclerotic /-sklərot′ik/ [Gk, *arteria* + *skleros*, hard], pertaining to a thickening and hardening of the arterial wall.

arteriosclerotic aneurysm, an aneurysm arising in a large artery, most commonly the abdominal aorta, as a result of weakening of the wall in severe atherosclerosis. Also called **atherosclerotic aneurysm**.

arteriosclerotic heart disease (ASHD), a thickening and hardening of the walls of the coronary arteries.

arteriosclerotic retinopathy [Gk, *arteria*, airpipe, *sklerosis*, hardening; L, *rete*, net; Gk, *pathos*, disease], a disorder of the retina associated with hardening and thickening of the arteries supplying that part of the eye. It often accompanies hypertension.

arteriospasm /ärtir′ē·ōspaz′əm/ [Gk, *arteria* + *spasmos*, spasm], a spasm of an artery.

arteriostenosis /-stənō′sis/, a narrowing of an artery.

arteriotomy /ärtir′ē·ot′əmē/, a surgical incision in an artery.

arteriovenous (AV) /-vē′nəs/ [Gk, *arteria* + L, *vena*, vein], pertaining to arteries and veins.

arteriovenous anastomosis [Gk, *arteria* + L, *vena*; Gk, *anastomoein*, to form a mouth], a communication between an artery and a vein, either as a congenital anomaly or as a surgically produced link between vessels.

arteriovenous aneurysm, a dilation affecting both an artery and a vein, often as an abnormal linkage of the two.

arteriovenous angioma of the brain, a congenital tumor consisting of a tangle of coiled, usually dilated arteries and veins, islets of sclerosed brain tissue, and, occasionally, cartilaginous cells. The lesion, which may be distinguished by an intracranial bruit, generally arises in the vascular system of the pia mater and may grow to project deeply into the brain, causing seizures and progressive hemiparesis.

arteriovenous fistula, an abnormal communication between an artery and vein. It may occur congenitally or result from trauma, infection, arterial aneurysm, or a malignancy. A continuous murmur and palpable thrill may be detected over the fistula and may be obliterated by compressing the feeding artery; this maneuver may slow the heartbeat (Branham's sign). Chronic arteriovenous fistulas may cause varicosities, cutaneous ulcers, and cardiac enlargement. A congenital fistula may result in a cavernous hemangioma. If an arteriovenous fistula is limited in size and is accessible, it can be treated by surgical excision. An arteriovenous fistula

is often created surgically to provide vascular access for hemodialysis.

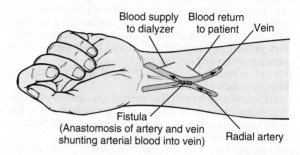

Arteriovenous fistula *(Lewis, Heitkemper, and Dirksen, 2004)*

arteriovenous oxygen (a-vo₂) difference, the arterial oxygen content minus the central venous oxygen content.

arteriovenous shunt (AV shunt), a passageway, artificial or natural, that allows blood to flow from an artery to a vein without going through a capillary network.

Arteriovenous shunt *(Sanders et al, 2000)*

arteritis /är′tərī′tis/ [Gk, *arteria* + *itis*], inflammation of the inner layers or the outer coat of one or more arteries. It may occur as a clinical entity or accompany another disorder, such as rheumatoid arthritis, rheumatic fever, polymyositis, or systemic lupus erythematosus. Kinds of arteritis include **infantile, rheumatic, Takayasu's,** and **temporal arteritis**. See also **endarteritis, periarteritis**.

arteritis obliterans. See **endarteritis obliterans**.

arteritis umbilicalis, septic inflammation of the umbilical artery in newborns, usually caused by the bacterium *Clostridium tetani*.

artery /är′tərē/ [Gk, *arteria*, airpipe], one of the large blood vessels carrying blood in a direction away from the heart to the tissues. See also **arterial wall, arteriole**. Compare **vein**.

artery forceps, any forceps used for grasping, compressing, and holding the end of an artery during ligation. Generally self-locking, its handles are scissorlike. Also called **hemostatic forceps**.

arthral. See **articular**.

arthralgia /ärthral′jə/ [Gk, *arthron,* joint, *algos,* pain], joint pain. —**arthralgic,** *adj.*

-arthria, suffix meaning a '(specified) condition involving the ability to articulate': *anarthria, dysarthria.*

-arthritic, -arthritical, suffix meaning 'arthritis': *antiarthritic, postarthritic.*

arthritis /ärthrī′tis/ [Gk, *arthron,* joint, *itis*], any inflammatory condition of the joints, characterized by pain, swelling, heat, redness, and limitation of movement. See also **osteoarthritis, rheumatoid arthritis.**

arthritis deformans. See **rheumatoid arthritis.**

arthro-, arthr-, combining form meaning 'joints, articulations': *arthralgia, arthrocentesis.*

arthrocentesis /är′thrōsintē′sis/ [Gk, *arthron + kentesis,* pricking], the puncture of a joint with a needle and the withdrawal of fluid, performed to obtain samples of synovial fluid for diagnostic purposes. It may also be used to instill medications and to remove fluid from joints to simply relieve pain. A local anesthetic is usually administered; surgical asepsis is observed in the procedure. Normal synovial fluid is a clear, straw-colored, slightly viscous liquid that forms a white, viscous clot when mixed with glacial acetic acid; if inflammation is present, as in rheumatoid arthritis, the fluid is watery and turbid, and its mixture with glacial acetic acid results in a flocculent, easily broken clot. The number of leukocytes, especially polymorphonuclear cells, and the protein content are increased, and the glucose level is decreased if inflammation is present. Synovial fluid samples are also cultured and examined microscopically to diagnose a septic process, such as bacterial arthritis.

Arthrocentesis *(Custalow, 2005)*

treatment. Also called **amyoplasia congenita** /əmī′ōplā′zhə/.

arthrokinematic /är′thrəkin′əmat′ik/, pertaining to the movement of bone surfaces within a joint.

arthron /är′thron/ [Gk], a joint or articulation, including its various components of bones, cartilaginous inserts, all soft tissue structures intervening between the rigid skeletal parts, and the adjacent muscular elements.

arthropathy /ärthrop′əthē/ [Gk, *arthron + pathos,* suffering], any disease or abnormal condition affecting a joint. —**arthropathic,** *adj.*

arthroplasty /är′thrəplast′ē/, [Gk, *arthron + plassein,* to mold], the surgical reconstruction or replacement of a painful, degenerated joint, to restore mobility in osteoarthritis or rheumatoid arthritis or to correct a congenital deformity. Either the bones of the joint are reshaped and soft tissue or a metal disk is placed between the reshaped ends, or all or part of the joint is replaced with a metal or plastic prosthesis. Preoperative care may include the typing and crossmatching of blood. After surgery the patient may be placed in traction to immobilize the affected limb. Physical therapy to increase muscle strength and range of motion is allowed in a slow, progressive schedule. When a lower extremity is involved, weight-bearing may or may not be allowed. Frequent checks of distal circulation are made and the nurse watches for bleeding, thrombophlebitis, pulmonary embolism, or fat embolism. Antibiotics are usually given to prevent infection, which is the most common cause of failure of the surgery. See also **osteoarthritis.**

arthropod /är′thrəpod′/ [Gk, *arthron + pous,* foot], a member of the Arthropoda, a large phylum of animal life that includes crabs and lobsters as well as mites, ticks, spiders, and insects. Arthropods generally are distinguished by a jointed exoskeleton (shell) and paired, jointed legs. They bite, sting, cause allergic reactions, and may serve as vectors for viruses and other disease-causing agents.

arthroscope /-skōp′/ [Gk, *arthron + skopein,* to watch], a type of endoscope used to examine joints.

arthroscopy /ärthros′kəpē/ [Gk, *arthron + skopein,* to watch], the examination of the interior of a joint, performed by inserting a specially designed endoscope through a small incision. The procedure, used chiefly in knee problems, permits biopsy of cartilage or synovium, diagnosis of a torn meniscus, and, in some instances, removal of loose bodies in the joint space. —**arthroscopic,** *adj.*

arthrodesis. See **ankylosis,** def. 2.

arthrodia. See **gliding joint.**

arthrogram /är′thrəgram/, **1.** a radiographic record after introduction of opaque contrast material into a joint. **2.** a nuclear medicine study used to detect the loosening of a prosthetic device.

arthrography [Gk, *arthron,* joint, *graphein,* to record], a method of radiographically visualizing the inside of a joint using a radiolucent or radiopaque contrast medium.

arthrogryposis multiplex congenita [Gk, *arthron + gryposis,* joint curve; L, *multus,* many, *plica,* fold, *congenitus,* born with], fibrous stiffness of one or more joints, present at birth. It is often associated with incomplete development of the muscles that move the involved joints and degenerative changes of the motor neurons that innervate those muscles. The cause of the condition, which is uncommon, is unknown. Physiotherapy to loosen the joints is the only

Arthroscopy *(Beare and Myers, 1998)*

arthrous /är′thrəs/ [Gk, *arthron*], **1.** pertaining to joints or the articulation of bones. **2.** pertaining to a disease of a joint.

Arthus reaction /ärtoōs′/ [Nicholas M. Arthus, French physiologist, 1862–1945], a rare, severe, immediate nonatopic hypersensitivity reaction to the injection of a foreign substance, that usually is not irritating but in certain individuals is antigenic. The reaction is thought to involve the formation of an antigen-antibody complex that activates complement. Acute local inflammation, usually in the skin and marked by edema, hemorrhage, and necrosis, occurs at the site of injection. Also called **Arthus phenomenon.** See also **serum sickness.**

articul-, combining form meaning 'joint, structure and function': *articular, articulatio.*

articular /ärtik′yələr/ [L, *articulare,* to divide into joints], relating to a joint or the involvement of joints.

articular capsule [L, *articulare,* to divide into joints], an envelope of tissue that surrounds a freely moving joint, composed of an external layer of white fibrous tissue and an internal synovial membrane. See also **fibrous capsule.**

articular cartilage [L, *articulare* + *cartilago*], a type of hyaline connective tissue that covers the articulating surfaces of bones within synovial joints. See also **cartilage.**

articular disk, the platelike cartilaginous end of certain bones in movable joints, sometimes closely associated with surrounding muscles or with cartilage.

articular fracture, a fracture involving the articulating surfaces of a joint.

articular head, a projection on a bone that forms a joint with another bone.

articular muscle, a muscle that is attached to the capsule of a joint.

articular process of vertebra, a bony outgrowth on a vertebra that forms a joint with an adjoining vertebra.

articulate /ärtik′yəlāt/ [L, *articulare,* to divide into joints], **1.** to form a joint. **2.** to use speech that is distinct and connected.

articulated /ärtik′yəlā′tid/, **1.** united by a movable joint. **2.** expressed in clear speech.

articulated partial denture. See **partial denture.**

articulatio cubiti. See **elbow joint.**

articulatio ellipsoidea. See **condyloid joint.**

articulatio genus. See **knee joint.**

articulation. See **joint.**

articulation of the pelvis /ärtik′yəlā′shən/, any one of the connections between the bones of the pelvis, involving four groups of ligaments. The first group connects the sacrum and the ilium; the second, the sacrum and the ischium; the third, the sacrum and the coccyx; and the fourth, the two pubic bones.

articulatio plana. See **gliding joint.**

articulatio sellaris. See **saddle joint.**

articulator /ärtik′yəlā′tər/ [L, *articulare,* to divide into joints], a mechanical device used in the fabrication and testing of dental prostheses. It represents the temporomandibular joints and jaw members to which maxillary and mandibular casts may be attached. Some articulators are adjustable, allowing movement of attached casts into various eccentric relationships.

articulus. See **joint.**

artifact /är′təfakt/ [L, *ars,* skill, *facere,* to make], anything artificially made; may be extraneous, irrelevant, or unwanted, such as a substance, structure, or piece of data or information. In radiologic imaging, spurious electronic signals may appear as an artifact in an image with as much strength as the signals produced by the real objects, thereby confusing the radiologist and the results of any examination.

artifactual modification /är′təfak′choo·əl/, a change in protein structure caused by in vitro manipulation.

artificial /är′tifish′əl/ [L, *artificium,* not natural], **1.** made by human work as a substitute for something that is natural. **2.** simulated, resulting from art in imitation of nature.

artificial abortion, an abortion that is produced deliberately.

artificial airway [L, *artificiosum,* skillfully made], a plastic or rubber device that can be inserted into the upper or lower respiratory tract to facilitate ventilation or the removal of secretions.

artificial airway management, a nursing intervention from the Nursing Interventions Classification (NIC) defined as maintenance of endotracheal and tracheostomy tubes and preventing complications associated with their use. See also **Nursing Interventions Classification.**

artificial ankylosis, a surgical procedure in which two or more parts of a joint are fixed so that the joint becomes immovable.

artificial anus, a surgical opening into the bowel, as in a colostomy.

artificial assists, any prosthetic devices or contrivances that may enable a physically challenged person to function. Examples include heart pacemakers, crutches, and artificial limbs.

artificial blood. See **perfluorocarbons.**

artificial classification of caries. See **classification of caries.**

artificial classification of cavities, any cavity that may be classified in one of six groups, the first five of which are those proposed by G.V. Black. Class 1: cavities associated with structural tooth defects in the occlusal surfaces of posterior teeth, and lingual surfaces of anterior teeth, such as pits and fissures; class 2: cavities in the proximal surfaces of premolars and molars; class 3: cavities in the proximal surfaces of the canines and incisors that do not involve removal and restoration of the incisal angle; class 4: cavities in the proximal surfaces of canines and incisors that require the removal and restoration of the incisal angle; class 5: cavities, except pit cavities, in the gingival third of the labial, buccal, or lingual surfaces of the teeth; class 6: (not included in Black's classification) cavities on the incisal edges and cusp tips of the teeth. See also **cavity classification, simple cavity, smooth surface cavity.**

artificial crown, a dental prosthesis that restores part or all of the crown of a natural tooth. Compare **anatomic crown, clinical crown, partial crown.**

artificial dentition. See **dentition.**

artificial eye, a prosthetic device resembling the anterior surface of a normal eyeball. It is fitted under the upper and lower eyelid of an eye that has been removed.

artificial fever, an elevated body temperature produced by artificial means, such as the injection of malarial parasites or a vaccine known to produce fever symptoms or application of heat to the body. An artificial fever may be prescribed for a patient to arrest a disease that is sensitive to elevated body temperatures. Also called **fever therapy.**

artificial genitourinary sphincter, an implantable prosthetic device for treating urinary incontinence caused by an incompetent or absent sphincter; an artificial sphincter is created with an inflatable cuff around the bladder neck or bulbar urethra.

artificial heart, a mechanical device of molded polyurethane, consisting of two ventricles implanted in the body and powered by an air compressor located outside the body. The first artificial heart for humans was implanted in December 1982 at the University of Utah Medical Center in Salt Lake City. It was attached to the atria and major blood vessels of the native heart with Dacron fittings and kept the patient alive for 112 days. See also **Jarvik-7.**

artificial homologous insemination. See **artificial insemination—husband (AIH).**

artificial impregnation. See **artificial insemination—husband.**

artificial insemination (AI), the introduction of semen into the vagina or uterus by mechanical or instrumental means rather than by sexual intercourse. The procedure is planned to coincide with the expected time of ovulation so that fertilization can occur. Kinds of artificial insemination are **artificial insemination—donor (AID)** and **artificial insemination—husband (AIH).** Also called **artificial impregnation.** See also **menstrual cycle.**

artificial insemination—donor (AID), artificial insemination in which the semen specimen is provided by an anonymous donor. The procedure is used primarily in cases where the husband is sterile. Also called **heterologous insemination.** Compare **artificial insemination—husband.**

artificial insemination—husband (AIH), artificial insemination in which the semen specimen is provided by the husband. The procedure is used primarily in cases of impotency, low sperm count, or a vaginal disorder or when the husband is incapable of sexual intercourse because of some physical disability. Also called **artificial homologous insemination.** Compare **artificial insemination—donor.**

artificial intelligence (AI), a system that makes it possible for a machine to perform functions similar to those performed by human intelligence, such as learning, reasoning, self-correcting, and adapting. Computer technology produces many instruments and systems that mimic and surpass some human capabilities, as speed of calculations, correlating, sensing, and deducing.

artificial kidney, a device used to remove the body waste, commonly excreted in urine, from circulating blood. It usually consists of a set of tubes or catheters that pass the blood through a dialysate solution where wastes are removed by osmosis and diffusion. Also called **dialyzer, hemodialyzer, kidney machine.** See also **hemodialysis, peritoneal dialysis.**

artificial labor [L, *artificiosum,* artificial, *labor,* work], induced labor, as when started with drugs or mechanical devices.

artificial limb. See **prosthesis.**

artificial lung. See **Drinker respirator.**

artificially acquired immunity. See **acquired immunity.**

artificial menopause [L, *artificiosus,* artificial, *men,* month; Gk, *pauein,* to cease], the termination of menstrual periods by surgery, radiation, or other methods. See also **menopause.**

artificial pacemaker. See **pacemaker.**

artificial pneumothorax. See **therapeutic pneumothorax.**

artificial respiration. See **artificial ventilation.**

artificial rupture of membranes. See **amniotomy.**

artificial saliva [L, *artificiosum,* artifice, *saliva,* spittle], a mixture of carboxymethylcellulose, sorbitol, sodium, and potassium chloride in an aqueous solution. It is available in a spray container for the treatment of xerostomia, or dry mouth.

artificial selection, the process by which the genotypes of successive plant and animal generations are determined through controlled breeding. See also **eugenics.** Compare **natural selection.**

artificial stone, a calcined gypsum derivative similar to but stronger than plaster of paris, used for making dental casts and dies. Also called **dental stone.**

artificial tears, a pharmaceutical preparation of various polymers that can be instilled in the eyes of patients suffering from dry eye or keratoconjunctivitis sicca.

artificial ventilation, the process of supporting respiration by manual or mechanical means when normal breathing is inefficient or has stopped. If artificial ventilation is unsuccessful, the patient is repositioned and the airway is tested for the presence of an obstruction. Also called **artificial respiration.** See also **cardiopulmonary resuscitation, resuscitation, ventilator.**

Art-line. See **arterial line.**

art therapist, a human service professional who uses art media and images, the creative process, and client responses to artwork in order to assess, treat, and rehabilitate patients with mental, emotional, physical, or developmental disorders. Through art, the therapist attempts to help the client access and express memories, trauma, and psychic conflict often not easily reached with words.

art therapy[1], the use of art media to reconcile emotional conflicts, foster self-awareness, and express unspoken and frequently unconscious concerns. Art therapy is often used when traditional forms of verbal psychotherapy have failed or been rejected by an individual and when individuals have difficulty expressing feelings or use verbalization as a defense mechanism.

art therapy[2], a nursing intervention from the Nursing Interventions Classification (NIC) defined as facilitation of communication through drawings or other art forms. See also **Nursing Interventions Classification.**

aryepiglottic folds /er′ē·ep′iglot′ik/, folds of mucous membrane that extend around the margins of the larynx from a junction with the epiglottis. They function as a sphincter during swallowing.

aryl-, prefix designating an alkyl monovalent radical derived from an aromatic hydrocarbon and used to denote aromatic groups.

aryl hydrocarbon hydroxylase (AHH), an enzyme that converts carcinogenic chemicals in tobacco smoke and in polluted air into active carcinogens within the lungs. Aryl hydrocarbon hydroxylase is the subject of numerous studies to determine why cancer develops in some smokers but not in others. Experimental blood tests indicate that the level of aryl hydrocarbon hydroxylase may be a factor in hereditary predisposition of a cigarette smoker to cancer.

arytenoid cartilage /ä·rit′ənoid kär′ti·ləj/ [Gk, *arytaina,* ladle + *eidos,* form; L, *cartilago*], one of the paired, pitcher-shaped cartilages of the back of the larynx at the upper border of the cricoid cartilage.

As, symbol for the element **arsenic.**

AS, abbreviation for **aortic stenosis.**

as-. See **ad-.**

a.s., abbreviation for **auris sinistra.**

ASA, 1. abbreviation for *American Society of Anesthesiologists.* 2. abbreviation for **aspirin** (acetylsalicylic acid).

5-ASA, 5-aminosalicylic acid.

ASAHP, 1. abbreviation for *American Society of Allied Health Professionals.* 2. abbreviation for *Association of Schools of Allied Health Professionals.*

ASAP, abbreviation for *as soon as possible.*

Artificial hearts

Pump type	Pump method	Ventricular support	Power & controller
Extracorporeal Biomedicus	• Centrifugal device—impeller inside cone that creates vortex • Can rotate to 5000 rpm • Maximum pump flow rate 10L/min	Right ventricle/left ventricle/ biventricular ECMO (extracorporeal membrane oxygenation)	• External motor and power console • Internal battery, 45 min
Abiomed's BVS 5000	• A pneumatic drive console • Can operate one or two blood pumps independently	Right ventricle/left ventricle/ biventricular	External power and control console
Paracorporeal Thoratec VAD System	• Blood flows to the VAD through an atrial or ventricular cannula • Sensor detects the VAD is full of blood and ejects blood from pump into the aorta (left side) or pulmonary artery (right side)	Right ventricle/left ventricle/ biventricular	*Dual Drive Console:* • Two independent and identical modules that provide alternating pulses of air pressure and vacuum to provide pulsatile flow *TLC-II Mobility Cart:* • Single driver unit: Univentricular Biventricular • 4 rechargeable batteries *TLC Docking Station:* • Serves as a home base for portable driver • Downloads data • Allows for pump parameters to be changed • Battery charger
Implantable Novacor, Heartmate	• Passive filling of the pump • Aortic valve does not open • Pump output depends on flow from the right side • Can track the natural heart rhythm	Left ventricular device only	• External microprocessor-based electronic controller powered by an AC external home unit as well as primary and secondary batteries • Life-threatening alarm systems cannot be muted • Can run in either auto or fixed rate mode • Battery charger

Courtesy Colleen Becker, RN, MSN, CCRN and Kathy Sue Rowland, RN, BS Educ., Barnes-Jewish Hospital.

Uses	Pump, console placement	Problems/issues
• Cardiopulmonary bypass short term (=5 days of circulatory support) • Postcardiotomy cardiogenic shock • Bridge to transplant	• External	• Can be used on newborns-adults • Non-pulsatile blood flow (kidneys, brain, endocardium require pulsatility to remain viable) • Anticoagulation • Needs intensive bedside management—nursing/perfusion • Emergency hand-crank pump • No CPR; can defibrillate • Patient on total bedrest • Anticoagulation • Infection control
• Only FDA-approved device for all patients with potentially reversible heart failure = 10 days • Bridge to transplant • Possible weaning from device as heart recovers	• External	• Pulsatile flow (kidneys, brain, endocardium require pulsatility to remain viable) • Managed at bedside; requires bedside specialty nursing care • Emergency foot pump • CPR and defibrillation possible • Bedrest, semi-Fowler's—surgeon preference • Anticoagulation • Infection control
• Used to support total or partial circulatory assistance • Possible wean from Thoratec to a less invasive device (i.e., IABP) • Bridge to transplant	• External	• Pulsatile flow (kidneys, brain, endocardium require pulsatility to remain viable) • Portable console • Small, battery-powered unit allows mobility • Patient can leave hospital for less acute facility near patient's home • Noncritical care personnel and family can be trained to care for basic functions and troubleshooting • Do not use povidone-iodine ointment for dressing • Emergency hand pump • Exposure to **ketoacetones** can destroy LVAD external housing—patient, family and health care personnel must be strongly cautioned against use. (printed signs in room) • Defibrillation possible • Anticoagulation • Infection control
• Bridge to transplant • Bridge to recovery • Chronic or "end stage" alternative therapy	Pump inside body with percutaneous lead cable tunneled to exit site (usually above the right iliac crest)	• Pulsatile flow (kidneys, brain, endocardium require pulsatility to remain viable) • Patient size a consideration for type of device that can be implanted • Must have good right-sided heart • Heartmate: no CPR and defibrillation with restrictions • Novacor: CPR and defibrillation can be performed • Possible infection of the drive line site • Patient can be mobile and at home, but with 24-hr supervision with noncritical personnel • Emergency hand pump • Novacor external equipment somewhat heavier (~10 lbs) than Heartmate • Abdominal scarring/previous surgeries may prevent implantation • MRI is contraindicated • Anticoagulation • Infection control

asbestos /asbes′təs/ [Gk, *asbestos,* unquenchable], a group of fibrous impure magnesium silicate minerals. Inhalation of the fibers can lead to pulmonary fibrosis if the fibers accumulate in terminal bronchioles. Continued exposure to asbestos fibers can result in lung cancer.

asbestos body, a structure found in the lungs of patients with asbestosis, consisting of an asbestos fiber engulfed by a macrophage or of a mass of asbestos spicules coated with calcium, iron salts, and other substances.

Asbestos bodies *(Silverberg, DeLellis, and Frable, 1997)*

asbestosis [Gk, *asbestos,* inextinguishable, *osis,* condition], a chronic lung disease caused by the inhalation of asbestos fibers that results in the development of alveolar, interstitial, and pleural fibrosis. Asbestos miners and workers are most frequently affected, but the disease sometimes occurs in other people who have been exposed to asbestos building materials. Chest x-ray films show the characteristic small linear opacities distributed throughout the lungs. The disease is progressive: Shortness of breath develops eventually into respiratory failure. Cigarette smoking and continuous exposure to asbestos aggravate the condition. Fatal mesothelial tumors sometimes occur. There is no treatment. See also **chronic obstructive pulmonary disease, inorganic dust.**

Asbestosis *(Kumar, Cotran, and Robbins, 2003)*

ASC, abbreviation for **altered state of consciousness.**

ascariasis /as′kərī′əsis/ [Gk, *askaris,* intestinal worm, *osis,* condition], an infection caused by a parasitic worm, *Ascaris lumbricoides,* that migrates through the lungs in its larval stage. The eggs are passed in human feces, contaminating the soil and allowing transmission to the mouths of others through hands, water, or food. After hatching in the small intestine, the larvae travel through the wall of the intestine and are carried by the lymphatics and blood to the lungs. Early respiratory symptoms of coughing, wheezing, hemoptysis, and fever are caused by the passage through the respiratory tract. The larvae are swallowed; they mature in the jejunum, where they release eggs; and the cycle is repeated. Intestinal infection may result in abdominal cramps and obstruction. In children migration of the adult worms into the liver, gallbladder, or peritoneal cavity may cause death. The infective eggs are readily identified in the feces. Piperazine citrate, pyrantel pamoate, mebendazole, and alberdazole are effective treatments. The disease can be prevented by educating people, especially children, about good hygiene such as handwashing.

ascaris, a nematode of the genus *Ascaris.*

Ascaris /as′kəris/, a genus of large parasitic intestinal roundworms, such as *Ascaris lumbricoides,* a cause of ascariasis, found throughout temperate and tropic regions.

Ascaris lumbricoides: adult worm
(Conlon and Snydman, 2000)

ascending aorta /asen′ding/ [L, *ascendere,* to climb], one of the four main sections of the aorta, branching into the right and left coronary arteries. See also **arch of the aorta.**

ascending colon, the segment of the colon that extends up the cecum in the lower right side of the colic fissure to the abdomen to the transverse colon at the hepatic flexure on the right side.

ascending current. See **centripetal current.**

ascending neuritis [L, *ascendere,* to rise; Gk, *neuron,* nerve, *itis,* inflammation], a nerve inflammation that begins on the periphery and moves upward along a nerve trunk.

ascending neuropathy, a disease of the nervous system that begins at a lower place in the body and spreads upward.

ascending paralysis, a condition in which there is successive flaccid paralysis of the legs, then the trunk and arms, and finally the muscles of respiration. Causes include poliomyelitis, Guillain-Barré syndrome, and exposure to toxic chemicals.

ascending pharyngeal artery, one of the smallest arteries that branch from the external carotid artery, deep in the neck. It supplies various organs and muscles of the head, such as the tympanic cavity, the longus capitis, and the longus colli. It divides into five branches: the pharyngeal, palatine, prevertebral, inferior tympanic, and posterior meningeal.

ascending poliomyelitis [L, *ascendere,* to rise; Gk, *polios,* gray, *myelos,* marrow, *itis,* inflammation], poliomyelitis that begins in the legs and spreads upward to involve the trunk and respiratory muscles. See also **ascending paralysis.**

ascending pyelonephritis, pyelonephritis caused by a urinary tract infection that has spread up the ureter into the kidney.

ascending testis, one that is in the scrotum in the infant boy but later ascends into cryptorchidism.

ascending tract [L, *tractus*], a nervous system pathway found in the spinal cord that carries impulses toward the brain. Also called **afferent tract.**

ascending urography. See **urography.**

asceticism /aset′isiz′əm/ [Gk, *askein,* to exercise], (in psychiatry) a defense mechanism that involves repudiation of all instinctual impulses. The concept is derived from the religious doctrine that material things are evil and only spiritual things are good.

Ascher's syndrome /äsh′ərz/ [Karl Wolfgang Ascher, Czech-born American ophthalmologist, 1887–1971], relaxation of the skin of the eyelid and redundancy of the mucous membrane and submucous tissue of the upper lip in goiter.

Aschoff bodies [Karl A.L. Aschoff, German pathologist, 1866–1942; AS, *bodig*], tiny rounded or spindle-shaped nodules containing multinucleated giant cells, fibroblasts, and basophilic cells. They are found in joints, tendons, the pleura, and the cardiovascular system of rheumatic fever patients.

Aschoff body
(Kumar, Cotran, and Robbins, 2003/courtesy Sid Murphree, MD, Department of Pathology, University of Texas Southwestern Medical School)

ascites /əsī′tēz/ [Gk, *askos,* bag], an abnormal intraperitoneal accumulation of a fluid containing large amounts of protein and electrolytes. Ascites may be detectable when more than 500 ml of fluid has accumulated. The condition may be accompanied by general abdominal swelling, hemodilution, edema, or a decrease in urinary output. Identification of ascites is made through palpation, percussion, and auscultation. Ascites is a complication, for example, of cirrhosis, congestive heart failure, nephrosis, malignant neoplastic disease, peritonitis, or various fungal and parasitic diseases. It is treated with dietary therapy and diuretic drugs; abdominal paracentesis may be performed to relieve pain and improve respiratory and visceral function by relieving the pressure of the accumulated fluid. A peritoneovenous shunt may be surgically inserted to drain the ascites via a tube from the peritoneal cavity to the superior vena cava. See also **paracentesis. —ascitic,** *adj.*

Ascites *(Lewis, Heitkemper, and Dirksen, 2004)*

ascites adiposus. See **chylous ascites.**

ascites praecox /prē′koks/ [Gk, *askos* + L, premature], an abnormal accumulation of fluid within the peritoneal cavity before the generalized edema associated with pericarditis. See also **ascites.**

ascitic fluid /əsit′ik/ [Gk, *askos,* bag], a watery fluid containing albumin, glucose, and electrolytes that accumulates in the peritoneal cavity in association with certain diseases, such as liver disease or congestive heart failure. The fluid occurs as leakage from the veins and lymphatics into extravascular spaces.

ASCO, abbreviation for *American Society of Clinical Oncology.*

ascorbemia /as′kôrbē′mē·ə/ [Gk, *a,* not; AS, *scurf,* scurvy; Gk, *haima,* blood], the presence of ascorbic acid in the blood in amounts greater than normal, usually reflecting only an excess of ascorbic acid intake. The condition is usually due to the use of ascorbic acid supplements.

ascorbic acid /əskôr′bik/ [Gk, *a,* not; AS, *scurf,* scurvy], a water-soluble, white crystalline vitamin present in citrus fruits, tomatoes, berries, potatoes, and fresh green and leafy vegetables, including broccoli, brussels sprouts, collards, turnip greens, parsley, sweet bell peppers, and cabbage. It is essential for the formation of collagen and fibrous tissue for normal intercellular matrices in teeth, bone, cartilage, connective tissue, and skin, and for the structural integrity of capillary walls. It also aids in fighting bacterial infections and interacts with other nutrients. Signs of deficiency are bleeding gums, tendency to bruise, swollen or painful joints, nosebleeds, anemia, lowered resistance to infections, and slow healing of wounds and fractures. Severe deficiency results in scurvy. A large excess of ascorbic acid may cause a burning sensation during urination, diarrhea, skin rash, and nausea and may disturb the absorption and metabolism of cyanocobalamin. Results of tests for glycosuria, uric acid, and iron may be inaccurate when the patient is receiving large amounts of the vitamin. Also called **antiscorbutic vitamin, vitamin C.** See also **ascorbemia, infantile scurvy, scurvy.**

ascorburia /as′kôrbyŏŏr′ē·ə/ [Gk, *a,* not; AS, *scurf,* scurvy; Gk, *ouron,* urine], the presence of ascorbic acid in the urine in amounts greater than normal. It usually reflects only an excess ascorbic acid intake, generally caused by the use of ascorbic acid supplements.

ascribed role /əskrībd′/, an assigned role in society, based on age, sex, or other factors about which the individual has no choice. See also **assumed role.**

ASD, abbreviation for **atrial septal defect.**

-ase, suffix used in naming enzymes; acts on the substance named in the word root (that precedes the suffix): *lipase, protease.*

Asendin, trademark for a tricyclic antidepressant (amoxapine).

asepsis /āsep′sis/ [Gk, *a, sepsis,* not decay], **1.** the absence of germs. **2. medical asepsis,** procedures used to reduce the number of microorganisms and prevent their spread. Examples include handwashing and "no touch" dressing technique. **3. surgical asepsis,** procedures used to eliminate any microorganisms; sterile technique. An example is sterilization of surgical instruments. **—aseptic,** *adj.*

aseptic /āsep′tik/ [Gk, *a,* without, *sepsis,* decay], pertaining to a condition free of living pathogenic organisms or infected material. See also **asepsis.**

aseptic-antiseptic, both aseptic and antiseptic.

aseptic body image, an awareness by operating room personnel of body, hair, makeup, clothing, jewelry, and placement with regard for maintenance of a sterile environment. The body image also includes an awareness of changing proximities between sterile and contaminated areas as a field becomes progressively contaminated.

aseptic bone necrosis, a type of bone and joint damage that may occur in people who repeatedly breathe compressed air, as in diving or tunneling occupations. The condition apparently results from occlusion of small arteries in the bone by nitrogen bubbles, followed by infarction of bone tissue. It may also occur in patients taking corticosteroids. The condition may be asymptomatic or, if joint surfaces are involved, marked by severe pain and joint collapse. It may also be associated with an injury to the joint. It typically occurs in the femoral head. See also **avascular necrosis.**

aseptic fever, a fever not associated with infection. Mechanical trauma, as in a crushing injury, can cause fever even when no pathogenic microorganism is present. Although the exact mechanism is not understood, fever in such cases is believed to result from the breakdown of leukocytes or the absorption of avascular tissue.

aseptic gauze, any gauze that is free of microorganisms.

aseptic meningitis, an inflammation of the meninges that is caused by one of a number of viruses, including coxsackieviruses, nonparalytic polioviruses, echoviruses, and mumps, or may be drug induced, such as with high-dose IV immunoglobulin. Viral meningitis is especially common in children during the late summer and early fall. In about one third of the cases no pathogen can be demonstrated, but analysis of cerebrospinal fluid reveals increased numbers of white blood cells, usually lymphocytes; normal glucose concentration; slightly elevated protein levels; and no bacteria. Symptoms vary, depending on the causative agent and may include fever, headache, stiff neck and back, nausea, and skin rash. No specific treatment is available. Supportive therapy is directed to maintaining hydration and controlling fever. Complete recovery, without complication or residual effect, is usual. See also **viral meningitis.**

aseptic necrosis [Gk, *a, sepsis,* without decay, *nekros,* dead, *osis,* condition], cystic and sclerotic degenerative changes

in tissues, as may follow an injury in the absence of infection.

aseptic peritonitis [Gk, *a, sepsis,* without decay, *peri,* near, *teinein,* to stretch, *itis,* inflammation], peritonitis in which inflammation of the peritoneum is caused by chemicals, radiation, or injury, rather than by an infectious agent.

aseptic surgery [Gk, *a, sepsis,* without decay, *cheirourgos,* surgeon], the prevention of contamination during surgical procedures.

aseptic technique, any health care procedure in which added precautions, such as use of sterile gloves and instruments, are used to prevent contamination of a person, object, or area by microorganisms.

Asepto syringe, trademark for a large bulb-fitted, blunt-tipped syringe used primarily for irrigating wounds.

asexual /āsek′shŏŏ·əl/ [Gk, *a,* not; L, *sexus,* male or female], **1.** not sexual. **2.** pertaining to an organism that has no sexual organs. **3.** pertaining to a process that is not sexual. **—asexuality,** *n.*

asexual dwarf, an adult dwarf whose genital organs are underdeveloped.

asexual generation. See **asexual reproduction.**

asexuality. See **asexual.**

asexualization /āsek′shŏŏ·əlīzā′shən/, the process of making one incapable of reproduction. Sterilization of an individual or animal by castration, vasectomy, removal of the ovaries, or use of chemicals.

asexual reproduction, any type of reproduction that occurs without the union of male and female gametes, such as fission, budding, sporulation, or parthenogenesis. Also called **asexual generation, direct generation, nonsexual generation.** Compare **sexual reproduction.**

ASHA, abbreviation for *American Speech, Language, and Hearing Association.*

ASHD, abbreviation for **arteriosclerotic heart disease.**

Asherman syndrome, secondary amenorrhea in a hormonally normal woman, caused by obliteration of the endometrial cavity by adhesions that form as a result of curettage or infection.

asialorrhea. See **hyposalivation.**

Asian flu. See **influenza.**

asiderosis /ā′sidərō′sis/, an iron deficiency and a cause of anemia.

-asis, suffix meaning an 'action, process, or result of': *metabasis, oxydasis.*

Ask-Upmark kidney, a hypoplastic kidney with fewer lobules than usual and fissures on its surface; most affected persons have severe hypertension, sometimes with hypertensive encephalopathy and retinopathy. The condition may be either congenital or a result of vesicoureteral reflux with pyelonephritis.

ASL, abbreviation for *American Sign Language.*

ASLT, abbreviation for **antistreptolysin-O test.**

ASMT, abbreviation for *American Society for Medical Technology.*

Asn, abbreviation for the amino acid **asparagine.**

asocial /āsō′shəl/ [Gk, *a,* without; L, *socius,* companion], withdrawn or disengaged from normal contacts with other individuals.

asoma /āsō′mə/ [Gk, *a,* not, *soma,* body], a fetus with an incomplete trunk and head.

ASOT, abbreviation for **antistreptolysin-O test.**

ASPAN, abbreviation for American Society of PeriAnesthesia Nurses.

asparaginase /aspar′əjinās/ [Gk, *asparagos,* asparagus], an enzyme that catalyzes the hydrolysis of asparagine to asparaginic acid and ammonia. Asparaginase is used as a chemotherapeutic agent in the treatment of acute lymphoblastic leukemia and lymphosarcoma.

asparagine (Asn) /aspar′əjin/, a nonessential amino acid found in many food and body proteins. It is easily hydrolyzed to aspartic acid and has diuretic properties. See also **amino acid, protein.**

Chemical structure of asparagine

aspartame /aspär′tām, as′pərtām/, a white, almost odorless crystalline powder that is used as an artificial sweetener. It is formed by binding the amino acids of phenylalanine and aspartic acid. Approximately 180 times as sweet as the same amount of sucrose, it is used mostly to sweeten cold or uncooked foods. Unprotected aspartame tends to lose its sweetness in the presence of heat, moisture, and alkaline media. Excessive use of this nonnutritive sweetener should be avoided by patients with phenylketonuria (PKU) because the substance hydrolyzes to form aspartate and phenylalanine.

aspartate aminotransferase (AST) /aspär′tāt/, an enzyme normally present in body serum and in certain body tissues, especially those of the heart and liver. This enzyme affects the intermolecular transfer of an amino group from aspartic acid to alpha-ketoglutaric acid, forming glutamic acid and oxaloacetic acid. The reaction is reversible. The enzyme is released into the serum because of tissue injury and thus may increase as a result of myocardial infarction and liver damage. Normal findings for adults are 8 to 20 U/L or 5 to 40 IU/L. Previously called **glutamic-oxaloacetic transaminase, serum glutamic oxaloacetic transaminase (SGOT).** Compare **alanine aminotransferase.**

aspartate aminotransferase test (AST, formerly called SGOT), a blood test used in the evaluation of suspected coronary occlusive heart disease or hepatocellular diseases. AST is one of several enzymes tested in the cardiac enzyme series to help diagnose myocardial infarction.

aspartate kinase, an enzyme that catalyzes the transfer of a phosphate group from adenosine triphosphate to aspartate to produce phosphoaspartate.

aspartate transaminase. See **aspartate aminotransferase.**

aspartic acid (Asp) /aspär′tik/, a nonessential amino acid present in sugar cane, beet molasses, and breakdown products of many proteins. Pure aspartic acid is a water-soluble, colorless crystalline substance. Aspartic acid is interconvertible with oxaloacetic acid from the citric acid cycle. Aspartic acid is used in culture media, dietary supplements, deter-

gents, fungicides, and germicides. Also called **aminosuccinic acid.** See also **amino acid, protein.**

Chemical structure of aspartic acid

aspastic /āspas′tik/, not characterized by spasms.

aspect [L, *aspectus,* a look], the appearance, look, facing, or fronting of a person or object.

Asperger's syndrome /äs′pər·gərz/ [Hans Asperger, Austrian psychiatrist, 20th century], a pervasive developmental disorder similar to autistic disorder, characterized by severe impairment of social interactions and by restricted interests and behaviors, but lacking the delays in development of language, cognitive function, and self-help skills that additionally define autistic disorder. It may be equivalent to a high-functioning form of autistic disorder.

aspergillic acid /as′pərjil′ik/, an antibiotic substance derived from *Aspergillus flavus,* an aflatoxin-producing mold found on corn, grain, and peanuts. See also **aflatoxins.**

aspergillosis /as′pərjilō′sis/ [L, *aspergere,* to sprinkle; Gk, *osis,* condition], an infection caused by inhalation of a fungus of the genus *Aspergillus* that can cause inflammatory, granulomatous lesions on or in any organ. The infection is relatively uncommon and typically occurs in an immunodeficient person already weakened by some other disorder. Topical fungicides can be used on the skin; amphotericin B is used to treat systemic aspergillosis, especially if it has spread to the lungs. Surgery may be required to remove a fungus ball. The prognosis, as for most systemic fungal infections, is poor. Compare **allergic bronchopulmonary aspergillosis.**

Aspergillus /as′pərjil′əs/ [L, *aspergere,* to sprinkle], a genus of fungi that is a common contaminant in the laboratory and a cause of nosocomial infection. The fungus has hyphae and spores, lives in the soil, is ubiquitous, and proliferates rapidly. Inhalation of the spores of the two pathogenic species, *Aspergillus fumigatus* and *A. flavus,* is common, but infection is rare.

aspermatic /ā′spurmat′ik/, unable to secrete or ejaculate semen.

aspermatogenesis /āspur′mətōjen′əsis/, failure of the testes to produce spermatozoa.

aspermia /āspur′mē·ə/ [Gk, *a, sperma,* without seed], lack of formation or ejaculation of semen.

asphyxia /asfik′sē·ə/ [Gk, *a + sphyxis,* without pulse], severe hypoxia leading to hypoxemia and hypercapnia, loss of consciousness, and, if not corrected, death. Some of the more common causes of asphyxia are drowning, electrical shock, aspiration of vomitus, lodging of a foreign body in

Aspergillus fumigatus (Murray et al, 1994)

the respiratory tract, inhalation of toxic gas or smoke, and poisoning. Oxygen and artificial ventilation are promptly administered to prevent damage to the brain. The underlying cause is then treated. See also **artificial ventilation. —asphyxiate,** v., **asphyxiated,** adj.

asphyxia livida /liv'ədə/, an abnormal condition in which a newborn's skin is cyanotic, the pulse is weak and slow, and the reflexes are slow or absent. Also called **blue asphyxia.**

asphyxia neonatorum, a condition in which a newborn does not breathe spontaneously. The asphyxia may develop before or during labor or immediately after delivery. The condition may involve placental or neonatal pulmonary dysfunction with underlying causes that can include abruptio placentae, umbilical compression, or uterine tetany. Other factors include congenital defects, such as a diaphragmatic hernia, or adverse effects of anesthetics or analgesics administered to the mother. Immediate resuscitation is required to prevent death or brain damage. Also called **perinatal asphyxia.** See also **asphyxia livida, asphyxia pallida.**

asphyxia pallida /pal'ədə/, an abnormal condition in which a newborn appears pale and limp, shows signs of apnea, and suffers from bradycardia as marked by a heartbeat of 80 beats/min or less.

asphyxiate /asfik'sē·āt/ [Gk, a + sphyxis, without pulse], to induce an inability to breathe. Causes may include circulatory congestion, chemical poisoning, electrical shock, or physical suffocation.

asphyxiated. See **asphyxia.**

asphyxiating thoracic dysplasia. See **Jeune's syndrome.**

asphyxiation [Gk, a + sphyxis, without pulse], a state of asphyxia or inability to breathe.

aspirant /as'pirənt/, the fluid, gas, or solid particles that are withdrawn from the body by aspiration methods.

aspirant maneuver, a procedure used in making x-ray films of the laryngopharyngeal area. The patient exhales completely, then slowly inhales while making a harsh, high-pitched sound. The maneuver adducts the vocal cords so the ventricle of the larynx is clearly visible in the x-ray.

aspirate /-rāt/ [L, aspirare, to breathe upon], to withdraw fluid or air from a cavity. The process is usually aided by use of a syringe or a suction device. See **paracentesis, thoracentesis.**

aspirating needle /-rā'ting/, a long hollow needle used to remove fluid from a cavity, vessel, or structure of the body.

aspirating syringe, a hypodermic syringe used to inject local anesthetics, especially in dentistry. Checking for blood in the syringe after pulling back slightly on the plunger ensures that the anesthetic solution will not be deposited in a blood vessel.

aspiration /as'pirā'shən/, **1.** drawing in or out by suction. **2.** the act of withdrawing a fluid, such as mucus or serum, from the body by a suction device. See also **aspiration pneumonia. —aspirate,** n.

aspiration biopsy, the removal of living tissue, for microscopic examination, by suction through a fine needle attached to a syringe. The procedure is used primarily to obtain cells from a lesion containing fluid or when fluid is formed in a serous cavity. See also **cytology, needle biopsy.**

aspiration biopsy cytology (ABC), a microscopic examination of cells obtained directly from living body tissue by aspiration through a fine needle. It is used primarily as a diagnostic procedure, generally as a technique for detecting nuclear and cytoplasmic changes in cancerous tissue. Compare **exfoliative cytology.**

aspiration control, a nursing outcome from the Nursing Outcomes Classification (NOC) defined as personal actions to prevent the passage of fluid and solid particles into the lung. See also **Nursing Outcomes Classification.**

aspiration drug abuse, the inhalation of a liquid, solid, or gaseous chemical into the respiratory system for nontherapeutic purposes. Examples include glue and solvent sniffing and cocaine snorting.

aspiration of vomitus, the inhalation of regurgitated gastric contents into the pulmonary system. See also **aspiration pneumonia.**

aspiration pneumonia, an inflammatory condition of the lungs and bronchi caused by inhaling foreign material or acidic vomitus. Compare **bronchopneumonia.** See also **pneumonia.**

■ OBSERVATIONS: Aspiration pneumonia may occur during anesthesia or recovery from anesthesia or during a seizure of acute alcoholic intoxication or other condition characterized by vomiting and a decreased level of consciousness. Patients receiving enteral feeding therapies may also be at risk.

■ INTERVENTIONS: Treatment consists of prompt suctioning of the bronchi and administration of 100% oxygen. Continued artificial ventilation may be required. As long as oxygen is administered, frequent analyses of blood gas levels may be indicated. Corticosteroids may be given to diminish inflammation. The sputum is cultured regularly, and any bacterial infection thus diagnosed is treated with an appropriate antibiotic.

■ NURSING CONSIDERATIONS: The pulse rate and quality of respirations, level of consciousness, and skin color are carefully monitored. An oral airway is left in place until the patient's condition improves, and secretions are removed by suction as necessary. Infection and respiratory failure are frequent complications. Aspiration pneumonia may be prevented by positioning unconscious patients with the head elevated 15 to 30 degrees and turned to the side and by paying careful attention to the maintenance of enteral feeding therapy and an adequate airway.

aspiration precautions, a nursing intervention from the Nursing Interventions Classification (NIC) defined as prevention or minimization of risk factors in the patient at risk for aspiration. See also **Nursing Interventions Classification.**

aspiration prevention, a nursing outcome from the Nursing Outcomes Classification (NOC) defined as personal actions to prevent the passage of fluid and solid particles into the lung.

aspiration, risk for, a nursing diagnosis accepted by the Eighth National Conference on the Classification of Nursing Diagnoses. Risk for aspiration is a state in which an individual is at risk for entry of gastric secretions, oropharyngeal secretions, or exogenous food or fluids into tracheobronchial

Aspiration pneumonia
(Mace and Kowalczyk, 2004/
courtesy Ohio State University Medical Center)

passages caused by dysfunction or absence of normal protective mechanisms.

■ RISK FACTORS: Risk factors include reduced level of consciousness, depressed cough and gag reflexes, presence of a tracheostomy or endotracheal tube, overinflated tracheostomy or endotracheal tube cuff, inadequate inflation of a tracheostomy or endotracheal tube cuff, GI tubes, and bolus tube feedings or medication administration. Other risk factors are situations hindering elevation of the upper body, increased intragastric pressure, increased gastric residual, decreased GI motility, delay in gastric emptying, impaired swallowing, wired jaws, and facial, oral, or neck surgery or trauma. See also **nursing diagnosis.**

aspirator /as′pirā′tər/ [L, *aspirare,* to breathe upon], any instrument that removes a substance from a body cavity by suction, such as a bulb syringe, piston pump, or hypodermic syringe.

aspirin (ASA) /as′pirin/, an analgesic, antipyretic, and antiinflammatory. Also called **acetylsalicylic acid** /əsē′təlsal′isil′ik, as′itəl-/, **(ASA).**

■ INDICATIONS: It is prescribed to reduce fever and relieve pain and inflammation.

■ CONTRAINDICATIONS: Bleeding disorders, peptic ulcer, pregnancy, concomitant use of anticoagulants, or known hypersensitivity to salicylates prohibits its use.

■ ADVERSE EFFECTS: Among the most serious adverse reactions are ulcers, occult bleeding, clotting defects, renal toxicities, tinnitus, dyspepsia, and allergic reactions. Reye's syndrome has been associated with aspirin use in children.

aspirin poisoning. See **salicylate poisoning.**

asplenia /āsplē′nē·ə/ [Gk, *a,* without, *spleen*], absence of a spleen. The condition may be congenital or result from surgical removal.

ASRT, abbreviation for *American Society of Radiologic Technologists.*

Assam fever. See **kala-azar.**

assault /əsôlt′/ [L, *assilirere,* to leap upon], **1.** an unlawful act that places another person, without that person's consent, in fear of immediate bodily harm or battery. **2.** the act of committing an assault. **3.** to threaten a person with bodily harm or injury. See **battery.**

assay /asā′, as′ā/ [Fr, *essayer,* to try], the analysis of the purity or effectiveness of drugs and other biologic substances, including laboratory and clinical observations.

assertion training. See **assertive training.**

assertiveness /əsur′tivnes/, behavior directed toward claiming one's rights without denying those of others.

assertiveness training, a nursing intervention from the Nursing Interventions Classification (NIC) defined as assistance with the effective expression of feelings, needs, and ideas while respecting the rights of others. See also **Nursing Interventions Classification.**

assertive training /əsur′tiv/ [L, *asserere,* to join to oneself], a therapeutic technique to help individuals become more self-assertive and self-confident in interpersonal relationships. It focuses on the direct, honest statement of feelings and beliefs, both positive and negative. The technique is learned by role playing in a therapeutic setting, usually in a group, followed by practice in actual situations. Also called **assertion training.**

assess. See **assessment.**

assessing /əses′ing/ [L, *assidere,* to sit beside] (in five-step nursing process) a category of nursing behavior that includes the gathering, verifying, and communicating of information related to the client. The nurse collects information from verbal interactions with the patient, the patient's family, and significant others; examines standard data sources for information; systematically checks for symptoms and signs; determines the patient's ability to perform self-care activities; assesses the patient's environment; and identifies reactions of the staff (including the nurse who is performing the assessment) to the patient and to the patient's family and significant others. To verify the data, the nurse confirms the observations and perceptions by gathering additional information; discusses the orders and decisions made by other members of the staff with them, when indicated; and personally evaluates and checks the patient's condition. The nurse reports the information that has been gathered and verified. Although assessing is the first of the five steps of the nursing process, preceding analyzing, in practice it is integral to effective nursing practice at all steps of the process. See also **analyzing, evaluating, implementing, nursing process, planning.**

assessment /əses′mənt/ [L, *assidere,* to sit beside], **1.** (in medicine and nursing) an evaluation or appraisal of a condition. **2.** the process of making such an evaluation. **3.** (in a problem-oriented medical record) an examiner's evaluation of the disease or condition based on the patient's subjective report of the symptoms and course of the illness or condition and the examiner's objective findings, including data obtained through laboratory tests, physical examination, medical history, and information reported by family members and other health care team members. See also **nursing assessment, problem-oriented medical record. —assess,** *v.*

assessment of the aging patient, an evaluation of the changes characteristic of advancing years exhibited by an elderly person.

■ METHOD: The patient is measured, weighed, examined, observed, and questioned about physical, functional, and behavioral changes; height normally diminishes 1 to 2 inches with aging, and weight steadily decreases in men over 65 years of age but increases in women. The skin is examined for dryness, wrinkles, sagging, thinning over the back of the hands, areas of vitiligo, keratoses, warts, changes in appearance of freckles and moles, skin tags, and senile telangiectases, and the hair for depigmentation, lack of luster, and thinning or loss on the scalp and in the axillary and pubic areas. Observations are made of enlargement of the nose and ears relative to face size, dryness of the eyes, opacity of the lens, discoloration of the sclera and iris, an opaque ring near the edge of the cornea (arcus senilis), decreased pupil size, and diminished peripheral vision. Tests are performed to determine whether there is hearing loss, especially of high-frequency tones; decreased tidal volume; diminished peripheral perfusion; exertional dyspnea; or deviation of the trachea, especially if scoliosis is present. Examination may reveal gum recession, loss of teeth and taste perception, and diminished salivation. It may also find decreased resting heart rate and cardiac output, increased diastolic and systolic blood pressure, and an easily palpable arterial pulse. The elderly patient may show decreased muscle mass, osteoarthritic joints, Heberden's or Bouchard's nodes at finger joints, contracture of lateral fingers, osteoporosis, a broad-based stance, and slow voluntary movements. The sense of position, of smell, and of touch and the sensitivity to heat and cold may be diminished, and deep tendon reflexes may be decreased. Signs of aging that may be found in women are pendulous, flaccid breasts; vaginal narrowing and shortening and diminished lubrication, causing painful coitus; and effects of long-term estrogen therapy. Signs of aging in men include decrease in the size and firmness of the testes and in the amount and viscosity of seminal fluid, increased diameter of the penis, and prostatic hypertrophy; libido and a sense of sexual satisfaction usually do not diminish.

■ NURSING CONSIDERATIONS: The nurse faces the patient during the evaluation, establishes eye contact, repeats questions if necessary, avoids shouting, and addresses the person by name. If the patient's visual perception and tactile sense are diminished, the nurse uses color contrasts and items of marked textural differences in the assessment.

■ OUTCOME CRITERIA: Aging does not progress at a uniform rate, and its effects may vary widely from one individual to the next, but, in many cases, changes once considered normal in elderly patients are disease processes that may respond to treatment. A thorough physical assessment distinguishes the effects of pathological disorders from those of aging and elucidates the care needed by the patient.

assimilate /əsim′əlāt/ [L, *assimilare,* to make alike], to absorb nutritive substances from the digestive tract to the circulatory system and convert them into living tissues.

assimilation [L, *assimulare,* to make alike], **1.** the process of incorporating nutritive material into living tissue. The end stage of the nutrition process, after digestion and absorption or simultaneous with absorption. **2.** (in psychology) the incorporation of new experiences into a person's pattern of consciousness. Compare **apperception. 3.** (in sociology) the process in which a person or a group of people of a different ethnic background become absorbed into a new culture. —**assimilate,** *v.*

assist-control mode, a system of mechanical ventilation in which the patient is allowed to initiate breathing, although the ventilator delivers a set volume with each breath. The ventilator can also be programmed to initiate breathing if the patient's breathing slows beyond a certain point or stops altogether.

assisted breech [L, *assistere,* to stand by], an obstetric operation in which a baby being born feet or buttocks first is permitted to deliver spontaneously as far as its umbilicus and is then extracted. Also called **partial breech extraction.** Compare **breech extraction.**

assisted circulation [L, *assistere,* to stand, *circulare,* to go around], a method of treating patients with severe circulatory deficiencies by introducing a mechanical pumping system to aid the blood flow.

assisted conception, assisted reproductive technology.

assisted death, a form of euthanasia in which an individual expressing a wish to die prematurely is helped to accomplish that goal by another person, either by counseling and/or by providing a poison or other lethal instrument. The assisted death may be regarded as a homicide or suicide by local authorities, and the person giving assistance may be held responsible for the death. See also **assisted suicide.**

assisted embryo hatching/embryo hatching, a micromanipulation technique.

assisted reproductive technology, the manipulation of egg and sperm in treating infertility. The processes include the administration of drugs to induce ovulation, fertilization, gamete intrafallopian transfer, zygote intrafallopian transfer, and cryopreservation of gametes. See also **in vitro fertilization.**

assisted suicide, a form of euthanasia in which a person wishes to commit suicide but feels unable to perform the act alone because of a physical disability or lack of knowledge about the most effective means. An individual who assists a suicide victim in accomplishing that goal may or may not be held responsible for the death, depending on local laws. The participation of health professionals, especially physicians, in assisted suicide is controversial. See also **euthanasia, suicide.**

assisted ventilation, the use of mechanical or other devices to help maintain respiration, usually by delivering air or oxygen under positive pressure. See also **IPPB, respiration.**

assistive listening device (ALD), a device other than a hearing aid that helps the deaf to hear. See also **hearing aid.**

associated antagonist, one of a pair of muscles or group of muscles that pull in opposite directions but whose combined action results in moving a part in one direction.

Associate Degree in Nursing (ADN) /əsō′shē·āt/ [L, *associare,* to unite], an academic degree awarded on satisfactory completion of a 2-year course of study, usually at a community or junior college. The recipient is eligible to take the national licensing examination to become a registered nurse. An associate degree in nursing is not available in Canada.

associated movement, a movement of parts that act together, as of the eyes. See **contralateral reflexes, synkinesis.**

associate nurse, **1.** (in primary nursing, United States) a nurse who is responsible for implementing a primary nurse's care plans. **2.** in some states, a registered nurse who holds a diploma from a hospital school of nursing or an associate degree.

association /əsō′shē·ā′shən/ [L, *associare,* to unite], **1.** a connection, union, joining, or combination of things. **2.** (in psychology) the connection of remembered feelings, emotions, sensations, thoughts, or perceptions with particular persons, things, or ideas. Kinds of association are **association of ideas, clang association, controlled association, dream association,** and **free association.**

association area, any part of the cerebral cortex involved in the integration of sensory information. Also called **association cortex.**

Association for Professionals in Infection Control and Epidemiology (APIC), a national professional organization of nurses working in the field of infection control.

Association for the Advancement of Medical Instrumentation (AAMI), a nonprofit organization involved in education and standards relating to biomedical engineering.

Association for the Care of Children's Health (ACCH), an international, interdisciplinary organization concerned with the psychosocial needs of children and their families in health care settings. A quarterly journal and a bimonthly newsletter are available to members. There are affiliate organizations throughout the United States and Canada.

associationist model of learning /əsō'shē·ā'shənist/, a theory that defines learning as behavioral change that is a result of reinforced practice. If the response has not been reinforced repeatedly, an alternative behavior may be substituted.

Association of Canadian Medical Colleges (ACMC), a Canadian organization of the deans and faculty members of the nation's 16 medical schools. It is concerned with all aspects of the education of physicians and acts as the liaison between the member schools and other professional organizations and governmental agencies. The official languages of the ACMC are English and French.

association of ideas, a mental connection established between similar or simultaneously occurring ideas, feelings, or perceptions.

Association of Operating Room Nurses (AORN), a national organization of operating room nurses.

Association of periOperative Registered Nurses (AORN), the professional organization of perioperative nurses, which supports registered nurses in achieving optimal outcomes for patients undergoing operative or other invasive procedures. Formerly called the **Association of Operating Room Nurses,** which accounts for the abbreviation.

Association of Women's Health, Obstetric, and Neonatal Nurses (AWHONN), an organization of nurses working in obstetrics and gynecology in the United States. Formerly called **Nurses Association of the American College of Obstetrics and Gynecology (NAACOG).**

association paralysis, a motor neuron disease in which wasting, weakness, and fasciculation of the tongue, facial muscles, pharynx, and larynx occur. Also called **progressive bulbar paralysis.**

association test, a technique used in psychiatric diagnosis and in educational and psychologic evaluation in which a person is asked to respond to a stimulus word with the first word that comes to mind. The time taken to respond and the associations offered are compared with pretested responses and are classified and enumerated for diagnostic significance. Also called **word association test.** See also **free association.**

associative looseness /əsō'shətiv/, a form of thought disorder in which the patient is unable to maintain consistent thought for more than a few minutes and jumps from thought to thought in a conversation. Fragmentation of thoughts is generally noted in patients with schizophrenia.

associative play, a form of play in which a group of children participate in similar or identical activities without formal organization, group direction, group interaction, or a definite goal. The children may borrow or lend toys or pieces of play equipment, and they may imitate others in the group, but each child acts independently, as on a playground or among a group riding tricycles or bicycles. Compare **cooperative play.** See also **parallel play, solitary play.**

assortive mating, the matching of males and females for reproduction in a manner that avoids random selection.

assumed role /əsoomd'/, a role in life that an individual usually selects or achieves by choice, such as one's role in marriage or employment. See also **ascribed role.**

AST, 1. abbreviation for **aspartate aminotransferase. 2.** less frequently, abbreviation for **angiotensin sensitivity test.**

-ast, combining form designating an antiasthmatic or antiallergic drug not acting primarily as an antihistamine.

astasia /astā'zhə/, a lack of motor coordination marked by an inability to stand or sit without assistance.

astasia-abasia [Gk, *a, stasis,* not stand, *a, basis,* not step], a form of ataxia in which the patient is unable to stand or walk because of lack of motor coordination although able to carry out natural leg movements when sitting or lying down. Also called **abasia-astasia.**

astatine (At) [Gk, *astasis,* unsteady], a very unstable, radioactive element that occurs naturally in tiny amounts. Its atomic number is 85; the atomic mass of its longest lived isotope is 210.

asteatosis /as'tē·ətō'sis/ [Gk, *a, stear,* without tallow, *osis,* condition], a dry skin condition caused by a deficiency of sebaceous gland secretions. Scales and fissures may result from the dryness. The condition is treated with creams and ointments that replace the missing skin oils.

Asteatotic eczema *(du Vivier, 1993)*

-aster, suffix meaning 'star-shaped': *diaster, oleaster.*

astereognosis /əstir'ē·og·nō'sis/, [Gk, *a, stereos,* not solid, *gnosis,* knowledge], an inability to identify objects or shapes by touch.

asterixis /as'tərik'sis/ [Gk, *a, sterixis,* not fixed position], a hand-flapping tremor, often accompanying metabolic disorders. The tremor is usually induced by extending the arm and dorsiflexing the wrist. Asterixis is seen frequently in hepatic encephalopathy. Also called **flapping tremor, liver flap.**

asteroid body [Gk, *aster,* star, *eidos,* form], an irregular star-shaped structure that develops in the giant cells in certain diseases, including sarcoidosis, actinomycosis, and nocardiosis.

asthenia /asthē'nē·ə/ [Gk, *a + sthenos,* without strength], **1.** the lack or loss of strength or energy; weakness; debility. **2.** (in psychiatry) lack of dynamic force in the personality. Kinds of asthenia include **myalgic asthenia** and **neurocirculatory asthenia.** See also **adynamia.** —**asthenic,** *adj.*

-asthenia, suffix meaning '(condition of) debility, loss of strength and energy, depleted vitality': *neurasthenia, phlebasthenia.*

asthenic /asthen'ik/ [Gk, *a + sthenos,* without strength], pertaining to a condition of weakness, feebleness, or loss of vitality.

asthenic fever. See **adynamic fever.**

asthenic habitus [Gk, *a + sthenos*, without strength; L, *habere*, to have], a body structure characterized by a slender build with long limbs, an angular profile, and prominent muscles or bones. Compare **athletic habitus, pyknic.** See also **ectomorph.**

asthenic personality, a personality characterized by low energy, lack of enthusiasm, depressed emotions, and oversensitivity to physical and emotional strain. A person who has this kind of personality may be easily fatigued and self-pitying and may place the burden of physical and emotional difficulties on others.

asthenopia /as′thənō′pē·ə/ [Gk, *a, sthenos + ops*, eye], a condition in which the eyes tire easily because of weakness of the ocular or ciliary muscles. Symptoms include pain in or around the eyes, headache, dimness of vision, dizziness, and slight nausea.

asthma /az′mə/ [Gk, panting], a respiratory disorder characterized by recurring episodes of paroxysmal dyspnea, wheezing on expiration and/or inspiration caused by constriction of the bronchi, coughing, and viscous mucoid bronchial secretions. The episodes may be precipitated by inhalation of allergens or pollutants, infection, cold air, vigorous exercise, or emotional stress. Treatment may include elimination of the causative agent, hyposensitization, aerosol or oral bronchodilators, beta-adrenergic drugs, methylxanthines, cromolyn, leukotriene inhibitors, and short- or long-term use of corticosteroids. Sedatives and cough suppressants may be contraindicated. Also called **bronchial asthma.** See also **allergic asthma, asthma in children, exercise-induced asthma, intrinsic asthma, organic dust, status asthmaticus.**

**Asthma: obstruction of airways
by excessive mucous production
and edema of respiratory mucosa**
(Thibodeau and Patton, 2003)

-asthma, suffix meaning '(condition of) labored breathing.'

asthma control, a nursing outcome from the Nursing Outcomes Classification (NOC) defined as personal actions to reverse inflammatory condition resulting in bronchial constriction of the airways. See also **Nursing Outcomes Classification.**

asthma crystal. See **Charcot-Leyden crystal.**

asthma in children, a chronic inflammatory disorder of the airways in which many cells, including mast cells and eosinophils play a part. The inflammation causes symptoms associated with obstructive airflow and characterized by recurring attacks of paroxysmal dyspnea, wheezing, prolonged expiration, and an irritative cough that is a common, chronic illness in childhood. Onset usually occurs between 3 and 8 years of age. Asthmatic attacks are caused by constriction of the large and small airways, resulting from bronchial smooth muscle spasm, edema or inflammation of the bronchial wall, or excessive production of mucus. It is a complex disorder involving biochemical, immunologic, infectious, endocrinologic, and psychologic factors. Asthma attacks in the past were classified as either extrinsic or intrinsic. Most extrinsic attacks in children were associated with an allergenic hypersensitivity to a foreign substance, such as airborne pollen, mold, house dust, certain foods, animal hair and skin, feathers, insects, smoke, and various chemicals or drugs. In infants, especially those with a family history of allergic reactions, food allergy is a common precipitating factor. Intrinsic attacks were associated with physical stress resulting from fatigue or exercise, exposure to cold air, or psychologic stress; this system of classification has been abandoned because many of the triggering factors overlap.

■ OBSERVATIONS: Asthma in children is often confused with acute middle and lower respiratory tract infections, congenital stridor, obstruction of the bronchi or trachea, bronchial or tracheal compression, and cystic fibrosis. The diagnosis is generally determined by observation during a physical examination, medical history, and familial allergic disease. Laboratory tests and x-ray studies may eliminate identification of other diseases. A diagnostic feature is the presence of large numbers of eosinophils and Charcot-Leyden crystals in the sputum. Pulmonary function tests are valuable for assessing the degree of airway obstruction and the volume of gas exchange. Asthmatic episodes vary greatly in frequency, duration, and degree of symptoms. They may range from occasional periods of wheezing, mild coughing, and slight dyspnea to severe attacks that can lead to total airway obstruction and respiratory tract failure (status asthmaticus). An attack may begin gradually or abruptly and is often preceded by an upper respiratory infection. Typically an attack begins with signs of air hunger, yawning, sighing, shortness of breath, paroxysms of wheezing, and a hacking, nonproductive cough. As secretions increase, the expiratory phase becomes prolonged. A large quantity of thick, tenacious mucoid sputum is produced as the attack subsides. The child appears apprehensive, speaks in a panting manner, and may assume a bent-over position to facilitate breathing. The prolonged expiratory phase is not as noticeable in infants and young children. In severe spasm or obstruction the respirations become shallow and irregular. A sudden increase in the rate of respiration, repeated hacking, and nonproductive coughing are indicative of lack of air movement with impending ventilatory failure and asphyxia.

■ INTERVENTIONS: Management of asthma in children is based on four stages of severity: intermittent, mild persistent, moderate persistent, and severe persistent. Clinical features of intermittent asthma include symptoms that occur less than once a week, brief exacerbations from a few hours to a few days, nighttime episodes that occur less than twice a month, and normal lung function between exacerbations. Mild persistent classification is characterized by symptoms that occur more than once a week but less than once a day

and nighttime episodes that occur more often than twice a month. Moderate persistent severity is manifested by daily symptoms with exacerbations that affect daily activities and sleep. Severe persistent asthma is characterized by continuous symptoms that limit physical activities, frequent exacerbations, and nighttime symptoms. Medications are classified as relievers and controllers to relieve symptoms immediately. A reliever may be a short-acting medication, such as a beta$_2$ agonist that serves as symptomatic therapy. Controllers such as inhaled and systemic corticosteroids and sustained-release theophylline are prescribed on a regular basis to keep symptoms under control. In the long-term management of asthma in children, an effort is made to control the symptoms with the minimum amount of medication, increasing the number and frequency of medications as symptoms increase and reducing the level as symptoms are brought under control. The major drugs used to relieve bronchospasm are the beta-adrenergic agents, including the relievers isoproterenol, metaproterenol, terbutaline, and salbutamol; the methylxanthines, including theophylline and aminophylline; corticosteroids; expectorants; and antibiotics for cases in which infection is the triggering mechanism. Rarely an acute attack does not respond to any of these measures, resulting in status asthmaticus. Hospitalization is required. The child is usually in a state of dehydration and acidosis with hypoxia and hypercapnia. Management consists of administration of IV fluids; humidified oxygen given by mask or cannula; administration of sodium bicarbonate or tromethamine to keep pH at acceptable levels; and use of bronchodilators to alleviate bronchospasm and of antibiotics to reduce risk of infection. Mild, intermittent episodes of asthma are treated with bronchodilators in aerosol sprays, which provide quick relief and are effective in controlling an attack; oral administration is preferred for younger children. Those with persistent chronic asthma receive daily oral doses of a bronchodilator, often theophylline, usually in combination with an expectorant and corticosteroids. Bronchospasm induced by exercise can be treated prophylactically with cromolyn sodium, a controller that inhibits the release of histamine in the lungs. Long-range management and treatment include physical training and exercises to induce physical and mental relaxation, improve posture, strengthen respiratory musculature, and develop better breathing patterns. Hyposensitization is recommended when an allergen is known and cannot be avoided. Prognosis varies considerably; many children lose their symptoms at puberty but the symptoms reappear in their 40s. The prognosis depends on the number and severity of symptoms, emotional factors, and the family history of allergy.
■ NURSING CONSIDERATIONS: The primary focus of nursing care for children with acute asthma is to relieve symptoms of respiratory distress by initiating IV infusion and oxygen therapy, correcting acidosis, and administering bronchodilators and corticosteroids. The nurse implements measures to promote physical comfort, induce rest, and reduce fatigue and anxiety. An especially important role is reassuring the child and parents about procedures, equipment, and prognosis. The nurse also plays a significant role in the long-term support of children with chronic asthma, primarily in teaching the child and parents about the disease and how to cope with the condition. Once an allergen is determined, the home environment must be modified to reduce or eliminate contact with possible causative agents, including presence of warm-blooded pets, tobacco smoke, cockroaches, dust mites, and fungi. The nurse teaches the child and parents how to use prescribed medications, especially nebulizers and aerosol devices, how to detect early signs of an attack so that it can

be controlled with medication, how to determine any adverse effects of the drugs, especially the dangers of overuse, and how to implement physical exercise and play activities as therapeutic measures, especially those that promote proper breathing techniques. Further educational support for families of children with asthma may be obtained from organizations such as the Asthma and Allergy Foundation of America and the American Lung Association.

asthma management, a nursing intervention from the Nursing Interventions Classification (NIC) defined as identification, treatment, and prevention of reactions to inflammation/constriction in the airway passages.

-asthmatic, suffix meaning 'asthma, its symptoms, or its treatment': *antiasthmatic, postasthmatic.*

asthmatic breathing /azmat'ik/ [Gk, *asthma,* panting; AS, *braeth*], breathing marked by prolonged wheezing on exhalation caused by spasmodic contractions of the bronchi.

asthmatic bronchitis, inflammation and swelling of the mucous membrane of the bronchi in a patient with asthma.

asthmatic cough [Gk, *asthma* + AS, *cohhetan*], a wheezing cough accompanied by signs of breathing difficulty.

asthmatic eosinophilia, a form of eosinophilic pneumonia, characterized by allergic bronchospasm, cough, fever, and expectoration of bronchial casts containing eosinophils and fungal mycelia. It is a result of hypersensitivity to the fungus *Aspergillus fumigatus* or *Candida albicans.* The condition usually occurs in the fourth or fifth decade of life and is twice as common in women as in men. Untreated, it may result in pleural effusion, pericarditis, ascites, encephalitis, hepatomegaly, and respiratory failure. Treatment is similar to that for asthma and includes administration of corticosteroids and antibiotics. Desensitization to the allergen is not usually effective. See also **allergic asthma, eosinophilic pneumonia.**

astigmatic /as'tigmat'ik/ [Gk, *a, stigma,* without point], pertaining to astigmatism, or an error of refraction in which a ray of light is not sharply focused on the retinal tissue but is spread over a more diffuse area. Astigmatism is due to differences in curvature in the various meridians of the cornea and lens of the eye.

astigmatic keratotomy, an operation in which the cornea is relaxed by a series of transverse incisions to flatten the meridian in which the incisions are made and increase the curvature in the meridian 90° away. It is done for the correction of astigmatism.

astigmatism /əstig'mətiz'əm/ [Gk, *a, stigma,* without point], an abnormal condition of the eye in which the light rays cannot be focused clearly in a point on the retina because the spheric curve of the cornea or lens is not equal in all meridians. Vision is typically blurred; if uncorrected, it often results in visual discomfort or asthenopia. The person cannot accommodate to correct the problem. The condition usually may be corrected with contact lenses or with eyeglasses ground to neutralize the condition.

-astine, combining form designating an antihistaminic.

Aston-Patterning, a bodywork technique to accommodate asymmetry and individual uniqueness of the human body to match human function to the environment. Appropriate alignment of the body provides the human structure with its most optimal support and adds the dynamic quality that facilitates motion. Alignment can be threatened by accidents, illnesses, or surgeries, and movement patterns are taught to include the asymmetric pattern rather than allowing a tension pattern to develop. This technique has been applied to fitness training and ergonomic product design.

astragalus[1], an herb that is grown throughout the world, most commonly in China, Japan, and Korea.

Astigmatism

Astrocyte (Monahan and Neighbors, 1998)

Astrocytoma (Kumar, Cotran, and Robbins, 2003)

■ USES: This herb is used as an immune stimulant; for viral infections, HIV/AIDS, cancer, and vascular disorders; to improve circulation; and to lower blood pressure. In most instances, there is insufficient reliable information regarding its effectiveness.

■ CONTRAINDICATIONS: Astragalus should not be used during pregnancy and lactation, in children, or during acute infections.

astragalus[2]. See **talus.**

astringent /əstrin'jənt/ [Gk, *astringere,* to tighten], **1.** a substance that causes contraction of tissues on application, usually used locally. **2.** having the quality of an astringent. —**astringency,** *n.*

astringent bath, a bath in which alum, tannic acid, or another astringent is added to the water. An astringent contracts body tissue and, therefore, stops capillary bleeding or loosens secretions.

astringent douche, a cleansing stream containing substances such as alum that can contract the mucous membrane of the vagina.

astro-, prefix meaning 'star or star-shaped': *astroblastoma, astrocytoma.*

astroblastoma *pl.* **astroblastomas, astroblastomata** /as'trōblastō'mə/ [Gk, *aster,* star, *blastos,* germ, *oma,* tumor], a malignant neoplasm of the brain and spinal cord. Cells of an astroblastoma lie around blood vessels or around connective tissue septa.

astrocyte /as'trōsīt'/ [Gk, *aster* + *kytos,* cell], a large, star-shaped neuroglial cell with many branches, found in certain tissues of the nervous system.

astrocytoma *pl.* **astrocytomas, astrocytomata** /as'trōsītō'mə/ [Gk, *aster, kytos* + *oma*], a primary tumor of the brain composed of astrocytes and characterized by slow growth, cyst formation, invasion of surrounding structures, and often development of a highly malignant glioblastoma, within the tumor mass. Complete surgical resection of an astrocytoma may be possible early in the development of the tumor. Also called **astrocytic glioma.**

astrocytosis /as'trōsītō'sis/ [Gk, *aster* + *kytos* + *osis,* condition], an increase in the number of neuroglial cells with fibrous or protoplasmic processes frequently observed in an irregular area adjacent to degenerative lesions, such as abscesses, certain brain neoplasms, and encephalomalacia. Astrocytosis represents a reparative process and in some cases may be diffuse in a large region.

astrophobia. See **tonitrophobia.**

asylum /əsī'ləm/ [Gk, *asylon,* inviolable], an institution for the care of physically or mentally challenged persons judged incapable of caring for themselves.

asymmetric /ā'simet'rik, as'imet'rik/ [Gk, *a* + *symmetria,* without proportion], **1.** (of the body or parts of the body) unequal in size or shape. **2.** different in placement or arrangement about an axis. Also called **asymmetrical.** Compare **symmetric.** —**asymmetry** /āsim'itrē, asim/, *n.*

asymmetric tonic neck reflex. See **tonic neck reflex.**

asymmetry. See **asymmetric.**

asymphytous /ə·sim'fə·təs/ [Gk, *a, symphysis,* not a growing together], separate or distinct; not grown together.

asymptomatic /āsimp'təmat'ik/ [Gk, *a,* without, *symptoma,* that which happens], without symptoms.

asymptomatic neurosyphilis [Gk, *a,* without, *symptoma, neuron,* nerve; Fr, *syphilide*], a form of neurosyphilis characterized by pathologic changes in the cerebrospinal fluid, although there are no symptoms of nervous system damage. Asymptomatic neurosyphilis may occur many years before actual nervous system damage is noticeable.

asynchronous /āsing'krənəs/ [Gk, *a* + *synchronos,* not simultaneous], (of an event or device) a computer operation in one command performed in response to a signal that the previous command has been completed. One operation is completed before the next is initiated.

asynclitism /āsing′klitiz′əm/ [Gk, *a* + *syn,* not together, *kleisis,* to lean], presentation of a parietal aspect of the fetal head to the maternal pelvic inlet in labor. The sagittal suture is parallel to the transverse diameter of the pelvis but anterior or posterior to it. In normal labor, the fetal head usually engages with some degree of asynclitism. **Anterior asynclitism,** in which the anterior part presents, is called Nägele obliquity. **Posterior asynclitism** is called Litzmann obliquity. See also **cardinal movements of labor, engagement.**

asyndesis /əsin′dəsis/, a mental disorder marked by an inability to assemble related ideas or thoughts into one coherent concept.

asynergy /āsin′ərjē/ [Gk, *a* + *syn* + *ergein,* to work], **1.** a condition characterized by faulty coordination among groups of organs or muscles that normally function harmoniously. **2.** the state of muscle antagonism found in cerebellar disease. See also **ataxia, cerebellum.**

asyntaxia /ā′sintak′sē-ə/ [Gk, *a* + *syn* + *taxis,* arrangement], any interference with the orderly sequence of growth and differentiation of the fetus during embryonic development, resulting in one or more congenital anomalies. A kind of asyntaxia is **asyntaxia dorsalis.** See also **developmental anomaly.**

asyntaxia dorsalis, failure of the neural tube to close during embryonic development. See also **neural tube defect.**

asystole /āsis′təlē/ [Gk, *a* + *systole,* not contraction], a life-threatening cardiac condition characterized by the absence of electrical and mechanical activity in the heart. Clinical signs include apnea and lack of pulse. Without cardiac monitoring, asystole cannot be distinguished from ventricular fibrillation. —**asystolic,** *adj.*

asystolic cardiac rhythm /ā′sistol′ik/, an electrocardiographic recording that appears as a flat line, indicating cardiac arrest.

At, symbol for the element **astatine.**

at-. See **ad-.**

atabrine stomatitis, an abnormal oral condition characterized by skin changes that resemble those of lichen planus. It may be associated with the use of Atabrine Hydrochloride. Compare **arsenic stomatitis, bismuth stomatitis.**

ataractic /at′ərak′tik/ [Gk, *ataraktos,* quiet], pertaining to a drug or other agent that has a tranquilizing or sedating effect.

Atarax, trademark for an antianxiety, antiemetic, and anticholinergic (hydroxyzine hydrochloride).

ataraxia /at′ərak′sē′ə/ [Gk, *a,* not, *tarakos,* disturbed], a vague state of mental tranquility.

atavism /at′əviz′əm/ [L, *atavus,* ancestor], the appearance in an individual of traits or characteristics more like those of a grandparent or earlier ancestor than of the parents. Atavistic data may offer clues to an examining physician of genetic or familial health factors. —**atavistic,** *adj.*

atavistic [L, *atavus,* ancestor], pertaining to the tendency for a genetic trait of a remote ancestor to be expressed in an individual as a result of a chance recombination of genes.

ataxia /ətak′sē-ə/ [Gk, without order], an impaired ability to coordinate movement. A staggering gait and postural imbalance are caused by a lesion in the spinal cord or cerebellum that may be the sequela of birth trauma, congenital disorder, infection, degenerative disorder, neoplasm, toxic substance stroke, or head injury. See also **hereditary ataxia.** —**ataxial, ataxic,** *adj.*

ataxiaphasia /-fā′zhə/ [Gk, *ataxia,* without order], a state in which a person is unable to connect words properly as needed to form a sentence.

ataxia-telangiectasia syndrome /təlan′jē-ektā′zhə/ [Gk, *ataxia* + *telos,* end, *angeion,* vessel, *ektasis,* expansion], a rare genetic disorder involving deficits in immunoglobulin metabolism that is transmitted as an autosomal recessive trait. It usually begins in infancy with impaired motor control (ataxia) and progresses slowly with increasing cerebellar degeneration to severe disability. Permanent dilation of superficial blood vessels (telangiectasias) are most prominent on skin surfaces exposed to the sun: ears, face, and bulbar conjunctiva. Intellectual ability seems to stop at the level of 10 years of age in many cases. Affected individuals are susceptible to upper and lower respiratory infections and have an increased risk of malignancy, especially lymphoma. Also called **Louis-Bar syndrome.**

ataxic. See **ataxia.**

ataxic aphasia. See **motor aphasia.**

ataxic breathing, a type of breathing associated with a lesion in the medullary respiratory center and characterized by a series of inspirations and expirations. See also **Biot's respiration.**

ataxic dysarthria, abnormal speech characterized by faulty formation of sounds because of neuromuscular dysfunction of the cerebellum. See also **cerebellar speech.**

ataxic gait. See **cerebellar gait.**

ataxic speech. See **cerebellar speech.**

atazanavir, an antiretroviral agent used to treat HIV-1 infection.

ATCC, abbreviation for **American Type Culture Collection.**

-ate, 1. suffix meaning 'acted upon or being in a (specified) state': *degenerate, enucleate.* **2.** suffix meaning 'possessing': *caudate, longipedate.* **3.** suffix meaning a 'chemical compound derived from a (specified) source': *silicate, opiate.* **4.** suffix meaning an 'acid compound': *oxalate, phosphate.*

atelectasis /at′ilek′təsis/ [Gk, *ateles,* incomplete, *ektasis,* expansion], an abnormal condition characterized by the collapse of alveoli, preventing the respiratory exchange of carbon dioxide and oxygen in a part of the lungs. Symptoms may include diminished breath sounds or aspiratory crackles, a mediastinal shift toward the side of the collapse, fever, and increasing dyspnea. As the remaining portions of the lungs eventually hyperinflate, oxygen saturation of the blood is often nearly normal. The condition may be caused by obstruction of the major airways and bronchioles, by compression of the lung as a result of fluid or air in the pleural space, or by pressure from a tumor outside the lung. Loss of functional lung tissue may secondarily cause increased heart rate, blood pressure, and respiratory rate. Secretions retained in the collapsed alveoli are rich in nutrients for bacterial growth, a condition often leading to stasis pneumonia in critically ill patients. See also **postoperative atelectasis, primary atelectasis.**

ateliosis /ətē′lē-ō′sis/ [Gk, *ateles,* incomplete, *osis,* condition], a form of dwarfism caused by the absence or destruction of eosinophil cells of the adenohypophysis. The person may appear childlike and have poorly developed muscles.

ateliotic dwarf /at′əlē-ot′ik/, a dwarf whose skeleton is incompletely formed as a result of the nonunion of the epiphyses and diaphyses during bone development.

atelo-, prefix meaning 'imperfect or incomplete': *ateloglossia, atelopodia.*

atelorachidia /at′əlôr′əkid′ē-ə/ [Gk, *ateles,* incomplete, *rhachis,* spine], a defective, incomplete formation of the spinal column. Also spelled **atelorhachidia.**

atenolol /aten′əlôl/, a beta₁ selective blocker.

Atelectasis *(Chabner, 2004)*

Atherectomy catheter *(Beare and Myers, 1998)*

■ INDICATION: It is prescribed for the treatment of hypertension.

■ CONTRAINDICATIONS: Sinus bradycardia, second- or third-degree atrioventricular block, cardiogenic shock, or cardiac failure prohibits its use.

■ ADVERSE EFFECTS: Among the more serious adverse reactions are bradycardia, dizziness, and nausea.

ATG, abbreviation for **antithymocyte globulin.**

athelia /āthē′lē·ə/ [Gk, *a,* not, *thele,* nipple], an absence of nipples.

atherectomy /ath′ərek′təmē/, surgical removal of an atheroma in a major artery.

atherectomy catheter, a specially designed catheter for cutting away atheromatous plaque from the lining of an artery. A tiny metal cone at the tip of the catheter has cutting edges for loosening the plaque and has openings through which the plaque fragments can be aspirated. The catheter is positioned and monitored by fluoroscopy.

atheroembolic renal disease /ath′ərō·embol′ik/, a condition of gradual or rapid kidney failure resulting from obstruction of the renal arteries by atheromas and emboli. It is associated with atherosclerosis and hypertension and occurs most frequently in persons over 60 years of age. The patient is usually azotemic and also experiences emboli in other body areas.

atheroembolism /ath′ərō·em′bəliz′əm/, obstruction of a blood vessel by a cholesterol-containing embolism originating from an atheroma in a major artery.

atherogenesis [Gk, *athere,* porridge, *oma,* tumor, *genein,* to produce], the formation of subintimal plaques in the lining of arteries.

atheroma *pl.* **atheromas, atheromata** /ath′ərō′mə/ [Gk, *athere,* meal, *oma,* tumor], an abnormal mass of fat or lipids, as in a sebaceous cyst or in deposits in an arterial wall. **—atheromatous,** *adj.*

atheromatosis /ath′ərōmətō′sis/, the development of many atheromas.

atheromatous [Gk, *athere,* meal, *oma,* tumor], pertaining to atheroma.

atheromatous plaque, a yellowish raised area on the lining of an artery formed by fatty deposits.

atherosclerosis /ath′ərō′sklərō′sis/ [Gk, *athere,* meal, *sklerosis,* hardening], a common disorder characterized by yellowish plaques of cholesterol, other lipids, and cellular debris in the inner layers of the walls of arteries. Atherosclerosis may be induced by injury to the arterial endothelium, proliferation of smooth muscle in vessel walls, or accumulation of lipids in hyperlipidemia. It usually occurs with aging and is often associated with tobacco use, obesity, hypertension, elevated low-density lipoprotein and depressed high-density lipoprotein levels, and diabetes mellitus. The condition begins as a fatty streak and gradually builds to a fibrous plaque or atheromatous lesion. The vessel walls become thick, fibrotic, and calcified, and the lumen narrows, resulting in reduced blood flow to organs normally supplied by the artery. The plaque eventually creates a risk for thrombosis and is one of the major causes of coronary heart disease, angina pectoris, myocardial infarction, and other cardiac disorders. Plaque rupture is usually provoked by activation of the sympathetic nervous system, such as sudden awakening, heavy physical exertion, or anger. Antilipemic agents do not reverse atherosclerosis. Segments of arteries obstructed or severely damaged by atheromatous lesions may be replaced by patch grafts or bypassed, as in coronary bypass surgery; the lesion may be removed from the vessel via endarterectomy; or obstructed arteries may be opened by balloon angioplasty or by the insertion of stents. A diet low in cholesterol, calories, and saturated fats, together with avoidance of smoking, stress, and a sedentary lifestyle, may help prevent the disorder. See also **arteriosclerosis.**

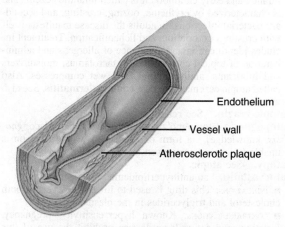

Endothelium

Vessel wall

Atherosclerotic plaque

Atherosclerosis: partial blockage of an artery by plaque
(Thibodeau and Patton, 2003)

Atherosclerosis
(Kumar, Cotran, and Robbins, 1997/courtesy Sid Murphree, MD, Department of Pathology, University of Texas Southwestern Medical School)

atherosclerotic aneurysm /-ot′ik/ [Gk, *athere* + *skleros,* hard, *aneurysma,* an arterial widening], a dilation that results from atherosclerotic weakening of the arterial wall.

atherothrombosis /ath′ərō′thrombō′sis/, a condition in which a thrombus originates in an atheromatous blood vessel.

athetoid /ath′ətoid/, pertaining to athetosis, as in the involuntary, purposeless weaving motions of the body or its extremities.

athetosis /ath′ətō′sis/ [Gk, *athetos,* not fixed], a neuromuscular condition characterized by slow, writhing, worm-like, continuous, and involuntary movement of the extremities, as seen in some forms of cerebral palsy and in motor disorders resulting from lesions in the basal ganglia, tabes dorsalis, or other conditions.

athiaminosis /əthī′əminō′sis/, a condition resulting from lack of thiamine in the diet. See also **beriberi, thiamin.**

athlete's foot. See **tinea pedis.**

athlete's heart /ath′lēts/, an enlarged but otherwise normal heart of an athlete trained for endurance. It is characterized by a low heart rate, an increased pumping capacity, and a greater ability to deliver oxygen to skeletal muscles. Also called **athletic heart syndrome (AHS).**

athletic habitus /athlet′ik/, a physique characterized by a well-proportioned, muscular body with broad shoulders, thick neck, deep chest, and flat abdomen. Compare **asthenic habitus, pyknic.** See also **mesomorph.**

athletic heart syndrome. See **athlete's heart.**

athletic trainer, an allied health professional who, with the consultation and supervision of attending physicians, is an integral part of the health care system associated with sports. Through both academic preparation and practical experience, the athletic trainer provides a variety of services, including injury prevention and recognition and immediate care, treatment, and rehabilitation of athletic trauma.

Ativan, trademark for a benzodiazepine antianxiety agent (lorazepam).

atlantal /ətlan′təl/, pertaining to the atlas, the first cervical vertebra.

atlantoaxial /ətlan′tō·ak′sē·əl/ [Gk, *atlas,* to bear, *axis,* pivot], pertaining to the first two cervical vertebrae.

atlantooccipital joint /-oksip′itəl/ [Gk, *atlas,* to bear; L, *ob,* against, *caput,* head], one of a pair of condyloid joints formed by the articulation of the atlas of the vertebral column with the occipital bone of the skull. It includes two articular capsules, two membranes, and two lateral ligaments. The atlantooccipital joint permits nodding and lateral movements of the head.

atlas [Gk, *atlas,* to bear, a mythical giant, compelled to uphold the world], the first cervical vertebra, articulating with the occipital bone and the axis.

Articular facet

Transverse foramen

Atlas *(Applegate, 2000)*

ATLS, abbreviation for *advanced trauma life support.*

atm, **1.** abbreviation for **atmosphere.** **2.** abbreviation for **atmospheric.**

atman /ät'män/, (in psychiatry) a concept derived from Eastern Indian philosophy that the highest value is knowledge of one's true self. The atman represents the most inward reality, the innermost spirit, and the highest controlling power of a person.

atmo-, prefix meaning 'steam or vapor': *atmolysis, atmotherapy.*

atmosphere (atm) /at'məsfir/ [Gk, *atmos,* vapor, *sphaira,* sphere], **1.** the natural body of air, composed of approximately 21% oxygen, 78% nitrogen, and 1% argon and other gases, including trace levels of carbon dioxide and water vapor that covers the surface of the earth. **2.** an envelope of gas, which may or may not duplicate the natural atmosphere in chemical components. **3.** a unit of gas pressure that is usually defined as being equivalent to the average pressure of the earth's atmosphere at sea level, or about 14.7 pounds per square inch or 760 mm Hg. —**atmospheric,** *adj.*

atmospheric pressure /-fer'ik/, the pressure exerted by the weight of the atmosphere. The average atmospheric pressure at sea level is approximately 14.7 pounds per square inch. With increasing altitude the pressure decreases: at 30,000 feet, approximately the height of Mt. Everest, the air pressure is 4.3 pounds per square inch. Also called **barometric pressure.**

ATN, abbreviation for **acute tubular necrosis.**

atom /at'əm/ [Gk, *atmos,* indivisible], **1.** (in chemistry and physics) the smallest division of an element that exhibits all the properties and characteristics of the element. It comprises neutrons, electrons, and protons. The number of protons in the nucleus of every atom of any given element is the same and is called its atomic number. **2.** *nontechnical,* the amount of any substance that is so small that further division is not possible. —**atomic,** *adj.*

atomic mass, the average mass, relative to an atom of carbon, of an atom of an element based on the natural isotopic mix of that element. Also called **atomic weight.** See also **atomic mass unit.**

atomic mass unit (amu) /ətom'ik/, the mass of a neutral atom of an element, expressed as 1/12 of the mass of the isotope carbon-12 which has a value of exactly 12. The energy equivalent of 1 amu is 931.2 MeV. The mass equivalent of 1 amu is $1.66 \ (10^{-24} \ g)$.

atomic number, the number of protons in the nucleus of an atom of a particular element. In a neutral atom, the atomic number equals the number of electrons. See also **atom, electron, proton.**

atomic theory [Gk, *atmos,* indivisible, *theoria,* speculation], the concept that all matter is composed of submicroscopic atoms that are in turn composed of protons, electrons, and neutrons. A chemical element is identified by the number of protons in its atoms.

atomic weight. See **atomic mass.**

atomize. See **nebulize.**

atomizer /at'əmī'zər/, a device used to reduce a liquid and eject it as a fine spray or vapor.

atomoxetine, a miscellaneous psychotherapeutic agent used to treat attention deficit hyperactivity disorder.

atonia /ātō'nē·ə/ [Gk, *a* + *tonos,* without tone], decreased or absent muscle tone. See also **atonic.**

atonic /əton'ik/, **1.** weak. **2.** lacking normal tone, as in the case of a muscle that is flaccid. **3.** lacking vigor, such as an atonic ulcer, which heals slowly. —**atony** /at'onē/, *n.*

atonic bladder. See **flaccid bladder.**

atonic constipation, constipation caused by failure of the colon to respond to the normal stimuli for evacuation, caused by loss of muscle tone. It may occur in elderly or bedridden patients or after prolonged dependence on laxatives. Also called **colon stasis, lazy colon.** See also **fecal impaction, fecalith, inactive colon, constipation.**

atonic impotence. See **impotence.**

atonicity. See **atonia.**

atony. See **atonic.**

atopic /ātop'ik/ [Gk, *a* + *topos,* not place], pertaining to a hereditary tendency to experience immediate allergic reactions such as asthma or vasomotor rhinitis because of the presence of an antibody (atopic reagin) in the skin and sometimes the bloodstream. —**atopy** /at'opē/, *n.*

atopic allergy [Gk, *a,* not, *topos,* place], a form of allergy that afflicts persons with a genetic predisposition to hypersensitivity to certain allergens. Examples include asthma, hay fever, and food allergies.

atopic asthma. See **allergic asthma.**

atopic dermatitis, an intensely pruritic, often excoriated inflammation commonly found on the face and antecubital and popliteal areas of allergy-prone (atopic) individuals. In infancy and early childhood it is called infantile eczema and is characterized by erythema, oozing, crusting, and secondary bacterial infections. In adults the disease manifests itself with crusting, excoriation, and lichenification. Treatment includes identification and avoidance of allergens and administration of topical corticosteroids, tacrolamus, moisturizers and lubricants, antihistamines, and wet compresses. Also called atopic eczema. Compare **contact dermatitis.** See also **atopic.**

atopic reagin, See **reagin.**

atopognosia /ātop'əgnō'zhə/ [Gk, *a, topos,* not place, *gnosis,* knowledge], a form of agnosia in which a person is unable to locate a tactile sensation correctly.

atopy. See **atopic.**

atorvastatin, an antihyperlipidemic.

■ INDICATIONS: This drug is used to lower the levels of both cholesterol and triglycerides in the plasma.

■ CONTRAINDICATIONS: Known hypersensitivity, pregnancy, lactation, and active liver disease prohibit the use of this drug.

■ ADVERSE EFFECTS: Liver dysfunction is a potentially life-threatening side effect of this drug. Other adverse effects include rash, pruritus, alopecia, dyspepsia, flatus, pancreatitis, lens opacities, myalgia, and headache.

atovaquone /ah-to'vah-kwōn/, an antibiotic used in treatment of mild to moderate *Pneumocystis* pneumonia and the prevention and treatment of falciparum malaria. It is administered orally.

atoxic. See **nontoxic.**

ATP, abbreviation for **adenosine triphosphate.**

ATPase, abbreviation for **adenosine triphosphatase.**

ATPD, abbreviation for **ambient temperature, ambient pressure.**

ATPS, abbreviation for **ambient temperature, ambient pressure.** See also **volume ATPS.**

atransferrinemic anemia /ā'transfer'inē'mik/, an iron-transport deficiency disease characterized by a failure of iron to move from the liver or other storage sites to tissues in which erythrocytes develop. The condition may be caused by a molecular defect in transferrin, an iron-binding protein. In addition to anemia, the patient usually suffers from hemosiderosis.

atraumatic /ā'trômat'ik/ [Gk, *a,* without, *trauma*], pertaining to therapies or therapeutic instruments and devices that are unlikely to cause tissue damage.

Infantile atopic dermatitis *(Callen et al, 2000)*

Atresia of the right external ear *(Zitelli and Davis, 1997)*

Atopic dermatitis *(Zitelli and Davis, 1997)*

atresia /ətrē′zhə/ [Gk, *a, tresis,* not perforation], the absence of a normal body opening, duct, or canal, such as of the anus, vagina, or external ear canal. **—atresic, atretic,** *adj.*

-atresia, suffix meaning a 'condition of abnormal occlusion' or congenital absence of an opening: *gynatresia, urethratresia.*

atresic teratism /ətrē′sik/ [Gk, *a, tresis + tera,* monster], a congenital anomaly in which any of the normal openings of the body, such as the mouth, nares, anus, or vagina, fails to form.

atretic. See **atresia.**

atreto-, prefix meaning 'closed, or lacking an opening': *atretoblepharia, atretorrhinia.*

atria. See **atrium.**

atrial appendix. See **auricle.**

atrial complex, the P wave of the electrocardiogram, representing electrical activity of the atria.

atrial extrasystole. See **premature atrial complex.**

atrial fibrillation (AF) /ā′trē·əl/, a cardiac arrhythmia characterized by disorganized electrical activity in the atria accompanied by an irregular ventricular response that is usually rapid. The atria quiver instead of pumping in an organized fashion, resulting in compromised ventricular filling and reduced stroke volume. Stasis of left atrial flow increases the risk of stroke. AF is associated with rheumatic heart disease (left atrial dilation), mitral stenosis, acute myocardial infarction, and heart surgery, or it may be idiopathic (lone AF). Treatment goals are to control the ventricular rate creating atrioventricular block, to prevent stroke through the use of anticoagulants, and to convert to sinus rhythm. Treatment categories are acute, subacute, and chronic. AF is called uncontrolled and controlled if ventricular response is less than 100. If ventricular response is 100 or more, it is called uncontrolled atrial fibrillation; less than 100, controlled.

atrial flutter (AF), a type of atrial tachycardia characterized by contraction rates between 230/min and 380/min. Two kinds, typical and atypical, have been identified and are distinguished from each other by their rates and electrocardiographic (ECG) patterns. During typical atrial flutter the atrial rate is between 290/min and 310/min and produces "fence post" or "sawtooth" ECG waves. During atypical atrial flutter the atrial rate is higher, and the ECG waves lack the sawtooth appearance, and are often sinusoidal. For both types, ventricular contractions usually follow atrial contractions in a 1:2, 1:3, 1:4, or variable ratio. Compare **atrial fibrillation.**

atrial gallop. See **S₄.**

atrial myxoma, a benign, pedunculated, gelatinous tumor that originates in the interatrial septum of the heart. The tumor is characterized by palpitations, disseminated neuritis, nausea, weight loss, fatigue, dyspnea, fever, and occasional sudden loss of consciousness. It is treated by surgical removal of the tumor.

Left atrial myxoma *(Fletcher, 2000)*

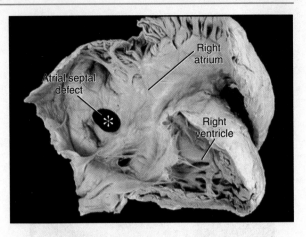

Atrial septal defect *(Damjanov and Linder, 2000)*

atrial natriuretic factor test (ANF), a blood test used to detect levels of ANF, which have been shown to be a marker of congestive heart failure (CHF) severity in patients with known CHF. ANF is also used to predict which cardiac patients are likely to develop CHF and to predict the chance of developing CHF after acute myocardial infarction.

atrial natriuretic peptide (ANP), a hormone involved in natriuresis and the regulation of renal and cardiovascular homeostasis. It is generally 28 amino acids in length but varies somewhat. It is synthesized as a prohormone in the granules of the myocytes of the atrium and is released into the circulation in response to atrial dilation or increased intravascular fluid volume. It causes natriuresis, diuresis, and renal vasodilation; reduces circulating concentrations of renin, aldosterone, and antidiuretic hormone; and thereby normalizes circulating blood pressure and volume. Also called **atrial natriuretic factor.**

atrial pacing. See **pacing.**

atrial premature complex (APC). See **premature atrial complex.**

atrial septal defect (ASD), a congenital cardiac anomaly characterized by an abnormal opening between the atria. The severity of the condition depends on the size and location of the opening, which are related to the stage at which embryonic development of the septum was arrested. ASDs are classified as **ostium primum defect,** in which there is inadequate development of the endocardial cushions of the first septum of the fetal heart; **ostium secundum defect,** in which the aperture in the second septum of the fetal heart fails to close; and **sinus venosus defect,** in which the superior portion of the atrium fails to develop. ASDs increase the flow of oxygenated blood into the right side of the heart, which is usually well tolerated, since the blood is delivered under much lower pressure than in ventricular septal defect. Clinical manifestations include a characteristic harsh, scratchy systolic murmur and a fixed splitting of the second heart sound, which does not vary with respiration. X-ray films and electrocardiograms generally show right atrial and right ventricular enlargement, although definitive diagnosis is made by cardiac catheterization or echocardiogram. Surgical closure is indicated in most cases but is usually postponed until later childhood, unless the defect is severe. See also **endocardial cushion defect.**

atrial septum [L, *atrium,* hall, *saeptum,* fence], a partition between the left and right atria of the heart.

atrial standstill, a condition of complete failure of the atria to contract. P waves are absent in all electrocardiogram surface leads, and A waves are absent in the jugular venous pulse and right atrial pressure tracings. Generally a junctional escape pacemaker maintains ventricular activity during atrial standstill.

atrial systole, the contraction of the atria of the heart, which precedes ventricular contraction by a fraction of a second.

atrial tachycardia [L, *atrium,* hall; Gk, *tachys,* quick, *kardia,* heart], rapid beating of the atria caused by abnormal automaticity, triggered activity, or intraatrial reentry. The atrial rate is usually less than 200/min; however, in cases of digitalis excess, the rate increases gradually to 130/min to 250/min as the digitalis is continued. When there is 2:1 conduction, the atrial rhythm is irregular in 50% of cases. The contour of the P′ waves is different from that of the sinus P wave except in cases of digitalis-induced atrial tachycardia, when the P′ wave is almost identical to the sinus P′ wave. Vagal maneuvers have no effect on atrial tachycardia, although they do cause atrioventricular block. Atrial tachycardia may be either nonparoxysmal (common) or paroxysmal (uncommon). Also called **auricular tachycardia.**

atrichia /ātrik′ē·ə/ [Gk, *a,* not, *thrix,* hair], **1.** pertaining to a group of bacteria that lack flagella. **2.** the absence of hair.

atrichosis /ā′trikō′sis/ [Gk, *a* + *trichia* without hair, *osis,* condition], a congenital absence of hair.

atrio-, prefix meaning "atrium of the heart" or entrance chamber: *atriocommissuropexy, atrionector.*

atrioventricular (AV) /ā′trē·ōventrik′yələr/ [L, *atrium,* hall, *ventriculus*], pertaining to a connecting conduction event or anatomic structure between the atria and ventricles.

atrioventricular block (AVB) [L, *atrium* + *ventriculus,* little belly], a disorder of cardiac impulse transmission that reflects prolonged, intermittent, or absent conduction of impulses between the atria and ventricles. It commonly occurs at the AV node or within the bundle branch system. Treatment depends on where the block is located and whether it is transient or permanent. Heart rate supporting drugs or pacemaker insertion are common options. See also **heart block, intraatrial block, intraventricular block, sinoatrial (SA) block.**

atrioventricular (AV) bundle, a band of atypical cardiac muscle fibers with few contractile units. It arises from the distal portion of the AV node and extends across the AV groove to the top of the intraventricular septum, where it divides into the bundle branches. Also called **bundle of His.**

atrioventricular (AV) dissociation, a breakdown in the normal conduction of excitation through the heart, allowing the atria and ventricles to beat independently under the control of their own pacemakers.

atrioventricular (AV) junction [L, *jungere,* to join], the region of the heart that separates the atria from the ventricles. It includes the AV bundle (bundle of His) and surrounds the AV node. See also **junctional extrasystole.**

atrioventricular (AV) node, an area of specialized cardiac muscle that receives the cardiac impulse from the sinoatrial (SA) node and conducts it to the AV bundle and thence to the Purkinje fibers and walls of the ventricles. The AV node is located in the septal wall between the left and right atria.

atrioventricular (AV) septum, a small portion of membrane that separates the atria from the ventricles of the heart.

atrioventricular (AV) valve, a valve in the heart through which blood flows from the atria to the ventricles. The valve between the left atrium and left ventricle is the mitral (bicuspid) valve; the right AV valve is the tricuspid valve.

at risk, the state of an individual or population being vulnerable to a particular disease or event. The factors determining risk may be environmental, psychosocial, psychologic, or physiologic. An example of an environmental factor is exposure to harmful substances or organisms. An example of a physiologic factor is genetic predisposition to a disease.

atrium *pl.* **atria** /ā′trē·əm/ [L, hall], a chamber or cavity, such as the right and left atria of the heart or the nasal cavity.

atrium of ear, the external part of the ear, including the auricle and the tubular portion of the external auditory meatus.

atrium of the heart, one of the two upper chambers of the heart. The right atrium receives deoxygenated blood from the superior vena cava, the inferior vena cava, and the coronary sinus. The left atrium receives oxygenated blood from the pulmonary veins. Blood is emptied into the ventricles from the atria during diastole.

Atromid-S, trademark for an antilipemic (clofibrate) used to lower plasma triglyceride (VLDL) levels.

-atrophia, **1.** suffix meaning a 'condition of nutrition and growth': *metatrophia, pantatrophia.* **2.** combining form meaning a 'progressive decline of a body part': *dermatrophia, neuratrophia.*

atrophic /ātrof′ik/ [Gk, *a,* without, *trophe,* nourishment], characterized by a wasting of tissues, usually associated with general malnutrition or a specific disease state. See also **dystrophic.**

atrophic acne, acne vulgaris in which, after the disappearance of small papular lesions, a stippling of tiny atrophic pits and scars remains.

atrophic arthritis. See **rheumatoid arthritis.**

atrophic catarrh [Gk, *a, trophe,* without nourishment, *kata,* down, *rhoia,* flow], an abnormal condition characterized by inflammation and discharge from the mucous membranes of the nose, accompanied by the loss of mucosal and submucosal tissue. Compare **hypertrophic catarrh.** See also **catarrh.**

atrophic cirrhosis [Gk, *a + trophe,* without nourishment, *kirrhos,* yellow-orange], a form of advanced portal cirrhosis with massive shrinking of the liver.

atrophic fracture, a spontaneous fracture caused by bone atrophy, as in the bones of a person with osteoporosis.

atrophic gastritis, a chronic inflammation of the stomach, associated with degeneration of the gastric mucosa. Seen in elderly patients and in persons with pernicious anemia, it rarely causes epigastric pain. See also **pernicious anemia.**

atrophic glossitis, a pathologic condition in which the various papillae are lost from the dorsum of the tongue, resulting in a very sore and highly sensitive surface that makes eating difficult. See also **glossitis.**

atrophic rhinitis [Gk, *a + trophe,* without nourishment, *rhis,* nose, *itis,* inflammation], a nasal condition in which there is atrophy of the mucous membrane of the nose, resulting in failure of the ciliary function and drying and crusting of the lining of the nasal passages. This may reduce the sense of smell.

atrophic vaginitis [Gk, *a + trophe,* without nourishment; L, *vagina,* sheath; Gk, *itis,* inflammation], degeneration of the vaginal mucous membrane after menopause due to decreased estrogen level thinning and dryness. See also **vaginitis.**

atrophied /at′rōfīd/ [Gk, *a + trophe,* without nourishment], decreased in size because of disuse or disease, as an organ, tissue, or body part.

atrophoderma /at′rōfədur′mə/ [Gk, *a + trophe + derma,* skin], the wasting away or decrease in thickness of the skin. The atrophy may affect the entire body surface or only localized areas. The condition is often associated with aging and may occur as a primary or secondary symptom of various diseases.

atrophy /at′rəfē/ [Gk, *a + trophe,* without nourishment], a wasting or decrease in size or physiologic activity of a part of the body because of disease or other influences. A skeletal muscle may undergo atrophy as a result of lack of physical exercise or neurologic or musculoskeletal disease. Cells of the brain and central nervous system may atrophy in old age because of restricted blood flow to those areas. See also **aging. —atrophic,** *adj.,* **atrophy,** *v.*

atrophy of aging, senile atrophy.

atrophy of disuse [Gk, *a, trophe* + L, *dis,* opposite of, *usus*], a shrinkage of tissues resulting from immobility or lack of exercise.

atropine /at′rōpin/ [Gk, *Atropos,* one of the three Fates], an alkaloid from *Atropa belladonna* and *Datura stramonium* plants. It is related to other drugs, such as scopolamine and hyoscyamine, and has a similar action of blocking parasympathetic stimuli by raising the threshold of response of effector cells to acetylcholine.

atropine sulfate, an antispasmodic and anticholinergic.
■ INDICATIONS: It may be prescribed in the treatment of GI hypermotility to decrease the tone of the detrusor muscle of the urinary bladder in urinary tract disorders, for cyclopegic refraction and dilation of the pupil in inflammation of the iris or the uvea, cardiac arrhythmias, and certain kinds of poisoning and as an adjunct to anesthesia.
■ CONTRAINDICATIONS: GI obstruction, glaucoma, hepatitis, liver or kidney dysfunction, porphyria, or known hypersensitivity to this drug or other anticholinergics prohibits its use.
■ ADVERSE EFFECTS: Among the more serious adverse reactions are tachycardia, angina, loss of taste, nausea, diarrhea, skin rash, blurred vision, and eye pain. Dry mouth and constipation are common effects.

atropine sulfate poisoning [Gk, *Atropos,* fate; L, *sulphur + potio,* drink], toxic effects of an overdose of a drug sometimes used as an adjunct to general anesthesia and to treat bradycardia. Symptoms include tachycardia, hot and dry flushed skin, dry mouth with thirst, restlessness and excitement, urinary retention, constipation, and a burning pain in the throat.

attached epithelial cuff.　See **junctional epithelium.**

attached gingiva,　gum tissue that covers and is firmly attached to the alveolar process in the maxilla and mandible. Also called **alveolar gingiva.**

attachment [Fr, *attachement*], **1.** the state or quality of being affixed or attached. **2.** (in psychiatry) a mode of behavior in which one individual relates in an affiliative or dependent manner to another; a feeling of affection or loyalty that binds one person to another. See also **bonding. 3.** (in dentistry) any device, such as a retainer or artificial crown, used to secure a partial denture to a natural tooth in the mouth.

attachment apparatus,　the various tissues that surround and support the teeth, including the cementum, the periodontal ligament, and the alveolar process. See also **masticatory system.**

attachment promotion,　a nursing intervention from the Nursing Interventions Classification (NIC) defined as facilitation of the development of the parent-infant relationship. See also **Nursing Interventions Classification.**

attack,　an episode in the course of an illness, usually characterized by acute and distressing symptoms.

attapulgite /at′ah-pul′jīt/, a clay mineral that contains aluminum silicate and is the main ingredient of Fuller's earth. *Activated attapulgite* is a heat-treated form that is administered orally in the treatment of diarrhea.

attending [L, *attendo,* to notice], (in psychology) pertaining to an aroused readiness to perceive, with an adjustment of the brain and sense organs to focus on a situation.

attending physician [L, *attendere,* to stretch], the physician who is responsible for a particular patient. In a university hospital setting, an attending physician often also has teaching responsibilities, holds a faculty appointment, and supervises residents and medical students. Also called *(informal)* **attending.**

attention [L, *attendere,* to stretch], the element of cognitive functioning in which the mental focus is maintained on a specific issue, object, or activity.

attention deficit disorder,　a syndrome affecting children, adolescents, and adults characterized by short attention span, hyperactivity, and poor concentration. The symptoms may be mild or severe and are associated with functional deviations of the central nervous system without signs of major neurologic or psychiatric disturbance. The people affected are usually of normal or above average intelligence. Other symptoms include impairment in perception, conceptualization, language, memory, and motor skills; decreased attention span; increased impulsivity; and emotional lability. The condition is 10 times more prevalent in boys than in girls and may result from genetic factors, biochemical irregularities, perinatal or postnatal injury, or disease. There is no known cure, and symptoms often subside or disappear with time. Medication with methylphenidate, pemoline, or the dextroamphetamines is frequently prescribed for children with hyperactive symptoms, and some form of psychotherapeutic counseling is often recommended. Some treatments include abstinence from certain foods and food additives. Also called **hyperactivity, hyperkinesis, minimal brain dysfunction.** See also **learning disability.**

attention deficit hyperactivity disorder (ADHD),　a childhood mental disorder with onset before 7 years of age and involving impaired or diminished attention, impulsivity, and hyperactivity. Also called **hyperactive child syndrome** in the twentieth century.

attenuated /ətenʹyo͞o-āʹtid/ [L, *attenuare,* to make thin], pertaining to the dilution of a solution or the reduction in

virulence or toxicity of a microorganism or a drug by weakening it.

attenuated virus [L, *attenuare,* to make thin, *virus,* poison], a strain of virus whose virulence has been lowered by physical or chemical processes, or by repeated passage through the cells of another species. Vaccines made by attenuated strains are used to prevent smallpox, measles, mumps, rubella, polio, yellow fever, and other viruses.

attenuation /ətenʹyo͞o-āʹshən/ [L, *attenuare,* to make thin], the process of reduction, such as the attenuation of an x-ray beam by reducing its intensity, the weakening of the degree of virulence of a disease organism, or culturing under unfavorable conditions.

attenuation coefficient,　in radiography or ultrasound, the difference between the energy that enters a body part and the energy that is not detected. The difference is caused by the absorption and scattering of energy within the body tissues.

attenuator /ətenʹyo͞o-āʹtər/ [L, *attenuare,* to make thin], an agent that weakens the toxicity of a poisonous substance or the virulence of a microorganism.

Attenuvax,　trademark for an active immunizing agent (live measles virus vaccine).

attic.　See **epitympanic recess.**

attitude /atʹətyo͞od, -to͞od/ [L, *aptitude,* fitness], **1.** a body position or posture, particularly the fetal position in the uterus, as determined by the degree of flexion of the head and extremities. **2.** (in psychiatry) any of the major integrative forces in the development of personality that gives consistency to an individual's behavior. Attitudes are cognitive in nature, formed through interactions with the environment. They reflect the person's innermost convictions about situations good or bad, right or wrong, desirable or undesirable.

attitudinal isolation /atʹətyo͞oʹdənəl/ [L, *attitudo,* posture], a type of social isolation that results from a person's own cultural or personal values.

attitudinal reflex,　any reflex initiated by a change in position of the head or by a change in position of the head with respect to the position of the body. Kinds of attitudinal reflexes include **tonic neck reflex** and **tonic labyrinthine reflex.** Also called **statotonic reflex.**

atto-,　a prefix in the metric system indicating a value of one quintillionth, or 10^{-18}.

attraction [L, *attrahere,* to draw to], a tendency of the teeth or other maxillary or mandibular structures to become elevated above their normal position.

ATTR amyloidosis,　the most common form of familial amyloidosis, in which any of numerous mutations of the gene encoding transthyretin cause systemic autosomal-dominant disorders characterized by polyneuropathies, cardiomyopathies, and variable organ involvement.

attrition /ətrishʹən/ [L, *atterere,* to wear away], the process of wearing away or wearing down by friction.

-ature,　noun-forming combining form: *ligature, tubulature.*

at. wt.,　abbreviation for **atomic weight.**

atypia /ātipʹē·ə/ [Gk, *a* + *typos,* without type], a condition of being irregular or nonstandard.

atypical /ātipʹəkəl/ [Gk, *a* + *typos,* without type], a condition or object that is not of a usual or standard type.

atypical measles syndrome (AMS),　a form of measles (rubeola) reported in persons immunized with a killed measles vaccine used in the United States from 1962 to 1967 and in Canada until 1970. Symptoms differ from those of typical measles, beginning with a sudden high fever, headache, abdominal pain, and coughing. The measles rash may appear only 1 or 2 days later, usually starting on the hands and feet, rather than the head and neck. The infection may be complicated by edema of the extremities and pneumonia.

atypical *Mycobacterium* [Gk, *a* + *typos,* without type, *mykes,* fungus, *bakterion,* small staff], a group of mycobacteria, including pathogenic and nonpathogenic forms, that are classified according to their ability to produce pigments, growth characteristics, and reactions to chemical tests. Mycobacteria, nontuberculosis (atypical) does not require isolation precautions.

atypical pneumonia [Gk, *a* + *typos,* without type, *pneumon,* lung, *ia,* condition], a group of relatively mild symptoms of chills, headache, muscular pains, moderate fever, and coughing, but without evidence of a bacterial infection. Chest x-ray film may show mottling at the bases of the lungs. Eaton agent, or *Mycoplasma pneumoniae,* may be the cause of the symptoms.

atypical polypoid adenomyoma, a rare and benign tumor that may be clinically and histologically mistaken for malignance.

atypical somatoform disorder, an abnormal condition marked by physical symptoms and complaints that appear related to a preoccupation with an imagined defect in one's personal appearance or ability.

Au, symbol for the element **gold.**

audible /ô'dəbəl/ [L, *audire,* to hear], capable of being heard. Some animals are able to hear sounds of higher or lower frequencies and different intensities than those audible to most humans.

audio-, combining form meaning 'hearing': *audiology.*

audioanalgesia /ô·dē·ō·an'əljē'sē·a/ [L, *audire,* to hear; Gk, *a, algos,* not pain], the use of music to enhance relaxation and to distract a patient's mind from pain, as during dentistry, during labor and childbirth, or during procedures with sedation or regional anesthetic techniques.

audiogenic epilepsy. See **auditory epilepsy.**

audiogram /ô'dē·əgram'/ [Gk, *audire* + *gramma,* record], a chart showing the faintest level at which an individual is able to detect sounds of various frequencies, usually in octaves from 125 Hz to 8000 Hz. See also **audiometry.**

audiologic. See **audiology.**

audiologist, a health professional with graduate education in normal hearing processes and hearing loss, who detects and evaluates hearing loss, and who determines how a client can best make use of remaining hearing. If a client can benefit from assistive learning devices such as hearing aids, the audiologist assists with the selection, fitting, and training in their use. See also **speech-language pathologist.**

audiology /-ol'əjē/ [L, *audire* + Gk, *logos,* science], a field of research and clinical practice devoted to the study of hearing disorders, assessment of hearing, hearing conservation, and aural rehabilitation. **—audiologic,** *adj.*

audiometer /ô'dē·om'ətər/ [L, *audire* + Gk, *metron,* measure], an electronic device for testing hearing. Earphones are placed over the ears (air-conduction testing), or a bone vibrator is placed on the mastoid (bone conduction testing). Hearing is tested by using tones from very low to very high frequencies at various decibels of intensity. The patient signals when a tone is heard, and the lowest level at which the patient hears is noted on an audiogram.

audiometrist /ô'dē·om'ətrist/, a technician who has received special training in the use of pure-tone audiometry equipment. An audiometrist conducts the hearing tests selected and interpreted by an audiologist, who supervises the process.

audiometry /ô'dē·om'ətrē/, the testing of the sensitivity of the sense of hearing. Various audiometric tests determine the lowest intensity of sound at which an individual can perceive auditory stimuli (hearing threshold) and distinguish different speech sounds. Pure tone audiometry assesses the person's ability to hear frequencies, usually ranging from 125 to 8000 hertz (Hz), and can indicate whether a hearing loss is caused by an outer ear, a middle ear, an inner ear, or an acoustic nerve problem. Speech audiometry tests the ability to understand selected words. Impedance audiometry is an objective method of assessing the resistance or compliance of the conducting mechanism of the middle ear with a probe inserted into the ear canal. **—audiometric,** *adj.*

audiovisual /ô'dē·ōvizh'əl/, pertaining to communication that uses both sight and sound messages.

audit /ô'dit/, **1.** a final statement of account. **2.** a review and evaluation of health care procedures and documentation.

auditory /ô'dətôr'ē/ [L, *auditorius,* hearing], pertaining to the sense of hearing and the hearing organs involved.

auditory amnesia [L, *auditorius,* hearing; Gk, *amnesia,* forgetfulness], a loss of memory for the meaning of sounds. Also called **word deafness.**

auditory area [L, *auditorium,* hearing], the sound perception area of the cerebral cortex. It is located in the floor of the lateral fissure and on the dorsal surface of the superior temporal gyrus.

auditory brainstem response (ABR), an electrophysiologic test used to measure hearing sensitivity and evaluate the integrity of ear structures from the auditory nerve through the brainstem. It is also used to screen hearing of newborns.

auditory canal. See **auditory meatus.**

auditory cortex. See **acoustic center.**

auditory epilepsy, a reflex form of epilepsy provoked by sounds. Also called **audiogenic epilepsy.**

auditory hair [L, *audire,* to hear; AS, *haer*], one of the cells with hairlike processes in the spiral organ of Corti. The hairs, or cilia, function as sensory receptors. Also called **acoustic hair cell, cell of Corti.**

auditory hallucination [L, *audire,* to hear, *alucinari,* a wandering mind], commonly seen in schizophrenia. It is a subjective experience of hearing voices or other sounds despite the absence of an actual reality based external stimulus to account for the phenomenon.

auditory meatus [L, *audire,* to hear, *meatus,* passage], **1.** the external auditory meatus, a tubelike channel of the external ear extending from the auricle to the tympanum of the middle ear. **2.** the internal auditory meatus, a short channel extending from the petrous part of the temporal bone to the fundus near the vestibule. It contains the eighth cranial nerve. Also called **auditory canal.**

auditory nerve. See **vestibulocochlear nerve.**

auditory ossicles [L, *audire* + *ossiculum,* little bone], the malleus, the incus, and the stapes, three small bones in the middle ear that articulate with each other. As the tympanic membrane vibrates, it transmits sound waves through the ossicles to the cochlea.

auditory system assessment, an evaluation of the patient's ears and hearing and an investigation of present and past diseases or conditions that may be responsible for an auditory impairment.

■ METHOD: The client is questioned in verbal or written form regarding previous ear problems, especially childhood problems of otitis media, perforations of the eardrum, and drainage, and history of measles, mumps, or scarlet fever. Information is obtained about past or present ototoxic medications, such as aspirin, chemotherapeutic drugs, NSAIDS. streptomycin, aminoglycerides, or diuretics. Previous ear surgeries as well as tonsillectomy and adenoidectomy or head injury are also documented. Use of a hearing aid and

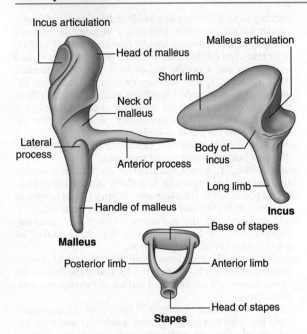

Incus articulation

Head of malleus

Malleus articulation

Short limb

Neck of malleus

Lateral process

Body of incus

Anterior process

Long limb

Handle of malleus

Incus

Base of stapes

Malleus

Posterior limb

Anterior limb

Head of stapes

Stapes

Auditory ossicles *(Drake, Vogl, and Mitchell, 2005)*

problems with compacted cerumin are noted. Symptoms of dizziness, ringing in the ears, and hearing loss are recorded. Information regarding allergies, prematurity, and family members with hearing loss is documented. Chronic medical conditions such as diabetes or cancer as well as occupational exposures to high-noise environments, with or without protection, are also important. Recreational ear hazards, such as swimming or chronic exposure to loud music, are noted. Physical examination includes inspection and palpation of the external ear including the mastoid area for tenderness, swelling, redness, nodules, or lesions. Otoscopic examination is then performed to assess the ear canal and tympanic membrane. Diagnostic procedures indicated by the history may include audiometry, a mastoid x-ray film, Rinne and Weber tuning-fork tests, and microbiologic studies for potential pathogens in smears of ear drainage.
■ NURSING CONSIDERATIONS: The nurse conducts the interview, makes the observations, and collects the pertinent background information and the results of the diagnostic procedures.
■ OUTCOME CRITERIA: A thorough assessment of the patient's auditory system is essential in establishing the diagnosis of an ear disorder.
auditory threshold [L, *audire,* to hear; AS, *threscold*], the lowest intensity at which a sound may be heard. An audiologist typically determines a patient's threshold for pure tones and speech.
auditory tube. See **eustachian tube.**
auditory vertigo [L, *audire,* to hear, *vertigo,* dizziness], vertigo associated with ear disease. It is characterized by sensations of gyration and, when severe, with prostration and vomiting.
Auerbach's plexus [Leopold Auerbach, German anatomist, 1828–1897; L, *plexus,* plaited], the myenteric plexus, a group of autonomic nerve fibers and ganglia located in the muscle tissue of the intestinal tract.
Auer rod /ou′ər/ [John Auer, American physiologist, 1875–

1948], an abnormal, needle-shaped or round, pink-staining inclusion in the cytoplasm of myeloblasts and promyelocytes in acute myelogenous, promyelocytic, or myelomonocytic leukemia. These inclusions contain enzymes such as acid phosphatase, peroxidase, and esterase and may represent abnormal derivatives of cytoplasmic granules. The finding of Auer rods in stained blood smears helps to differentiate acute myelogenous leukemia from acute lymphoblastic leukemia. Also called **Auer body.**

Auer rod *(Carr and Rodak, 1999)*

augmentation /ôg′məntā′shən/ [L, *augmentare,* to increase], **1.** stimulation of an increased rate of biologic activity, such as faster cell division or heartbeat. **2.** breast enlargement through mammoplasty.
augmentation mammoplasty, a surgical procedure to enlarge the breasts.
aur-, auri-, prefix meaning 'ear': *auricle, aural.*
aura /ôr′ə/ [L, breath], **1.** *pl.* **aurae** /ôr′ē/, a sensation, as of light, warmth, or emotion (such as fear) that may precede an attack of migraine or an epileptic seizure. **2.** *pl.* **auras,** an emanation of light or color surrounding a person as seen in Kirlian photography and studied in current nursing research in healing techniques.
aural[1] /ôr′əl/, pertaining to the ear or hearing. —**aurally,** *adv.*
aural[2], pertaining to an aura.
aural forceps, a dressing forceps with fine, bent tips used in surgery.
aurally. See **aural.**
aural rehabilitation, a form of therapy in which hearing-impaired individuals are taught to improve their ability to communicate. Methods taught include, but are not limited to, speech-reading, auditory training, use of hearing aids, and use of assistive listening devices such as telephone amplifiers.
auramine /ôr′əmēn/, a yellow aniline dye used in the manufacture of paints, textiles, and rubber products. The experimental carcinogen in animals has been identified as a cause of bladder cancer in humans. Also called **dimethylaniline.**
auramine O, a fluorescent, yellow aniline dye used as a stain for the tubercle bacillus and for deoxyribonucleic acid (DNA).
auranofin /ôr′ənof′in/, an oral gold disease-modifying antirheumatoid drug.
■ INDICATIONS: It can be prescribed for the treatment of rheumatoid arthritis, but is generally not first line therapy.
■ CONTRAINDICATIONS: Auranofin is contraindicated for patients who have disorders that are caused by or aggravated by medicines containing gold or who have impaired kidney function.
■ ADVERSE EFFECTS: Among the most severe adverse effects

are diarrhea, loose stools, abdominal pain, nausea, vomiting, rash, pruritus, stomatitis, anemia, leukopenia, granulocytopenia, thrombocytopenia, eosinophilia, proteinemia, hematuria, and elevated liver enzyme levels.

aurantiasis cutis /ôr′əntī′əsis/ [L, *aurantium,* orange; Gk, *osis,* condition; L, *cutis,* skin], a yellowish skin pigmentation that results from eating excessive amounts of foods containing carotene, such as carrots.

auras. See **aura.**

auriasis. See **chrysiasis.**

auricle /ôr′ikəl/ [L, *auricula,* little ear], **1.** the external ear. Also called **pinna. 2.** the left or right cardiac atrium, so named because of its earlike shape. Also called **atrial appendix.**

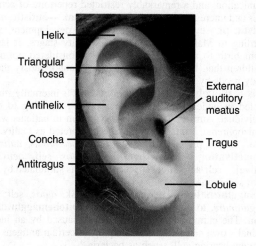

Auricle *(Seidel et al, 1999)*

auricular /ôrik′yələr/, **1.** pertaining to the auricle of the ear. **2.** otic.

auricular acupuncture, acupuncture performed using points on the ear that have been mapped to specific anatomic areas of the body.

auricular cervical nerve reflex. See **Snellen's reflex.**

auricularis anterior, one of three extrinsic muscles of the ear. It functions to move the auricula forward and upward. Some people can voluntarily contract the auricularis anterior to move the ears. Compare **auricularis posterior, auricularis superior.**

auricularis posterior, one of three extrinsic muscles of the ear. It serves to draw the auricula backward. Compare **auricularis anterior, auricularis superior.**

auricularis superior, a thin, fan-shaped muscle that is one of three extrinsic muscles of the ear. It acts to draw the auricula upward. Compare **auricularis anterior, auricularis posterior.**

auricular line, a hypothetical line passing through the external auditory meatuses and perpendicular to the Frankfort horizontal plane.

auricular point, the center of the external auditory meatus.

auricular tachycardia. See **atrial tachycardia.**

auricular tubercle, a small projection sometimes found on the edge of the helix of the ear, conjectured by some to be a relic of a simian ancestry. Also called **darwinian tubercle, Darwin's tubercle.**

Auricularis anterior, auricular posterior, and auricularis superior
(Thibodeau and Patton, 2003)

auriculin /ôrik′yəlin/, a hormonelike substance with diuretic activity produced in the atria of the heart.

auriculocranial /-krā′nē-əl/, pertaining to the auricle of the ear and the cranium.

auriculotemporal /-tem′pərəl/, pertaining to the auricle of the ear and the temporal area of the skull.

auriculoventriculostomy /ôrik′yəlōventrik′yəlos′təmē/ [L, *auricula* + *ventriculus,* little belly; Gk, *stoma,* opening], a surgical procedure that directs cerebrospinal fluid into the general circulation in the treatment of hydrocephalus, usually in the newborn. In this procedure a polyethylene tube is passed from the lateral ventricle through a burr hole in the parietal skull area under the scalp and into the jugular vein or abdomen for the discharge of cerebrospinal fluid. The tube, which has valves, is inserted to prevent reflux of the blood into the ventricles and to maintain the draining of excess cerebrospinal fluid when ventricular pressure increases. This procedure is performed to correct the communicating and the obstructive forms of hydrocephalus. Also called **ventriculoatrial shunt, ventriculoatriostomy.**

auris dextra (a.d.), the Latin term for right ear.

auris sinistra (a.s.), the Latin term for left ear.

auromine-rhodamine stain, a fluorescent dye consisting of auramine O, rhodamine B, and phenal that is used in the fluorochrome acid-fast staining method. The dye binds to mycolic acids in the cell wall of bacteria and resists decolorization with acid alcohol.

aurothioglucose /ôr′ōthī′ōglooˈkōs/, an organic gold compound used as a disease-modifying antirheumatoid drug.

■ INDICATION: It is prescribed for adjunctive treatment of adult and juvenile rheumatoid arthritis, but generally no longer considered first line therapy.

■ CONTRAINDICATIONS: Severe uncontrolled diabetes, renal or hepatic dysfunction, a history of infectious hepatitis, hypertension, heart failure, systemic lupus erythematosus, agranulocytosis, hemorrhagic diathesis, pregnancy, urticaria, eczema, colitis, or known hypersensitivity to this drug prohibits its use.

■ ADVERSE EFFECTS: Among the most serious adverse effects are kidney and liver damage and allergic reactions. Dermatitis and lesions of mucous membranes are common.

auscultate /ôs′kəltāt/ [L, auscultare, to listen], to practice auscultation, or to listen and interpret sounds produced within the body.

auscultation /ôs′kəltā′shən/ [L, *auscultare,* to listen], the act of listening for sounds within the body to evaluate the condition of the heart, blood vessels, lungs, pleura, intestines, or other organs or to detect the fetal heart sound. Auscultation may be performed directly with the unaided ear, but most commonly a stethoscope is used to determine the frequency, intensity, duration, and quality of the sounds. **—auscultate,** *v.,* **auscultatory** /ôskul′tətôr′ē/, *adj.*

Auscultation *(Seidel et al, 2003)*

auscultatory gap, time in which sound is not heard in the auscultatory method of measuring blood pressure with a sphygmomanometer, occurring particularly in hypertension and in aortic stenosis.

auscultatory percussion. See **auscultation, percussion.**

Austin Flint murmur [Austin Flint, American physiologist, 1812–1886], a low-pitched sound characteristic of severe aortic regurgitation without mitral valve disease. It is typically heard during ventricular middiastole at the mitral valve area. Amyl nitrate may help differentiate this murmur from that of mitral valve stenosis.

Australia antigen, hepatitis B surface antigen (HBsAg), found present in acute or chronic hepatitis B. See also **hepatitis.**

Australian lift, a type of shoulder lift used to move a patient who is unable to assume a sitting position on a bed or other surface. The lift is executed by two persons, one on each side of the patient, who place their shoulders near the patient under the patient's axillae. At the same time, the two lifters grasp each other's hands under the patient's thighs and make coordinated movements needed to lift the patient onto or from a bed or wheelchair.

Australian Q fever. See **Q fever.**

autacoid /ô′təkoid/, any one of the substances produced locally by one group of cells that exerts effects on other types of cells in the same region.

authenticity /ô′thəntis′itē/, (in psychiatry) emotional and behavioral openness; a quality of being genuine and trustworthy.

authoritarian personality, a group of behavioral traits characteristic of one who advocates obedience and strict adherence to rules.

authority /ôthôr′ətē/, a relationship between two or more persons or groups characterized by the influence one may exercise over the other through ideas, commands, suggestions, or instructions.

authority figure, a person who by virtue of status, strength, knowledge, or other recognized superiority exerts influence over others.

autism [Gk, *autos,* self], a mental disorder characterized by extreme withdrawal and an abnormal absorption in fantasy, accompanied by delusion, hallucination, and inability to communicate verbally or otherwise relate to people. Schizophrenic children are often autistic. See also **infantile autism. —autistic,** *adj.*

autistic disorder /ôtis′tik/ [Gk, *autos,* self], a pervasive developmental disorder with onset in infancy or childhood, characterized by impaired social interaction, impaired communication, and a remarkably restricted repertoire of activities and interests. See also **infantile autism. —autistic,** *adj.*

autistic phase, a period of preoedipal development, according to Mahler's system of personality stages. It lasts from birth to around 1 month and is considered normal. Children then become aware that they cannot satisfy their body needs by themselves.

autistic thought, a form of thinking that is internally stimulated in which the ideas have a private meaning to the individual. Autistic thinking is a symptom in patients with schizophrenia. Fantasy life may be interpreted as reality.

auto-, aut-, prefix meaning 'self': *autocatharsis, autism.*

autoactivation /-ak′tivā′shən/ [Gk, *autos,* self, *activus,* active], self-activation, as when a gland is stimulated by its own secretions.

autoagglutination /-əglo͞o′tənā′shən/ [Gk, *autos,* self; L, *agglutinare,* to glue], **1.** also called **autohemagglutination.** The clumping of red blood cells caused by an individual's own serum. **2.** the clumping of certain antigens or antigen-bearing cells, such as bacteria.

Autoagglutination *(Carr and Rodak, 1999)*

autoamputation /-amp′yo͞otā′shən/, the spontaneous detachment of a body part, usually the fourth or fifth toe, as occurs among the males of some African peoples. A depression develops across the digitoplantar fold of the toe and gradually progresses until the toe falls off. The condition is usually painless and has no other symptoms. Also called **ainhum** /ān′hŏŏm, īnyoon′/.

autoantibody /ô′tō·an′tibod′ē/ [Gk, *autos* + *anti,* against; AS, *bodig,* body], an immunoglobulin produced by a person that recognizes an antigen on that person's own tissues. Several mechanisms may trigger the production of autoantibodies: an antigen, formed during fetal development and then sequestered, may be released as a result of infection, chemical exposure, or trauma, as occurs in autoimmune thyroiditis, sympathetic uveitis, and aspermia; there may be disorders of immune regulatory or surveillance function; antibodies produced against certain streptococcal antigens during infection may cross-react with myocardial tissue, causing rheumatic heart disease, or with glomerular basement membrane, causing glomerulonephritis; and normal body proteins may be converted to autoantigens by chemicals, infectious organisms, or therapeutic drugs. Some examples of autoantibodies are those found against gastric parietal cells in pernicious anemia, against platelets in autoimmune thrombocytopenia, and against antigens on the surface of erythrocytes in autoimmune hemolytic anemia. There is growing evidence that genetic factors increase the incidence and severity of autoimmune diseases.

autoantigen /ô′tō·an′tijin/ [Gk, *autos* + *anti,* against, *genein,* to produce], an endogenous body constituent that stimulates the production of autoantibodies and an autoimmune reaction. An autoantigen associated with **Addison's disease** has been identified as the enzyme 17 α-hydroxylase. Also called **self-antigen.** See also **antibody-specific model, autoantibody, autoimmune disease.**

autoantitoxin /-an′titok′sin/, an antibody produced as protection against a toxin resulting from infection in the same individual, such as *Escherichia coli* endotoxin.

autoaugmentation /-ôg′məntā′shən/, a surgical procedure in which the detrusor muscle of the bladder is removed, leaving the bladder epithelium otherwise intact.

autoblast /ô′təblast/, a free-living unicellular microorganism.

autocatheterization /-kath′ərizā′shən/, the insertion of a catheter by the patient, usually referring to urinary catheterization. See also **self-catheterization.**

autochthonous /ôtok′thənəs/ [Gk, *autos,* self, *chthon,* earth], **1.** relating to a disease or other condition that appears to have originated in the part of the body in which it was discovered. **2.** (in psychology) describing the sudden appearance of a system of delusions.

autochthonous idea [Gk, *autos* + *chthon,* earth], an idea that originates in the unconscious and arises spontaneously in the mind, independent of the conscious train of thought.

autoclassis /ôtok′ləsis/ [Gk, *autos,* self, *klassis,* breaking], the rupturing or breaking of a part of the body caused by a force or agent arising from within the body itself.

autoclave /ô′təklāv/, an appliance used to sterilize medical instruments or other objects with steam under pressure.

autocoid, local hormone.

autocrine /ô′təkrin/, denoting the effect of a hormone on cells that produce it.

autodermic graft. See **autogenous graft.**

autodigestion, a condition in which gastric juices in the pancreas or stomach digest the organ's own tissues.

autodiploid /ô′tōdip′loid/ [Gk, *autos* + *diploos,* double, *eidos,* form], **1.** an individual, organism, strain, or cell containing two genetically identical or nearly identical chromosome sets that are derived from the same ancestral species and result from the duplication of the haploid set. **2.** pertaining to such an individual, organism, strain, or cell. Also

Autoclave *(Sorrentino, 2000)*

autodiploidic. Compare **allodiploid.** See also **autopolyploid.**

autodiploidy /ô′tōdip′loidē/, the state or condition of having two genetically identical or nearly identical chromosome sets from the same ancestral species. Such a state enables cell division to occur in a normal manner. Compare **allodiploidy.**

autoeroticism /-irot′əsiz′əm/ [Gk, *autos* + *eros,* love], **1.** sensual, sexual gratification of the self, usually obtained through the stimulus of one's own body without the participation of another person. It is derived from such acts as stroking, masturbation, and fantasy, or from other oral, anal, or visual sources of stimulation. **2.** sexual feeling or desire occurring without any external stimulus. **3.** (in Freudian psychoanalytic theory) an early phase of psychosexual development, occurring in the oral and the anal stages. Also called **autoerotism.** Compare **heteroeroticism. —autoerotic,** *adj.*

autoerythrocyte sensitization /ô′tō·ərith′rəsīt/ [Gk, *autos* + *erythros,* red, *kytos,* cell], hypersensitivity to one's own red blood cells. It results in the spontaneous appearance of painful, hemorrhagic spots on the anterior aspects of the arms and legs. Autoimmune hemolytic anemia, an extreme example of the condition, may cause fulminant hemolysis, fever, abdominal pain, hyperbilirubinemia, thrombosis, and shock. Psychoneurotic disorders also may be associated with the condition.

autoerythrocyte sensitization syndrome. See **Gardner-Diamond syndrome.**

autogenesis /ô′tōjen′əsis/ [Gk, *autos* + *genein,* to produce], **1.** abiogenesis. **2.** a self-produced condition; a condition originating from within the organism. Also called **autogeny** /ôtoj′ənē/. Compare **heterogenesis, homogenesis. —autogenetic, autogenic,** *adj.*

autogenic therapy /-jen′ik/, a mental health therapy introduced by Wolfgang Luthe. It is based on the concept that natural forces in the brain are able to remove disturbing influences so that functional harmony can be restored in the mind and body. It was developed from research on sleep and hypnosis and involves biofeedback exercises.

autogenic training, a nursing intervention from the Nursing Interventions Classification (NIC) defined as assisting with self-suggestions about feelings of heaviness and warmth for the purpose of inducing relaxation. See also **Nursing Interventions Classification.**

autogenous /ôtoj'ənəs/, **1.** self-generating. **2.** originating from within the organism, as a toxin or vaccine.

autogenous graft [Gk, *autos*, self, *genein*, to produce, *graphion*, stylus], a skin graft transplanted from one site to another in the same individual.

autogenous vaccine [Gk, *autos*, self, *genein*, to produce; L, *vacca*, cow], a vaccine prepared from cultures of an infectious agent taken from the patient to be treated.

autogeny. See **autogenesis.**

autograft /ô'təgraft'/ [Gk, *autos* + *graphion*, stylus], surgical transplantation of any tissue from one part of the body to another location in the same individual. Autografts are used in several kinds of plastic surgery, most commonly to replace skin lost in severe burns. Compare **allograft, isograft, xenograft.** See also **graft.**

Autograft *(Black and Hawks, 2005)*

autographism. See **dermatographia.**

autohemagglutination. See **autoagglutination.**

autohemolysis /-hēmol'isis/ [Gk, *autos*, self, *haima*, blood, *lysein*, to loosen], the destruction of erythrocytes by hemolytic agents found in an individual's own blood.

autohexaploid, autohexaploidic. See **autopolyploid.**

autohypnosis [Gk, *autos*, *hypnos*, sleep], the self-induction of hypnosis by an individual who concentrates on one subject to attain an altered state of consciousness. It may also occur in a person who has become habituated to the process by undergoing hypnosis a number of times.

autoimmune /-imyoon'/ [Gk, *autos* + L, *immunus*, exempt], pertaining to an immune response to one's own tissues. See also **autoimmune disease.**

autoimmune disease, one of a large group of diseases characterized by altered function of the immune system of the body, resulting in the production of antibodies against the body's own cells. Antigens normally present on the body's cells stimulate the development of autoantibodies, which, unable to distinguish those antigens from external antigens, act against the body's cells to cause localized and systemic reactions. These reactions can affect almost any cell or tissue and cause a variety of diseases, including systemic lupus erythematosus (SLE) and autoimmune thyroiditis. Some au-

toimmune disorders, such as Hashimoto's disease, are tissue specific, whereas others, such as SLE, affect multiple organs and systems.

■ OBSERVATIONS: The manifestations and clinical characteristics depend on the specific disease and on the organ or organ systems affected. See specific diseases.

■ INTERVENTIONS: Therapy includes corticosteroid, antiinflammatory, and immunosuppressive drugs. Symptoms are treated specifically.

■ NURSING CONSIDERATIONS: Many autoimmune diseases are characterized by periods of crisis interrupted by periods of remission. During a crisis, the patient may be hospitalized and require extensive nursing care, with relief from pain, applications of heat or cold, range of motion exercises, or assistance in movement and ambulation. It is important also to teach the patient and the family the side effects of the drugs being prescribed and how the drugs are to be taken. See also **autoantibody, autoantigen.**

autoimmune hypothesis, a concept that defects occur in the body's immune system as one ages. As a result of the defects, a person's antibody-producing cells can no longer distinguish between "self" and "nonself" tissues. The body's own cells are then misidentified as foreign and are attacked by antibodies.

autoimmune polyglandular syndromes. See **polyglandular autoimmune syndromes.**

autoimmune response. See **indirect anaphylaxis.**

autoimmunity /-imyoo'nitē/, an abnormal condition in which the body reacts against constituents of its own tissues. Autoimmunity may result in hypersensitivity and autoimmune disease. Also called **acute immune disease.** See also **antibody-specific model, autoantibody, autoantigen, autoimmune disease.**

autoimmunization /-im'yənizā'shən/, the process whereby a person's immune system develops antibodies against one or more of the person's own tissues. See also **autoantibody, autoantigen, autoimmune disease.**

autoinfection, an infection by disease organisms already present in the body but developing in a different body part.

autoinfusion /-infyoo'zhən/, a technique for forcing blood from the extremities to the body core by applying bandages. It may be used to control bleeding and, in surgery, to create a relatively bloodless surgical field.

autoinoculation /-inok'yəlā'shən/ [Gk, *autos* + L, *inoculare*, to graft], the inoculation of a microorganism obtained by contact with a lesion on one's own body, producing a secondary infection.

autointoxication /-intok'sikā'shən/ [Gk, *autos* + L, *in;* Gk, *toxikon*, poison], a condition of poisoning by substances generated by one's own body, as by toxins resulting from a metabolic disorder.

autokeratoplasty /-ker'ətōplas'tē/, the surgical transfer of corneal tissue from one eye of a patient to repair the cornea of the other.

autokinesia /-kinē'zhə/, voluntary movement.

autolesion /-lē'zhən/, a self-inflicted injury.

Autolet /ô'tōlet/, trademark for a small, sharp instrument, as a lancet, that is used to obtain a capillary blood specimen.

autologous /ôtol'əgəs/ [Gk, *autos* + *logos*, ratio], pertaining to a tissue or structure occurring naturally and derived from the same individual such as blood donated by a patient before surgery to be returned to the patient during or after surgery.

autologous graft [Gk, *autos*, *logos*, *graphion*, stylus], the transfer of tissue from one site to another on the same body.

autologous stem cell transplantation (ASCT), a treatment for advanced or refractory solid tumors, such as neuroblastomas, lymphomas, and Ewing's sarcoma. Stem cells from the bone marrow or blood are withdrawn before high-dose irradiation or chemotherapy that destroys many of the remaining cells; afterwards the removed cells are reinfused to form a new population of blood cells.

autologous transfusion, a procedure in which blood is removed from a donor and stored for a variable period before it is returned to the donor's circulation.

autologous transplantation, autotransplantation.

autolysis /ôtol′isis/, the spontaneous destruction of tissues by intracellular enzymes. It generally occurs in the body after death.

automated external defibrillator (AED), a portable apparatus used to restart a heart that has stopped. It is programmed to analyze cardiac rhythms automatically and indicate to a health professional when to deliver a defibrillating shock after the health professional has determined that no one is in contact with the patient.

automated reagin test (ART), a modification of the rapid plasma reagin (RPR) test for use with automated analyzers. It is used in clinical chemistry.

automatic behavior. See **automatism.**

automatic bladder. See **spastic bladder.**

automatic external defibrillator (AED), a portable defibrillator designed to be automated such that it can be used by persons without substantial medical training who are responding to a cardiac emergency.

automatic implanted cardioverter defibrillator (AICD), a surgically implanted device that automatically detects and corrects potentially fatal arrhythmias.

automatic infiltration detector /ô′təmat′ik/ [Gk, *automatismos,* self-action], a temperature-sensitive device that activates an alarm and automatically stops an IV infusion when the IV fluid passes into tissue. The device detects any cooling of the skin at the IV site, a common sign of infiltration. The detector is usually secured to the skin with tape and attaches by a small cable to the fluid-monitoring circuit of an IV pump.

automaticity /ô′tōmətis′itē/, a property of specialized excitable tissue that allows self-activation through spontaneous development of an action potential, as in the pacemaker cells of the heart.

automatic mallet condenser. See **mechanical condenser.**

automatic speech, speech composed of or containing words or phrases spoken without much conscious thought, often consisting of expletives, profanities, and greetings.

automation /ô′təmā′shən/, use of a machine designed to follow a predetermined sequence of individual operations repeatedly and automatically.

automatism /ôtom′ətiz′əm/ [Gk, *automatismos,* self-action], **1.** (in physiology) involuntary function of an organ system independent of apparent external stimuli, such as the beating of the heart, or dependent on external stimuli but not consciously controlled, such as the dilation of the pupil of the eye. **2.** (in philosophy) the theory that the body acts as a machine and that the mind, whose processes depend solely on brain activity, is a noncontrolling adjunct of the body. **3.** (in psychology) mechanical, repetitive, and undirected behavior that is not consciously controlled, as seen in psychomotor epilepsy, hysterical states, and such acts as sleepwalking. Kinds of automatism include **ambulatory automatism, command automatism,** and **immediate post-traumatic automatism.** Also called **automatic behavior.**

automnesia /ô′tōmnē′zhə/, the recollection of a previous experience.

autonomic /ô′tənom′ik/ [Gk, *autos* + *nomos,* law], **1.** hav-

ing the ability to function independently without outside influence. **2.** pertaining to the autonomic nervous system.

autonomic bronchodilators, a category of drugs with actions that dilate bronchiolar smooth muscle tissue by acting on the autonomic nervous system. Examples include adrenergic drugs, such as epinephrine, and anticholinergic products, such as atropine sulfate.

autonomic drug, any of a large group of drugs that mimic or modify the function of the autonomic nervous system.

autonomic dysreflexia, a syndome affecting persons with a spinal cord lesion above the midthoracic level (quadriplegics and some paraplegics) that is characterized by hypertension, bradycardia, severe headaches, pallor below and flushing above the cord lesions, and convulsions. It is the result of impaired function of the autonomic nervous system caused by simultaneous sympathetic and parasympathetic activity, such as may occur with bowel or bladder distension pain or a pressure ulcer. A cerebrovascular accident and death may occur during an attack. See also **autonomic hyperreflexia.**

autonomic epilepsy. See **vasomotor epilepsy.**

autonomic ganglion [Gk, *autos,* self, *nomos,* law, *ganglion,* knot], a physical grouping of autonomic neuron cell bodies. It can be near the target organ, as in the parasympathetic division, or more distant, as in the sympathetic division. See also **sympathetic ganglion.**

autonomic hyperreflexia, a neurologic disorder characterized by a discharge of sympathetic nervous system impulses as a result of stimulation of the bladder, large intestine, or other visceral organs. It occurs in persons with certain spinal cord injuries. Symptoms may include bradycardia, profuse sweating, headache, and severe hypertension.

autonomic imbalance [Gk, *autos,* self, *nomos,* law; L, *in,* not, *bilanx,* having two scales], a disruption of a segment of the autonomic nervous system, as in autonomic ataxia.

autonomic nerve [Gk, *autos,* self, *nomos,* law, *neuron,* nerve], a nerve of the autonomic nervous system, which includes both the sympathetic and parasympathetic nervous systems. It possesses the ability to function independently and spontaneously as needed to maintain optimal status of body activities.

autonomic nervous system, the part of the nervous system that regulates involuntary body functions, including the activity of the cardiac muscle, smooth muscles, and glands. It has two divisions: The **sympathetic nervous system** accelerates heart rate, constricts blood vessels, and raises blood pressure; the **parasympathetic nervous system** slows heart rate, increases intestinal peristalsis and gland activity, and relaxes sphincters.

autonomic reflex, any of a large number of normal reflexes governing and regulating the functions of the viscera. Autonomic reflexes control such activities of the body as blood pressure, heart rate, peristalsis, sweating, and urination.

autonomous /ôton′əməs/ [Gk, *autos,* self, *nomos,* law], being functionally independent.

autonomous bladder. See **flaccid bladder.**

autonomy /ôton′əmē/ [Gk, *autos* + *nomos,* law], the quality of having the ability or tendency to function independently. **—autonomous,** *adj.*

autonomy drive, a behavioral trait characterized by the attempt of an individual to master the environment and to impose his or her purposes on it.

auto-PEEP /aw′to-pēp′/, intrinsic positive end-expiratory pressure.

autopentaploid, autopentaploidic. See **autopolyploid.**

autophagia /-fā′jə/, **1.** a mental disorder characterized by the biting or eating of one's own flesh, as may occur in Lesch-Nyan syndrome. **2.** the automatic consumption of one's own tissues by fasting or dieting. **3.** the metabolic action of catabolism.

autoplastic maneuver /-plas'tik/, (in psychology) a process that is part of adaptation, involving an adjustment within the self. Compare **alloplastic maneuver.**

autoplasty /ô'təplas'tē/ [Gk, *autos* + *plassein*, to mold], a plastic surgery procedure in which autografts, or parts of the patient's own tissues, are used to replace or repair body areas damaged by disease or injury.

autoploid /ô'təploid/, having homologous chromosome sets, or two or more copies of a single haploid set.

autopodium /-pō'dē·əm/, the distal major subdivision of a hand or foot.

autopolymer resin. See **self-curing resin.**

autopolyploid /ô'tōpol'iploid/ [Gk, *autos* + *polyploos,* many times, *eidos* form], **1.** an individual, organism, strain, or cell that has more than two genetically identical or nearly identical sets of chromosomes that are derived from the same ancestral species. They result from the duplication of the haploid chromosome set and are referred to as autotriploid, autotetraploid, autopentaploid, autohexaploid, and so on, depending on the number of multiples of the haploid chromosomes they contain. Also called **autopolyploidic. 2.** pertaining to such an individual, organism, strain, or cell. Compare **allopolyploid.** See also **allodiploid.**

autopolyploidy /ô'tōpol'iploi'dē/, the state or condition of having more than two identical or nearly identical sets of chromosomes. Compare **allopolyploid.**

autopsy /ô'topsē/ [Gk, *autos* + *opsis,* view], a postmortem examination performed to confirm or determine the cause of death. Also called **necropsy** /nek'ropsē/, **thanatopsy** /than'ətop'sē/. —**autopsic, autopsical,** *adj.,* **autopsist,** *n.*

autopsy pathology, the study of disease by the examination of the body after death by a pathologist. The organs and tissues are first described by their appearance at the time of dissection, then by their appearance in the microscopic examination or laboratory analysis of small representative samples of tissue taken for their diagnostic value.

autoregulation [Gk, *autos,* self; L, *regula,* rule], an intrinsic capacity of organs to regulate their own blood flow or metabolic activity. The former process results from the contraction or relaxation of self-excitable smooth muscle, which causes the constriction or dilation vessels. It allows organs to maintain constant blood flow and meet their metabolic needs despite variations in systemic arterial pressure.

autosensitization /-sen'sətīzā'shən/ [Gk, *autos,* self; L, *sentire,* to feel], the sensitization of an individual by humoral antibodies or by a delayed cellular reaction to substances in his or her own body tissues.

autosepticemia /-sep'tisē'mē·ə/, a systemic infection in which pathogens are present in the circulating bloodstream, developing from an infection within the body.

autoserous treatment /ô'təsir'əs/ [Gk, *autos* + L, *serum,* whey], therapy of an infectious disease by inoculating the patient with the patient's own serum.

autosite /ô'təsīt/ [Gk, *autos* + *sitos,* food], the larger, more normally formed member of unequal or asymmetric conjoined twins on whom the other smaller fetus depends for various physiologic functions and for nutrition and growth. Compare **parasitic fetus. —autositic.** *adj.*

autosmia /ôtoz'mē·ə/ [Gk, *autos,* self, *osme,* smell], awareness of one's own body odor.

autosomal /ô'təsō'məl/ [Gk, *autos* + *soma,* body], **1.** pertaining to or characteristic of an autosome. **2.** pertaining to any condition transmitted by an autosome.

autosomal-dominant inheritance, a pattern of inheritance in which the transmission of a dominant allele on an autosome causes a trait to be expressed. Males and females are usually affected with equal frequency. If both parents are heterozygous *(Aa),* each of their children has a 50% chance of being heterozygous, a 25% chance of being homozygous for the dominant allele *(AA),* and a 25% chance of being homozygous for the recessive allele *(aa);* children with either of the first two genotypes will express the trait of the dominant allele. If one parent is homozygous for the dominant allele, all of the children will express the trait. Achondroplasia, osteogenesis imperfecta, polydactyly, Marfan's syndrome, and some neuromuscular disorders are transmitted through autosomal-dominant inheritance. Compare **autosomal-recessive inheritance.** See also **dominance.**

autosomal inheritance, a pattern of inheritance in which the transmission of traits depends on the presence or absence of certain alleles on the autosomes. The pattern may be dominant or recessive, and males and females are usually affected with equal frequency. The majority of hereditary disorders are the result of a defective gene on an autosome. Kinds of autosomal inheritance are **autosomal-dominant inheritance** and **autosomal-recessive inheritance.** See also **inheritance.**

autosomal-recessive inheritance, a pattern of inheritance resulting from the transmission of a recessive allele on an autosome. Males and females are usually affected with equal frequency. If both parents are heterozygous *(Aa),* each of their children has a 25% chance of expressing the trait of the recessive allele. If both parents are homozygous recessive *(aa),* all of the children will express the trait. If one parent is homozygous recessive and the other is homozygous dominant *(AA),* none of the children will express the trait, but all will be carriers *(Aa).* There may be no family history of the trait; it becomes manifest when two carriers have a child who is homozygous recessive. Cystic fibrosis, phenylketonuria, and galactosemia are examples of traits that result from autosomal-recessive inheritance. Compare **autosomal-dominant inheritance.** See also **recessive.**

autosomatognosis /-sō'mətognō'sis/, a phantom sensation that an amputated part of the body is still attached.

autosome /ô'təsōm/, any chromosome that is not a sex chromosome and that appears as a homologous pair in a somatic cell. Humans have 22 pairs of autosomes, which transmit all genetic traits and conditions other than those that are sex-linked. Also called **euchromosome** /yoo'krəsōm/. Compare **sex chromosome. —autosomal,** *adj.*

autosplenectomy /ô'tōsplinek'təmē/ [Gk, *autos* + *splen,* spleen, *ektomē,* excision], a progressive shrinking of the spleen that may occur in sickle cell anemia. The spleen is replaced by fibrous tissue and becomes nonfunctional.

autosuggestion [Gk, *autos* + L, *suggerere,* to suggest], an idea, thought, attitude, or belief suggested to oneself, often as a formula or incantation, as a means of controlling one's behavior. Compare **suggestion.**

autotetraploid, autotetraploidic. See **autopolyploid.**

autotopagnosia /ô'tōtop'əg·nō'zhə/ [Gk, *autos* + *topos,* place, *a* + *gnosis,* without knowledge], the inability to recognize or localize the various body parts because of organic brain damage. It is associated generally with lesions of the dominant hemisphere and may be an effect of some cases of cerebrovascular accident (CVA). It is also characterized by a loss of ability to distinguish left from right, manifested during a neurologic examination when the patient is unable to perform a task such as touching the right ear with the left thumb. Retraining involves touching various parts of the patient's body and asking the patient to identify the area touched and by having the patient assemble human figure puzzles. Also called **body-image agnosia, body-scheme disorder.** See also **agnosia, proprioception.**

autotoxemia /-tokse̅'me̅·ə/, a form of poisoning caused by substances generated within the body as a result of the pathologic alteration of the person's own tissues.

autotoxic, pertaining to autotoxins.

autotransfusion[1] /-transfyoo̅'zhən/, the collection, anticoagulation, filtration, and reinfusion of blood from an active bleeding site. It may be used in cases of major trauma or in major surgery when blood can be collected from a sterile site. Collection devices can be attached to drains following orthopedic or chest procedures.

autotransfusion[2], a nursing intervention from the Nursing Interventions Classification (NIC) defined as collecting and reinfusing blood that has been lost intraoperatively or postoperatively from clean wounds. See also **Nursing Interventions Classification.**

autotransplantation. See **autograft, autoplasty.**

autotriploid, autotriploidic. See **autopolyploid.**

autovaccination, a second vaccination in which a virus from the first vaccine sore is used.

autozygous /-zī'gəs/, pertaining to genes in a homozygote that are copies of the same ancestral gene as a result of a mating between related individuals.

autumn fever. See **leptospirosis.**

aux-. See **auxo-.**

auxanology /ôks'ənol'əje̅/ [Gk, *auxein,* to grow, *logos,* science], the scientific study of growth and development. **—auxanologic,** *adj.*

auxcardia [Gk, *auxein,* increase, *kardia,* heart], an enlarged heart.

auxesis, growth from increase in cell size without cell division. See also **hypertrophy.**

auxiliary /ôksil'yəre̅/ [L, *auxilium,* aid], an individual or group serving in assistive, supporting, or complementary tasks in a clinical setting.

auxiliary enzyme [L, *auxilium,* assist], an enzyme that links the enzyme being measured with an indicator enzyme. It is a component of the coupled assay system.

auxiliary storage, a storage device for adding to the main storage of the computer, using such media as floppy disks, hard disks, compact disks, zip (a brand name by Iomega zip™) disks, or tapes.

auxo-, aux-, prefix meaning 'growth, acceleration, or stimulation': *auxochrome, auxesis.*

auxotonic /ôk'so̅ton'ik/, pertaining to muscle contractions that increase in force as the muscle shortens.

auxotox [Gk, *auxein,* increase, *toxikon,* poison], a chemical with a particular atomic grouping that, if added to a relatively benign substance, increases the toxic characteristics of the mixture.

AV, abbreviation for **arteriovenous, atrioventricular.**

available arch length /əva̅'ləbəl/ [ME, *availen,* to be of use], the length or space in a dental arch that is available for all the natural teeth of an individual. See also **arch length, arch length deficiency, arch width.**

avalvular /āvalv'yələr/ [Gk, *a,* without; L, *valva,* valve], pertaining to an absence of one or more valves.

Avandia, trademark for an oral antidiabetic (rosiglitazone).

avantin. See **isopropyl alcohol.**

avascular /āvas'kyələr/ [Gk, *a,* without; L, *vasculum,* vessel], **1.** pertaining to a tissue area that is not receiving a sufficient supply of blood. The reduced supply may be the result of blockage by a blood clot or of the deliberate stoppage of flow during surgery or during control of a hemorrhage. **2.** pertaining to a kind of tissue that does not have blood vessels.

avascular graft [Gk, *a,* without; L, *vasculum,* vessel; Gk, *graphion,* stylus], a tissue graft in which there is no infiltration of blood vessels.

avascularization [Gk, *a,* without; L, *vasculum,* vessel], a diversion of blood flow away from tissues.

avascular necrosis. See **coagulation necrosis.**

AVB, abbreviation for **atrioventricular block.**

average, (in mathematics) a value established by dividing the sum of a series by the number of its units.

aversion therapy /əvur'zhən/ [L, *aversus,* a turning away], a form of behavior therapy in which punishment or unpleasant or painful stimuli, such as electric shock or drugs that induce nausea, are used to suppress undesirable behavior. The procedure is used in treating such conditions as drug abuse, alcoholism, gambling, overeating, smoking, and various sexual deviations. Also called **aversive conditioning.** See also **behavior therapy.**

aversive stimulus /əvur'siv/, an undesirable stimulus, such as electric shock, that causes psychic or physical pain. See also **aversion therapy.**

avian flu. See **avian influenza.**

avian influenza, a highly contagious viral disease of birds caused by an influenza A virus; it occurs in both mild and severe forms. It may be transmitted to humans through contact with bird droppings or surfaces contaminated by them or through intermediate hosts such as pigs. Person-to-person transmission appears to be rare. Symptoms of avian influenza in humans range from typical influenza-like symptoms to eye infections, pneumonia, acute respiratory distress, and other severe and life-threatening complications. The only means of control when avian influenza has been observed in a flock of domestic fowl is destruction of infected birds and disinfection of the farm. Also called **bird flu** or **avian flu.**

avian tuberculosis /ā'vē·ən/, a strain of tuberculosis in birds, caused by *Mycobacterium avium.* The organism is also pathogenic in humans and is especially problematic in the immunocompromised, such as those with human immunodeficiency virus infection.

aviation medicine /āv'ē·ā'shən/, a branch of medicine that is concerned with the health effects of travel by aircraft, including such aspects as jetlag, restricted body movement for long periods, and reaction to violent aircraft movement in turbulent weather. Also called **aerospace medicine.** See also **aviation physiology.**

aviation physiology, a branch of physiology that is concerned with the effects on humans and animals exposed for long periods to pressurized cabins, radiation hazards at high altitudes, weightlessness, disturbances of biologic rhythms, acceleration, and mental functions under stressful flying conditions.

avidin, a glycoprotein in raw egg white that interacts with biotin to make it unavailable to the body. Cooking destroys avidin.

avidity /avid'ite̅/ [L, *avidus,* eager], an inexact measure of the binding strength of antibodies to multiple antigenic determinants on natural antigens.

A-V interval [L, *intervallum,* space between ramparts], the time between an atrial polarization and the next ventricular polarization. In His bundle electrograms (HBEs), the A-V interval is the time between the A wave and the V deflection. The A wave is the first deflection on the HBE and represents low right atrial activation. The V deflection is the last deflection on the HBE and represents ventricular activation; it is concurrent with the QRS complex on a surface electrocardiogram.

avirulent /āvir'yələnt/ [Gk, *a,* not; L, *virus,* poison], not virulent; not pathogenic.

avitaminosis /āvī'təminō'sis/ [Gk, *a,* not; L, *vita,* life, amine, *osis,* condition], a condition resulting from a deficiency of or lack of absorption or use of one or more dietary vitamins. Also called **hypovitaminosis.** Compare **hypervitaminosis.** See also specific vitamins.

AV nicking, a vascular abnormality in the retina of the eye, visible on ophthalmologic examination, in which a vein is compressed by an arteriovenous crossing. The vein appears "nicked" as a result of constriction or spasm. It is a sign of hypertension, arteriosclerosis, or other vascular conditions.

AV nicking *(Lemmi and Lemmi, 2000)*

avobenzone /av'o-ben'zōn/, a sunscreen that absorbs light in the UVA range.

Avogadro's constant, Avogadro's number.

Avogadro's law /av'ōgad'rōz/, [Amedeo Avogadro, Italian physicist, 1776–1856], a law in physics stating that equal volumes of all gases at a given temperature and pressure contain the identical number of particles.

Avogadro's number [Amedeo Avogadro], the number of atoms in exactly 12 g of the isotope of carbon ^{12}C, or 6.02 × 10^{23}. One mole of any monoatomic element contains this number of atoms and one mole of any polyatomic element or molecule contains this number of molecules.

avoidance [ME, *avoiden,* to empty], (in psychiatry) a conscious or unconscious defense mechanism, physical or psychologic, by which an individual tries to avoid or escape from unpleasant stimuli, conflicts, or feelings, such as anxiety, fear, pain, or danger.

avoidance-avoidance conflict, a conflict resulting from the confrontation of two or more alternative goals or desires that are equally aversive and undesirable. Also called **double-avoidance conflict.** See also **conflict.**

avoidance conditioning, the establishment of certain patterns of behavior to avoid unpleasant or painful stimuli.

avoidant personality, a personality disorder characterized by hypersensitivity to rejection and a reluctance to start a relationship because of a fear of not being accepted uncritically. The person has a strong desire for affection and acceptance and may be distressed by an inability to relate comfortably with others.

avoirdupois weight /av'ərdəpoiz'/, [OF, *avoir de pois,* to have weight], the English system of weights in which there are 7000 grains, 256 drams, or 16 ounces to 1 pound. One ounce in this system equals 28.35 g, and 1 pound equals 453.59 g. Compare **apothecaries' weight.** See also **metric system.**

Avonex, trademark for an antiviral and immune system regulator (interferon beta-1a) useful for treating multiple sclerosis.

avulse. See **avulsion.**

avulsed tooth /əvulst/ [L, *avulsio,* a pulling away], a tooth that has been forcibly displaced from its normal position. In some cases, if attended to early, it can be surgically reimplanted. Also spelled **evulsed tooth.** See also **avulsion.**

Avulsed teeth *(Zitelli and Davis, 1997)*

avulsion /əvul'shən/ [L, *avulsio,* a pulling away], the separation, by tearing, of any part of the body from the whole. —**avulse,** *v.*

avulsion fracture, a fracture caused by the tearing away of a fragment of bone where a strong ligamentous or tendinous attachment forcibly pulls the fragment away from osseous tissue.

awake anesthesia [ME, *awakenen*], an anesthetic procedure in which analgesia and anesthesia are accomplished without loss of consciousness. Dental procedures, surgery on a limb or an extremity, scopic examinations, and certain kinds of head surgery are performed using awake anesthesia. With the patient awake or sedated, muscle relaxation is not required. Various combinations of sedatives, tranquilizers, and low concentrations of anesthetic gas may be used. Also called **conscious sedation,** monitored anesthesia care.

AWHONN, abbreviation for **Association of Women's Health, Obstetric, and Neonatal Nurses.**

AWOL /ā'wôl/, abbreviation for **absent without leave.**

axenic culture, a pure culture of microorganisms, i.e., one free from contaminating microorganisms or, in the case of parasites, without the presence of the host.

axetil, contraction for *l-acetoxyethyl.*

axi-, axio-, axo-, prefix meaning 'axis': *axial, axolysis.*

axial (A) /ak'sē-əl/ [Gk, *axon,* axle], **1.** pertaining to or situated on the axis of a body structure or part. **2.** (in dentistry) relating to the long axis of a tooth.

axial current, the central part of the blood current.

axial gradient, **1.** the variation in metabolic rate in different parts of the body. **2.** the development toward the body axis or its parts in relation to the metabolic rate in the various parts.

axial illumination, light transmitted along the axis of a microscope. See also **illumination.**

axial neuritis. See **parenchymatous neuritis.**

axial resolution, the ability of an ultrasound system to separate two objects lying along the axis of an ultrasound beam.

axial skeleton [L, *axis,* axle; Gk, *skeletos,* dried up], the bones forming the axis of the skeleton, including the skull, vertebrae, ribs, and sternum. See also **appendicular skeleton.**

axial spillway, a groove that crosses a cusp ridge or a marginal ridge and extends onto an axial surface of a tooth. Compare **interdental spillway, occlusal spillway.**

Axid, trademark for an antiulcerative H_2-receptor agent (nizatidine).

axifugal /aksif′yəgəl/ [L, *axis,* axle, *fugere,* to flee], extending away from an axis or axion. Also called **axofugal.** See also **centrifugal.**

axilla *pl.* **axillae** /aksil′ə/ [L, wing], a pyramid-shaped space forming the underside of the shoulder between the upper arm and the side of the chest. Also called **armpit.** —**axillary,** *adj.*

axillary /ak′siler′ē/ [L, *axilla,* wing], pertaining to the armpit.

axillary abscess [L, *axilla,* wing, *abscedere,* to go away], an abscess in the armpit.

axillary artery [L, *axilla,* wing], one of a pair of continuations of the subclavian arteries that starts at the outer border of the first rib and ends at the distal border of the teres major, where it becomes the brachial artery. It has three parts and six branches, supplying various chest and arm muscles.

axillary block anesthesia. See **brachial plexus block.**

axillary dissection. See **axillary node dissection.**

axillary line, an imaginary vertical line on the body wall, passing through a point midway between the anterior and posterior folds of the axilla.

axillary nerve, one of the last two branches of the posterior cord of the brachial plexus before the posterior cord becomes the radial nerve. It divides into a posterior branch and an anterior branch. The posterior branch innervates the teres minor, part of the deltoideus, and part of the skin overlying the deltoideus; the anterior branch innervates the deltoideus. Some fibers of the nerve also supply the capsule of the shoulder joint.

axillary node, one of the lymph glands of the axilla that help fight infections in the chest, armpit, neck, and arm and drain lymph from those areas. The 20 to 30 axillary nodes are divided into the lateral group, the anterior group, the posterior group, the central group, and the medial group. See also **lymphatic system, lymph node.**

axillary node dissection, surgical removal of axillary nodes, through an incision in the axilla, or may be done as part of modified radical mastectomy. Also called **axillary dissection.**

axillary region, the area of the upper chest surrounding the axilla, lateral to the pectoral region.

axillary temperature [L, *axilla,* wing, *temperatura*], the body temperature as recorded by a thermometer placed in the armpit. The reading is generally 0.5° to 1° F less than the oral temperature.

axillary vein, one of a pair of veins of the upper limb that becomes the subclavian vein at the outer border of the first rib. It receives deoxygenated blood from the venous tributaries. Compare **subclavian vein.**

axillofemoral bypass graft /ak′silōfem′ərəl/, a synthetic artery that is surgically anastomosed to the axillary and common femoral arteries in cases of peripheral arterial insufficiency. The graft shunts blood between those arteries, increasing blood flow to the lower extremities.

axio-. See **axi-.**

Axillary temperature measurement
(Elkin, Perry, and Potter, 2004)

axion /ak′sē·on/, **1.** the brain and spinal cord. **2.** the cerebrospinal axis.

axioplasm. See **axoplasm.**

axis *pl.* **axes** /ak′sēz/ [Gk, *axon,* axle], **1.** (in anatomy) a line that passes through the center of the body, or a part of the body, such as the frontal axis, binauricular axis, and basifacial axis. **2.** the second cervical vertebra, about which the atlas rotates, allowing the head to be turned, extended, and flexed. Also called **epistropheus odontoid vertebra.**

axis artery, one of a pair of extensions of the subclavian arteries, running into and supplying the upper limb, continuing into the forearm as the palmar interosseous artery.

axis cylinder. See **axon.**

axis deviation, an electrocardiogram trace in which the QRS axis of the heart in the frontal plane lies outside the

Axis *(Applegate, 2000)*

usual range of -30 to 110 degrees. It represents an abnormal direction of ventricular depolarization.

axis traction, **1.** the process of pulling a baby's head with obstetric forceps in a direction in line with the path of least resistance, following the curve of Carus through the mother's birth canal. **2.** *informal.* any mechanical device attached to obstetric forceps to facilitate pulling in the proper direction.

axo-. See **axi-.**

axoaxonic synapse /ak′sō-akson′ik/ [Gk, *axon*, axle (to) *axon*, axle], a synapse in which the axon of one neuron comes in contact with the axon of another neuron.

axodendritic synapse /-dendrit′ik/ [Gk, *axon* + *dendron*, tree], a synapse in which the axon of one neuron comes in contact with the dendrites of another neuron.

axodendrosomatic synapse /-den′drōsōmat′ik/, a synapse in which the axon of one neuron comes in contact with both the dendrites and the cell body of another neuron.

axofugal. See **axifugal.**

axolysis /aksol′isis/, the degeneration of the axon of a nerve cell.

axon /ak′son/ [Gk, axle], an extension, usually long and slender, of a neuron capable of conducting action potentials or self-propagating nervous impulses. Axons can conduct impulses over great distances away from the cell body. Only ends of axons (terminals) can release neurotransmitters and stimulate other neurons/effectors. Also called **axone.** /ak′sōn/, **axis cylinder.** Compare **dendrite.** See also **action potential, neurotransmitter.**

axon flare, vasodilation, reddening, and increased sensitivity of the skin surrounding an injured area, caused by an axon reflex. It is considered part of a triple response in which injury or stroking of the skin results in local reddening, the release of histamine or a histamine-like substance, a surrounding flare, and wheal formation. A pinprick in the involved area causes more intense pain than a similar stimulus before injury.

axonography /ak′sənog′rəfē/, the recording of electrical activity in the axon of a nerve cell. Also called **electroaxonography.**

axonotmesis /ak′sənotmē′sis/ [Gk, *axon* + *temnein*, to cut], an interruption of the axon from nerve injury, with subsequent wallerian degeneration of the distal nerve segment. Connective tissue of the nerve, including the Schwann cell basement membranes, may remain intact.

axon reflex [Gk, *axon*, axle], a neuron reflex in which an afferent impulse travels along a nerve fiber away from the cell body until it reaches a branching, where it is diverted to an end organ without entering the cell body. It does not involve a complete reflex arc, and therefore it is not a true reflex.

axon sheath [Gk, *axon* + AS, *scaeth*], a laminated myelin sheath that is interrupted at intervals by nodes of Ranvier.

axoplasm /ak′sōplaz′əm/, cytoplasm of an axon which encloses the neurofibrils.

axoplasmic flow /ak′sōplaz′mik/ [Gk, *axon* + *plassein*, to shape], the continuous pulsing, undulating movement of the cytoplasm between the cell body of a neuron, where protein synthesis occurs, and the axon fiber to supply it with the substances vital for the maintenance of activity and for repair. The nerve fiber depends totally on the cell body for metabolites, and any interruption in the axoplasmic flow caused by disease or trauma results in the degeneration of the unsupplied areas of the axon.

axosomatic synapse /ak′sōsōmat′ik/ [Gk, *axon* + *soma*, body], a synapse in which the axon of one neuron comes in contact with the cell body of another neuron.

axotomy /ak′sōplaz′əm/, surgical transection of an axon.

Aygestin, trademark for an oral progestin (norethindrone acetate).

ayurveda, a major health care system that emphasizes a preventive approach to health, focusing on an inner state of harmony and spiritual realization for self-healing. It includes special types of diets, herbs, minerals, and changes based on a system of constitutional categories in lifestyle. Enemas and purgation are used to cleanse the body of excess toxins. Ayurveda emphasizes lifestyle analysis and change as the most significant aspects of the healing process.

azatadine maleate /azat′ədēn/, an antihistamine with antiserotonin, anticholinergic, and sedative effects. It is used for treating allergic rhinitis and chronic urticaria.

azathioprine /az′əthī′ōprēn/, an immunosuppressive.

■ INDICATIONS: It is prescribed to prevent organ rejection after transplantation and to treat lupus erythematosus and other systemic inflammatory diseases, such as rheumatoid arthritis unresponsive to other agents.

■ CONTRAINDICATION: Known hypersensitivity to this drug prohibits its use. It is contraindicated in rheumatoid arthritis and in pregnant women.

■ ADVERSE EFFECTS: Among the most serious adverse reactions are bone marrow depression and hepatotoxicity. Nausea and fever are common.

azelaic acid /az′ĕ-la′ik/, a dicarboxylic acid occurring in whole grains and animal products. It has antibacterial effects on both aerobic and anaerobic organisms, particularly *Propionibacterium acnes* and *Staphylococcus epidermidis;* normalizes keratinization, and has a cytotoxic effect on malignant or hyperactive melanocytes. It is applied topically in the treatment of acne vulgaris.

azelastine, an H1-selective antihistamine that also inhibits leukotriene and platelet activating factor (PAF) synthesis and release.

■ INDICATIONS: This drug is used to treat seasonal allergic rhinitis and seasonal allergic conjuctivitis.

■ CONTRAINDICATIONS: Known hypersensitivity, acute asthma attacks, and lower respiratory tract disease prohibit this drug's use.

■ ADVERSE EFFECTS: Side effects include sedation (more common with increased doses), increased drowsiness, weight increase, and myalgia.

Azelex /az-ĕ-leks/, trademark for a preparation of azelaic acid used for treating acne.

-azepam, combining form designating a diazepam-type antianxiety agent.

azidothymidine. See **zidovudine.**

azithromycin, a macrolide antibiotic that suppresses the formation of protein by bacteria, retards bacterial growth, or causes death of the microorganisms. It does not suppress hepatic metabolism of other drugs like the macrolides prototype erythromycin and has a very long half-life, which makes it an appealing therapy against susceptible microorganisms.

■ INDICATIONS: It is prescribed in the treatment of mild to moderate infections by certain bacteria in adults, including respiratory tract infections, skin disorders, and sexually transmitted diseases.

■ CONTRAINDICATIONS: The drug should not be given to patients with allergies to erythromycin or any macrolide antibiotics or with kidney or liver diseases. Its safety has not been established for women who are pregnant or breast-feeding.

■ ADVERSE EFFECTS: The side effects most often reported include diarrhea, loose stools, nausea, stomach pains, or vomiting.

azlocillin sodium /az′lōsil′in/, a semisynthetic penicillin antibiotic.

■ INDICATIONS: It is prescribed for lower respiratory tract, urinary tract, skin, bone, and joint infections, and bacterial septicemia caused by susceptible strains of microorganisms, mainly *Pseudomonas aeruginosa.*

■ CONTRAINDICATION: Hypersensitivity to any of the penicillins prohibits its use.

■ ADVERSE EFFECTS: The most serious adverse reactions are anaphylactic reactions, convulsive seizures, epigastric pain, reduction in blood elements, and elevation in hepatic and renal parameters.

azo-, az-, prefix meaning 'containing nitrogen': *azotemia, azine.*

-azocine, combining form designating a narcotic agonist or antagonist.

azo compounds /ā′zō/ [Fr, *azote,* nitrogen], one of many organic aromatic compounds containing the divalent chromophore, —N═N—. They are produced by the alkaline reduction of nitro compounds among other methods.

azo dye, a type of nitrogen-containing compound used in commercial coloring materials. Some forms of the chemical are potential carcinogens.

azoic /āzō′ik/ [Gk, *a,* not, *zoe,* life], devoid of life.

azole antifungal, any of a group of antifungals characterized by the presence of an azole ring structure, which includes the triazoles and the imidazoles (qq.v.). They are usually fungistatic but can be fungicidal at higher concentrations and act by interfering with the enzyme activity of cytochrome P-450, decreasing the production of ergosterol and so damaging the cell membrane by altering its permeability and functions.

-azoline, combining form designating an antihistaminic or local vasoconstrictor.

azoospermia /āzō′əspur′mē·ə/ [Gk, *a, zoon,* not animal, *sperma* seed], lack of spermatozoa in the semen. It may be caused by testicular dysfunction, cancer chemotherapy, or blockage of the tubules of the epididymis, or it may be induced by vasectomy. Infertility, but not impotence, is associated with azoospermia. Compare **oligospermia.**

azoprotein /ā′zōpro′tēn/, a protein coupled to another substance through a diazo (—N═N—) linkage. Azoproteins are often used in immunochemical procedures.

Azorean disease. See **Machado-Joseph disease.**

-azosin, combining form designating a prazosin-type antihypertensive agent.

azotemia /az′ōtē′mē·ə/ [Fr, *azote,* nitrogen; Gk, *haima,* blood], retention of excessive amounts of nitrogenous compounds in the blood. This toxic condition is caused by failure of the kidneys to remove urea from the blood and is characteristic of uremia. Also spelled **azotaemia.** See also **uremia. —azotemic,** *adj.*

azoturia /az′ōtŏŏr′ē·ə/ [Fr, *azote,* nitrogen; Gk, *ouron,* urine], an excess of nitrogenous compounds including urea in the urine.

AZT, trademark for a human immunodeficiency virus inhibitor (Zidovudine). Also called **Retrovir.**

azul, azula. See **pinta.**

Azulfidine, trademark for a sulfonamide antibacterial (sulfasalazine) used to treat ulcerative colitis and rheumatoid arthritis.

azure /āz′hər/, one of a group of basic blue methylthionine or phenothiazine dyes used in staining blood and cell nuclei.

azurophil, a substance that stains readily with an azure blue aniline dye.

azurophilia /āzh′ŏŏrəfil′yə/, a condition in which the blood contains some cells that have granules that stain readily with azure (blue) dye.

azygography /az′īgog′rəfē/, the radiographic imaging of the azygos venous system after injection of a radiopaque contrast medium.

azygos. See **azygous.**

azygospore /az′igəspôr/ [Gk, *a + zygon,* not yoke, *sporos,* seed], a spore that is produced directly from a gamete that has not undergone conjugation, as in certain algae and fungi.

azygous /az′əgəs/ [Gk, *a + zygon,* not yoke], occurring as a single entity or part, such as any unpaired anatomic structure; not part of a pair. Also **azygos. —azygos** /az′əgos′/, *n.*

azygous lobe, a congenital anomaly of the lung caused by a fold of pleural tissue carried by the azygous vein during descent into the thorax during embryonic development. It produces an extra lobe in the right upper lung and may appear on x-ray film as a fissure in the shape of an upside-down comma.

azygous vein, one of the seven veins of the thorax. Beginning opposite the first or second lumbar vertebra, it rises through the aortic hiatus in the diaphragm and passes to the right of the vertebral column to the fourth thoracic vertebra, then arches ventrally over the root of the right lung, and ends in the superior vena cava. It receives numerous veins, such as the hemiazygous veins, several esophageal veins, and the right bronchial vein. In cases of obstruction to the inferior vena cava it is the principal vein that returns blood to the heart. Compare **internal thoracic vein, left brachiocephalic vein, right brachiocephalic vein.**

B, symbol for the element **boron**.

B. See **oxalic acid**.

B, β. See **beta**.

B6 bronchus sign, an artifact in a lung radiograph in which an air bronchogram appears in the lower lobe as a result of consolidation of atelectasis.

B19 virus, a strain of human parvovirus associated with a number of diseases, including hemolytic anemia, erythema infectiosum, fifth disease, and symptoms of arthritis and arthralgia.

Ba, symbol for the element **barium**.

BA, **1.** abbreviation for *Bachelor of Arts.* **2.** abbreviation for blood alcohol.

babbling, a stage in speech development characterized by the production of strings of speech sounds in vocal play, such as "ba-ba-ba."

Babcock's operation [William W. Babcock, American surgeon, 1872–1963], the removal of a varicosed saphenous vein by insertion of an acorn-tipped sound, tying the vein to the sound, and drawing it out. Also called **subcutaneous stripping**.

Babès-Ernst body, metachromatic granule.

babesiosis /bəbē′sē-ō′sis/ [Victor Babès, Romanian bacteriologist, 1854–1926], an infection caused by protozoa of the genus *Babesia*. The parasite is introduced into the host through the bite of ticks of the species *Ixodes dammini* and infects red blood cells. In the United States, incidence of the disease is highest in the Northeast and North Central regions. Symptoms include headache, fever, chills, vomiting, hepatosplenomegaly, hemolytic anemia, fatigue, myalgia, and hemolysis. Treatment is clindamycin or quinone. Also called **babesiasis** /bab′əsī′əsis/.

Babesiosis *(Carr and Rodak, 1999)*

Babinski's reflex /bəbin′skēz/ [Joseph F.F. Babinski, French neurologist, 1857–1932], dorsiflexion of the big toe with extension and fanning of the other toes elicited by firmly stroking the lateral aspect of the sole of the foot. The reflex is normal in newborns and abnormal in children and adults, in whom it may indicate a lesion in the pyramidal tract.

Babinski's sign [Joseph Babinski], a series of partial responses that are pathognomonic of different degrees of upper motor neuron disease, including (1) absence of an ankle

Babinski's reflex in an adult *(Seidel et al, 2003)*

jerk in sciatica; (2) an extensor plantar response, with an extension of the great toe and adduction of the other toes; (3) a more pronounced concentration of platysma on the unaffected side during blowing or whistling; (4) pronation that occurs when an arm affected by paralysis is placed in supination; and (5) when a patient in a supine position with arms crossed over the chest attempts to assume a sitting position, the thigh on the affected side is flexed, and the heel is raised, while the leg on the unaffected side remains flat.

baby [ME, *babe*], **1.** an infant or young child, especially one who is not yet able to walk or talk. **2.** to treat gently or with special care.

baby bottle caries, early childhood caries.

baby bottle tooth decay, a dental condition that occurs in children between 12 months and 3 years of age as a result of being given a bottle at bedtime, resulting in prolonged exposure of the teeth to milk or juice. Caries are formed because pools of milk or juice in the mouth break down to lactic acid and other decay-causing substances. Preventive measures include elimination of the bedtime feeding or substitution of water for milk or juice in the nighttime bottle. Formerly called **nursing bottle caries**.

Baby Jane Doe regulations, rules established in 1984 by the U.S. Health and Human Services Department requiring state governments to investigate complaints about parental decisions involving the treatment of handicapped infants. The rules also allowed the federal government to have access to children's medical records and required hospitals to post notices urging physicians and nurses to report any suspected cases of denial of proper medical care to infants. The controversial regulations have been found illegal by a federal court. The popular name for the federal rules was taken from the name "Jane Doe" given to an infant born in New

Baby bottle tooth decay
(Seidel et al, 2003/courtesy Drs. Abelson and Cameron)

infectious agent is associated with contact with young cats infected with fleas and is also the cause of cat-scratch fever. It is manifested in persons with cellular immunodeficiency such as human immunodeficiency virus (HIV)-infected patients as small hemangioma-like lesions of the skin but may also involve the lymph nodes and viscera. The skin lesions are often mistaken for Kaposi's sarcoma.

Bacillary angiomatosis *(Stone and Gorbach, 2000)*

York with an open spinal column and other defects who became the object of a campaign to force lifesaving surgery for the child over parental objections. Also called **Baby Doe rules.**

baby talk, **1.** the speech patterns and sounds of young children learning to talk, characterized by mispronunciation, imperfect syntax, repetition, and phonetic modifications, such as lisping or stuttering. See also **lallation. 2.** the intentionally oversimplified manner of speech, imitative of young children learning to talk, used by adults in addressing children or pets. **3.** the speech patterns characteristic of regressive stages of various mental disorders, especially schizophrenia.

BAC, abbreviation for **bronchoalveolar carcinoma.**

bacampicillin hydrochloride, a semisynthetic penicillin.
- INDICATIONS: It is prescribed in the treatment of respiratory tract, urinary tract, skin, and gonococcal infections.
- CONTRAINDICATIONS: Known sensitivity to this drug or other penicillins prohibits its use.
- ADVERSE EFFECTS: Among the most serious adverse reactions are hypersensitivity reactions, gastritis, enterocolitis, and transient blood disorders.

Bachelor of Science in Nursing (BSN) /bach′ələr/, an academic degree awarded on satisfactory completion of a 4-year course of study in a college or university. The recipient is eligible to take the national certifying examination to become a registered nurse. A BSN degree is a prerequisite to advancement in nursing education and in most systems and institutions that employ nurses. Compare **Associate Degree in Nursing, diploma program in nursing.**

Bach remedies, a set of 38 flower essences, developed as a milder alternative to homeopathic remedies, that produce mental or emotional but not physical symptoms upon proving; they are used to treat mental and emotional complaints and have no direct effect on physical symptoms.

bacill-, combining form meaning "rod-shaped bacterium": **bacillemia, bacillosis.**

Bacillaceae /bas′əlā′si·ē/ [L, *bacillum,* small rod], a family of Schizomycetes of the order Eubacteriales, consisting of gram-positive, rod-shaped cells that can produce cylindric, ellipsoid, or spheric endospores situated terminally, subterminally, or centrally. These cells are chemoheterotrophic and mostly saprophytic, commonly appearing in soil. Some are parasitic on insects and animals and are pathogenic. The family includes the genus *Bacillus,* which is aerobic, and the genus *Clostridium,* which is facultatively anaerobic.

bacillary angiomatosis /bas′əler′ē/, a condition of multiple angiomata caused by an infection of *Bartonella.* The

bacillary dysentery. See **shigellosis.**
bacillary white diarrhea, pullorum disease.
bacille /bah-sēl′/, bacillus.
bacille Calmette-Guérin (BCG) /kalmet′gāran′/ [Léon C.A. Calmette, French bacteriologist, 1863–1933; Camille Guérin, French bacteriologist, 1872–1961], The bacillus of Calmette and Guerin (BCG) is an attenuated strain of mycobacterium bovis that is given as a live bacterial vaccine to prevent the development of TB. An attenuated strain of tubercle bacilli, used in many countries as a vaccine against tuberculosis, most often administered intradermally, with a multiple-puncture disk. When administered to infants in high-prevalence areas, there is some evidence that it prevents the more serious forms of tuberculosis. It may have some efficacy against leprosy. BCG is also instilled into the bladder as a treatment for bladder cancer to stimulate the immune response in people who have certain kinds of malignancy. It induces a positive tuberculin reaction and may mask early, active infection by removing the diagnostic sign of conversion from the negative to the positive skin reaction. See also **tuberculin test, tuberculosis.**

bacille Calmette-Guérin vaccine, an active immunizing agent prepared from an attenuated bacille Calmette-Guérin strain of *Mycobacterium bovis.*
- INDICATION: It is prescribed most commonly for immunization against tuberculosis. It is instilled intravesically to treat carcinoma in situ of the urinary bladder in certain situations. It is seldom administered in the United States as an immunizing agent, but is often given in many countries to infants, caregivers, etc., who are at high risk for intimate and prolonged exposure to people with active tuberculosis.
- CONTRAINDICATIONS: Hypogammaglobulinemia, immunosuppression, or concomitant use of corticosteroids or isoniazid prohibits its use. It is not given after a vaccination for smallpox, nor is it given to patients with a positive tuberculin reaction or a burn.
- ADVERSE EFFECTS: Among the most serious adverse reactions are anaphylaxis and disseminated pulmonary tuberculosis. Pain, inflammation, and granuloma may develop at the site of injection.

bacillemia /bas′əlē′mē·ə/, a condition in which bacilli are circulating in the blood. See also **bacteremia, sepsis, septicemia.**

bacilli /bəsil´ī/, *sing.* **bacillum** [L, *bacillum,* small rod], any rod-shaped bacteria. See **bacillus.**

bacilliform /bəsil´ifôrm/, rod-shaped, like a bacillus.

bacillosis /bas´əlō´sis/, a condition in which bacilli have invaded tissues, inducing symptoms of an infection.

bacillum. See **bacilli.**

bacilluria /bas´əlŏŏr´ē·ə/ [L, *bacillum* + Gk, *ouron,* urine], the presence of bacilli in the urine.

Bacillus /bəsil´əs/, a genus of aerobic, gram-positive, or facultatively anaerobic, spore-bearing, rod-shaped microorganism of the family Bacillaceae, order Eubacteriales. The genus includes 33 species, 3 of which are pathogenic and the rest saprophytic soil forms. Some species are nonpathogenic, but others cause a wide variety of diseases, ranging from anthrax to tuberculosis. Many microorganisms formerly classified as *Bacillus* are now classified in other genera. See also **Bacillaceae, acid-fast bacillus.**

Bacillus anthracis, a species of gram-positive, facultative anaerobe that causes anthrax, a disease primarily of cattle and sheep. The spores of this organism, if inhaled, can cause a pulmonary form of anthrax; spores can live for many years in animal products, such as hides and wool, and in soil. See also **anthrax, woolsorter's disease.**

Bacillus cereus, a species of bacilli found in the soil. It causes food poisoning (an emetic type and a diarrheal type) by the formation of an enterotoxin in contaminated foods. It can also cause infections, such as ocular infections.

bacitracin /bas´itrā´sin/ [L, *bacillum* + *Tracy,* surname of patient in whom toxin-producing bacillus species was isolated], an antibacterial.

■ INDICATION: A common component of topical antibiotic ointments used for treating skin infections.

■ CONTRAINDICATION: Known hypersensitivity to this drug prohibits its use.

■ ADVERSE EFFECTS: Skin rash.

back [AS, *baec*], the posterior or dorsal portion of the trunk of the body between the neck and the pelvis. The back is divided by a middle furrow that lies over the tips of the spinous processes of the vertebrae. The skeletal portion of the back includes the thoracic and the lumbar vertebrae and both scapulae. The nerves that innervate the various muscles of the back arise from the segmental spinal nerves.

backache /bak´āk/ [AS, *baec* + ME, *aken*], a pain in the lumbar, lumbosacral, or cervical region of the back, varying in sharpness and intensity. Causes may include muscle strain or other muscular disorders or pressure on the root of a nerve, such as the sciatic nerve, caused in turn by a variety of factors, including a herniated vertebral disk. Treatment may include heat, ultrasound, and devices to provide support for the affected area while the individual is in bed or standing or sitting, bed rest, surgical intervention, and medications to relieve pain and relax spasm of the muscle of the affected area.

back-action condenser, an instrument for compacting dental amalgams that has a U-shaped shank, which develops the condensing force from a pulling motion rather than from the more common pushing motions.

backboard, a long, flat, rigid piece of wood or other material that is placed under an accident victim with possible spinal injury. It is used to transport the patient to a hospital or as a firm surface for CPR.

backbone, the vertebral column.

backcross [AS, *baec* + *cruc,* cross], **1.** a mating (cross) between a heterozygote and a homozygote. **2.** an organism or strain produced by such a cross. See also **testcross.**

Long backboard *(Chapleau, 2004)*

background level, the usual intensity of a chemical or other stimulus in the environment.

background radiation [AS, *baec* + OE, *grund,* ground], naturally occurring radiation emitted by soil, groundwater, building materials, radioactive substances in the body (especially potassium 40, and cosmic rays from outer space. Each year the average person is exposed to 44 millirad (mrad) of external terrestrial radiation, 18 mrad of naturally occurring internal radioaction, and 44 mrad of cosmic radiation. Background radiation levels may vary in different locales.

backing /bak´ing/ [AS, *baec*], in dentistry, the piece of metal that supports a porcelain or resin facing on a fixed or removable partial denture.

back knee. See **genu recurvatum.**

back pressure [AS, *baec* + L, *premere,* to press], pressure that builds in a vessel or a cavity as fluid accumulates. The pressure increases and extends backward if the normal mechanism for egress or passage of the fluid is not restored.

backscatter radiation. See **scattered radiation.**

backup, 1. a duplicate computer, data file, equipment, or procedure for use in the event of equipment failure. **2.** The act of creating another copy of a file, group of files, or an entire computer hard drive.

baclofen, an antispastic agent.

■ INDICATION: It is prescribed to reduce the spasticity associated with multiple sclerosis, cerebal palsy, and spinal cord injury; not effective against spasticity caused by stroke.

■ CONTRAINDICATION: Known hypersensitivity to this drug prohibits its use.

■ ADVERSE EFFECTS: Among the more serious adverse reactions are confusion, hypotension, dyspnea, impotence, nausea, and transient drowsiness.

-bactam, combining form designating a beta-lactamase inhibitor.

bacter-. See **bacterio-.**

bacteremia /bak´tirē´mē·ə/ [Gk, *bakterion,* small staff, *haima,* blood], the presence of bacteria in the blood. Undocumented bacteremias occur frequently and usually abate spontaneously. Bacteremia is demonstrated by blood culture. Antibiotic treatment, if given, is specific for the organism found and appropriate to the locus of infection. Also called **bacteriemia.** Also spelled **bacteraemia.** Compare **septicemia.** See also **septic shock. —bacteremic,** *adj.*

bacteremic shock, septic shock caused by the release of

toxins by bacteria, usually gram-negative bacteria, in the blood.

bacteria /baktir′ē·ə/, *sing.* **bacterium** [Gk, *bakterion,* small staff], the small unicellular microorganisms of the class Schizomycetes. The genera vary morphologically, being spheric (cocci), rod-shaped (bacilli), spiral (spirochetes), or comma-shaped (vibrios). The nature, severity, and outcome of any infection caused by a bacterium are characteristic of that species.

-bacteria, suffix meaning "genus of microscopic plants forming the class Schizomycetes": *lysobacteria, streptobacteria.*

bacterial adherence /baktir′ēəl/, the process whereby bacteria attach themselves to cells or other surfaces before proliferating.

bacterial aneurysm, a localized dilation in the wall of a blood vessel caused by the growth of bacteria. It often follows septicemia or bacteremia and usually occurs in peripheral vessels. See also **mycotic aneurysm.**

bacterial cholangitis, the most common type of cholangitis, caused by bacterial infection; if bacteria invade the liver they can enter the bloodstream and cause septicemia that can be fatal.

bacterial count. See **count.**

bacterial endocarditis, an acute or subacute bacterial infection of the endocardium or the heart valves or both. The condition is characterized by heart murmur, prolonged fever, bacteremia, splenomegaly, and embolic phenomena. The acute variety progresses rapidly and is usually caused by staphylococci. The subacute variety is usually caused by lodging of *Streptococcus viridans* in heart valves damaged by rheumatic fever. Prompt treatment of both types with antibiotics, such as penicillin, cephalosporin, or gentamicin given intravenously, is essential to prevent destruction of the valves and cardiac failure. See also **endocarditis, subacute bacterial endocarditis.**

Acute bacterial endocarditis
(Kumar, Cotran, and Robbins, 2003)

bacterial enteritis, enteritis caused by bacterial infection; the most common types in humans are *Campylobacter* enteritis, *Salmonella* enteritis, *Shigella* enteritis, and *Yersinia* enteritis.

bacterial enzyme, an enzyme produced by a bacterium.

bacterial food poisoning, a toxic condition resulting from the ingestion of food contaminated by certain bacteria. Acute infectious gastroenteritis caused by various species of *Sal-*

monella is characterized by fever, chills, nausea, vomiting, diarrhea, and general discomfort beginning 8 to 48 hours after ingestion and continuing for several days. Similar symptoms caused by *Staphylococcus,* usually *S. aureus,* appear much sooner and rarely last more than a few hours. Food poisoning caused by the neurotoxin of *Clostridium botulinum* is characterized by GI symptoms, disturbances of vision, weakness or paralysis of muscles, and, in severe cases, respiratory failure. See also **botulism.**

bacterial inflammation [L, *bacterium* + *inflammare,* to set afire], any inflammation that is part of a body's response to a bacterial infection.

bacterial kinase, **1.** a kinase of bacterial origin. **2.** a bacterial enzyme that activates plasminogen, the precursor of plasmin.

bacterial laryngitis, a form of laryngitis caused by a bacterial infection and usually associated with rhinosinusitis or laryngotracheal bronchitis. Signs of a bacterial infection are a cough and purulent rhinorrhea. The infection is treated with any of several antibiotics. See also **laryngitis.**

bacterial meningitis. See **meningitis.**

bacterial overgrowth syndrome. See **stasis syndrome.**

bacterial plaque, a dense, nonmineralized complex composed primarily of colonies of bacteria embedded in a gelatinous matrix. It contains amino acids, carbohydrates, proteins, lipids, and salts from saliva and gingival fluid; soluble food substances; shed leukocytes and epithelial cells; and products of bacterial metabolism. Plaque is the major causitive factor in most dental diseases, including dental caries and inflammatory periodontal diseases. Also called **dental plaque.**

bacterial pneumonia, pneumonia caused by bacteria, such as *Klebsiella pneumoniae, Mycoplasma pneumoniae, Staphylococcus aureus, Streptococcus pneumoniae, Streptococcus pyogenes,* and others.

bacterial prostatitis, a bacterial infection of the prostate. Acute bacterial infections usually involve gram-negative bacilli, such as *Escherichia coli.* Most cases are treated with broad-spectrum antimicrobial drugs. Abscesses may be associated with anaerobic bacteria. Chronic bacterial prostatitis is usually caused by gram-negative bacilli. It is less common and characterized by low back pain, dysuria, and perineal discomfort. See also **prostatitis.**

bacterial protein, a protein produced by a bacterium.

bacterial resistance, the ability of certain strains of bacteria to develop a tolerance to specific antibiotics to which they once were susceptible.

bacterial toxin [Gk, *bakterion,* small staff, *toxikon,* poison], any poisonous substance produced by a bacterium. Kinds of bacterial toxins include **endotoxins** and **exotoxins.**

bacterial vaccine, a saline solution suspension of a strain of attenuated or killed bacteria prepared for injection into a patient to stimulate development of active immunity to that strain and against similar bacteria.

bacterial vaginosis [Gk, *bakterion,* small staff; L, *vagina,* sheath; Gk, *osis,* condition], a chronic inflammation of the vagina caused by a bacterium, *Gardnerella vaginalis.* Vaginal flora commonly includes lactobacilli, streptococci, gardnerella vaginalis, strains of enterobacteriaceae, and anaerobes. Also called **vulvovaginitis.**

bacterial virus, a virus with the ability to infect and/or destroy bacteria. See also **bacteriophage.**

bactericidal /baktir′isī′dəl/, bringing death to bacteria. Also **bacteriocidal.** Compare **bacteriostatic.**

bactericidal antibiotic [Gk, *bakterion* + *caedere,* to kill; Gk, *anti,* against, *bios,* life], an antibiotic drug that kills bacteria.

Bacterial vaginosis (*Zitelli and Davis, 1997*)

bactericide /baktir'əsīd/ [GK, *bakterion* + L, *caedere,* to kill], any drug or other agent that kills bacteria.

bactericidin [Gk, *bakterion* + L, *caedere,* to kill], an antibody that kills bacteria in the presence of complement. Also called **bacteriocidin.**

bacteriemia. See **bacteremia.**

bacterio-, bacter-, bacteri-, combining form meaning "bacterial microorganism": *bacteriogenic, bacteriod, bactericide.*

bacteriocidal. See **bactericidal.**

bacteriocidal antibiotic. See **bactericide.**

bacteriocidin. See **bactericidin.**

bacteriocin /baktir'ē·əsin/, protein produced by certain species of bacteria that are toxic to related strains of those bacteria. Also called **protein antibiotic.**

bacteriocinogenic /baktir'ē·əsin'əjen'ik/, pertaining to an organism capable of producing bacteriocins.

bacteriogenic /baktir'ē·əjen'ik/, **1.** capable of producing bacteria. **2.** derived from or originating in bacteria.

bacterioidal. See **bacteroid.**

bacteriologic /baktir'ē·əloj'ik/ [Gk, *bakterion*], pertaining to **bacteriology.** Also **bacteriological.**

bacteriologic sputum examination, a laboratory procedure to determine the presence or absence of bacteria in a sputum specimen. Part of the specimen is stained and examined microscopically on a glass slide, and part is inoculated on a culture medium and allowed to incubate for more specific examination later. Also called a **sputum culture** and **smear.**

bacteriologist /baktir'ē·ol'əjist/, a specialist in the scientific study of bacteria.

bacteriology /-ol'əjē/ [Gk, *bakterion* + *logos,* science], the scientific study of bacteria.

bacteriolysin /baktir'ē·əlī'sin/ [Gk, *bakterion* + *lyein,* to loosen], an antibody that causes the breakdown of a particular species of bacterial cell. Complement is usually also necessary for this reaction. See also **bacteriolysis.**

bacteriolysis /baktir'ē·ol'əsis/, the intracellular or extracellular breakdown of bacteria. See also **bacteriolysin. —bacteriolytic,** *adj.*

bacteriophage /baktir'ē·əfāj'/ [Gk, *bakterion* + *phagein,* to eat], any virus that causes lysis of host bacteria, including the blue-green algae. Bacteriophages resemble other viruses in that each is composed of either ribonucleic acid (RNA) or deoxyribonucleic acid (DNA). They vary in structure from simple fibrous bodies to complex forms with contractile "tails." Bacteriophages associated with temperate bacteria may be genetically intimate with the host and are named for the bacterial strain for which they are specific, such as coliphage and corynebacteriophage. **—bacteriophagic,** *adj.,* **bacteriophagy** /-of'əjē/, *n.*

bacteriophage typing, the process of identifying a species of bacterium according to the type of virus that attacks it.

bacteriophagic, bacteriphagy. See **bacteriophage.**

bacteriospermia /baktir'ēəspur'mē·ə/, the presence of bacteria in semen.

bacteriostasis /baktir'ē·os'təsis/ [Gk, *bakterion* + Gk, *stasis,* standing still], a state of suspended growth and/or reproduction of bacteria.

bacteriostatic /baktir'ē·əstat'ik/ [Gk, *bakterion* + *statikos,* standing], tending to restrain the development or the reproduction of bacteria. Compare **bactericidal.**

bacterium. See **bacteria.**

bacteriuria /baktir'ēyŏŏr'ē·ə/, the presence of bacteria in the urine. The presence of more than 100,000 pathogenic bacteria per milliliter of urine is usually considered significant and diagnostic of urinary tract infection. See also **urinary tract infection.**

bacteroid /bak'təroid/, **1.** pertaining to or resembling bacteria. **2.** a structure that resembles a bacterium. Also **bacterioid** /baktir'ē-oid/. **—bacteroidal, bacterioidal,** *adj.*

Bacteroides /bak'təroi'dēz/ [Gk, *bakterion,* small staff, *eidos,* form], a genus of obligate anaerobic bacilli normally found in the colon, mouth, genital tract, and upper respiratory system. Severe infection may result from the invasion of the bacillus through a break in the mucous membrane into the venous circulation, where thrombosis and bacteremia may occur. Foul-smelling abscesses, gas, and putrefaction are characteristic of infection with this organism. Of the 30 species, *Bacteroides fragilis* is the most common and most virulent.

Bactrim, trademark for a fixed-combination drug containing two antibiotics (sulfamethoxazole and trimethoprim) commonly prescribed to treat urinary tract infection.

BAER, abbreviation for **brainstem auditory evoked response.**

baffling, the process of removing large water particles from suspension in a jet nebulizer so that the particles entering the patient's airways are of a uniform therapeutic size. The function may be performed in part by a perforated plate against which liquid particles impinge and fracture and are reflected into the vapor chamber of the nebulizer.

bag [AS, *baelg*], a flexible or dilatable sac or pouch designed to contain gas, fluid, or semisolid material such as crushed ice. An Ambu bag or breathing bag is used to control the flow of respiratory gases entering the lungs of a patient. Several types of bags are used in medical or surgical procedures to dilate the anus, vagina, or other body openings.

bagasse /bəgas'/ [Fr, cane trash], the crushed fibers or the residue of sugarcane, a source of the thermophilic actinomycetes antigen that is a cause of bagassosis hypersensitivity pneumonitis.

bagassosis /bag'əsō'sis/, a self-limited lung disease caused by an allergic response to bagasse, the fungi-laden, dusty debris left after the syrup has been extracted from sugarcane. It is characterized by fever, dyspnea, and malaise.

bagging, *informal.* the artificial ventilation performed with a ventilator or respirator bag, such as an Ambu bag or the reservoir bag on an anesthesia machine. The bag is squeezed to deliver air to the patient's lungs through a mask or an endotracheal tube. During general anesthesia the anesthetist may also use this technique to assist or control the respiration of an unconscious patient.

bag lady/man, a homeless indigent woman or man who carries all personal possessions in a portable container.

bag of waters, the membranous sac of amniotic fluid surrounding the fetus in the uterus of a pregnant woman. See **amnion.**

bag-valve-mask resuscitator, a device consisting of a manually compressible container with a plastic bag of oxygen at one end and at the other a one-way valve and mask that fit over the mouth and nose of the person to be resuscitated. See also **Ambu bag.**

Bag-valve-mask resuscitators *(Sanders et al, 2000)*

Bainbridge reflex [Francis A. Bainbridge, English physiologist, 1874–1921], a cardiac reflex in which stimulation of stretch receptors in the wall of the left atrium causes an increased pulse rate. It may be triggered by the infusion of large amounts of IV fluids or by backflow of blood in congestive heart failure.

Baker's cyst [William M. Baker, British surgeon, 1839–1896], a synovial cyst that forms at the back of the knee. It is often associated with rheumatoid arthritis and may appear only when the leg is straightened.

Baker's cyst *(Moll, 1997)*

baker's itch [AS, *giccan,* to bake], a rash that may develop on the hands and forearms of bakery workers, probably as an allergic reaction to flours or other ingredients in bakery products.

BAL, **1.** abbreviation for **British antilewisite.** See **dimercaprol. 2.** abbreviation for **bronchoalveolar lavage.**

balance[1] [L, *bilanx,* having two scales], **1.** an instrument for weighing. **2.** a normal state of physiologic equilibrium. **3.** a state of mental or emotional equilibrium. **4.** to bring into equilibrium.

balance[2], a nursing outcome from the Nursing Outcomes Classification (NOC) defined as ability to maintain body equilibrium. See also **Nursing Outcomes Classification.**

balanced anesthesia, a highly variable technique of general anesthesia in which large doses of narcotic analgesics, muscle relaxation, and minimal inhalation, usually in the form of nitrous oxide only, render the patient unconscious.

balanced articulation, simultaneous contact between the upper and lower teeth as they glide over each other when the mandible is moved laterally. See also **balanced occlusion.**

balanced diet, a diet containing adequate energy and all of the essential nutrients that cannot be synthesized in adequate quantities by the body, in amounts adequate for growth, energy needs, nitrogen equilibrium, repair, and maintenance of normal health.

balanced forearm orthosis (BFO). See **mobile arm support.**

balanced occlusion, simultaneous contact between the upper and lower teeth on both sides and in the anterior and posterior occlusal areas of the jaws. An appropriate dental prosthesis develops such as an occlusion to prevent the denture base from tipping or rotating in relation to the supporting structures. This term is primarily associated with the mouth but may also be used in relation to testing the occlusion of denture casts with an articulator. See also **balanced articulation.**

balanced polymorphism, in a population, the occurrence of a certain proportion of homozygotes and heterozygotes for specific genetic traits, which is maintained from generation to generation by the forces of natural selection. Compare **genetic polymorphism.**

balanced suspension, a system of splints, ropes, slings, pulleys, and weights for suspending the lower extremities of the body, used as an aid to realignment and healing from fractures or from surgical intervention. See also **lower extremity suspension, upper extremity suspension.**

balanced traction, a system of balanced suspension that supplements traction in the treatment of fractures of the lower extremities or after various operations affecting the lower parts of the body that require traction.

balanced translocation, the transfer of segments between nonhomologous chromosomes in such a way that the configuration and total number of chromosomes change but each cell contains the normal amount of diploid or haploid genetic material. Usually the long arm of an acrocentric chromosome is transferred to another chromosome, and the small fragment containing the centromere is lost, leaving only 45 chromosomes. A person with a balanced translocation is phenotypically normal but may produce children with trisomies. Compare **reciprocal translocation, robertsonian translocation.**

balancing side, the side of the mouth opposite the working side of dentition or a denture.

balanic /bəlan′ik/ [Gk, *balanos,* acorn], pertaining to the glans penis or the glans clitoridis.

balanic hypospadias. See **glandular hypospadias.**

Balanced suspension *(Elkin, Perry, and Potter, 2004)*

Balanitis xerotica obliterans *(du Vivier, 1993)*

Balanitis xerotica obliterans *(Callen et al, 2000)*

balanitis /bal'ənī'tis/ [Gk, *balanos* + *itis*], inflammation of the glans penis.

Balanitis *(Callen et al, 2000)*

balanitis diabetica, an inflammation of the glans penis or glans clitoridis caused by the sugar content of the urine and commonly seen in diabetics.

balanitis xerotica obliterans /zirot'ikə oblit'ərans/ [Gk, *balanos* + *itis* + *xeros*, dry, *tokos*, labor; L, *obliterare*, to efface], a chronic skin disease of the penis, characterized by a white indurated area surrounding the meatus. Local antibacterial and antiinflammatory agents are used to treat it.

balano-, balan-, combining form meaning "the head of the penis in males; may also mean the glans clitoris in females": *balanoplasty, balanitis*.

balanoplasty /bal'ənōplas'tē/ [Gk, *balanos* + *plassein*, to mold], an operation involving plastic surgery of the glans penis to correct a congenital defect or to serve an aesthetic purpose.

balanoposthitis /bal'ənōposthī'tis/ [Gk, *balanos* + *posthe*, penis, foreskin, *itis*], a generalized inflammation of the glans penis and prepuce. It is characterized by soreness, irritation, and discharge, which occurs as a complication of bacterial or fungal infection. Smear and culture can determine the causative agent—often a common venereal disease—so that specific antimicrobial therapy can then be instituted. Circumcision may be considered in severe cases. To relieve discomfort, the inflamed area can be irrigated with a warm saline solution several times a day.

balanopreputial /bal'ənōpripyoo'shəl/ [Gk, *balanos* + L, *praeputium*, foreskin], pertaining to the glans penis and the prepuce.

balanorrhagia /bal'ənōrā'jē·ə/ [Gk, *balanos* + *rhegnynai*, to burst forth], balanitis in which pus is discharged copiously from the penis.

balantidiasis /bal'əntidī'əsis/, an infection caused by ingestion of cysts of the protozoan *Balantidium coli*. Pigs are the animal reservoir. In some cases the organism is a harmless inhabitant of the large intestine, but infection with *B. coli* usually causes diarrhea. Infrequently the infection progresses, and the protozoan invades the intestinal wall and produces ulcers or abscesses, which may cause dysentery and death. Diagnosis is made by identification of trophozoites in the stool or in sampled colonic tissue. Tetracycline, iodoquinol, or metronidazole is usually prescribed to treat the infection.

Balantidium coli /bal'əntid'ē·əm/ [Gk, *balantidion,* little bag, *kolon,* colon], the largest and the only ciliated protozoan species that is pathogenic to humans, causing balantidiasis. The organism is seen in two life stages: the motile trophozoite and the encysted cercaria. It is a normal inhabitant of the domestic hog and is transmitted to humans by the ingestion of cysts excreted in hog feces.

baldness [ME, *balled*], absence of hair, especially from the scalp. See also **alopecia.**

BAL in Oil, trademark for a heavy metal antagonist (dimercaprol).

Balint's syndrome [Rudolph Balint, Hungarian neurologist, 1874–1929], a group of visual symptoms characterized by agnosia and optic ataxia. The patient experiences nystagmus, or loss of control of eye movements, simultaneously with loss of perceptive ability. The patient may begin to follow a moving object but lose it. The cause is bilateral disease of the parietotemporal areas of the brain.

Balkan traction frame, an overhead, rectangular frame attached to the bed and used for attaching splints, suspending or changing the position of immobilized limbs, or providing continuous traction with weights and pulleys.

Balkan tubulointerstitial nephritis /too'byəlō· in'tərstish'-əl/, a chronic kidney disorder marked by renal insufficiency, proteinuria, tubulointerstitial nephritis, and anemia. The onset is gradual, but end-stage disease occurs within 5 years after the first signs. About one third of the patients also suffer from urinary tract cancers. The disease is endemic in the Balkans but is not hereditary.

ball [ME, *bal*], spherical object, such as one of the collagen balls embedded in hyaline cartilage.

Ballance's sign [Charles A. Ballance, English surgeon, 1856–1936], a dull percussion resonance sound heard on the right flank of a patient lying in the left decubitus position. The sound may shift with the patient's change of position. The condition is attributed to rupture of the spleen, which causes an accumulation of liquid blood on the right side and coagulated blood on the left.

ball-and-socket joint, a synovial or multiaxial joint in which the globular (ball-shaped) head of an articulating bone is received into a cuplike cavity, allowing the distal bone to move around an indefinite number of axes with a common center, such as in hip and shoulder joints. Also called **enarthrosis, spheroidea.** Compare **condyloid joint, pivot joint, saddle joint.** See also **joint.**

ball-bearing feeder. See **mobile arm support.**

ball-catcher position, a position of the hands used in making a radiograph to diagnose rheumatoid arthritis. The hands are held with the palms upward and the fingers cupped, as if to catch a ball.

Baller-Gerold syndrome /bä'lər ga'rōlt/ [Friedrich Baller, German physician, 20th century; M. Gerold, German physician, 20th century], an autosomal recessive syndrome characterized by craniosynostosis and absence of the radius.

ballism. See **ballismus.**

ballismus /bôl'iz'məs/ [Gk, *ballismo,* dancing], an abnormal neuromuscular condition characterized by uncoordinated swinging of the limbs and jerky movements. Ballism is associated with extrapyramidal disorders such as Sydenham's chorea. The condition may occur in a unilateral form as hemiballismus. Also called **ballism.**

ballistic movement /bəlis'tik/, a high-velocity musculoskeletal movement, such as a tennis serve or boxing punch,

requiring reciprocal coordination of agonistic and antagonistic muscles.

ballistics /bəlis'tiks/ [Gk, *ballein,* to throw], the study of the motion, trajectory, and impact of projectiles, including bullets and rockets.

ballistocardiograph [Gk, *ballein,* to throw, *kardia,* heart, *graphein,* to record], an apparatus for recording body movements caused by the thrust of the heart during systolic ejection of the blood into the aorta and the pulmonary arteries. It has been used in measuring cardiac output and the force of contraction of the heart.

ballistocardiography /balis'tōkär'dē·og'rəfē/, the recording of body movements in reaction to the beating of the heart and the circulation of the blood.

ball of the foot, the part of the foot composed of the distal heads of the metatarsals and their surrounding fatty fibrous tissue pad.

balloon angioplasty /bəloon'/, a method of dilating or opening an obstructed blood vessel by threading a small, balloon-tipped catheter into the vessel. The balloon is inflated to compress arteriosclerotic lesions against the walls of the vessel, leaving a larger lumen, through which blood can pass. It is used in treating arteriosclerotic heart disease.

Balloon angioplasty *(Thibodeau and Patton, 2003)*

balloon bezoar [Fr, *ballon,* a large ball; Ar, *bazahr,* counterpoison], a balloon that is inserted into the stomach and inflated to create a sensation of fullness, used as a therapy for obesity. It is rarely used now because of complications and improved results with gastric bypass.

balloon compression, a percutaneous therapy for trigeminal neuralgia. A balloon is inflated to compress the gasserian ganglion and produce trigeminal injury.

balloon flower, *Platycodon grandiflorum.*

balloon septostomy. See **Rashkind procedure.**

balloon tamponade [Fr, tamponnade], a procedure in which a device consisting of a flexible tube and two balloons is inserted into a passageway and the balloons are expanded to restrict the flow of blood or to force open a stenosis. See also **balloon angioplasty.**

balloon-tip catheter, a catheter bearing a nonporous inflatable sac around its far end. After insertion of the catheter the sac can be inflated with air or sterile water, introduced via injection into a special port at the near end of the catheter. The inflated sac secures the catheter in the correct position. See also **Foley catheter, Swan-Ganz catheter.**

ballottable /bəlot′əbəl/ [Fr, *balloter,* a shaking about], pertaining to a use of palpation to detect movement of objects suspended in fluid, such as a fetus in amniotic fluid, or the patella bumping against the femur. See **ballottement.**

ballottable head [Fr, *ballotage,* shaking up], a fetal head that has not descended and has not become fixed in the maternal bony pelvis.

ballottement /bä′lôtmäN′, bəlot′ment/ [Fr, tossing], a technique of palpating an organ or floating structure by bouncing it gently and feeling it rebound. Ballottement of a fetus within a uterus is a probable objective sign of pregnancy. In late pregnancy a fetal head that can be ballotted is said to be **floating** or **unengaged,** as differentiated from a fixed or an engaged head, which cannot be easily dislodged from the pelvis.

ball thrombus, a relatively round, coagulated mass of blood, containing platelets, fibrin, and cellular fragments, that may obstruct a blood vessel or an orifice, usually the mitral valve of the heart.

ball-valve action, the intermittent opening and closing of an orifice by a buoyant, ball-shaped mass, which acts as a valve. Some kinds of objects that may act in this manner are kidney stones, gallstones, and blood clots.

balm /bäm/ [Gk, *balsamon,* balsam], 1. a healing or a soothing substance, such as any of various medicinal ointments. 2. an aromatic plant of the genus *Melissa* that relieves pain. Also called **balsam.**

balneology /bal′nē·ol′əjē/ [L, *balneum,* bath; Gk, *logos,* science], a field of medicine that deals with the chemical compositions of various mineral waters and their healing characteristics, especially in baths. —**balneologic,** *adj.*

balneotherapy /bal′nē·ōther′əpē/ [L, *balneum* + Gk, *therapeia,* treatment], use of baths in the treatment of many diseases and conditions.

balneum pneumaticum. See **air bath.**

balsalazide /bal-sal′ah;-zīd/, a prodrug of the antiinflammatory mesalamine, to which it is converted in the colon; administered orally as the disodium salt in the treatment of ulcerative colitis.

balsam /bôl′səm/ [Gk, *balsamon*], 1. any of a variety of resinous saps, generally from evergreens, usually containing benzoic or cinnamic acid. Balsam is sometimes used in rectal suppositories and dermatologic agents as a counterirritant. 2. See **balm.**

Baltimore Longitudinal Study of Aging (BLSA), a long-range examination of interrelations between multiple correlates of aging. Although men of varied backgrounds were selected for the original study (1955) in order to explore uncontrolled factors that might lead to new knowledge regarding aging, the BLSA now includes both men and women.

-bamate, combining form designating a propanediol or pentanediol derivative.

Bamberger's sign [Heinrich Bamberger, Austrian physician, 1822–1888], 1. a neural disorder characterized by the feeling of a tactile stimulation at a corresponding point on the opposite side of the body (known as allochiria). 2. pericardial effusion signs at the level of the scapula that disappear when the patient leans forward.

bamboo spine /bamboo′/ [Malay, *bambu*], a rigid spine characteristic of advanced ankylosing spondylitis. Also called **poker spine.** See also **ankylosing spondylitis.**

band [ME, *bande,* strip], 1. (in anatomy) a bundle of fibers, as seen in striated muscle, that encircles a structure or binds one part of the body to another. 2. (in dentistry) a strip of metal that fits around a tooth and serves as an attachment for orthodontic components. 3. also called **stab form.** *informal,*

the immature form of a segmented granulocyte characterized by a sausage-shaped nucleus. It is the only immature leukocyte normally found in the peripheral circulation. Bands represent 3% to 5% of the total white cell volume. An increase in the relative number of bands indicates bacterial infection or acute stress to the bone marrow.

band adapter, an instrument for aiding in the fitting of a circumferential orthodontic band to a tooth.

bandage /ban′dij/ [ME, *bande* strip], 1. a strip or roll of cloth or other material that may be wound around a part of the body in a variety of ways to secure a dressing, maintain pressure over a compress, or immobilize a limb or other part of the body. See also **cravat bandage.** 2. to apply a bandage.

Circular

Spiral

Spiral reverse

Figure-eight

Recurrent

Types of bandage turns *(Potter and Perry, 2005)*

bandage shears, a sturdy pair of scissors used to cut through bandages. The blades of most bandage shears are angled to the shaft of the instrument, and the lower blade is rounded and blunt to facilitate insertion under the bandage without harming the patient's skin. Also called **bandage scissors.**

band cell, a developing granular (immature) leukocyte in circulating blood, characterized by a curved or indented nucleus. Band cells are intermediate leukocytic forms between metamyelocytes and adult leukocytes with segmented nuclei.

band heterotopia, an anomaly of the cerebral cortex in which a heterotopic band of gray matter is found between the lateral ventricles and the cortex; affected patients may have mental retardation or epilepsy.

banding [ME, *bande,* strip], any of several techniques of staining chromosomes with fluorescent stains or chemical dyes that produce a series of transverse light and dark areas whose intensity and position are characteristic of each chromosome. Banding patterns are identified as C-banding, G-banding, Q-banding, or R-banding according to the staining technique used. Also called **chromosome banding.**

Bandl's ring. See **pathologic retraction ring.**

bandpass, (in radiology) a measure of the number of times per second an electron beam can be modulated, expressed as Hertz (Hz). It is a factor that influences horizontal resolution on a cathode-ray tube. The higher the bandpass, the greater the horizontal resolution. Also called **bandwidth.**

band pusher, an instrument used for adapting metal circumferential orthodontic bands to the teeth.

band remover, an instrument used to help take circumferential orthodontic bands off teeth.

bandwidth, 1. the range of frequencies that can be satisfactorily transmitted or processed by a system. 2. See **bandpass.**

bang. See **bhang.**

Bangkok hemorrhagic fever. See **dengue fever.**

bank blood [It, *banca,* bench; AS, *blod*], anticoagulated preserved blood collected from donors usually in units of 500 ml and stored under refrigeration for future use. Dated and identified as to blood type, it is stored for a usual maximum period of 21 days. Bank blood may be used in transfusion after crossmatching against the recipient's blood or for the extraction and preparation of any of its components. See also **packed cells, pooled plasma, whole blood.**

Banting, Sir Frederick G. [Canadian physician, 1891–1941], co-winner, with John J. Macleod, of the 1923 Nobel prize for medicine and physiology for their research, with the Canadian physiologist Charles H. Best, showing the link between the pancreas and insulin in the control of diabetes. See also **Macleod, John J.**

Banti's syndrome /ban'tēz/ [Guido Banti, Italian pathologist, 1852–1925], a chronic, progressive disorder involving several organ systems, characterized by portal hypertension, splenomegaly, anemia, leukopenia, GI tract bleeding, and cirrhosis of the liver. Obstruction of the blood vessels that lie between the intestines and the liver leads to venous congestion, enlargement of the spleen, and abnormal destruction of red and white blood cells. Early symptoms are weakness, fatigue, and anemia. Surgical removal of the spleen and creation of a portacaval shunt to improve portal circulation are sometimes necessary. Since the syndrome is often a complication of alcoholic cirrhosis of the liver, medical treatment includes prescribing improved nutrition, vitamins, abstinence from alcohol, and rest. Also called **Banti's disease.** See also **congestive splenomegalia, cirrhosis, portacaval shunt, portal hypertension.**

BAO, abbreviation for **basal acid output.**

bar, (in physical science) a measure of air pressure. It is equal to 1000 millibars, or 10^6 dyne/cm^2, or approximately 1 standard atmosphere (1 atm). Also called **barye.**

bar-. See **baro-.**

baralyme /ber'əlīm/ [Gk, *barys,* heavy; AS, *lim,* lime], a mixture of calcium and barium compounds used to absorb exhaled carbon dioxide in an anesthesia rebreathing system.

Bárány's test. See **caloric test.**

-barb, combining form designating a barbituric acid derivative.

Barbados cherry. See **acerola.**

barber's itch. See **sycosis barbae.**

barbiturate /bärbich'ōōrāt, -ərit/ [Saint Barbara, drug discovered on day of the saint, 1864], a derivative of barbituric acid that acts as a sedative or hypnotic. These derivatives act by depressing the respiratory rate, blood pressure, temperature, and central nervous system. They have great addiction potential. Some barbiturates are used in anesthesia and in treatment of seizures.

barbiturate coma [Ger, Saint Barbara's Day, Gk, *koma,* deep sleep], an effect of barbituric acid or its derivatives, which may be rapid-acting sedatives, hypnotics, and respiratory depressants. Barbituate coma may be intentionally induced for the treatment of some neurologic conditions. Death may result from intentional or accidental overdosage.

barbiturate poisoning. See **barbiturism.**

-barbituric, combining form used to designate compounds derived from barbituric acid: *dibromobarbituric, isobarbituric.*

barbiturism /bärbich'əriz'əm/, 1. acute or chronic poisoning by any of the derivatives of barbituric acid. Ingestion of such preparations in excess of therapeutic quantities may be fatal or may produce physiologic, pathologic, and psychologic changes, such as depressed respiration, cyanosis, disorientation, and coma. Sometimes referred to as **barbiturate poisoning.** 2. addiction to a barbiturate.

bar clasp arm, (in prosthetic dentistry) a clasp arm that originates from a denture base and serves as an extracoronal retainer.

Bardeleben's bone. See **os trigonum.**

Bard-Pic syndrome /bärd'pik'/ [Louis Bard, French anatomist, 1857–1930; Adrian Pic, French physician, b. 1863], a condition characterized by progressive jaundice, enlarged gallbladder, and cachexia, associated with advanced pancreatic cancer.

Bard's sign [Louis Bard], the increased oscillations of the eyeball in organic nystagmus when the patient tries to visually follow a target moved from side to side across the line of sight. Such oscillations usually cease during the same test if the patient has congenital nystagmus.

bare lymphocyte syndrome, an immune deficiency condition caused by defective beta-2 microglobulin, one of the major histocompatibility antigens on cell surfaces. It is inherited as an autosomal recessive trait.

baresthesia /bär'esthē'zhə/, sensitivity to weight or pressure.

bar graph [OF, *barre*], a graph in which frequencies are represented by bars extending from the ordinate or the abscissa, allowing the distribution of the entire sample to be seen at once.

bariatrics /ber'ē·at'riks/ [Gk, *baros,* weight, *iatros,* physician], the field of medicine that focuses on the treatment and control of obesity and diseases associated with obesity.

bariatric surgery, surgery on part of the GI tract as a treatment for morbid obesity.

baritosis /ber'ətō'sis/, a benign form of pneumoconiosis caused by an accumulation of barium dust in the lungs. Barium does not cause fibrosis and is not a common cause of functional impairment. The condition is most likely to affect persons involved in the mining and processing of barite, a barium-containing compound used in the manufacture of paints.

barium (Ba) /ber′ē·əm/ [Gk, *barys,* heavy], a pale yellow, metallic element classified with the alkaline earths. Its atomic number is 56; its atomic mass is 137.36. The acid-soluble salts of barium are poisonous. Barium carbonate, formerly used in medicine, is now used to prepare the cardiac stimulant barium chloride; fine, milky barium sulfate is used as a contrast medium in radiographic imaging of the digestive tract.

barium enema, a rectal infusion of barium sulfate, a radiopaque contrast medium, which is retained in the lower intestinal tract during roentgenographic studies for diagnosis of obstruction, tumors, or other abnormalities, such as ulcerative colitis. The procedure is used therapeutically in children to reduce nonstrangulated intussusception. Also called **contrast enema.**

Barium enema
(Mace and Kowalczyk, 2004/
courtesy Ohio State University Medical Center)

barium enema with air contrast. See **double-contrast barium enema.**

barium meal, the ingestion of barium sulfate, a radiopaque contrast medium, for the radiographic examination of the esophagus, stomach, and intestinal tract in the diagnosis of such conditions as dysphagia, peptic ulcer, and fistulas. The movement of the barium through the GI tract is followed by fluoroscopy, x-ray studies, or both. Before the test, the patient receives nothing by mouth for at least 8 hours. See also **barium swallow.**

barium poisoning, a condition characterized by a severe, rapid decrease in plasma potassium levels and a shift of potassium into cells caused by the ingestion of soluble barium salts. The patient may experience nausea, vomiting, abdominal cramps, bloody diarrhea, dizziness, dysrhythmias, ringing in the ears, cardiac arrest, and respiratory failure.

barium sulfate, a radiopaque medium used as a diagnostic aid in radiology.

■ INDICATION: It is prescribed for x-ray examination of the GI tract.

■ CONTRAINDICATION: Known hypersensitivity to this drug prohibits its use.

■ ADVERSE EFFECTS: Among the more serious complications is severe constipation.

barium swallow [Gk, *barys,* heavy; AS, *swelgan,* to swallow], the oral administration of a radiopaque barium sulfate suspension given to radiographically demonstrate possible defects in the esophagus and abnormal borders of the posterior aspects of the heart. See also **barium meal.**

Barlow's disease. See **infantile scurvy.**

Barlow's syndrome [John B. Barlow, South African cardiologist, b. 1924], an abnormal cardiac condition characterized by an apical systolic murmur, a systolic click, and an electrocardiogram indicating inferior ischemia. These signs are associated with mitral regurgitation caused by prolapse of the mitral valve. Also called **floppy-valve syndrome.** See also **mitral valve prolapse.**

Barnard, Kathryn E., a nursing theorist who developed the Child Health Assessment Interaction Model. Her model and theory were the outcome of the Nursing Child Assessment Project (1976–1979). Barnard believes that the parent-infant system is influenced by individual characteristics of each member. Those characteristics are modified to meet the needs of the system by adaptive behavior. The interaction between parent (or caregiver) and child is shown in Barnard's model to take place with five cues and activities: (1) the infant's clarity in sending cues, (2) the infant's responsiveness to the parent, (3) the parent's sensitivity to the child's cues, (4) the parent's ability to recognize and alleviate the infant's distress, and (5) the parent's social, emotional, and cognitive growth-fostering activities. A major issue in Barnard's theoretic assertions is that the nurse gives support to the mother's sensitivity and response to her infant's cues rather than trying to change her characteristics or mothering style.

baro-, bar-, bari- combining form meaning "pressure, heaviness, weight": *baresthesia, barognosis, bariatrics.*

barognosis /ber′əgnō′sis/, *pl.* **barognoses** [Gk, *baros,* weight, *gnosis,* knowledge], the ability to perceive and evaluate weight, especially that held in the hand.

barograph /ber′əgraf′/ [Gk, *baros* + *graphein,* to record], an instrument that continually monitors barometric pressure and records pressure changes on paper.

barometer /bərom′ətər/ [Gk, *baros* + *metron,* measure], an instrument for measuring atmospheric pressure, commonly consisting of a slender tube filled with mercury, sealed at one end, and inverted into a reservoir of mercury. At sea level the normal height of mercury in the tube is 760 mm. At higher elevations the mercury column height (barometric pressure) is less. Fluctuations in barometric pressure may precede major changes in weather, making a barometer useful in meteorologic forecasting. **—barometric,** *adj.*

barometric pressure. See **atmospheric pressure.**

baroreceptor /ber′ōrisep′tər/ [Gk, *baros* + L, *recipere,* to receive], one of the pressure-sensitive nerve endings in the walls of the atria of the heart, the aortic arch, and the carotid sinuses. Baroreceptors stimulate central reflex mechanisms that allow physiologic adjustment and adaptation to changes in blood pressure via changes in heart rate, vasodilation, or vasoconstriction. Baroreceptors are essential for homeostasis. Also called **pressoreceptor.**

barosinusitis. See **aerosinusitis.**

Barosperse, trademark for a radiopaque medium (barium sulfate).

barotitis. See **aerotitis.**

barotitis media. See **aerotitis media.**

barotrauma /ber'ōtrô'mə, -trou'mə/ [Gk, *baros + trauma,* wound], physical injury sustained as a result of exposure to changing air pressure, or rupture of the tympanic membranes, as may occur among scuba divers or caisson workers or anyone near nuclear or atomic blasts. Barotrauma may be iatrogenic as in the case of excessive ventilator pressures leading to lung injury. Compare **decompression sickness.**

Barr body. See **sex chromatin.**

barrel chest, a large, rounded thorax, as in the inspiratory phase, considered normal in some stocky individuals and certain others who live in high-altitude areas and consequently have increased vital capacity. Barrel chest may also be a sign of pulmonary emphysema. Also called **emphysematous chest.**

Barrel chest *(Zitelli and Davis, 1997/courtesy Dr. Meyer B. Marks)*

barrel distortion, outward bowing of gridded straight lines in an image, resulting from lens distortion such that the lateral magnification at the center of the image is greater than that at the edges.

Barr-Epstein virus. See **Epstein-Barr virus.**

Barré's pyramidal sign /bärāz'/ [Jean A. Barré, French neurologist, 1880–1971], a diagnostic sign indicating a disease of the pyramidal tracts. The patient lies face down and the legs are flexed at the knee. The patient is unable to maintain this position.

Barrett's syndrome [Norman R. Barrett, English surgeon, 1903–1979], a disorder of the lower esophagus marked by a benign ulcerlike lesion in columnar epithelium, resulting most often from chronic irritation of the esophagus by gastric reflux of acidic digestive juices. Major symptoms include dysphagia, decreased lower esophageal (LES) pressure, and heartburn. Symptoms may be relieved by eating frequent small meals, avoiding foods that produce gas, taking antacid medication, and elevating the head of the bed to prevent passive reflux when lying down. Also called **Barrett's esophagus.**

Barrett's syndrome *(Goldman et al, 2004)*

barrier /ber'ē·ər/ [ME, *barrere*], **1.** a wall or other obstacle that can restrain or block the passage of substances. Barrier methods of contraception, such as the condom or cervical diaphragm, prevent the passage of spermatozoa into the uterus. Membranes and cell walls of body tissues function as screenlike barriers to permit the movement of water or certain other molecules from one side to the other while preventing the passage of other substances. Skin is an important barrier that protects against the entry of microorganisms and the exit of body fluids. Barriers in kidney tissues adjust automatically to regulate the retention or excretion of water and other substances according to the needs of organ systems elsewhere in the body. **2.** something nonphysical that obstructs or separates, such as barriers to communication or compliance. **3.** (in radiography) any device that intercepts beams of x-rays. A primary barrier is one that blocks the passage of the useful x-ray beam, such as the walls and floor. A secondary barrier is one that intercepts only leakage and scattered x-ray emissions. An example is the ceiling.

barrier creams, ointments, lotions, and similar preparations applied to exposed areas of the skin to protect skin cells from exposure to various allergens, irritants, and carcinogens, including sunlight.

barrier-free design [AS, *freo,* barreres; L, *designare,* to mark out], the design of homes, workplaces, and public buildings that allows physically challenged individuals to make regular use of such structures.

barrier methods, contraceptive methods, such as condoms and diaphragms, in which a plastic or rubber barrier blocks passage of spermatozoa through the vagina or cervix. See discussion under **contraception.**

Barsony-Koppenstein method, a procedure for making radiographic images of the cervical intervertebral foramina.

Barthel Index (BI) [D.W. Barthel, twentieth century American psychiatrist], a disability profile scale developed by D.W. Barthel in 1965 to evaluate a patient's self-care abilities in 10 areas, including bowel and bladder control. The patient is scored from 0 to 15 points in various categories, depending on his or her need for help, such as in feeding, bathing, dressing, and walking.

bartholinian abscess. See **Bartholin's abscess.**

bartholinitis /bär′təlini′tis/ [Caspar T. Bartholin, Danish anatomist, 1655–1738; Gk, *itis*], an inflammatory condition of one or both Bartholin's glands, caused by bacterial infection. Usually the causative microorganism is a species of *Streptococcus* or *Staphylococcus* or a strain of gonococcus. The condition is characterized by swelling of one or both glands, pain, and development of an abscess in the infected gland. A fistula may develop from the gland to the vagina, anus, or perineum. Treatment includes local application of heat, often by soaking in hot water; antibiotics; or, if necessary, incision of the gland and drainage of the purulent material or excision of the entire gland and its duct.

Bartholin's abscess /bär′təlinz/ [Caspar T. Bartholin; L, *abscedere,* to go away], an abscess of the greater vestibular gland of the vagina. Also called **bartholinian abscess.**

Bartholin's cyst *(Greer et al, 2001)*

Bartholin's abscess *(Swartz, 2002)*

Bartholin's cyst [Caspar T. Bartholin], a cyst that arises from one of the vestibular glands or from its ducts and fills with clear fluid that replaces the suppurative exudate characteristic of chronic inflammation.

Bartholin's duct [Caspar T. Bartholin], the major duct of the sublingual salivary gland.

Bartholin's gland [Caspar T. Bartholin], one of two small mucus-secreting glands located on the posterior and lateral aspect of the vestibule of the vagina. Also called **greater vestibular gland.**

Bartholin's gland carcinoma [Caspar T. Bartholin], a rare malignancy that occurs deep in the labia majora. The tumor has overlying skin and some normal glandular tissue. The treatment and prognosis are the same as for squamous cell cancer of the vulva.

Barton, Clara (1821–1912), an American philanthropist, humanitarian, and founder of the American National Red Cross. During the U.S. Civil War, she was a volunteer nurse, often on the battlefield, and at its end she organized a bureau of records to help in the search for missing men. When the Franco-Prussian War erupted, she assisted in the organization of military hospitals in Europe in association with the International Red Cross. This experience led to her advocacy of establishment of an American Red Cross organization, of which she became the first president.

Bartonella /bär′tənel′ə/ [Alberto Barton, Peruvian bacteriologist, 1871–1950], a genus of small gram-negative flagellated pleomorphic coccobacilli. Members of the genus infect red blood cells and the epithelial cells of the lymph nodes, liver, and spleen. They are transmitted at night by the bite of a sandfly of the genus *Phlebotomus. B. bacilliformis,* causes bartonellosis. Because of its distinctive appearance, it is easily identified on microscopic examination of a smear of blood stained with Wright's stain. *B. henselae* is the causative agent of cat-scratch fever and bacillary angiomatosis.

Bartonella henselae, the etiologic agent of cat-scratch fever. Feline infection results in chronic asymptomatic bacteremia which may last up to 17 months. Approximately 40% of cats are infected with the organism. Most human infections occur between September and February and follow a cat bite or scratch.

bartonellosis /bär′tənəlō′sis/, an acute infection caused by *Bartonella bacilliformis,* transmitted by the bite of a sandfly. It is characterized by fever, severe anemia, bone pain, and, several weeks after the first symptoms are observed, multiple nodular or verrucose skin lesions. The disease is endemic in the valleys of the Andes in Peru, Colombia, and Ecuador. The treatment usually includes chloramphenicol, penicillin, streptomycin, or tetracycline. Untreated, the infection is often fatal. Also called **Carrión's disease, Oroya fever, verruga peruana.**

Barton forceps. See **obstetric forceps.**

Barton's fracture [John R. Barton, American surgeon, 1794–1871], a break in the distal articular surface of the radius, which may be accompanied by the dorsal dislocation of the carpus on the radius.

Bartter's syndrome /bär′tərz/ [Frederick C. Bartter, American physiologist, 1914–1983], a rare hereditary disorder, characterized by hyperplasia of the juxtaglomerular area and secondary hyperaldosteronism. Renin and angiotensin levels may be elevated, but blood pressure usually remains normal. Early signs in childhood are abnormal physical growth and mental retardation, often accompanied by chronic hypokalemia and alkalosis.

bary-, combining form meaning "heavy or difficult": *baryphonia.*

barye. See **bar.**

basal /bā′səl/ [Gk, *basis,* foundation], pertaining to the fundamental or the basic, as basal anesthesia, which produces the first stage of unconsciousness, and the basal metabolic rate, which indicates the lowest metabolic rate; basal membrane.

basal acid output (BAO), the minimum volume of gastric fluid produced by an individual in a given period. Normal adult volume is 2 to 5 mEq/hr. It is used infrequently in the diagnosis of various diseases of the stomach and intestines, such as gastric ulcers and Zollinger-Ellison syndrome.

basal anesthesia [Gk, *basis,* foundation, *anaisthesia,* lack of feeling], **1.** a state of unconsciousness just short of complete surgical anesthesia in depth, in which the patient does not respond to words but reacts to pinprick or other noxious stimuli. **2.** narcosis produced by injection or infusion of potent sedatives alone, without added narcotics or anesthetic agents. **3.** also called **narcoanesthesia.** Any form of anesthesia in which the patient is completely unconscious, in contrast to awake anesthesia.

basal body temperature, the temperature of the body under conditions of absolute rest, taken orally or rectally, after sleep and before the patient does anything, including getting out of bed, smoking a cigarette, moving around, talking, eating, or drinking.

basal body temperature method of family planning, a natural method of family planning that relies on identification of the fertile period of the menstrual cycle by noting the rise in basal body temperature that occurs with ovulation. The progesterone-mediated rise is 0.5° to 1° F; rate and pattern vary greatly from woman to woman, and to some extent from cycle to cycle in any one woman. The woman keeps careful records over several cycles, taking her temperature at the same time every morning, before getting out of bed or doing anything else. She may take her temperature orally or rectally in the same way every day. Talking, getting up, smoking a cigarette, eating, or even moving about in bed may change the temperature. Many other factors may also affect the reading, including infection, stress, a bad night's sleep, medica-

tion, or environmental temperature. If any of these factors is present, the woman notes them on her record. The days after that period are considered "safe" infertile days. Abstinence is required to avoid pregnancy from 6 days before the earliest day that ovulation was noted to occur during the preceding 6 months until the third day after the rise in temperature in the current cycle. Another way of calculating the possible beginning of the fertile days is to subtract 19 days from the shortest complete menstrual cycle of the preceding 6 months. The basal body temperature method is more effective when used with the ovulation method than is either method used alone. The combination of these methods is called the symptothermal method of family planning. Compare **calendar method of family planning, ovulation method of family planning.**

basal bone, 1. (in prosthodontics) the osseous tissue of the mandible and the maxilla, except for the rami and the processes, which provides support for artificial dentures. **2.** (in orthodontics) the fixed osseous structure that limits the movement of teeth in the creation of a stable occlusion.

basal cell, any one of the cells in the deepest layer of stratified epithelium; the base.

basal cell acanthoma. See **basal cell papilloma.**

basal cell carcinoma [Gk, *basis* + L, *cella,* storeroom; Gk, *karkinos,* crab, *oma,* tumor], a malignant epithelial cell tumor that begins as a papule and enlarges peripherally, developing a central crater that erodes, crusts, and bleeds. Metastasis is rare, but local invasion destroys underlying and adjacent tissue. In 90% of cases the lesion occurs between the hairline and the upper lip. The primary known cause of the cancer is excessive exposure to the sun or to radiation. Treatment is eradication of the lesion, often by electrodesiccation or cryotherapy. Also called **basal cell epithelioma, basaloma, basiloma, carcinoma basocellulare, hair matrix carcinoma.** See also **rodent ulcer.**

Basal cell carcinoma *(Swartz, 2002)*

basal cell papilloma. See **seborrheic keratosis.**

basal energy expenditure (BEE). See **basal metabolic rate.**

basal ganglia [Gk, *basis* + *ganglion,* knot], the islands of gray matter, largely composed of cell bodies, within each cerebral hemisphere. The most important are the caudate nucleus, the putamen, and the pallidum. The basal ganglia are surrounded by the rings of the limbic system and lie between the thalamus of the diencephalon and the white matter of the hemisphere.

Basaljel, trademark for an antacid (aluminum carbonate gel).

basal lamina [Gk, *basis* + L, *lamina,* plate], a thin, non-cellular layer of ground substance lying just under epithelial surfaces. Constituting the uppermost layer of the basement membrane, it can be examined with an electron microscope. Also called **basement lamina.**

basal layer. See **stratum basale.**

basal layer of endometrium, the deepest layer of the endometrium, which contains the blind ends of the uterine glands; the cells of this layer undergo minimal change during the sexual cycle.

basal layer of epidermis, stratum basale.

basal membrane, a sheet of tissue that forms the outer layer of the choroid and lies just under the pigmented layer of the retina. It is composed of elastic fibers in an otherwise thin homogenous layer.

basal metabolic rate (BMR), the amount of energy used in a unit of time by a fasting, resting subject to maintain vital functions. The rate, determined by the amount of oxygen used, is expressed in Calories consumed per hour per square meter of body surface area or per kilogram of body weight. Also called **basal energy expenditure (BEE).** See also **Calorie (Cal).**

basal metabolism [Gk, *basis* + *metabole,* change], the amount of energy needed to maintain essential body functions, such as respiration, circulation, temperature, peristalsis, and muscle tone. Basal metabolism is measured when the subject is awake and at complete rest, has not eaten for 14 to 18 hours, and is in a comfortable, warm environment. It is expressed as a basal metabolic rate, according to Calories per hour per square meter of body surface. See also **Calorie (Cal).**

basal narcosis [Gk, *basis,* foundation, *narkosis,* a benumbing], a narcosis induced with sedatives in a surgical patient before general anesthetic is administered. It is less profound than that of general anesthesia. The patient is unresponsive to verbal stimuli but may respond to noxious stimuli. Also called **basis narcosis.**

basaloid carcinoma /bā'səloid/ [Gk, *basis* + *eidos,* form, *karkinos* crab, *oma* tumor], a rare transitional malignant neoplasm of the anal canal containing areas that resemble basal cell carcinoma of the skin. Basaloid carcinoma is rapidly invasive. Tumor may spread to the skin of the perineum.

Basaloid carcinoma *(Fletcher, 2000)*

basaloma. See **basal cell carcinoma.**

basal seat, (in dentistry) the oral structures that support a denture. See also **basal seat outline.**

basal seat area, the portion of the oral structures that is available to support a denture. Also called **denture-bearing area, stress-bearing area.**

basal seat outline, a profile on the oral mucous membrane or on a cast of the entire oral area to be covered by a denture. See also **basal seat.**

basal temperature. See **basal body temperature.**

basal temperature chart [Gk, *basis,* foundation; L, *temperatura* + *charta,* paper], a daily temperature chart, usually including the temperature on awakening. A basal temperature chart is sometimes used by women to establish a date of ovulation, when the temperature may show a sudden increase.

basal tidal volume, the amount of air inhaled and exhaled by a healthy person at complete rest, with all bodily functions at a minimal level of activity, adjusted for age, weight, and sex. See also **tidal volume (TV).**

base [Gk, *basis,* foundation], **1.** a chemical compound that increases the concentration of hydroxide ions in aqueous solution. Compare **alkali. 2.** a molecule or radical that takes up or accepts hydrogen ions. **3.** an electron pair donor. **4.** the major ingredient of a compounded material, particularly one that is used as a medication. Petroleum jelly is frequently used as a base for ointments. **5.** (in radiology) the rigid but flexible foundation of a sheet of x-ray film. The base is essentially transparent but is given a bluish tint during manufacture to reduce eyestrain of the radiologist viewing x-ray films.

base analog [Gk, *basis* + *analogos,* proportionate], a chemical analog of one of the purine or the pyrimidine bases normally found in RNA or DNA.

Basedow's goiter /bä'sədōz/ [Karl A. von Basedow, German physician, 1799–1854], a name for colloid goiter, which is an enlargement of the thyroid gland, characterized by the hypersecretion of thyroid hormone after iodine therapy. The condition causes increased basal metabolic rate, insomnia, and fine motor tremor.

base excess, a measure of metabolic alkalosis or metabolic acidosis (negative value of base excess) expressed as the amount of acid or alkali needed to titrate 1 L of fully oxygenated blood to a pH of 7.40, the temperature being held at a constant 37° C and the PCO_2 at 40 mm Hg.

base-forming food, a food that increases the pH of the urine. Base-forming foods mainly are fruits, vegetables, and dairy products, which are sources of sodium and potassium. Some foods that are acidic in their natural state may be converted to alkaline metabolites.

baseline /bās'līn/ [Gk, *basis* + L, *linea*], **1.** a known value or quantity with which an unknown is compared when measured or assessed. **2.** (in radiology) any of several basic anatomic planes or locations used for positioning purposes. They include the orbitomeatal, infraorbitomeatal, acanthomeatal, and glabellomeatal lines.

baseline behavior, a specified frequency and form of a particular behavior during preexperimental or pretherapeutic conditions.

baseline condition, an environmental condition during which a particular behavior reflects a stable rate of response before the introduction of experimental or therapeutic conditions.

baseline fetal heart rate, the fetal heart rate pattern between uterine contractions. An electronic fetal monitor is used to detect abnormally rapid or slow rates (less than 110 or more than 160 beats/min) at term.

baseline pain, the average intensity of pain experienced for 12 or more hours in a 24-hour period.

basement lamina. See **basal lamina.**

basement membrane [Fr, *soubassement,* under base], the fragile noncellular layer that secures the overlying epithelium to the underlying tissue. It is the deepest layer, may contain reticular fibers, and can be selectively stained with silver stains. Also called **basal lamina, basement lamina.**

base of gastric gland, the main part of a gastric gland interior to the neck.

base of renal pyramid, the part of a renal pyramid that is directed away from the renal sinus.

base of the heart, the portion of the heart opposite the apex. It is superior and medially located. It forms the upper border of the heart, lies just below the second rib, and primarily involves the left atrium, part of the right atrium, and the proximal portions of the great vessels.

base of the skull, the floor of the skull, containing the anterior, middle, and posterior cranial fossae and numerous foramina, such as the optic foramen, foramen ovale, foramen lacerum, and foramen magnum.

base pair, a pair of nucleotides in the complementary strands of a DNA molecule that interact through hydrogen bonding across the axis of the helix. One of the nucleotides in each pair is a purine (either adenine or guanine), and the other is a pyrimidine (either thymine or cytosine). Because of their spatial configuration, adenine always pairs with thymine, and guanine always pairs with cytosine.

base pairing, the formation of base pairs in DNA.

baseplate [Gk, *basis* + ME, *plate*], a temporary form that represents the base of a denture, used for making records of maxillomandibular relationships, for arranging artificial teeth, or for ensuring a precise fit of a denture by trial placement in the mouth. Also called **record base, temporary base.**

baseplate wax, a dental wax containing about 75 percent paraffin or ceresin with additions of beeswax and other waxes and resins; used chiefly to establish the initial arch form in making trial plates for the construction of complete dentures.

base plus fog, the optical density of a processed film in the absence of any radiation exposure.

base ratio, the ratio of the molar quantities of purine and pyrimidine bases in DNA and RNA.

bas-fond /bäfôN′/ [Fr, bottom], the bottom or fundus of any structure, especially the fundus of the urinary bladder.

basi-, basio-, bas-, baso-, prefix meaning "a foundation or a base": *basicranial, basiotribe, basal, basophil.*

-basia /bā′zhə/, suffix meaning "ability to walk": *brachybasia, dysbasia.*

BASIC /bā′sik/, abbreviation for *b*eginner's *a*ll-purpose *s*ymbolic *i*nstruction *c*ode, a computer programming language.

-basic, suffix meaning "relating to or containing alkaline compounds": *ammonobasic, polybasic.*

basic aluminum carbonate gel, an aluminum hydroxide aluminum carbonate gel, used as an antacid, for treatment of hyperphosphatemia in renal insufficiency and to prevent phosphate urinary calculi.

basic amino acid, an amino acid that has a positive electric charge in solution at a pH of 7. The basic amino acids are arginine, histidine, and lysine.

basic group identity, (in psychiatry) the shared social characteristics, such as world view, language, values, and ideologic system, that evolve from membership in an ethnic group.

basic health services, the minimum degree of health care considered to be necessary to maintain adequate health and protection from disease.

basic human needs, the elements required for survival and normal mental and physical health, such as food, water, shelter, protection from environmental threats, and love.

basic life support (BLS) [Gk, *basis,* foundation; AS, *lif* + L, *supportare,* to bring up to], emergency treatment of a victim of cardiac or respiratory arrest through cardiopulmonary resuscitation and emergency cardiac care.

basic salt, a salt that contains an unreplaced hydroxide ion from the base generating it, such as Ca(OH)Cl.

basifacial /bā′sifā′shəl/ [Gk, *basis* + L, *facies,* face], pertaining to the lower portion of the face.

basilar /bas′ilər/ [Gk, *basis,* foundation], pertaining to a base or a basal area.

basilar artery, the single posterior arterial trunk formed by the junction of the two vertebral arteries at the base of the skull. It extends from the inferior to the superior border of

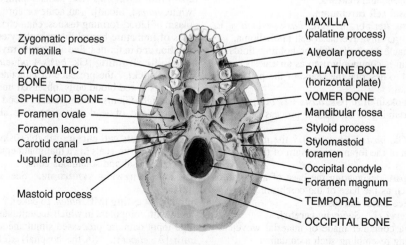

Zygomatic process of maxilla

ZYGOMATIC BONE

SPHENOID BONE

Foramen ovale

Foramen lacerum

Carotid canal

Jugular foramen

Mastoid process

MAXILLA (palatine process)

Alveolar process

PALATINE BONE (horizontal plate)

VOMER BONE

Mandibular fossa

Styloid process

Stylomastoid foramen

Occipital condyle

Foramen magnum

TEMPORAL BONE

OCCIPITAL BONE

Base of the skull *(Applegate, 2000)*

the pons before dividing into the left and right posterior cerebral arteries. It supplies the internal ear and parts of the brain. Its branches are the pontine, labyrinthine, anterior inferior cerebellar, superior cerebellar, and posterior cerebral.

basilar artery insufficiency syndrome, the composite of clinical indicators associated with insufficient blood flow through the basilar artery, a condition that may be caused by arterial occlusion. Common signs of this syndrome include dizziness, blindness, numbness, depression, dysarthria, dysphagia, and weakness on one side of the body.

basilar artery occlusion, an obstruction of the basilar artery, resulting in dysfunction involving cranial nerves III through XII, cerebellar dysfunction, hemiplegia or quadriplegia, and loss of proprioception.

basilar membrane, the cellular structure that forms the floor of the cochlear duct and is supported by bony and fibrous projections from the cochlear wall. It provides a fibrous base for the spiral organ of Corti.

basilar plexus [Gk, *basis* + L, braided], the venous network interlaced between the layers of the dura mater over the basilar portion of the occipital bone. It connects the two petrosal sinuses and communicates with the anterior vertebral venous plexus.

basilar sulcus [Gk, *basis* + L, furrow], the sulcus that cradles the basilar artery in the midline of the pons.

basilar vertebra, the lowest or last of the lumbar vertebrae.

basilic vein /bəsil′ik/, one of the four superficial veins of the arm, beginning in the ulnar part of the dorsal venous network and running proximally on the posterior surface of the ulnar side of the forearm. It is often chosen for blood testing. Compare **dorsal digital vein, median antebrachial vein.**

basiliximab, a monoclonal antibody used for immunosuppression.

■ INDICATIONS: This drug is used in combination with cyclosporine and corticosteroids to treat acute allograft rejection in renal transplant patients.

■ CONTRAINDICATIONS: Known hypersensitivity to this drug contraindicates its use.

■ ADVERSE EFFECTS: Life-threatening effects of this drug include pulmonary edema and cardiac failure. Other adverse effects include hypotension, headache, constipation, abdominal pain, infection, and moniliasis. Common side effects include pyrexia, chills, tremors, dyspnea, wheezing, chest pain, vomiting, nausea, and diarrhea.

basiloma. See **basal cell carcinoma.**

basiloma terebrans /ter′əbrənz/ [Gk, *basis* + *oma* + L, *terebare,* to bore], an invasive basal cell epithelioma.

basin, 1. a receptacle for collecting or holding fluids. A kidney-shaped basin is commonly used as an emesis receptacle. **2.** term used to describe the shape of the pelvis.

basio-. See **basi-.**

basioccipital /bā′si·ok·sip′ətəl/ [Gk, *basis* + L, *occiput,* back of the head], pertaining to the basilar process of the occipital bone.

basion /bā′sē·on/ [Gk, *basis,* foundation], the midpoint on the anterior margin of the foramen magnum of the occipital bone.

basis, the lower part, designating the base of an organ or other structure, such as the base of the cerebrum.

basis narcosis. See **basal narcosis.**

basis pedunculi cerebri. See **crus cerebri.**

basket /bas·ket/, a container made of material woven together, or something resembling such a container.

basket cell [L, *bascauda,* dishpan], deep stellate cells (neu-

rons) of the cerebral cortex with a horizontal axon that sends out branches. Each axon branch or collateral breaks up into a basketlike mesh that surrounds a Purkinje cell.

Basle Nomina Anatomica (BNA), an international system of anatomic terminology adopted at Basel, Switzerland.

basolateral membrane, the layer of plasma membrane of epithelial cells that is adjacent to the basement membrane and separated from the apical membrane by the zonula occludens.

basophil /bā′səfil/ [Gk, *basis* + *philein,* to love], a granulocytic white blood cell characterized by cytoplasmic granules that stain blue when exposed to a basic dye. Basophils represent 1% or less of the total white blood cell count. The relative number of basophils increases in myeloproliferative diseases and decreases in severe allergic reactions. An increase in number is seen during the healing phase of inflammation. Also called **basophilic erythrocyte.** Compare **eosinophil, neutrophil.** See also **agranulocyte, differential white blood cell count, granulocyte, leukocyte, polymorphonuclear leukocyte.**

Basophil *(Carr and Rodak, 1999)*

basophilic adenoma [Gk, *basis* + *philein,* to love, *aden,* gland, *oma*], a tumor of the pituitary gland composed of cells that can be stained with basic dyes. Compare **acidophilic adenoma, chromophobic adenoma.**

basophilic erythrocyte. See **basophil.**

basophilic leukemia [Gk, *basis* + *philein,* to love, *leukos,* white, *haima,* blood], an acute or chronic malignant neoplasm of blood-forming tissues, characterized by large numbers of immature basophilic granulocytes in peripheral circulation and in tissues. See also **acute myelocytic leukemia.**

basophilic stippling [Gk, *basis* + *philein,* to love; D, *stippen,* to prick], the presence of punctate blue nucleic acid remnants in red blood cells, observed under the microscope on a Wright-Giemsa-Gram-stained blood smear. Stippling is characteristic of lead poisoning. See also **basophil, lead poisoning.**

basosquamous cell carcinoma /bā′sōskwā′məs/ [Gk, *basis* + L, *squamosus,* scaly], a malignant epidermal tumor composed of basal and squamous cells.

Bassen-Kornzweig syndrome. See **abetalipoproteinemia.**

batch processing [ME, *baten,* to bake], a processing mode used with computers in which accumulated similar programs and input data are processed simultaneously.

bath [AS, *baeth*], (in the hospital) a cleansing procedure performed by or for patients, as needed for hygienic or ther-

Basophilic stippling *(Carr and Rodak, 1999)*

apeutic purposes, to help prevent infection, preserve the unbroken condition of the skin, stimulate circulation, promote oxygen intake, maintain muscle tone and joint mobility, and provide comfort.

■ METHOD: The bath may be a bed or tub bath, a shower, or a partial bath, depending on the patient's condition and preference and the room temperature. The bath period may be used to instruct the patient on hygienic measures, range of motion exercises, and general measures to promote skin health. Observations are made of the general cleanliness and odor of the patient's body; the color, dryness, turgor, and elasticity and integrity of the skin; and the condition of the hair, hands, joints, feet, fingernails, and toenails. Any discoloration, abrasion, rash, discharge, perineal or rectal irritation, clubbing of the digits, hair loss, or evidence of lice infestation is carefully noted. Mild soap and warm water are used for the bath, and a lanolin-based lotion may be used for an after-bath massage. The patient's hair is combed daily and shampooed as needed; fingernails and toenails are cleaned and trimmed whenever required. The diabetic client may require specialized care of the nails.

■ INTERVENTIONS: The nurse gives the bed bath in a setting that provides privacy for the patient. Firm, gentle strokes are used to wash, dry, and massage the person; vigorous rubbing is avoided. The partial bath is given with the patient seated in or on the side of the bed or in a chair. Self-help is encouraged, and the procedure is completed as quickly as possible to prevent chilling. In preparation for a tub bath, the nurse checks the safety strips in the bottom of the tub and the water temperature and assists the patient into the tub. Precautions are taken to prevent chilling, and on completion of the bath the nurse may help the patient out of the tub. In preparation for a shower, the nurse explains the operation of the dials regulating water temperature and provides a bath mat.

■ OUTCOME CRITERIA: A bath provides an opportunity to assess external signs of disease, effects of therapy, and signs of pressure ulcer development and supports the patient's sense of well-being and self-esteem.

bath blanket, a thin, lightweight cloth used to cover a patient during a bath. It absorbs moisture while keeping the patient warm. See also **blanket bath.**

bathesthesia /bath′əsthē′zhə/ [Gk, *bathys,* deep, *aisthesia,* feeling], sensitivity to deep structures in the body. Also called **bathyesthesia.** /bathē-əs-/.

bathing, a nursing intervention from the Nursing Interventions Classification (NIC) defined as cleaning of the body for the purposes of relaxation, cleanliness, and healing. See also **Nursing Interventions Classification.**

bathmic evolution. See **orthogenic evolution.**

bathy-, batho-, prefix meaning "depth, deep": *bathycentesis, bathomorphic.*

bathyanesthesia /bath′ēan′esthē′zhə/ [Gk, *bathys,* deep, *anaisthesia,* loss of feeling], a loss of deep feeling, such as that associated with organs or structures beneath the body surface, or muscles and joints; a loss of sensitivity to deep structures in the body.

bathycardia /bath′ēkär′dē·ə/ [Gk, *bathys,* deep, *kardia,* heart], a condition in which the heart is located at an abnormally low site in the thorax.

bathyesthesia. See **bathesthesia.**

Batten disease /bat′en/, **1.** Vogt-Spielmeyer disease. **2.** more generally, any or all of the group of disorders constituting neuronal ceroid lipofuscinosis.

Batten's disease [Frederick E. Batten, English opthalmologist neurologist, 1865–1918], a progressive childhood encephalopathy characterized by disturbed metabolism of polyunsaturated fatty acids. It occurs in children between 5 and 10 years of age. The child experiences sudden blindness and progressive mental deterioration. Also called neuronal ceroid lipofuscinosis.

battered baby syndrome. See **child abuse.**

battered woman syndrome (BWS), repeated episodes of physical assault on a woman by the person with whom she lives and with whom she has a relationship, often resulting in serious physical and psychologic damage to the woman. Not limited to live-in mates. Such violence tends to follow a predictable pattern. The violent episodes usually follow verbal argument and accusation and are accompanied by verbal abuse. Almost any subject—housekeeping, money, childrearing—may begin the episode. Over time, the violent episodes escalate in frequency and severity. Most battered women report that they thought that the assaults would stop; unfortunately, studies show that the longer the women stay in the relationship the more likely they are to be seriously injured. Less and less provocation seems to be enough to trigger an attack once the syndrome has begun. The use of alcohol may increase the severity of the assault. The man is more likely to be abusive as the alcohol wears off. Battering occurs in cycles of violence. In the first phase the man acts increasingly irritable, edgy, and tense. Verbal abuse, insults, and criticism increase, and shoves or slaps begin. The second phase is the time of the acute, violent activity. As the tension mounts, the woman becomes unable to placate the man, and she may argue or defend herself. The man uses this as the justification for his anger and assaults her, often saying that he is "teaching her a lesson." The third stage is characterized by apology and remorse on the part of the man, with promises of change. The calm continues until tension builds again. Battered woman syndrome occurs at all socioeconomic levels, and one half to three quarters of female assault victims are the victims of an attack by a lover or husband. It is estimated that in the United States between 1 and 2 million women a year are beaten by their husbands. Men who grew up in homes in which the father abused the mother are more likely to beat their wives than are men who lived in nonviolent homes. Personal and cultural attitudes also affect the incidence of battering. Aggressive behavior is a normal part of male socialization in most cultures; physical aggression may be condoned as a means of resolving a conflict. A personality profile obtained by psychologic testing reveals the typical battered woman to be reserved, withdrawn, depressed, and anxious, with low self-esteem, a poorly integrated self-image, and a general inability to cope with life's demands. The parents of such women encouraged compliance, were not physically affectionate, and socially restricted their daughters' independence, preventing the widening of social contact that normally occurs in adolescence. Victims of the battered woman syndrome are often afraid to leave the man and the situation; change, loneliness, and the unknown are perceived as more painful than the beatings. Nurses are in an excellent position to offer assistance to battered women in several ways, because encouraging a woman to talk about the battering and the injuries may help her to admit what she may have been too embarrassed to reveal even to her parents. A realistic appraisal of the situation is then possible; the woman wants to hear that the nurse thinks the battering will not recur, but the nurse can tell her only that the usual pattern is for the abuse to continue and to become more severe. The woman may be referred to the social service department or given directions for contacting community agencies such as a battered women's shelter or a hotline to a counseling service. Caring for and counseling a battered woman often require great patience because she is usually ambivalent about her situation and may be confused to the point of believing that she deserves the assaults she has suffered. Written and photographic records are maintained to document the extent of the problem, including the form of abuse reported, the injuries sustained, and a summary of similar incidents and previous admissions.

battery [Fr, *batterie*], **1.** a device of two or more electrolytic cells connected to form a single source providing direct current or voltage. **2.** a series or a combination of tests to determine the cause of a particular illness or the degree of proficiency in a particular skill or discipline. **3.** the unlawful use of force on a person. See **assault.**

Battey bacillus /bat′ē/ [Battey Hospital, in Rome, Georgia, where bacteria strain first isolated], any of a group of atypical mycobacteria, including *Mycobacterium avium* and *M. intracellulare,* that cause a chronic pulmonary disease resembling tuberculosis. These organisms are resistant to most of the common bacteriostatic and antibiotic medications but may be treated with multiple drug regimens. Surgical resection of involved lung tissue may be necessary and may improve the outcome in serious cases. Rest, good nutrition, and general supportive care are usually recommended. Compare **tuberculosis.**

battledore placenta /bat′əldôr′/ [ME, *batyldoure,* a beating instrument; L, *placenta,* flat cake], a condition in which the umbilical cord is attached at the margin of the placenta. It rarely occurs and does not affect placental functioning. Also called **placenta battledore.**

Battle's sign [William H. Battle, English surgeon, 1855–1936], a bogginess of the area behind the ear. It may indicate a fracture of a bone of the lower skull.

batyl alcohol /bat′əl/, an alcohol found in fish liver oil that is used to treat bracken poisoning in cattle.

baud /bôd/ [J.M.E. Baudot, French inventor, b. 1845], a measure of data flow or the speed with which a computer device transmits information.

Baudelocque's diameter. See **external conjugate.**

bay, an anatomic depression or recess, usually containing fluid, as the lacrimal bay of the eye.

Bayes' theorem /bāz′/ [Thomas Bayes, British mathematician, 1702–1761], a mathematic statement of the relationships of test sensitivity, specificity, and the predictive value of a positive test result. The predictive value of the test is the number that is useful to the clinician. A positive result demonstrates the conditional probability of the presence of a disease.

Bayley Scales of Infant Development [Nancy Bayley, twentieth century American psychologist], a three-part scale for assessing the development of children between the ages of 2 months and 2-1/2 years. Infants are tested for perception, memory, and vocalization on the mental scale; sitting, stair climbing, and manual manipulation on the mo-

tor scale; and attention span, social behavior, and persistence on the behavioral scale.

Baylisascaris /bā′lis·as′kä·ris/, a genus of nematodes found in the intestines of mammals. *B. columnaris,* infests the central nervous system of dogs. *B. procyonis* is usually found in raccoons and rodents, but fecal contamination from those animals can cause spread to domestic animals and humans, resulting in nervous system infection or larva migrans.

bayonet angle former. See **angle former.**

bayonet condenser [Fr, *baionette*], an instrument used in dentistry for compacting restorative material. It has an offset nib and a shank with right-angle bends, used primarily for varying the line of force in the compaction of gold. There are many variations in angle, length, and diameter of the nib.

BBB, **1.** abbreviation for **bundle branch block. 2.** abbreviation for **blood-brain barrier.**

BBT, abbreviation for **basal body temperature.**

BCAA, abbreviation for **branched-chain amino acids.**

B cell, a type of lymphocyte that originates in the bone marrow. A precursor of the plasma cell, it is one of the two lymphocytes that play a major role in the body's immune response. Compare **T cell.** See also **plasma cell.**

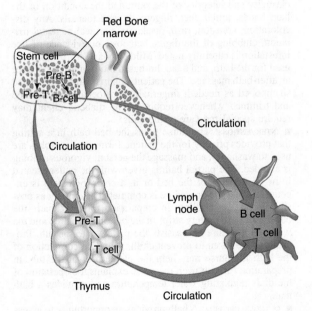

Development of B and T cells *(Thibodeau and Patton, 2003)*

B cell–growth/differentiation factor, one of several substances, such as interleukins IL-4, IL-5, and IL-6, that are derived from T-cell cultures and are necessary for the differentiation, growth, and maturation of plasma cells and B memory cells.

B-cell lymphoma, any in a large group of non-Hodgkin's lymphomas characterized by malignant transformation of the B lymphocytes. See also **non-Hodgkin's lymphoma.**

B cell–mediated immunity, the ability to produce an immune response induced by B lymphocytes. Contact with a foreign antigen stimulates B cells to differentiate into plasma cells, which release antibodies. Plasma cells also generate memory cells, which provide a rapid response if the same antigen is encountered again.

B-cell stimulating factor-1. See **interleukin-4.**

BCG, abbreviation for **bacille Calmette-Guérin.**

BCG solution, an aqueous suspension of bacille Calmette-Guérin for instillation into the bladder to activate the immune system in treatment of superficial bladder cancers. It reduces the risk of a subsequent bladder cancer developing, although the exact mechanism of action is unknown.

BCG vaccine. See **bacille Calmette-Guérin vaccine.**

BCHC diet, abbreviation for **Bristol Cancer Help Center diet.**

BCNU. See **carmustine.**

B complex vitamins, a large group of water-soluble nutrients that includes thiamine (vitamin B_1), cyanocobalamin (vitamin B_{12}), niacin (vitamin B_3), pyridoxine (vitamin B_6), riboflavin (vitamin B_2), biotin, folic acid, and pantothenic acid. The B complex vitamins are essential, for example for the conversion of simple carbohydrates like glucose and the carbon skeletons of amino acids into energy, and for the metabolism of fats and proteins. Good sources include brewer's yeast, liver, whole grain cereals, nuts, eggs, meats, fish, and vegetables. Because some B complex vitamins are produced by intestinal bacteria, taking antibiotics may destroy these bacteria. Symptoms of vitamin B deficiency include nervousness, depression, insomnia, neuritis, anemia, alopecia, acne or other skin disorders, and hypercholesterolemia. See also specific vitamins.

b.d. See **b.i.d.**

B-DNA, a long, thin form of deoxyribonucleic acid in which the helix is right-handed.

Be, symbol for the element **beryllium.**

beaded /bē'did/ [ME, *bede*], **1.** having a resemblance to a row of beads. **2.** pertaining to bacterial colonies that develop along the inoculation line in various stab cultures. **3.** pertaining to stained bacteria that develop more deeply stained beadlike granules.

beak, **1.** any pointed anatomic structure, as the beak of the sphenoid bone. **2.** a pair of dental pincers used in shaping prostheses. **3.** a radiographic image of a bony protuberance adjacent to a degenerative intervertebral disk.

beaker cell. See **goblet cell.**

beak sign, the appearance of abnormal structures on radiographic images of the GI tract: of the distal esophagus in achalasia and of the proximal pyloric canal in pyloric stenosis.

Beals' syndrome /bēlz/ [Rodney Kenneth Beals, American orthopedic surgeon, b. 1931], a congenital type of bone dysplasia with contractures and arachnodactyly. An autosomal dominant syndrome characterized by long thin extremities with arachnodactyly, multiple joint contractures, kyphoscoliosis, and malformed auricles of the ears; it is a form of hereditary bone dysplasia.

beam [ME, *beem*, tree], **1.** a bedframe fitting for pulleys and weights, used in the treatment of patients requiring weight traction. See **Balkan traction frame. 2.** (in radiology) the primary beam of radiation emitted from the x-ray tube.

BEAM /bēm, bē'ē'ā'em'/, abbreviation for **brain electrical activity map.**

beam alignment, in radiography, the process of positioning the radiographic tube head so it is aligned properly with the x-ray film.

beam collimation, the restriction of x-radiation to the area being examined or treated by confining the beam with metal diaphragms or shutters with high radiation-absorption power. In addition to protecting the patient and others from scatter radiation, beam collimation reduces radiographic density.

beam hardening, the process of increasing the average energy level of an x-ray beam by filtering out the low-energy photons.

BE amputation, abbreviation for **below-elbow amputation.**

beam quality, the energy of an x-ray beam.

beam restrictor, a device that reduces scatter radiation from x-ray equipment. Three basic types of restrictors are variable-aperture collimators, cones or cylinders, and aperture diaphragms.

beam splitter, a device that reflects light from the output phosphor of an image intensifier to a photographic recording. Also called *image distributor*.

beam-splitting mirror, a device that allows a radiologist to view a fluoroscopic examination of a patient while the same view is being recorded on film. The mirror can be adjusted to reflect from 10% to 90% of the x-ray beam to the fluorescent screen while the rest is directed to the film.

beam therapy. See **chromotherapy, external beam radiotherapy.**

bean [ME, *bene*], the pod-enclosed flattened seed of numerous leguminous plants. Beans used in pharmacologic preparations are alphabetized by specific name.

bearing down /ber'ing/ [OE, *beran*, to bear, *adune*, down], a voluntary effort by a woman in the second stage of labor to aid in the expulsion of a fetus. By applying the Valsalva maneuver, the mother increases intraabdominal pressure.

bearing down pains [OE, *beran*, to bear, *adune*, down; L, *poena*, penalty], the pains experienced by a woman during the second stage of labor while performing the Valsalva maneuver to help expel the fetus.

beat, the mechanical contraction or electrical activity of the heart muscle, which may be detected and recorded as the pulse or on the electrocardiogram, respectively.

Beau's lines /bōz'/ [Joseph H.S. Beau, French physician, 1806–1865], transverse depressions that appear as white lines across the fingernails as a sign of an acute severe illness such as malnutrition, a systemic disease, trauma, or coronary occlusion.

Beau's lines *(Callen et al, 2000)*

becaplermin /bĕ-kap′ler-min/, a recombinant platelet-derived growth factor used in treatment of chronic severe dermal ulcers of the lower limbs in diabetes mellitus.

Beck depression inventory (BDI). See **Beck's Diagnostic Inventory.**

Becker's muscular dystrophy [Peter E. Becker, German geneticist, b. 1908], a chronic degenerative disease of the muscles, characterized by progressive weakness. It occurs in childhood between 8 and 20 years of age. It occurs less frequently, progresses more slowly, and has a better prognosis than the more common pseudohypertrophic form of muscular dystrophy. The pathophysiologic characteristics of the disease are not understood; it is transmitted genetically as an autosomal recessive trait. Also called **benign pseudohypertrophic muscular dystrophy.** Compare **Duchenne's muscular dystrophy.**

Beck's Diagnostic Inventory (BDI) [Aaron T. Beck, American psychiatrist, b. 1921], a system of classifying a total of 18 criteria of depressive illness. It was developed by A.T. Beck in the 1970s as a diagnostic and therapeutic tool for the treatment of childhood affective disorders. The BDI is similar to the 21-criteria DSM-IV diagnostic system of the 1980s except that the DSM-IV scale includes loss of interest, restlessness, and sulkiness, which are missing from the BDI; the Beck inventory lists somatic complaints and loneliness, which are criteria not included in the DSM-III inventory. Also called **Beck depression inventory (BDI).** See also **DSM.**

Beck's triad [Claude Schaeffer Beck, American surgeon, 1894–1971], a combination of three symptoms that characterize cardiac tamponade: high central venous pressure, low arterial pressure, and a small, quiet heart. Also called acute compression syndrome.

Beckwith's syndrome [John B. Beckwith, American pathologist, b. 1933], a hereditary disorder of unknown cause associated with neonatal hypoglycemia and hyperinsulinism. Clinical manifestations include gigantism, macroglossia, omphalocele or umbilical hernia, visceromegaly, hyperplasia of the kidney and pancreas, and extreme enlargement of the cells of the adrenal cortex. Treatment consists of adequate glucose, diazoxide, and glucocorticoid therapy. Subtotal pancreatectomy is often necessary in cases of beta cell hyperplasia, nesidioblastosis, or beta cell tumor of the pancreas.

Beckwith-Wiedemann syndrome. See **EMG syndrome.**

beclomethasone dipropionate, a glucocorticoid.

■ INDICATION: It is prescribed in a metered-dose inhaler in the maintenance treatment of bronchial asthma as prophylactic therapy and as an aerosol for inhalation to treat chronic rhinitis.

■ CONTRAINDICATIONS: Status asthmaticus, acute asthma, or known hypersensitivity to this drug prohibits its use.

■ ADVERSE EFFECTS: Among the more serious adverse reactions of systemic administration are the symptoms of adrenal insufficiency. Hoarseness, sore throat, and fungal infections of the oropharynx and larynx may occur. Good oral and dental hygiene after each use is requisite.

becquerel (Bq) /bekrel′, bek′ərel′/ [Antoine H. Becquerel, French physicist, 1852–1908], the SI unit of radioactivity, equal to one radioactive decay per second. See also **curie.**

bed [AS, *bedd*], (in anatomy) a supporting matrix of tissue, such as the nailbeds of modified epidermis over which the fingernails and the toenails move as they grow.

bed board, a board that is placed under a mattress to give added support to a patient with back problems.

bedbug [AS, *bedd* + ME, *bugge,* hobgoblin], a blood-sucking arthropod of the species *Cimex lectularius* or the species

C. hemipterus that feeds on humans and other animals. The bedbug can be removed after covering it with petrolatum. The bite, which causes itching, pain, and redness, can be treated with a lotion or cream containing a corticosteroid or other topical antiinflammatory or analgesic preparation.

Bedbug bites *(Callen et al, 2000)*

bed cradle, a frame placed over a bed to prevent sheets or blankets from touching the patient. See also **footboard.**

Bedford finger stall, a removable finger splint that holds the injured and an adjacent finger in a brace or cast. It can be worn for prolonged periods.

Bednar's aphthae /bed′närz/ [Alois Bednar, Austrian pediatrician, 1816–1888], the small, yellowish, slightly elevated ulcerated patches that occur on the posterior portion of the hard palate of infants who place infected objects in their mouths. It is also associated with marasmus. Compare **Epstein's pearls, thrush.**

bed pan, a vessel, made of metal or plastic, used to collect feces and urine of bedridden patients.

bed rest, the restriction of a patient to bed for therapeutic reasons for a prescribed period.

bed rest care, a nursing intervention from the Nursing Interventions Classification (NIC) defined as promotion of comfort and safety and prevention of complications for a patient unable to get out of bed. See also **Nursing Interventions Classification.**

bedridden, describing a person who is unable or unwilling to leave the bed because of illness or injury.

Bed pans (Potter and Perry, 2005)

bedside laboratory testing, a nursing intervention from the Nursing Interventions Classification (NIC) defined as performance of laboratory tests at the bedside or point of care. See also **Nursing Interventions Classification.**

bedside manner, the behavior of a nurse or doctor as perceived by a patient or peers.

bedside thermometer. See **clinical thermometer.**

bedsore. See **pressure ulcer.**

bedwetting. See **enuresis.**

BEE, abbreviation for **basal energy expenditure.**

bee cell pessary. See **pessary.**

beef tapeworm. See *Taenia saginata.*

beef tapeworm infection [OF, *buef,* cow; AS, *taeppe, wyrm*], an infection caused by the tapeworm *Taenia saginata,* transmitted to humans when they eat contaminated beef. The adult worm can live for years in the intestine of humans without causing any symptoms. The infection is rarely found in North America and Western Europe, where beef is carefully inspected before being made available and is often thoroughly cooked before eating, but it is common in other parts of the world. See **tapeworm infection.**

bee sting [AS, *beo + stingan*], an injury caused by the venom of bees, usually accompanied by pain and swelling. The stinger of the honeybee usually remains implanted and should be removed. Pain may be alleviated by application of an ice pack or a paste of sodium bicarbonate and water. Serious reactions may result from multiple stings, stings on some areas of the head, or the injection of venom directly into the circulatory system. In a hypersensitive person, a single bee sting may result in death through anaphylactic shock and airway obstruction. Hypersensitive individuals are encouraged to carry emergency treatment supplies, including epinephrine, with them when the possibility of bee sting exists. Compare **wasp.**

beet sugar, sucrose from sugar beets.

behavior /bihā′vyər/ [ME, *behaven*], **1.** the manner in which a person acts or performs. **2.** any or all of the activities of a person, including physical actions, which are observed directly, and mental activity, which is inferred and interpreted. Kinds of behavior include **abnormal behavior, automatic behavior, invariable behavior,** and **variable behavior.**

behavioral isolation /behā′vyərəl/, social isolation that results from a person's socially unacceptable behavior.

behavioral marital therapy, a form of marital therapy using principles and techniques from behavior therapy; it attempts to alleviate marital distress by increasing positive, pleasant interactions between the members of a couple.

behavioral medicine, a segment of psychosomatic medicine focused on psychological means of influencing physical symptoms, such as biofeedback or relaxation.

behavioral objective, a goal in therapy or research that concerns an act or a specific behavior or pattern of behaviors.

behavioral science, any of the various interrelated disciplines, such as psychiatry, psychology, sociology, and anthropology, that observe and study human activity, including psychologic and emotional development, interpersonal relationships, values, and mores.

behavioral systems model, a conceptual framework describing factors that may affect the stability of a person's behavior. The model examines systems of behavior, not the behavior of an individual at any particular time. In one model, behavior is defined as an integrated response to stimuli. Several subsystems of behavior form the eight human microsystems, which are ingestion, elimination, dependency, sex, achievement, affiliation, aggression, and restoration. Each subsystem comprises several structural components called *imperatives,* which are goal, set, choice, action, and support. The goal of nursing care is to attain, maintain, or restore balance of the subsystems of behavior for the stability of the patient.

behavior disorder, any of a group of antisocial behavior patterns occurring primarily in children and adolescents, such as overaggressiveness, overactivity, destructiveness, cruelty, truancy, lying, disobedience, perverse sexual activity, criminality, alcoholism, and drug addiction. Treatment may include psychotherapy, milieu therapy, medication, and family counseling. See also **antisocial personality disorder.**

behaviorism, a school of psychology founded by John B. Watson that studies and interprets behavior by observing measurable responses to stimuli without reference to consciousness, mental states, or subjective phenomena, such as ideas and emotions. See also **neobehaviorism.**

behaviorist, an advocate of the school of behaviorism.

behavioristic psychology. See **behaviorism.**

behavior management, a nursing intervention from the Nursing Interventions Classification (NIC) defined as helping a patient to manage negative behavior. See also **Nursing Interventions Classification.**

behavior management: overactivity/inattention, a nursing intervention from the Nursing Interventions Classification (NIC) defined as provision of a therapeutic milieu that safely accommodates the patient's attention deficit and/or overactivity while promoting optimal function. See also **Nursing Interventions Classification.**

behavior management: self-harm, a nursing intervention from the Nursing Interventions Classification (NIC) defined as assisting the patient to decrease or eliminate self-mutilating or self-abusive behaviors. See also **Nursing Interventions Classification.**

behavior management: sexual, a nursing intervention from the Nursing Interventions Classification (NIC) defined as delineation and prevention of socially unacceptable sexual behaviors. See also **Nursing Interventions Classification.**

behavior modification[1]. See **behavior therapy.**

behavior modification[2], a nursing intervention from the Nursing Interventions Classification (NIC) defined as promotion of a behavior change. See also **Nursing Interventions Classification.**

behavior modification: social skills, a nursing intervention from the Nursing Interventions Classification (NIC) defined as assisting the patient to develop or improve interpersonal social skills. See also **Nursing Interventions Classification.**

behavior reflex. See **conditioned response.**

behavior therapy, a kind of psychotherapy that attempts to modify observable maladjusted patterns of behavior by substituting a new response or set of responses to a given stimulus. The treatment techniques involve the methods, concepts, and procedures derived from experimental psychology; they include assertiveness training, aversion therapy, contingency management, flooding, modeling, operant conditioning, and systemic desensitization. Also called **behavior modification.** See also **biofeedback.**

behaviour. See **behavior.**

Behçet's disease /bā′sets/ [Hulusi Behçet, Turkish dermatologist, 1889–1948], a rare and severe illness of unknown cause, mostly affecting young males and characterized by severe uveitis and retinal vasculitis. Some other signs are optic atrophy and aphthous lesions of the mouth and the genitals, indicating diffuse vasculitis. Also called Behçet's syndrome.

Behçet's disease conjunctivitis
(Regezi, Sciubba, and Jordan, 2003)

Behla's bodies. See **Plimmer's bodies.**

BEI, abbreviation for **butanol-extractable iodine.**

bejel /bej′əl/ [Ar, *bajal*], a nonvenereal form of syphilis prevalent among children in the Middle East and North Africa, caused by the spirochete *Treponema pallidum* subsp. *endemicum.* It is transmitted by person-to-person contact and by the sharing of drinking and eating utensils. The primary lesion is usually on or near the mouth, appearing as a mucous patch, followed by the development of pimplelike sores on the trunk, arms, and legs. Chronic ulceration of the nose and soft palate occurs in the advanced stages of the infection. Destructive changes in the tissues of the heart, central nervous system, and mouth, often associated with the venereal form of syphilis, rarely develop. Intramuscular injection of penicillin is effective in curing the infection, but if extensive tissue destruction has occurred, scar tissue forms and may be permanently disfiguring.

Békésy audiometry /bek′əsē/ [George von Békésy, Hungarian-American physicist and Nobel laureate, 1899–1972], a type of hearing test in which the subject controls the intensity of the stimulus by pressing a button while listening to a pure tone whose frequency slowly moves through the entire audible range. The intensity diminishes as long as the button is pressed. When the intensity is too low for the

subject to hear the tone, the button is released and the intensity begins to increase. When the subject again hears the tone, the button is again pressed, yielding a zigzag tracing. Continuous and interrupted tones are used, and the tracings of the two are compared. The test may be used to differentiate between hearing losses of cochlear and neural origins.

Bekhterev-Mendel reflex. See **Mendel's reflex.**

bel [Alexander G. Bell, Canadian inventor, 1847–1922], a unit that expresses intensity of sound. It is the logarithm (to the base 10) of the ratio of the power of any specific sound to the power of a reference sound. The most common reference sound has a power of 10^{-16} watts per square centimeter, or the approximate minimum intensity of sound at 1000 cycles per second that is perceptible to the human ear. An increase of 1 bel approximately doubles the intensity or loudness of most sounds. See also **decibel.**

belching. See **eructation.**

belladonna /bel′ədon′ə, belädôn′ä/ [It, fair lady], the dried leaves, roots, and flowering or fruiting tops of *Atropa belladonna,* a common perennial called deadly nightshade, containing the alkaloids hyoscine and hyoscyamine. Hyoscyamine has anticholinergic and antispasmodic properties.

belladonna alkaloids, a group of anticholinergic alkaloids occurring in belladonna *(Atropa belladonna).*

belladonna and atropine poisons [It, *belladonna,* fair lady; Gk, *Atropos,* one of three Fates; L, *potio,* drink], two powerful poisons obtained from solanaceous plants. Atropine, derived from *Atropa belladonna,* blocks the effects of acetylcholine in effector organs supplied by postganglionic cholinergic nerves. Belladonna is obtained from the dried leaves of *Atropa belladonna,* also known as deadly nightshade, or of *Atropa acuminata,* a source of alkaloids that are converted to atropine. Atropine sulfate is commonly used in ophthalmologic applications and as an antispasmodic.

Bell-Magendie law. See **Bell's law.**

bellows murmur /bel′ooz/ [AS, *belg,* bag; L, humming], a blowing sound, such as that of air moving in and out of a bellows.

bellows ventilator, a respiratory care device in which oxygen and other gases are mixed in a mechanism that contracts and expands. The system pressure is increased or decreased in the chamber surrounding the bellows. The gases are moved into the patient circuit when the system pressure increases. As the patient exhales, the bellows contracts and fills again with gases from air and oxygen intakes.

bell-shaped curve, the curve of the probability density function of the normal distribution. Also called **normal curve.**

Bell's law [Charles Bell, Scottish surgeon, 1774–1842], an axiom stating that the anterior spinal nerves contain only motor and the posterior spinal roots are sensory. Also called **Bell-Magendie law, Magendie's law.**

Bell's palsy [Charles Bell, Scottish Surgeon, 1774-1842], a unilateral paralysis of the facial nerve. It results from trauma to the nerve, compression of the nerve by a tumor, or, possibly, an unknown infection. Most frequent infection associated is herpes simplex virus. Any or all branches of the nerve may be affected. The person may not be able to close an eye or control salivation on the affected side. The condition is usually unilateral and can be transient or permanent. Also called **Bell's paralysis.**

Bell's phenomenon [Charles Bell], a sign of peripheral facial paralysis, manifested by the upward and outward rolling of the eyeball when the affected individual tries to close the eyelid. It occurs on the affected side in peripheral facial paralysis.

Bell's spasm [Charles Bell], a convulsive facial tic.

Forehead not wrinkled
Eyeball rolls up, eyelid does not close

Flat nasolabial fold, paralysis of lower face

Bell's palsy *(Lewis, Heitkemper, and Dirksen, 2004)*

belly [AS, *beig*, bag], **1.** the fleshy central bulging portion of a muscle. **2.** Informal term for **abdomen.**

belly button. See **umbilicus.**

belonephobia /bel′ənəfō′bē·ə/ [Gk, *belone*, needle, *phobos*, fear], a morbid fear of sharp-pointed objects, especially needles and pins.

below-elbow (BE) amputation, an amputation of the arm below the elbow.

belt restraint, a device used around the waist to secure a patient on a stretcher or in a chair.

Belt restraint *(Courtesy Medline Industries)*

Benadryl, trademark for a first-generation antihistamine (diphenhydramine hydrochloride).

Benassi method /bənas′ē/, a positioning procedure for producing x-ray images of the liver. With the patient in a prone position so that the liver is closer to the x-ray film, two radiographs are made from the angles of 25 degrees caudad and 10 degrees cephalad.

Bence Jones protein /bens/ [Henry Bence Jones, English physician, 1814–1873], a protein found almost exclusively in the urine of patients with multiple myeloma. The protein constitutes the light chain component of myeloma globulin; it coagulates at temperatures of 45° to 55° C and redissolves completely or partially on boiling. See also **multiple myeloma, protein.**

Bence Jones protein test, a urine test whose positive result most commonly indicates multiple myeloma. The test is used to detect and monitor the treatment and clinical course of multiple myeloma and similar diseases.

bench research, *informal,* (in medicine) any research done in a controlled laboratory setting using nonhuman subjects.

-bendazole, combining form designating a tibendazole-type anthelmintic.

Bender's Visual Motor Gestalt test [Lauretta Bender, American psychiatrist, 1897–1987; L, *visus,* vision, *movere,* to move; Ger, *Gestalt,* form; L, *testum,* crucible], a standard psychologic test in which the subject copies a series of patterns.

bending fracture, a fracture indirectly caused by the bending of an extremity, such as the foot or the big toe.

bendrofluazide. See **bendroflumethiazide.**

bendroflumethiazide /ben′drōfloo′məthī′əzīd/, a diuretic and antihypertensive.

■ INDICATIONS: It is prescribed in the treatment of hypertension and edema.

■ CONTRAINDICATIONS: Anuria or known hypersensitivity to this drug, to other thiazide medication, or to sulfonamide derivatives prohibit its use.

■ ADVERSE EFFECTS: Among the more serious are hypokalemia, hyperglycemia, hyperuricemia, and hypersensitivity reactions.

bends. See **decompression sickness.**

Benedict's qualitative test [Stanley R. Benedict, American biochemist, 1884–1936], a test for sugar in the urine based on the reduction by glucose of cupric ions. Formation of an orange or red precipitate indicates more than 2% sugar (called 4+), yellow indicates 1% to 2% sugar (called 3+), olive green indicates 0.5% to 1% sugar (called 2+), and green indicates less than 0.5% sugar (called 1+). It is not in common use. Also called **Benedict's method.**

Benedict's solution [Stanley R. Benedict], a term referring to two reagents (a qualitative and a quantitative) used in the examination of urine specimens. Both solutions contain cupric sulfate dissolved in a solution of sodium sulfate and sodium citrate in two different concentrations. When the solution is heated, the color of the resulting mixture depends on the concentration of glucose in the urine. See also **Benedict's qualitative test.**

beneficiary /ben′əfish′ərē/, a person or group designated to receive certain profits, benefits, or advantages, as the recipient of a will or insurance policy.

beneficiary member. See **enrollee.**

benefit. See **covered benefit.**

Benemid, trademark for a uricosuric (probenecid).

benign /binīn′/ [L, *benignus,* kind], (of a tumor) non-cancerous and therefore not an immediate threat, even though treatment eventually may be required for health or cosmetic reasons. See also **benign neoplasm.** Compare **malignant.**

benign congenital hypotonia, a condition marked by signs of weakness and floppiness in babies, resulting from nonprogressive weakness of skeletal muscles from birth.

benign cystic nephroma, multilocular cyst of kidney.

benign essential tremor. See **essential tremor.**

benign familial chronic pemphigus [L, *benedicere,* to bless, *familia,* household; Gk, *pemphix,* bubble], a hereditary condition of the skin characterized in the early stages by blisters that break, leaving red, eroded areas followed by crusts. Also called **Hailey-Hailey disease.**

Benign familial chronic pemphigus *(Callen et al, 2000)*

benign familial hematuria, a rare, usually benign disorder characterized by abnormally thin basement membranes of the glomerular capillaries and persistent hematuria; autosomal dominant inheritance is suspected.

benign forgetfulness, a temporary memory block in which some fact from the recent or remote past is forgotten but later recalled.

benign hypertension, a misnomer implying a harmless elevation of blood pressure. Because any sustained elevation of blood pressure may adversely affect health, it is incorrect to refer to the condition as "benign." See also **essential hypertension.**

benign intracranial hypertension. See **pseudotumor cerebri.**

benign juvenile melanoma, a noncancerous pink or fuchsia raised papule with a scaly surface, usually on a cheek. Occurring most commonly in children between 9 and 13 years of age, it may be mistaken for a malignant melanoma. Also called **compound melanocytoma, spindle cell nevus, Spitz nevus.**

Benign juvenile melanoma *(Callen et al, 2000)*

benign lymphocytic meningitis. See **sterile meningitis.**

benign lymphoreticulosis. See **cat-scratch fever.**

benign mesenchymoma [L, *benignare* + Gk, *meso,* middle, *egchyma,* infusion, *oma,* tumor], a benign neoplasm that has two or more definitely recognizable mesenchymal elements in addition to fibrous tissue.

benign migratory glossitis. See **geographic tongue.**

benign mucosal pemphigoid. See **cicatricial pemphigoid.**

benign myalgic encephalomyelitis. See **postviral fatigue syndrome.**

benign neoplasm [L, *benignare* + Gk, *neos,* new, *plasma,* formation], a localized tumor that has a fibrous capsule, limited potential for growth, a regular shape, and cells that are well differentiated. A benign neoplasm does not invade surrounding tissue or metastasize to distant sites. Some kinds of benign neoplasms are **adenoma, fibroma, hemangioma,** and **lipoma.** Also called **benign tumor.** Compare **malignant neoplasm.**

benign nephrosclerosis, a renal disorder marked by arteriolosclerotic (arteriosclerosis affecting mainly the arterioles) lesions in the kidney. It is associated with hypertension.

benign paroxysmal peritonitis. See **familial Mediterranean fever.**

benign paroxysmal positional vertigo, recurrent vertigo and nystagmus occurring when the head is placed in certain positions. It is usually not associated with central nervous system lesions.

■ OBSERVATIONS: A sensation of disorientation in space combined with a sensation of motion accompanied by nystagmus, nausea and/or vomiting, perspiration, pallor, increased salivation, and general malaise. Diagnosis is made by history and clinical exam in conjunction with ENG and positional testing. Audiology, ABR, CT, or MRI may be used to rule out other causes of vertigo.

■ INTERVENTIONS: Treatment is focused on a series of vestibular exercises, including gait training, sets of visual vestibular head and eye movements, Epley maneuvers, Brandt-Daroff maneuvers. If exercises provoke nausea, premedication with antiemetics may be necessary. Surgical plugging of the posterior semicircular canal may be done in individuals with an intractable recurrent pattern of vertigo attacks that are unresponsive to exercise therapy.

■ NURSING CONSIDERATIONS: Nursing care focuses on demonstration and return demonstration of prescribed exercises.

benign prostatic hyperplasia (BPH), nonmalignant, noninflammatory enlargement of the prostate, most common among men over 50 years of age. BPH is usually progressive and may lead to urethral obstruction and to interference with urine flow, urinary frequency, nocturia, dysuria, and urinary tract infections. Treatment may include medication, localized application of heat, balloon dilation, laser vaporization, and microwave hyperthermia. Surgical resection of the enlarged prostate is sometimes necessary. Compare **prostatitis.** See also **prostatectomy.**

benign prostatic hypertrophy. See **benign prostatic hyperplasia.**

benign pseudohypertrophic muscular dystrophy. See **Becker's muscular dystrophy.**

benign stupor, a state of apathy or lethargy, such as occurs in severe depression.

benign thrombocytosis. See **thrombocytosis.**

benign tumor. See **benign neoplasm.**

benne oil. See **sesame oil.**

Benner, Patricia, a nursing theorist who confirmed the levels of skill acquisition in nursing practice in *From Novice* to Expert: Excellence and Power in Clinical Nursing Practice (1984). Benner used systematic descriptions of five stages: novice, advanced beginner, competent, proficient, and expert. Thirty-one competencies emerged from an analysis of actual patient care episodes. From this work seven areas of nursing practice having a number of competencies with similar intents, functions, and meanings developed. They are identified as (1) the helping role, (2) the teaching-coaching function, (3) the diagnostic and patient-monitoring function, (4) effective management of rapidly changing situations, (5) administering and monitoring therapeutic interventions and regimens, (6) monitoring and ensuring the quality of health care practices, and (7) organizational work-role competencies. Benner's work describes nursing practice in the context of what nursing actually is and does rather than from context-free theoretic descriptions.

Bennet's small corpuscle. See **Drysdale's corpuscle.**

Bennett angle [Norman G. Bennett, English dentist, 1870–1947], the angle formed by the sagittal plane and the path of the advancing condyle during lateral mandibular movement, as viewed in the horizontal plane.

Bennett hand tool test, a test used in occupational therapy and prevocational testing to measure hand function and coordination and speed in performance.

Bennett's fracture [Edward H. Bennett, Irish surgeon, 1837–1907], a fracture that runs obliquely through the base of the first metacarpal bone and into the carpometacarpal joint, detaching the greater part of the articular facet. Bennett's fracture may be associated with dorsal subluxation or with dislocation of the first metacarpal.

Benoquin, trademark for a depigmenting agent (monobenzone).

benserazide /ben-ser'ah-zīd/, an inhibitor of the decarboxylation of peripheral levodopa to dopamine, having actions similar to those of carbidopa. When given with levodopa, benserazide produces higher brain concentrations of dopamine with lower doses of levodopa, thus lessening the side effects seen with higher doses. It is used orally in conjunction with levodopa as an antiparkinsonian agent.

bent fracture. See **greenstick fracture.**

bentiromide test, (for pancreatic function) bentiromide is administered orally, and its cleavage into benzoyl-tyrosyl and p-aminobenzoic acid is monitored as a measure of pancreatic production of chymotrypsin.

bentonite [Fort Benton, Montana], colloidal, hydrated aluminum silicate that, when added to water, swells to approximately 12 times its dry size. It is used as a bulk laxative and as a base for skin care preparations. Also called **mineral soap.**

bentonite test, a flocculation test for the presence of rheumatoid factor in patient blood samples. After sensitized bentonite particles are added to the serum, the test result is considered positive for rheumatoid arthritis if adsorption has occurred with 50% of the particles.

bentoquatam /ben'to-kwah'tam/, a topical skin protectant used to prevent or reduce allergic contact dermatitis from contact with poison ivy, oak, and sumac.

Bentyl, trademark for an anticholinergic antispasmodic (dicyclomine hydrochloride).

benz, abbreviation for a benzoate carboxylate anion.

benzalkonium chloride, a disinfectant and fungicide prepared in an aqueous solution in various strengths.

benzathine penicillin G. See **penicillin G benzathine.**

benzene /ben'zēn/, a colorless, highly flammable liquid hydrocarbon (C_6H_6) derived by fractional distillation of coal tar. The prototypical aromatic compound, it is used in the production of various organic compounds, including pharmaceuticals.

benzene poisoning, a toxic condition caused by ingestion of benzene, inhalation of benzene fumes, or exposure to benzene-related products such as toluene or xylene, characterized by nausea, headache, dizziness, and incoordination. In acute cases respiratory failure or ventricular fibrillation may cause death. Chronic exposure may result in aplastic anemia (a form of leukemia). See also **nitrobenzene poisoning.**

benzethonium chloride /ben'zəthō'nē-əm/, a topical antiinfective used for disinfecting the skin and for treating some infections of the eye, nose, and throat. It is also used as a preservative in some pharmaceutical preparations.

benzhexol hydrochloride. See **trihexyphenidyl hydrochloride.**

benzo[a]pyrene dihydrodiol epoxide (BPDE-I), a carcinogenic derivative of benzo[a]pyrene associated with tobacco smoke.

benzocaine /ben'zəkān/, an ester-type, local anesthetic agent derived from aminobenzoic acid that is most useful when applied topically. It is used in many over-the-counter compounds for pruritus and pain. Benzocaine has a low incidence of toxicity, but sensitization to it may result from prolonged or frequent use. Topical application of benzocaine may cause methemoglobinemia in infants and small children. A minimum of 5% benzocaine is required in a compound to be effective.

benzodiazepine derivative /ben'zōdī-az'əpin/, one of a group of psychotropic agents, including the tranquilizers chlordiazepoxide, diazepam, oxazepam, lorazepam, and chlorazepate, prescribed to alleviate anxiety, and the hypnotics flurazepam and triazolam, prescribed in the treatment of insomnia. Tolerance and physical dependence occur with prolonged high dosage. Withdrawal symptoms, including seizures, may follow abrupt discontinuation. Adverse reactions to the benzodiazepines include drowsiness, ataxia, and a paradoxic increase in aggression and hostility; these reactions are not common with the usual recommended dosage.

benzoic acid /benzō'ik/, a keratolytic agent, usually used with salicylic acid as an ointment in the treatment of athlete's foot and ringworm of the scalp. It has little antifungal action but makes deep infections accessible to more potent preparation. Mild irritation may occur at the site of application.

benzonatate /benzō'nətāt/, a nonopiate antitussive.
■ INDICATION: It is prescribed to suppress the cough reflex.
■ CONTRAINDICATION: Known hypersensitivity to this drug prohibits its use.
■ ADVERSE EFFECTS: Hypersensitivity reactions, such as bronchospasm, laryngospasm, and cardiovascular collapse, may occur and may be serious. Vertigo, sedation, headache, and constipation may sometimes occur.

benzoyl peroxide /benzō'il/, an antibacterial, keratolytic drying agent.
■ INDICATION: It is prescribed in the treatment of acne.
■ CONTRAINDICATIONS: Known hypersensitivity to this drug prohibits its use. It is not used in the eye, on inflamed skin, or on mucous membranes.
■ ADVERSE EFFECTS: Among the more serious adverse reactions are excessive drying and allergic contact sensitization.

benzquinamide /benzkwin'əmīd/, an antiemetic.
■ INDICATIONS: It is prescribed in the treatment of postoperative nausea and vomiting.
■ CONTRAINDICATIONS: Known hypersensitivity to this drug prohibits its use. It is not usually administered to children or to pregnant women.

■ ADVERSE EFFECTS: Among the most serious adverse reactions are sudden increase in blood pressure and cardiac arrhythmia. Drowsiness, chills, and shivering are commonly noted.

benzthiazide /benzthī'əzid/, a diuretic and antihypertensive.

■ INDICATIONS: It is prescribed in the treatment of hypertension and edema.

■ CONTRAINDICATIONS: Anuria or known hypersensitivity to this drug, to other thiazide medication, or to sulfonamide derivatives prohibits its use.

■ ADVERSE EFFECTS: Among the more serious adverse effects are hypokalemia, hyperglycemia, hyperuricemia, and hypersensitivity reactions.

benztropine mesylate /benztrō'pēn/, an anticholinergic and antihistaminic agent.

■ INDICATIONS: It may be prescribed as adjunctive therapy in the treatment of all forms of parkinsonism.

■ CONTRAINDICATIONS: Known sensitivity to this drug prohibits its use, and it is not administered to children less than 3 years of age.

■ ADVERSE EFFECTS: Among the most serious adverse reactions are blurred vision, xerostomia, nausea and vomiting, constipation, depression, and skin rash.

benzyl alcohol /ben'zil/, a clear, colorless, oily liquid, derived from certain balsams, used as a topical anesthetic and as a bacteriostatic agent in solutions for injection. Also called **phenyl carbinol, phenyl methanol.**

benzyl benzoate /benzō'āt/, a clear, oily liquid with a pleasant, pervasive aroma. It is used as an agent to destroy lice and scabies, as a solvent, and as a flavor for gum.

benzyl carbinol. See **phenylethyl alcohol.**

bepridil /bep'rĭ-dil/, a calcium channel blocking agent used orally as the hydrochloride salt in treatment of chronic angina pectoris.

beractant /ber-ak'tant/, a substance obtained from bovine lungs, containing mostly phospholipids; it mimics the action of human pulmonary surfactant and is used in prevention and treatment of respiratory distress syndrome of the newborn. Administered by endotracheal intubation.

Berdon syndrome, megacystis-microcolon-intestinal hypoperistalsis.

bereavement /bərēv'mənt/ [ME, *bereven,* to rob], a form of grief with anxiety symptoms that is a common reaction to the loss of a loved one. It may be accompanied by insomnia, hyperactivity, and other effects. Although bereavement does not necessarily lead to depressive illness, it may be a triggering factor in a person who is otherwise vulnerable to depression. See also **grief, mourning.**

Berger's disease [Jean Berger, twentieth century French nephrologist], a kidney disorder characterized by recurrent episodes of macroscopic hematuria, proteinuria, and a granular deposition of immunoglobulin A (IgA) from the glomerular mesangium. The condition may or may not progress to renal failure over a period of many years. A spontaneous remission occurs in some cases. The onset of disease is usually in childhood or early adulthood, and males are affected twice as often as females. Treatment is similar to that of other renal diseases. Also called **mesangial IgA nephropathy** /mesan'jē·əl/.

Berger's paresthesia [Oskar Berger, nineteenth century German neurologist; Gk, *para,* near, *aisthesia,* sensation], a condition of tingling, prickliness, or weakness and a loss of feeling in the legs without evidence of organic disease. The condition affects young people.

Berger wave. See **alpha wave.**

Bergonié-Tribondeau law /ber'gônē'tribôdō'/ [Jean A. Ber-

gonié, French radiologist, 1857–1925; Louis F.A. Tribondeau, French physician, 1872–1918], a rule stating that the radiosensitivity of a tissue depends on the number of undifferentiated cells in the tissue, their mitotic activity, and the length of time they are actively proliferating.

beriberi /ber'ēber'ē/ [Sinhalese, *beri,* weakness], a disease of the peripheral nerves caused by a deficiency of or an inability to assimilate thiamine. It frequently results from a diet limited to polished white rice, and it occurs in endemic form in eastern and southern Asia. Rare cases in the United States are associated with stressful conditions, such as hypothyroidism, infections, pregnancy, lactation, and chronic alcoholism. Symptoms are fatigue, diarrhea, appetite and weight loss, disturbed nerve function causing paralysis and wasting of limbs, edema, and heart failure. Kinds of beriberi include alcoholic beriberi, atrophic beriberi, cardiac beriberi, and cerebral beriberi. Administration of thiamine prevents and cures most cases of the disease. Also called **athiaminosis.** See also **thiamine.**

Cardiac beriberi *(McLaren, 1992)*

berkelium (Bk) /burk'lē·əm/ [Berkeley, California], an artificial radioactive transuranic element. Its atomic number is 97; the atomic mass of its longest-lived isotope is 247.

berlock dermatitis [Fr, *breloque,* bracelet charm], a temporary skin condition, characterized by hyperpigmentation and skin lesions. It is caused by a unique reaction to psoralen-type photosynthesizers, commonly used in perfumes, colognes, and pomades, such as oil of bergamot. Also spelled **berloque dermatitis.**

■ OBSERVATIONS: Berlock dermatitis commonly produces an acute erythematous reaction, similar to that associated with sunburn. The area affected becomes hyperpigmented and surrounded by darker pigmentation. Areas of the neck where perfume containing oil of bergamot is applied often become affected by pendantlike lesions. Diagnosis is based on the appearance of such signs and on patient history, which may include recent exposure to psoralens.

■ INTERVENTIONS: Treatment seeks to identify and eliminate the cause of the condition. Topical steroids may be administered to relieve discomfort.

■ NURSING CONSIDERATIONS: Patients benefit from advice about the complications of prolonged exposure to sunlight and ultraviolet light. They also appreciate the reassurance that the lesions will vanish within a few months.

Berlock dermatitis *(Callen et al, 2000)*

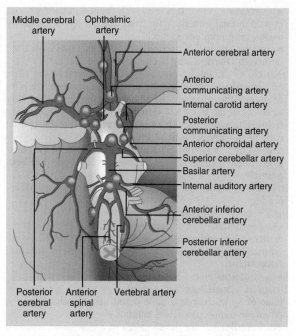

Middle cerebral artery
Ophthalmic artery
Anterior cerebral artery
Anterior communicating artery
Internal carotid artery
Posterior communicating artery
Anterior choroidal artery
Superior cerebellar artery
Basilar artery
Internal auditory artery
Anterior inferior cerebellar artery
Posterior inferior cerebellar artery
Posterior cerebral artery
Anterior spinal artery
Vertebral artery

Berry aneurysm *(Goldman et al, 2004)*

Bernard-Soulier syndrome /bernär′sōōlyā′/ [Jean A. Bernard, French hematologist, b. 1907; Jean-Pierre Soulier, French hematologist, b. 1915], a coagulation disorder characterized by an absence of or a deficiency in the ability of the platelets to aggregate because of the relative lack of an essential glycoprotein in their membranes. On microscopic examination the platelets appear large and dispersed. The use of aspirin may provoke hemorrhage. After trauma or surgery, loss of blood may be greater than normal and a transfusion may be required.

Bernoulli's principle /bərnōō′lēz/ [Daniel Bernoulli, Swiss scientist, 1700–1782], (in physics) the principle stating that the sum of the velocity and the kinetic energy of a fluid flowing through a tube is constant. The greater the velocity, the less the lateral pressure on the wall of the tube. Thus, if an artery is narrowed by an atherosclerotic plaque, the flow of blood through the constriction increases in velocity and decreases in lateral pressure. Also called **Bernoulli's law.**

Bernoulli theorem /bər·nōō′lē/, in an experiment involving probability, the larger the number of trials, the closer the observed probability of an event approaches its theoretical probability.

berry aneurysm [ME, *berye* + Gk, *aneurysma,* widening], a small, saccular dilation of the wall of a cerebral artery. It occurs most frequently at the junctures of vessels in the circle of Willis. A berry aneurysm may be the result of a congenital developmental defect and may rupture without warning, causing intracranial hemorrhage. Smoking and hypertension increase the likelihood of rupture.

Bertel method /bur′təl/, a positioning procedure for producing x-ray images of the inferior orbital fissures. The central x-ray beam is directed through the nasion at an angle of 20 to 25 degrees cephalad.

Bertin's column hypertrophy, congenital enlargement of renal columns (columns of Bertin), a benign condition sometimes mistaken for a renal tumor. Also called *renal column h.*

berylliosis /bəril′ē·ō′sis/, poisoning that results from the inhalation of dusts or vapors containing beryllium or beryllium compounds. The substance also may enter the body through or under the skin. It is characterized by granulomas throughout the body and by diffuse pulmonary fibrosis, resulting in a dry cough, shortness of breath, and chest pain. Symptoms may not appear for several years after exposure. See also **inorganic dust.**

beryllium (Be), a steel-gray, lightweight metallic element. Its atomic number is 4; its atomic mass is 9.012. Beryllium occurs naturally as beryl and is used in metallic alloys and in fluorescent powders. Inhalation of beryllium fumes or particles may cause the formation of granulomas in the lungs, skin, and subcutaneous tissues. See also **berylliosis.**

bestiality /bes′chē·al′itē/ [L, *bestia,* beast], **1.** a brutal or animal-like character or nature. **2.** conduct or behavior characterized by beastlike appetites or instincts. **3.** also called **zooerastia.** sexual relations between a human being and an animal. **4.** sodomy. See also **zoophilia.**

besylate, a contraction for benzenesulfonate.

beta /bē′tə, bā′tə/, B, β, the second letter of the Greek alphabet, used in scientific notation to denote position of a carbon atom in a molecule, a type of protein configuration, or identification of a type of activity, as beta blocker, beta particle, or beta rhythm. It is used in statistics to define an error in the interpretation of study results.

beta-adrenergic antagonist, beta-adrenergic blocking agent.

beta-adrenergic blocking agent. See **antiadrenergic.**

beta-adrenergic receptor. See **beta receptor.**

beta-adrenergic stimulating agent. See **adrenergic.**

beta-alaninemia /-al′əninē′mē·ə/, an inherited metabolic disorder marked by a deficiency of an enzyme, beta-alanine-alpha-ketoglutarate aminotransferase. The clinical signs include seizures, drowsiness, and, if uncorrected, death. The condition is sometimes treated with vitamin B_6 (pyridoxine).

beta-blocker, a popular term for beta-adrenergic blocking (or beta receptor antagonist) agent. See **antiadrenergic.**

beta-carotene [Gk, beta; L, *carota,* carrot], a vitamin A precursor and ultraviolet screening agent.

■ INDICATION: It is prescribed to ameliorate photosensitivity in patients with erythropoietic protoporphyria.

■ CONTRAINDICATIONS: It is used with caution in patients with impaired renal or hepatic function. Known hypersensitivity to this drug prohibits its use.

■ ADVERSE EFFECTS: No serious adverse reactions have been observed. Diarrhea may occur.

beta cells, 1. insulin-producing cells situated in the islets of Langerhans. Their insulin-producing function tends to accelerate the movement of glucose, amino acids, and fatty acids out of the blood and into the cellular cytoplasm, countering glucagon function of alpha cells. 2. the basophilic cells of the anterior lobe of the pituitary gland.

beta decay, a type of radioactivity that results in the emission of beta particles, either electrons or positrons. See **beta particle.**

Betadine, trademark for a topical antiinfective (povidone-iodine).

beta error. See **type II error.**

beta-fetoprotein, a protein found in fetal liver and in some adults with liver disease. It is now known to be identical with normal liver ferritin. See also **alpha-fetoprotein, ferritin, fetoprotein.**

beta-galactosidase. See **lactase.**

Betagan, trademark for a topical glaucoma drug (levobunolol hydrochloride); same brand name is also used for povidone-iodine germicidal solutions.

beta hemolysis, the development of a clear zone around a bacterial colony growing on blood agar medium, characteristic of certain pathogenic bacteria. Compare **alpha hemolysis.**

beta-hemolytic streptococci, the pyogenic streptococci of groups A, B, C, E, F, G, H, K, L, M, and O that cause hemolysis of red blood cells in blood agar in the laboratory. These organisms cause most of the acute streptococcal infections seen in humans, including scarlet fever, many cases of pneumonia and sepsis syndrome, and streptococcal sore throat. Penicillin is usually prescribed to treat these infections when they are suspected, even before the results of the bacteriologic culture are available, because it is known that these organisms as a group are usually sensitive to the effects of penicillin and because the sequelae of untreated streptococcal infection may include glomerulonephritis and rheumatic fever.

betahistine /ba′tah-his′tēn/, a histamine analogue used as the hydrochloride salt and as a vasodilator to reduce the frequency of attacks of vertigo in Meniere's disease, especially in patients having a high frequency of such attacks; administered orally.

17β-hydroxycorticosterone, cortisol.

beta-hydroxyisovaleric aciduria, an inherited metabolic disease caused by a deficiency of an enzyme needed to metabolize the amino acid leucine. The condition results in an accumulation of leucine in the tissues, causing maple sugar odor to the urine, ketoacidosis, retardation, and muscle atrophy. See also **maple syrup urine disease.**

beta₂-interferon. See **interleukin-6.**

beta-ketobutyric acid. See **acetoacetic acid.**

beta-lactam antibiotic, any of a group of antibiotics, including the cephalosporins and the penicillins, whose chemical structure contains a β-lactam ring.

beta-lactamase /-lak′təmāz/ [*lactam,* a cyclic amide, *ase,* enzyme], a bacterial enzyme that catalyzes the hydrolysis of the beta-lactam ring of some penicillins and cephalosporins, producing penicilloic acid and rendering the antibiotic ineffective. Also called **cephalosporinase, penicillinase.**

beta-lactamase resistance. See **beta-lactamase-resistant antibiotics.**

beta-lactamase-resistant antibiotics, antibiotics that are resistant to the enzymatic effects of **beta-lactamase.**

beta-lactamase-resistant penicillin. See **beta-lactamase-resistant antibiotics.**

betamethasone, a glucocorticoid.

■ INDICATION: It is prescribed for topical corticosteroid-responsive dermatoses and injected directly into lesions (bursitis, rheumatoid arthritis, etc.) to help control pain and inflammation.

■ CONTRAINDICATIONS: Systemic fungal infections, dermatologic viral and fungal infections, impaired circulation, or known hypersensitivity to this drug prohibits its use.

■ ADVERSE EFFECTS: Among the more serious adverse reactions associated with prolonged use of the drug are GI, endocrine, neurologic, and fluid and electrolyte disturbances.

beta-naphthylamine /-nafthil′əmēn/, an aromatic amine used in aniline dyes and a cause of bladder cancer in humans.

beta-oxidation, a catabolic process in which fatty acids are used by the body as a source of energy. The fatty acid molecules are converted through a series of intermediates into acetylcoenzyme A molecules, which then enter the tricarboxylic acid (TCA) cycle along with metabolites of carbohydrates and proteins.

Betapar, trademark for a glucocorticoid (meprednisone).

beta particle, an electron emitted from the nucleus of an atom during radioactive decay of the atom. Beta particles have a range of 10 m in air and 1 mm in soft tissue. Also called **beta ray.**

Betapen-VK, trademark for an antibiotic (penicillin V potassium).

beta phase, the period immediately following the alpha, or redistribution, phase of drug administration. During the beta phase the blood level of the drug falls more slowly as it is metabolized and excreted from the body.

beta rays, a stream of beta particles, as emitted from atoms of disintegrating radioactive elements. Normally, when the element is a nuclide with a high ratio of neutrons to protons, the beta particle is an electron.

beta receptor, any one of the postulated adrenergic (sympathetic fibers of autonomic nervous system) components of receptor tissues that respond to epinephrine and such blocking agents as propranolol. Activation of beta receptors causes various physiologic reactions such as relaxation of the bronchial muscles and an increase in the rate and force of cardiac contraction. Also called **beta-adrenergic receptor.** Compare **alpha receptor.**

beta rhythm. See **beta wave.**

beta-thalassemia, an anemia that is caused by diminished synthesis of beta chains of hemoglobin. The homozygous form is known as thalassemia major and the heterozygous form is known as thalassemia minor. See **thalassemia.**

betatron /bā′tətron/, a cyclic accelerator that produces high-energy electrons for radiotherapy. The magnetic field of the betatron deflects electrons into a circular orbit, and an increasing magnetic orbital flux produces an induced circumferential electric field that accelerates them.

beta wave, one of the four types of brain waves, characterized by relatively low voltage and a frequency of more than 13 Hz. Beta waves are the "busy waves" of the brain, recorded by electroencephalograph from the frontal and the central areas of the cerebrum when the patient is awake and alert with eyes open. Also called **beta rhythm.** Compare **alpha wave, delta wave, theta wave.**

betaxolol hydrochloride /betak′səlol/, a topical drug for open-angle glaucoma (Betoptic). An oral preparation (Kerlone) is indicated for the management of hypertension.

■ INDICATIONS: It is prescribed for the relief of ocular hypertension and chronic open-angle glaucoma (ophthalmic) and for the management of hypertension (oral).

■ CONTRAINDICATIONS: Betaxolol hydrochloride is contraindicated in patients with sinus bradycardia, greater than first-degree atrioventricular (AV) block, cardiogenic shock, and overt heart failure. The ophthalmic preparation is used with caution by patients who are also receiving oral beta-adrenergic blocking drugs.

■ ADVERSE EFFECTS: Adverse reactions include stinging and tearing of the eyes. Systemic effects are rare. Adverse effects of the oral preparation are bradycardia, fatigue, dyspnea, and lethargy.

bethanechol chloride /bethan′əkol/, a cholinergic.

■ INDICATIONS: It is prescribed in the treatment of fecal and urinary retention and neurogenic atony of the bladder.

■ CONTRAINDICATIONS: Uncertain strength of the bladder, obstruction of the GI or urinary tract, hyperthyroidism, peptic ulcer, bronchial asthma, cardiovascular disease, epilepsy, Parkinson's disease, hypotension, or known hypersensitivity to this drug prohibits its use. It is not given during pregnancy. It is never given intramuscularly or intravenously.

■ ADVERSE EFFECTS: Among the more serious adverse reactions are flushing, headache, GI distress, diarrhea, excessive salivation, sweating, and hypotension.

Betopic, trademark for a topical glaucoma medication (betaxolol hydrochloride).

Betz cells [Vladimir A. Betz, Russian anatomist, 1834–1894; L, *cella,* storeroom], large pyramidal neurons of the motor cortex with axons that form part of the pyramidal tract associated with voluntary movements.

bevel /bev′əl/ [OFr, *baif,* open mouth angle], 1. any angle, other than a right angle, between two planes or surfaces. 2. (in dentistry) any angle other than 90 degrees between a tooth cut and a cavity wall in the preparation of a tooth cavity. Compare **cavosurface bevel, contra bevel.**

bexarotene, a second-generation retinoid.

■ INDICATIONS: This drug is prescribed for cutaneous T-cell lymphoma. Investigational uses include treatment of breast cancer.

■ CONTRAINDICATIONS: Pregnancy and known hypersensitivity to retinoids prohibit bexarotene's use.

■ ADVERSE EFFECTS: Life-threatening adverse reactions include acute pancreatitis, leukopenia, and neutropenia. Other serious side effects include asthenia, infection, anemia, and hypothyroidism. Among the drug's common side effects are headache, nausea, abdominal pain, and diarrhea.

bezoar /bē′zôr/ [Ar, *bazahr,* protection against poison], a hard ball of hair or vegetable fiber that may develop within the stomach of humans. More often it is found in the stomachs of ruminants. In some societies it was formerly considered a useful medicine and possessed of certain magical properties. It is apparently still used as a therapeutic and mystical device by some, especially in the Far East.

B/F, abbreviation for *black female,* often used in the initial identifying statement in a patient record.

Bg blood group, a blood group consisting of the erythrocytic HLA antigens Bg[a], Bg[b], Bg[c], DBG, Ho, Ho-like, Ot, and Sto.

Bh, symbol for the element **Bohrium.**

bhang /bang/ [Hindi, *bag*], an Asian Indian hallucinogenic, composed of dried leaves and the young stems of uncultivated *Cannabis sativa.* It is usually ingested as a boiled mixture with milk, sugar, or water; it produces euphoria. It also may be smoked or chewed. Also spelled **bang.** See also **cannabis.**

BHC, benzene hexachloride.

Bezoar *(Kumar, Abbas, and Fausto, 2005)*

Bi, symbol for the element **bismuth.**

bi-, prefix meaning "twice, two": *biarticular, bicaudal.*

BIA, abbreviation for **bioelectric impedance analysis.**

-bia, suffix meaning "creature possessing a mode of life": *aerobia.*

biarticular. See **diarticular.**

bias /bī′əs/ [MFr, *biais*], 1. an oblique or a diagonal line. 2. a prejudiced or subjective attitude. 3. (in statistics) the distortion of statistical findings. There can be many kinds of bias; some may be caused by the sampling process, but bias can be caused by other factors. 4. (in electronics) a voltage applied to an electronic device, such as a vacuum tube or a transistor, to control operating limits. See also **detection bias.**

biased sample /bī′əst/ [OFr, *biais,* slant; L, *exemplum,* sample], (in research) a sample of a group in which all factors or participants are not equally balanced or objectively represented.

biasing /bī′əsing/, a method of treating neuromuscular dysfunction by contracting a muscle against resistance, causing the muscle spindles to readjust to the shorter length and the muscle tissue to be more responsive and sensitive to stretching.

biauricular /bī′aw·rik′yōō·lər/ [L, *bis,* twice + *auriculus,* little ear], pertaining to the two auricles of the ears. Also called **binauricular.**

Biavax, trademark for a rubella and mumps vaccine.

bibliotherapy[1], a type of group therapy in which books, poems, and newspaper articles are read in the group to help stimulate thinking about events in the real world and to foster relations among group members.

bibliotherapy[2], a nursing intervention from the Nursing Interventions Classification (NIC) defined as use of literature to enhance the expression of feelings and the gaining of insight. See also **Nursing Interventions Classification.**

bicalutamide, an anticancer chemotherapy agent.

■ INDICATIONS: It is prescribed in the treatment of metastatic prostate cancer. The drug acts by binding to androgen receptors within target cells, preventing androgens from binding to them.

■ CONTRAINDICATIONS: The drug should not be given to patients who have an allergic reaction to it. Bicalutamide should be used with caution in patients with moderate to severe liver dysfunction.

■ ADVERSE EFFECTS: The side effects most often reported include hot flashes, general body pain, asthenia, constipation, nausea, and diarrhea.

bicameral /bī′·kam′ər·əl/ [L, *bis,* twice + *camera,* vaulted chamber], having two chambers.

bicameral abscess /bīkam′ərəl/, an abscess with two pockets.

bicapsular /bī·kap′syoo·lər/ [L, *bis*, twice + *capsula*, little box], having two capsules, as an articular capsule.

bicarbonate (HCO₃⁻) /bīkär′bənāt/ [L, *bis*, twice, *carbo*, coal], an anion of carbonic acid in which only one of the hydrogen atoms has been removed, as in sodium bicarbonate (NaHCO₃). It is also called hydrogencarbonate.

bicarbonate of soda. See **sodium bicarbonate.**

bicarbonate precursor, an injection of sodium lactate used in the treatment of metabolic acidosis. It is metabolized in the body to sodium bicarbonate.

bicarbonate therapy, a procedure to increase a patient's stores of bicarbonate when there are signs of severe acidosis. It is usually performed only in certain cases and as a stopgap measure to neutralize acidosis partially when the patient's blood pH has fallen to levels that may be hazardous to the survival of vital tissues.

bicarbonate transport, the route by which most of the carbon dioxide is carried in the bloodstream. Once dissolved in the blood plasma, carbon dioxide combines with water to form carbonic acid, which immediately ionizes into hydrogen and bicarbonate ions. The bicarbonate ions serve as part of the alkaline reserve.

bicellular /bī·sel′yoo·lər/ [L, *bis*, twice + *cella*, storeroom], made up of two cells, or having two cells.

biceps brachii /bī′seps brā′kē·ī/ [L, *bis*, twice, *caput*, head, *bracchii*, arm], the long fusiform muscle of the upper arm on the anterior surface of the humerus, arising in two heads from the scapula. It flexes the arm and the forearm and supinates the hand. Also called **biceps, biceps flexor cubiti.** Compare **brachialis, triceps brachii.**

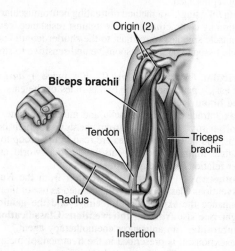

Biceps brachii *(Herlihy and Maebius, 2003)*

biceps femoris [L, *bis*, twice, *caput*, head, *femoris*, thigh], one of the posterior femoral muscles. It has two heads at its origin. The biceps femoris flexes the leg and rotates it laterally and extends the thigh, rotating it laterally. It is one of the **hamstring muscle** group and lies on the posterior, lateral side of the thigh.

Biceps femoris

biceps flexor cubiti. See **biceps brachii.**

biceps reflex, a contraction of a biceps muscle produced when the tendon is tapped with a percussor in testing deep tendon reflexes. See also **deep tendon reflex.**

Biceps reflex testing *(Seidel et al, 2003)*

Bichat's membrane /bishäz′/ [Marie F.X. Bichat, French anatomist, 1771–1802], an elastic lining beneath the endothelium of an arterial wall.

Bicillin C-R /bi-sil′in/, trademark for combination preparations of the antibiotics penicillin G benzathine and penicillin G procaine.

bicipital groove /bīsip′ətəl/ [L, *bis*, twice, *caput*, head; D, *groeve*], a groove between the greater and lesser tubercles of the humerus for passage of the tendon of the long head of the biceps muscle.

Bickerdyke /bik′ərdīk/, **Mary Ann** (1817–1901), an American nurse who, after taking a short course in homeopathy, cared for the sick and wounded on battlefields during the U.S. Civil War. She insisted on cleanliness, good food, and the best of medical care for her patients. At night she searched the battlefield with a lantern for survivors.

biclor /bī′klôr/, abbreviation for *two chloride anions* in a salt.

biconcave /bīkon′kāv/ [L, *bis,* twice, *concavare,* to make hollow], concave on both sides, especially as applied to a lens. —**biconcavity,** *n.*

biconvex /bīkon′veks/ [L, *bis* + *convexus,* vaulted], convex on both sides, especially as applied to a lens. —**biconvexity,** *n.*

bicornate /bīkôr′nāt/ [L, *bis* + *cornu,* horn], having two horns or processes.

bicornate uterus, an abnormal uterus that may be either a single or a double organ with two horns, or branches. The anomaly is believed to result from an embryonic development error and is associated with a high incidence of preterm birth, spontaneous abortion, and infertility.

bicornuate. See **bicornate.**

bicuspid /bīkus′pid/ [L, *bis* + *cuspis,* point], **1.** having two cusps or points. **2.** See **premolar.**

bicuspid valve. See **mitral valve.**

bicycle ergometer [L, *bis,* twice; Gk, *kyklos,* circle, *ergon,* work, *metron,* measure], a stationary bicycle dynamometer that measures the strength of an individual's muscle contraction.

b.i.d., (in prescriptions) abbreviation for *bis in die* /dē′ā/, a Latin phrase meaning 'twice a day.'

bidactyly /bīdak′tilē/ [L, *bis* + Gk, *daktylos,* finger], an abnormal condition in which the second, third, and fourth digits on a hand are missing and only the first and fifth are present. Also called **lobster claw deformity.** —**bidactylous,** *adj.*

Bidactyly
(Zitelli and Davis, 1997/ courtesy Dr. Christine L. Williams, New York Medical College)

bidermoma /bī′dərmō′mə/, *pl.* **bidermomas, bidermomata** [L, *bis* + Gk, *derma,* skin, *oma,* tumor], a teratoid neoplasm composed of cells and tissues originating in two germ layers.

bidet /bidā′/ [Fr, pony], a fixture resembling a toilet bowl, with a rim to sit on and usually equipped with plumbing implements for cleaning the genital and rectal areas.

biduotertian fever /bī′doo-ətur′shən/ [L, *bis* + *dies,* day, *tertius,* three], a form of malaria characterized by overlapping paroxysms of chills, fever, and other symptoms. It is caused by infection with two strains of *Plasmodium,* each having its own cycle of symptoms, such as in quartan and tertian malaria. Compare **double quartan fever.** See also **malaria.**

Bier block /bēr blok/ [August Karl Gustav Bier, German surgeon, 1861–1949], regional anesthesia by IV injection of a local anesthesia such as lidocain. Used for surgical procedures on the arm below the elbow or the leg below the knee; performed in a bloodless field maintained by a pneumatic tourniquet that also prevents the anesthetic from entering the systemic circulation.

bifid /bī′fid/ [L, *bis* + *findere* to cleave], cleft, or split into two parts, as in the spinous processes of the cervical vertebrae.

bifid scrotum, separation of the two halves of the scrotum, as in penoscrotal transposition.

bifid tongue [L, *bis* + *findere,* to cleave; AS, *tunge*], a tongue divided by a longitudinal furrow. Also called **cleft tongue.**

bifid ureter, one in which proximal segments come from two different collecting systems but join to form one ureter before reaching the bladder.

bifid uvula, bifurcation of the uvula, an incomplete form of cleft palate.

bifocal /bīfō′kəl/ [L, *bis* + *focus,* hearth], **1.** pertaining to the characteristic of having two foci. **2.** (of a lens) having two areas of different focal lengths.

bifocal contact lens, a contact lens that contains corrections for both near and far vision.

bifocal glasses [L, *bis,* twice, *focus,* hearth; AS, *glaes*], eyeglasses in which each lens is made up of two segments of different refractive powers or strength. Generally, the upper part of the lens is used for ordinary or distant vision, and the smaller, lower section for near vision for close work, such as reading or sewing. Bifocal eyeglasses may be prescribed for presbyopia, which often occurs with aging.

biforate /bīfôr′āt/ [L, *bis* + *forare,* to pierce twice], having two perforations or foramina.

bifrontal suture /bīfron′təl/ [L, *bis* + *frons,* front, *sutura*], the interlocking lines of fusion between the frontal and parietal bones of the skull.

bifurcate /bīfur′kāt/ [L, *bis,* twice, *furca,* fork], pertaining to the division or branching of an object into two branches, as the branching of blood vessels or bronchi. —**bifurcated,** *adj.*

bifurcation /bī′fərkā′shən/ [L, *bis* + *furca,* fork], a splitting into two branches, such as the trachea, which branches into the two bronchi.

Bigelow's lithotrite /big′əlōz/ [Henry J. Bigelow, American surgeon, 1818–1890; Gk, *lithos,* stone; L, *terere,* to rub], a long-jawed instrument, passed through the urethra, for crushing a calculus in the bladder.

bigeminal /bījem′inəl/ [L, *bis,* twice, *geminus,* twin], pertaining to pairs, twins, or dual events, as a bigeminal pulse, which is characterized by two beats in rapid succession. See also **bigeminy.**

bigeminal pregnancy, a twin pregnancy.

bigeminal pulse, an abnormal pulse in which two beats in close succession are followed by a pause during which no pulse is felt. See also **trigeminal pulse, trigeminy.**

bigeminal rhythm [L, *bis* + *geminus,* twin; Gk, *rhythmos*], an abnormal heartbeat in which ectopic ventricular or atrial beats alternate with and are precisely coupled to sinus beats, or in which ventricular ectopic, beats occur in pairs, as in ventricular tachycardia with 3:2 exit block. Also called **bigeminy, coupled rhythm.**

bigeminy /bījem′inē/ [L, *bis* + *geminus,* twin], **1.** an association in pairs. **2.** See **bigeminal rhythm.** —**bigeminal,** *adj.*

bilabe /bī′lāb/ [L, *bis* + *labium,* lip], a narrow forceps used to remove small calculi from the bladder by way of the urethra.

bilabial /bī·lā′bē·əl/, a consonantal speech sound produced using the two lips, such as *b, p,* or *m.* Also called **labial.**

bilaminar /bīlam′ənər/ [L, *bis* + *lamina*, plate], pertaining to or having two layers, such as the basal lamina and the reticular lamina that constitute the basement membrane of the epithelium.

bilaminar blastoderm, the stage of embryonic development before mesoderm formation in which only the ectoderm and entoderm primary germ layers have formed. Compare **trilaminar blastoderm.**

bilateral /bilat′ərəl/ [L, *bis* + *lateralis*, side], **1.** having two sides. **2.** occurring or appearing on two sides. A patient with bilateral hearing loss may have partial or total hearing loss in both ears. **3.** having two layers.

bilateral carotid artery [L, *bis*, twice, *latus*, side; Gk, *karos*, heavy sleep], a main artery to the head and neck that divides into left and right branches and again into external and internal branches.

bilateral lithotomy [L, *bis*, twice, *latus*, side; Gk, *lithos*, stone, *temnein*, to cut], a surgical procedure for removing urinary tract stones from the bladder by making transverse perineal incisions through the lateral lobes of the prostate.

bilateral long-leg spica cast, an orthopedic device of plaster of paris, fiberglass, or other casting material that encases and immobilizes the trunk cranially as far as the nipple line and both legs caudally as far as the toes. A horizontal crossbar to improve immobilization connects the parts of the cast encasing both legs at ankle level. It is used to aid the healing of fractures of the hip, the femur, the acetabulum, and the pelvis and to correct hip deformities. Compare **one-and-a-half spica cast, unilateral long-leg spica cast.**

bilateral strabismus [L, *bis* + *latus*, side; Gk, *strabismos*], an eye disorder, characterized by bilateral squint, which is caused by a failure of ocular accommodation.

bilateral symmetry [L, *bis* + *latus*, side; Gk, *syn*, together, *metron*, measure], similar structure of the halves of an organism.

Bilbao tube /bilbō′ə/, a long, thin, flexible tube that is used to inject barium into the small intestine. The tube is guided with a stiff wire from the mouth to the end of the duodenum under fluoroscopic control.

bilberry, an herb found in the central, Northern, and Southeastern regions of Europe.

■ USES: This herb is used for diabetic retinopathy, macular degeneration, glaucoma, cataract, capillary fragility, varicose veins, hemorrhoids, and mild diarrhea; possibly effective for some indications but controlled clinical trials do not support its use for improving vision.

■ CONTRAINDICATIONS: Bilberry should not be used during pregnancy and lactation or in children until more research is available.

bile /bīl/ [L, *bilis*], a bitter, yellow-green secretion of the liver. Stored in the gallbladder, bile receives its color from the presence of bile pigments such as bilirubin. Bile passes from the gallbladder through the common bile duct in response to the cholecystokinin (CCK) produced in the duodenum in the presence of a fatty meal. Bile emulsifies these fats (breaks them into smaller particles and lowers the surface tension), preparing them for further digestion and absorption in the small intestine. Any interference in the flow of bile will result in the presence of unabsorbed fat in the feces and in jaundice. Also called **gall.** See also **biliary obstruction, jaundice. —biliary,** *adj.*

bile acid, a steroid acid of the bile, produced during the metabolism of cholesterol. On hydrolysis, bile acid yields glycine and choleic acid.

bile acid breath test, a breath test for overgrowth of bacteria in the intestine: the patient is given a dose of a conjugated bile acid labeled with carbon 14 and the amount of radioactively labeled carbon dioxide in the breath is measured at hourly intervals. Excessive labeled carbon dioxide in the breath indicates excessive bacteria in the intestine breaking down the bile acids.

bile acid therapy, administration of bile acids for treatment of hyperliposis.

bile duct. See **biliary duct.**

bile duct abscess, a cavity containing pus and surrounded by inflamed tissue in the bile duct.

bile pigments, a group of substances that contribute to the colors of bile, which may range from a yellowish green to brown. A common bile pigment is bilirubin, which contains a reddish iron pigment derived from the breakdown of old red blood cells.

bile salts [L, *bilis*, bile; AS, *sealt*], a mixture of sodium salts of the bile acids and chollic and chenodeoxycholic acids synthesized in the liver as a derivative of cholesterol. Their low surface tension contributes to the emulsification of fats in the intestine and their absorption from the GI tract.

bile solubility test, a bacteriologic test used in the differential diagnosis of pneumococcal and streptococcal infection. A broth culture of each organism is placed into two tubes. Ox bile is added to one and salt to the other. Pneumococci dissolve in ox bile, producing a clear solution; because streptococci do not dissolve, the resulting solution is cloudy. The tube with salt is used for comparative purposes.

Bilharzia. See *Schistosoma.*

bilharziasis. See **schistosomiasis.**

bili-, prefix meaning "bile": *biliary, bilifuscin.*

biliary /bil′ē·er′ē/, pertaining to bile or to the gallbladder and bile ducts, which transport bile. These are often called the **biliary tract** or the **biliary system.** Also **bilious.** See also **bile, biliary calculus.**

biliary abscess, an abscess of the gallbladder or liver.

biliary atresia, congenital absence or underdevelopment of one or more of the biliary structures, causing jaundice and early liver damage. As the condition worsens, the child's growth may be retarded, and portal hypertension may develop. Surgery can correct the defective ducts in only a small percentage of cases. Liver transplantation is an option. Most infants die in early childhood from biliary cirrhosis. It is essential to distinguish between this condition and neonatal hepatitis, which is treatable. See also **biliary cirrhosis.**

biliary calculus [L, *bilis*, bile, *calculus*, pebble], a stone formed in the biliary tract, consisting of cholesterol or bile pigments and calcium salts. Biliary calculi may cause jaundice, right upper quadrant pain, obstruction, and inflammation of the gallbladder. If stones cannot pass spontaneously into the duodenum, cholangiography or similar processes will reveal their location, and they can be removed surgically. Also called **choledocholithiasis, gallstones.** See also **cholangitis, cholecystitis, cholelithiasis.**

biliary cirrhosis [L, *bilis* + *kirrhos*, yellow-orange, *osis*, condition], an inflammatory condition in which the flow of bile through the ductules of the liver is obstructed. Primary biliary cirrhosis most commonly affects women in their middle years, and its cause is unknown. It is characterized by itching, jaundice, steatorrhea, and enlargement of the liver and spleen. The disease is slowly progressive. There is no specific medical or surgical treatment. Care must be taken to rule out secondary biliary cirrhosis caused by obstruction of the biliary structures outside the liver, because the latter condition can be treated successfully. Compare **biliary calculus, biliary obstruction.**

biliary colic [L, *bilis* + *kolikos*, colon pain], a type of smooth muscle or visceral pain specifically associated with

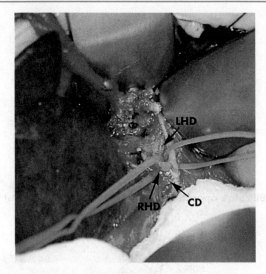

Biliary atresia: *LHD,* **left hepatic duct;**
RHD, **right hepatic duct**
(Greig and Garden, 1996)

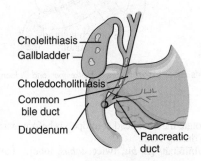

Common locations of biliary calculi
(Beare and Myers, 1998)

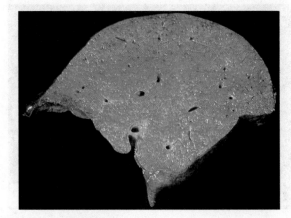

Biliary cirrhosis *(Kumar, Cotran, and Robbins, 2003)*

the passing of stones through the bile ducts. Also called
cholecystalgia. See also **biliary calculus.**

biliary duct, one of the muscular ducts through which bile
passes from the liver and gallbladder to the duodenum. See
also **common bile duct.**

biliary dyskinesia, an abnormal condition caused by a
dysfunction of the sphincter of Oddi, disrupting the flow of
bile from the gallbladder.

biliary dyspepsia, a digestive upset caused by an inadequate flow of bile into the duodenum.

biliary fistula, an abnormal passage from the gallbladder, a bile duct, or the liver to an internal organ or the
surface of the body. Biliary fistulae into the duodenum
may complicate cholelithiasis; a gallstone may become impacted, usually in the ileocecal valve, and cause intestinal
obstruction.

biliary glands. See **glands of bile duct.**

biliary obstruction, blockage of the common or cystic
bile duct, usually caused by one or more gallstones. It impedes bile drainage and produces an inflammatory reaction.
Less common causes of biliary obstruction include chole-
dochal cysts, pancreatic and duodenal tumors, Crohn's disease, pancreatitis, echinococcosis, ascariasis, and sclerosing
cholangitis. Stones, consisting chiefly of cholesterol, bile
pigment, and calcium, may form in the gallbladder and in the
hepatic duct in persons of either sex at any age but are more
common in middle-aged women. Increased amounts of serum cholesterol in the blood, such as occurs in obesity, diabetes, hypothyroidism, biliary stasis, and inflammation of
the biliary system, promote gallstone formation. Cholelithiasis may be asymptomatic until a stone lodges in a biliary
duct, but the patient usually has a history of indigestion and
discomfort after eating fatty foods.

■ OBSERVATIONS: Biliary obstruction is characterized by severe epigastric pain, often radiating to the back and shoulder,
nausea, vomiting, and profuse diaphoresis. The dehydrated
patient may have chills; fever; jaundice; clay-colored stools;
dark, concentrated urine; an electrolyte imbalance; and a
tendency to bleed because the absence of bile prevents the
synthesis and absorption of fat-soluble vitamin K.

■ INTERVENTIONS: The patient is placed in bed in a semi-
Fowler's position and is usually administered intermittent
nasogastric suctioning, parenteral fluids with electrolytes
and fat-soluble vitamins, and medication for pain. Antibiotics, anticholinergic and antispasmodic drugs, and a chole-
cystogram or ultrasound scan may be ordered. The blood
pressure, temperature, pulse, and respirations are monitored,
and the patient is helped to turn, cough, and deep breathe
every 2 to 4 hours. Fluid intake and output are measured, and
the color and character of urine and stools are noted. When
the nasogastric tube is removed, the patient initially receives
a low-fat liquid diet and progresses to a soft or normal diet,
as tolerated; up to 2500 ml of fluids a day are encouraged or
administered intravenously, unless contraindicated. Cholecystectomy is usually the definitive treatment, but in most
cases surgery is delayed until the patient's condition is sta-
bilized and any prothrombin deficiency (caused by vitamin
K malabsorption) is corrected.

biliary pseudolithiasis, pain in the bile ducts with symptoms resembling those of cholelithiasis but in the absence of
gallstones.

biliary system. See **biliary.**

biliary tract [L, *bilis,* bile, *tractus*], the pathway for bile
flow from the canaliculi in the liver to the opening of the bile
duct into the duodenum.

biliary tract cancer, a rare adenocarcinoma in a bile duct
often causing jaundice, pruritus, and weight loss. The lesion

may be papillary or flat and ulcerated. The tumor is often unresectable at diagnosis.

biligenesis /bil'ijen'əsis/, the process by which bile is produced.

bilingulate /bīling'gyəlit/ [L, *bis*, twice, *lingula*, little tongue], having two tongues or two tonguelike structures.

biliopancreatic diversion, a surgical treatment for morbid obesity consisting of resection of the distal two thirds of the stomach and attachment of the ileum to a stoma so that the entire duodenum and jejunum are bypassed; the duodenum and jejunum empty their secretions into the distal ileum through a new stoma. Also called *biliopancreatic bypass*.

bilious /bil'yəs/ [L, *bilis*, bile], **1.** pertaining to bile. **2.** characterized by an excessive secretion of bile. **3.** characterized by a disorder affecting bile.

bilious vomiting, the vomiting of bile. Also called *cholemesis*.

bilirubin /bil'iroo'bin/ [L, *bilis* + *ruber*, red], the orange-yellow pigment of bile, formed principally by the breakdown of hemoglobin in red blood cells after termination of their normal lifespan. Water-insoluble unconjugated bilirubin normally travels in the bloodstream to the liver, where it is converted to a water-soluble, conjugated form and excreted into the bile. In a healthy person about 250 mg of bilirubin is produced daily. The majority of bilirubin is excreted in the stool. The characteristic yellow pallor of jaundice is caused by the accumulation of bilirubin in the blood and in the tissues of the skin. Testing for bilirubin in the blood provides information for diagnosis and evaluation of liver disease, biliary obstruction, and hemolytic anemia. Normal levels of total bilirubin are 0.1 to 1 mg/dl or 5.1 to 17 μmol/L. See also **jaundice, van den Bergh's test.**

bilirubin blood test, a blood test performed in cases of jaundice to help determine whether the jaundice is caused by hepatocellular dysfunction (as in hepatitis) or extrahepatic obstruction of the bile ducts (as with gallstones or tumor blocking the bile ducts). Total serum bilirubin is made up of conjugated (direct) and unconjugated (indirect) bilirubin, with varying ratios of each characterizing different diseases.

bilirubin cast, a cast containing bilirubin, giving it a yellow-brown color, as seen with obstructive jaundice.

bilirubin diglucuronide, a conjugated water-soluble form of bilirubin, formed in the liver by esterification of two molecules of glucuronide to the bilirubin molecule; this is the usual form in which bilirubin is found in the bile.

bilirubinemia /-ē'mē-ə/ [L, *bilis*, bile, *ruber*, red; Gk, *haima*, blood], the presence of bilirubin in the blood.

bilirubinuria /-ōōr'ē-ə/, the presence of bilirubin in urine.

biliuria /bil'iyōōr'ē-ə/ [L, *bilis* + Gk, *ouron*, urine], the presence of bile pigments in the urine.

biliverdin /bil'ivur'din/ [L, *bilis* + *virdis*, green], a greenish bile pigment formed in the breakdown of hemoglobin and converted to bilirubin. See also **bile, bilirubin.**

billing limit. See **limiting charge.**

Billings method, a way of estimating ovulation time by changes in the cervical mucus that occur during the menstrual cycle. See also **ovulation method of family planning.**

Billroth's operation I [Christian A. Billroth, Austrian surgeon, 1829–1894], the surgical removal of the pylorus in the treatment of gastric cancer or peptic ulcer. The proximal end of the duodenum is anastomosed to the stomach.

Billroth's operation II [Christian A. Billroth], the surgical removal of the pylorus and duodenum. The cut end of the stomach is anastomosed to the jejunum through the transverse mesocolon. Also called **gastrojejunostomy.**

Bill's maneuver [Arthur H. Bill, American obstetrician, 1877–1961], an obstetric procedure in which a forceps is

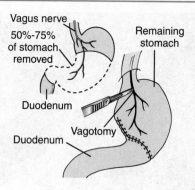

Billroth's operation I *(Lewis, Heitkemper, and Dirksen, 2004)*

Billroth's operation II *(Lewis, Heitkemper, and Dirksen, 2004)*

used to rotate the fetal head at midpelvis before extraction of the head during birth.

bilobate /bīlō'bāt/ [L, *bis*, twice, *lobus*, lobe], having two lobes.

bilobate placenta [L, *bis*, twice, *lobus*, lobe, *placenta*, flat cake], a placenta with two connected lobes. Also called **bilobed placenta, placenta bipartitia.**

Bilobate placenta *(Carlson, 2004)*

bilobulate /bīlob′yəlāt/, having two lobules. Also **bilobular.**

bilocular /bīlok′yələr/ [L, *bis* + *loculus,* compartment], **1.** divided into two cells. **2.** containing two cells. Also **biloculate.**

Biltricide, trademark for an anthelmintic (praziquantel).

bimanual /bīman′yŏŏ·əl/ [L, *bis* + *manus,* hand], with both hands.

bimanual examination [L, *bis* + *manos,* hand], an examination that requires the use of two hands.

bimanual palpation, the examination of a woman's pelvic organs in which the examiner places one hand on the abdomen and one or two fingers of the other hand in the vagina.

Bimanual palpation *(Swartz, 2002)*

bimanual percussion [L, *bis,* twice, *manus,* hand, *percutere,* to strike through], a diagnostic technique of producing sound vibrations in body cavities by the use of two hands, one serving as the plexor, or "hammer," and the other as the pleximeter, or striking plate. See also **percussion.**

bimastoid /bīmas′toid/, pertaining to the two mastoid processes of the temporal bone.

bimatoprost /bĭ-mat′o-prost/, a synthetic prostaglandin analogue that acts as an ocular hypotensive; applied topically to the conjunctiva in the treatment of open-angle glaucoma and ocular hypertension.

bimaxillary /bīmak′siler′ē/ [L, *bis* + *maxilla,* jawbone], pertaining to the right and left maxillae. The term is also used in some clinical situations to refer to both the upper and lower jaws.

bimodal distribution /bīmo′dəl/ [L, *bis* + *modus,* measure], the distribution of quantitative data into two clusters. It is suggestive of two separate normally distributed populations from which the data are drawn.

bimolecular reaction (E^2) /bī′molek′yələr/, a reaction in which more than one molecule is involved in the slow step. An enzyme-catalyzed reaction usually consists of a series of bimolecular reactions. It may follow second-order, or more complicated chemical kinetics.

bin-, prefix meaning "twice, two": *binocular, binovular.*

binangle /bin′ang·gəl/ [L, *bini,* twofold, *angulus,* angle], a double-ended surgical or operative instrument that has a shank with two offsetting angles to keep the cutting edge of the instrument within 3 mm of the shaft axis.

binary fission /bī′nərē/ [L, *bini,* twofold, *fissionis,* splitting], the division of a cell or nucleus into two equal parts. It is the common form of asexual reproduction among bacteria, protozoa, and other unicellular organisms. Also called **simple fission.** Compare **multiple fission.**

binary number, a number in base 2 represented by 0s and 1s. For example, the number 2 in the decimal form is written as 10 in the binary form, the decimal number 3 is written as 11, the decimal number 4 is written as 100 in the binary form, and so on.

binaural /bī·naw′rəl/ [L, *bis,* twice + *auris,* ear], pertaining to both ears.

binaural stethoscope. See **diaphragm stethoscope.**

binauricular. See **biauricular.**

bind [AS, *binden*], **1.** to bandage or wrap in a band. **2.** to join together with a band or with a ligature. **3.** (in chemistry) to combine or unite molecules by using reactive groups within the molecules or by using a binding chemical. Binding is especially associated with chemical bonds that are fairly easily broken, such as in the bonds between toxins and antitoxins.

binder, a bandage made of a large piece of material to fit and support a specific body part.

Abdominal binder *(Harkreader and Hogan, 2004)*

binding energy, **1.** the amount of energy required to separate a nucleus into its individual nucleons. **2.** the energy released as the nucleus forms from nucleons.

binding site [ME, *binden* + L, *situs*], the location on the surface of a cell or a molecule where other cell fragments or molecules attach to initiate a chemical or physiologic action.

Binet age /binā′/ [Alfred Binet, French psychologist, 1857–1911], the mental age of an individual, especially a child, as determined by the Binet-Simon tests, which are evaluated on the basis of tested intelligence of the "normal" individual at any given age. The Binet age corresponding to "profoundly retarded" is 1 to 2 years; to "severely retarded," 3 to 7 years; and to "mildly retarded," 8 to 12 years.

binge eating. See **bulimia.**

binocular /bīnok′yələr, bin-/ [L, *bini* + *oculus,* eye], **1.** pertaining to both eyes, especially regarding vision. **2.** a microscope, telescope, or field glass that can accommodate viewing by both eyes.

binocular fixation, the process of having both eyes directed at the same object at the same time, which is essential for good depth perception.

binocular ophthalmoscope, an ophthalmoscope having two eyepieces used for stereoscopic examination of the eye.

binocular parallax /per'əlaks/ [L, *bini* + *oculus* + Gk, *parallax,* in turn], the difference in the angles formed by the sight lines to two objects situated at different distances from the eyes. Binocular parallax is a major factor in depth perception. Also called **stereoscopic parallax.**

binocular perception, the visual ability to judge depth or distance by virtue of having two eyes.

binocular vision, the simultaneous use of both eyes so that the images perceived by each eye are combined to appear as a single image. Compare **diplopia.**

binomial /bīnō'mē·əl/, containing two names or terms.

binomial nomenclature [L, *bis,* twice; Gk, *nomos,* law; L, *nomenclatio,* calling by name], a system of classification of animals, plants, and other life forms (developed by Carl Linné) that assigns a two-part Latinized name to each species, such as *Homo sapiens* for humans.

binovular /bīnov'yələr/ [L, *bini* + *ovum,* egg], developing from two distinct ova, as in dizygotic twins. Also **diovular.** Compare **uniovular.**

binovular twins. See **dizygotic twins.**

Binswanger's disease /bin'swäng·ərz/ [Otto Binswanger, German neurologist, 1852–1929], a degenerative dementia of presenile onset caused by thinning of the subcortical white matter of the brain; some have attributed it to sclerotic changes of blood vessels. Associated with multiple subcortical strokes.

binuclear /bīnoo'klē·ər/ [L, *bis,* twice, *nucleus,* nut kernel], having two nuclei, as in the example of a heterokaryon or binucleate hybrid cell. Also **binucleate** /bīnoo'klē·āt/.

bio- /bī'ō-/, prefix meaning "life": *bioassay, biopsy.*

bioactive [Gk, *bios,* life; L, *activus,* with energy], having an effect on or causing a reaction in living tissue.

bioactivity /-aktiv'itē/, any response from or reaction in living tissue. —**bioactive,** *adj.*

bioassay /bī'ō·as'ā, -əsā'/ [Gk, *bios* + Fr, *assayer,* to try], the laboratory determination of the concentration of a drug or other substance in a specimen by comparing its effect on an organism, an animal, or an isolated tissue with that of a standard preparation. Also called **biologic assay.**

bioastronautics /-as'trōnôt'iks/, the science dealing with the biologic aspects of space travel.

bioavailability /-əvā'libil'itē/ [Gk, *bios* + ME, *availen,* to serve], the degree of activity or amount of an administered drug or other substance that becomes available for activity in the target tissue.

biocenosis /-sənō'sis/ [Fk, *bios,* life, *koinos,* common], an ecologic community.

biochemical genetics. See **molecular genetics.**

biochemical marker /-kem'ikəl/ [Gk, *bios* + *chemeia,* alchemy], any hormone, enzyme, antibody, or other substance that is detected in the urine or other body fluids or tissues that may serve as a sign of a disease or other abnormality. An example is the **Bence Jones protein** that appears in the urine of multiple myeloma patients.

biochemistry /-kem'istrē/, the chemistry of organisms and life processes. Also called **biologic chemistry, physiologic chemistry.**

biochemorphics /-kemôr'fik/, the study of the relationship between chemical structure and biologic function.

biochromatic analysis /-krōmat'ik/ [Gk, *bios* + *chroma,*

color], the spectrophotometric monitoring of a reaction at two wavelengths. It is used to correct for background color.

bioclimatology /-klī'mətol'əjē/, the study of the relationship and interactions between climate and organisms.

biocybernetics /-sī'bərnet'iks/, the science of communication and control within and among organisms and of the interaction between organisms and mechanical or electronic systems.

biodegradable /-digrā'dəbəl/ [Gk, *bios,* life; L, *de,* away, *gradus,* step], the natural ability of a chemical substance to be broken down into less complex compounds or compounds having fewer carbon atoms by bacteria or other microorganisms.

biodynamics /-dīnam'iks/, the study of the effects of dynamic processes, such as radiation, on organisms.

bioelectric impedance analysis (BIA) /-ilek'trik/, a method of measuring the fat composition of the body, compared to other tissues, by its resistance to electricity. Fat tissue does not conduct electricity; muscle and bone are poor conductors. The method is reported to be 95% accurate, depending on body water content, which may fluctuate with exercise, diet, sweating, and use of alcohol or drugs. See also **total body electric conductivity (TOBEC).**

bioelectricity /-ilektris'itē/ [Gk, *bios* + *elektron,* amber], electrical current that is generated by living tissues, such as nerves and muscles. The electrical potentials of human tissues, recorded by electrocardiograph, electroencephalograph, and similar sensitive devices, are used in diagnosing the condition of various vital organs.

bioenergetics /-en'ərjet'iks/ [Gk, *bios* + *energein,* to be active], a system of exercises based on the concept that natural healing will be enhanced by bringing the patient's body rhythms and the natural environment into harmony.

bioequivalent /bī'ō·ikwiv'ələnt/ [Gk, *bios* + L, *aequus,* equal, *valere,* to be strong], **1.** (in pharmacology) pertaining to a drug that has the same effect on the body as another drug, usually one nearly identical in its chemical formulation but possibly requiring a different amount to see the same effect. **2.** going in and out of the body at the same rate. —**bioequivalence,** *n.*

bioethics /bī'ō·eth'iks/ [Gk, *bios,* life + *ethos,* the habits of humans or animals], obligations of a moral nature relating to biological research and its applications.

biofeedback[1] /-fēd'bak/ [Gk, *bios* + AS, *faedan,* food, *baec,* back], a process providing a person with visual or auditory information about the autonomic physiologic functions of his or her body, such as blood pressure, muscle tension, and brain wave activity, usually through use of instruments. By trial and error, the person learns consciously to control these processes, which were previously regarded as involuntary. Biofeedback may be used clinically to treat many conditions, such as pain, anxiety, hypertension, insomnia, and migraine headache.

biofeedback[2], a nursing intervention from the Nursing Interventions Classification (NIC) defined as assisting the patient to modify a body function using feedback from instrumentation. See also **Nursing Interventions Classification.**

biofilm /bi'ō-film'/, a thin layer of microorganisms adhering to the surface of a structure, which may be organic or inorganic, together with the polymers that they secrete.

bioflavonoid /bī'ōflā'vənoid/ [Gk, *bios* + L, *flavus,* yellow; Gk, *eidos,* form], a generic term for any of a group of colored flavones found in many fruits. Once believed to reduce capillary bleeding, bioflavonoids are now considered nonessential nutrients. Several are being investigated as possible low-calorie sweeteners.

biogenesis /bī'ōjen'əsis/ [Gk, *bios* + *genein,* to produce], **1.**

also called **biogeny** /bī·oj'ənē/, the doctrine that living material can originate only from preexisting life and not from inanimate matter. **2.** the origin of life; ontogeny and phylogeny. **—biogenetic,** *adj.*

biogenetic law. See **recapitulation concept.**

biogenic /bī'ōjen'ik/, **1.** produced by the action of a living organism, such as fermentation. **2.** essential to life and the maintenance of health, such as food, water, and proper rest.

biogenic amine, one of a large group of naturally occurring biologically active compounds, most of which act as neurotransmitters. The most dominant, norepinephrine, is involved in such physiologic functions as emotional reactions, memory, sleep, and arousal from sleep. Other biochemicals of the group include three catecholamines: histamine, serotonin, and dopamine. These substances are active in regulating blood pressure, elimination, body temperature, and many other centrally mediated body functions.

biogenous /bī·oj'ənəs/, **1.** biogenetic. **2.** biogenic.

biogeny. See **biogenesis.**

biogravics /-grav'iks/, the study of the effects of gravity, including reduced and increased gravitational forces, on organisms.

biohazard /-haz'ərd/ [Gk, *bios,* life; OFr, *hasard*], anything that is a risk to organisms, such as ionizing radiation or harmful bacteria or viruses.

Biohazard label *(Zakus, 2001)*

bioimpedance analysis, a method for analyzing the water content of the body through variations in bioimpedance between different types of tissue.

bioinstrument, a sensor or other device implanted into or attached to a living organism for the purpose of recording physiologic data, such as brain activity or heart function.

biokinetics /-kinet'iks/ [Gk, *bios,* life, *kinetikos,* moving], the study of the movements within developing organisms.

biologic /-loj'ik/ [Gk, *bios* + *logos,* science], **1.** pertaining to organisms and their products. **2.** any preparation made from organisms or their products and used as a diagnostic, preventive, or therapeutic agent. Kinds of biologics include **antigens, antitoxins, sera,** and **vaccines.** Also called **biological.**

biologic activity, the inherent capacity of a substance, such as a drug or toxin, to alter one or more chemical or physiologic functions of a cell, tissue, organ, or organism. The biologic activity of a substance is determined not only by the substance's physical and chemical nature but also by its concentration and the duration of cellular exposure to it. Biologic activity may reflect a "domino effect," in which the alteration of one function disrupts the normal activity of one or more other functions.

biological. See **biologic.**

biologic armature, the connective tissue-rich aggregate of larger ducts, vessels, and autonomic nerves that in many mammalian exocrine glands serves as an internal framework whose function of support, and often anchorage, resembles that of the armature within a clay sculpture.

biologic assay. See **bioassay.**

biologic chemistry. See **biochemistry.**

biologic death, death attributed to natural causes. In CPR terms, *biologic death* refers to permanent cellular damage, resulting from lack of oxygen, that is not reversible.

biologic dressing, a dressing for burn injuries that is made from pigskin or synthetic materials with characteristics like those of human skin. The dressing is most effective in treating burns that are of uniform depth and of superficial partial thickness. It should be applied as soon as possible after the injury and should adhere to the wound during healing. Once adherence is established the wound can be left open and the patient can bathe and wear clothing over it.

biologic half-life, the time required for the body to eliminate half of an administered dose of any substance by regular physiologic processes. The biologic half-life is approximately the same for stable and radioactive isotopes of a specific element. Also called **metabolic half-life.** See also **effective half-life, half-life.**

biologic monitoring, **1.** a process of measuring the levels of various physiologic substances, drugs, or metabolites within a patient during diagnosis or therapy. **2.** the measurement of toxic substances in the environment and the identification of health risks to the population. Biologic monitoring often uses indirect methods of identifying and measuring substances, such as analyses of samples of blood, urine, feces, hair, nails, sweat, saliva, or exhaled air and extrapolation from metabolic effects.

biologic plausibility, a method of reasoning used to establish a cause-and-effect relationship between a biologic factor and a particular disease.

biologic psychiatry, a school of psychiatric thought that stresses the physical, chemical, and neurologic causes of and treatments for mental and emotional disorders.

biologic rhythm [Gk, *bios,* life, *logos,* science, *rhythmos*], the periodic recurrence of a biologic phenomenon, such as the respiratory cycle, the sleep cycle, or the menstrual cycle. Also called **biorhythm.**

biologic vector. See **vector.**

biologist /bī·ol'əjist/ [Gk, *bios,* life, *logos,* science], a person who studies life sciences.

biology /bī·ol'əje/, the scientific study of life. Some branches of biology are **biometry, cytology, ecology, evolution, genetics, molecular biology,** and **physiology.**

biolysis /bī·ol'isis/ [Gk, *bios,* life, *lysis,* loosening], the disintegration or dissolution of organic matter resulting from the activity of organisms, such as bacterial action on living tissue.

biome /bī'ōm/ [Gk, *bios* + *oma,* tumor, mass], the collection of biologic communities existing in and characteristic of a broad geographic region, such as desert, tropical forest, or savanna. A biome includes all organisms of a particular region.

biomechanic. See **biomechanics.**

biomechanic adaptation, a process in which a patient with a physical disability adjusts to the use of an orthotic device, such as an ankle-foot brace or a patellar-tendon-bearing prosthesis. Adaptation requires the central nervous system input received during therapeutic exercises with the orthotic appliance.

biomechanics [Gk, *bios* + *mechane,* machine], the study of mechanical laws and their application to living organisms, especially the human body and its locomotor system. —**biomechanic,** biomechanical, *adj.*

biomedical, pertaining to the biologic aspects of medicine.

biomedical engineering /-med′ikəl/ [Gk, *bios* + L, *medicare,* to heal], a system of scientific techniques that is applied to biologic processes to solve practical medical problems or answer questions in biomedical research.

biometry /bī·om′ətrē/, the application of statistical methods in analyzing data obtained in biologic or anthropologic research. See also **biology.**

biomicroscopy /-mīkros′kəpē/, **1.** microscopic examination of living tissue in the body. **2.** ophthalmic examination of the eye by use of a slit lamp and a magnifying lens. See also **slit lamp, slit-lamp microscope.**

bionics /bī·on′iks/, the science of applying electronic principles and devices, such as computers and solid-state miniaturized circuitry, to medical problems. An example of the application of bionics is the development of artificial pacemakers to correct abnormal heart rhythms. —**bionic,** *adj.*

biopharmaceutics /-fär′məsoo′tiks/, the study of the chemical and physical properties of drugs, their components, and their activities in living organisms.

biophore /bī′əfôr′/ [Gk, *bios* + *phora,* bearer], according to the German biologist A.F.L. Weismann (1834-1914), the basic hereditary unit contained in the germ plasm from which all living cells develop and all inherited characteristics are transmitted. Compare **gemma.**

biophysics, the application of physical laws to life processes of organisms.

biopotentials /-pəten′shəl/, a voltage produced by a tissue of the body, particularly muscle tissue during a contraction. Electrocardiography depends on measurement of changing potentials in contracting heart muscle; electromyography and electroencephalography function similarly in the diagnosis of neuromuscular and brain disorders, respectively.

biopsy /bī′opsē/ [Gk, *bios* + *opsis,* view], **1.** the removal of a small piece of living tissue from an organ or other part of the body for microscopic examination to confirm or establish a diagnosis, estimate prognosis, or follow the course of a disease. **2.** the tissue excised for examination. **3.** *informal,* to excise tissue for examination. Kinds of biopsy include **aspiration biopsy, needle biopsy, punch biopsy,** and **surface biopsy.** —**bioptic** /bī·op′tik/, *adj.*

biopsychic /bī′ōsī′kik/ [Gk, *bios* + *psyche,* mind], pertaining to mental factors as they relate to living organisms.

biopsychology. See **psychobiology.**

biopsychosocial /bī′ōsī′kōsō′shəl/ [Gk, *bios* + *psyche,* mind; L, *socius,* companion], pertaining to the complex of biologic, psychologic, and social aspects of life.

bioptic. See **biopsy.**

bioptome tip catheter /bī·op′tōm/, a catheter with a special end designed for obtaining endomyocardial biopsy samples. It is threaded through a guiding catheter to the right ventricle, where it snips small tissue samples from the septal wall for pathologic examination. The bioptome tip device is used to monitor heart transplantation patients for early signs of tissue rejection.

biorhythm. See **biologic rhythm.**

biosafety, a system for the safe handling of toxic and dangerous biologic and chemical substances. Guidance in biosafety is offered by the U.S. Centers for Disease Control, Occupational Safety and Health Administration, and National Institute for Occupational Safety and Health.

-biosis, suffix meaning "a specific way of living": *macrobiosis, otobiosis.*

biostatistics /-stətis′tiks/, numeric data on births, deaths, diseases, injuries, and other factors affecting the general health and condition of human populations. Also called **vital statistics.**

biosynthesis /-sin′thəsis/ [Gk, *bios* + *synthesis,* putting together], any one of thousands of chemical processes continually occurring throughout the body in which less complex molecules form more complex biomolecules, especially the carbohydrates, lipids, proteins, nucleotides, and nucleic acids. Biosynthetic reactions constitute the anabolism of the body. —**biosynthetic,** *adj.*

biosystem, any organism or complex system of organisms.

biotaxis /bī′ōtak′sis/ [Gk, *bios* + *taxis,* arrangement], the ability of cells to develop into certain forms and arrangements. See also **cytoclesis. —biotactic,** *adj.*

biotaxy /bī′ōtak′sē/, **1.** biotaxis. **2.** the systematic classification of organisms according to their phenotypic characteristics; taxonomy.

biotechnology /-teknol′əjē/ [Gk, *bios* + *techne,* art, *logos,* science], **1.** the study of the relationships between humans or other living organisms and machinery, such as the health effects of computer equipment on office workers or the ability of airplane pilots to perform tasks when traveling at supersonic speeds. **2.** the industrial application of the results of biologic research, particularly in fields such as recombinant deoxyribonucleic acids (DNA) or gene splicing, which permits the production of synthetic hormones or enzymes by combining genetic material from different species. See **recombinant DNA.**

biotelemetry /-təlem′ətrē/, the transmission of physiologic data, such as electrocardiographic (ECG) and electroencephalographic (EEG) recordings, heart rate, and body temperature by radio or telephone systems. Transmission of such data uses sophisticated electronic devices developed for the study of the effects of space travel on animals and humans; it has progressed to the use of communication satellites for relaying such data from one part of the world to another.

bioterrorism, the calculated use, or threatened use, of biologic agents against civilian populations in order to attain political or ideological goals by intimidation or coercion.

bioterrorism preparedness, a nursing intervention from the Nursing Interventions Classification (NIC) defined as preparing for an effective response to bioterrorism events or disaster.

biotherapy, a system of cancer therapy that uses alpha- and beta-interferons and mitogen-stimulated lymphocytes.

-biotic, suffix meaning "life": *anabiotic, microbiotic;* also, meaning "possessing a (specified) mode of life": *endobiotic, photobiotic.*

biotic factor /bī·ot′ik/, an environmental influence on living things, as distinguished from climatic or geologic factors.

biotic potential, the possible growth rate of a population of organisms under ideal conditions, which include an absence of predators and an unlimited availability of nutrients and space for expansion.

biotin /bī′ətin/ [Gk, *bios*, life], a colorless, crystalline, water-soluble B complex vitamin that acts as a coenzyme in fatty acid production and in the oxidation of fatty acids and carbohydrates. It also aids in the use of protein, folic acid, pantothenic acid, and vitamin B_{12}. Rich sources are egg yolk, beef liver, kidney, unpolished rice, brewer's yeast, peanuts, cauliflower, and mushrooms. Previously called **vitamin H.** See also **avidin.**

biotin deficiency syndrome, an abnormal condition caused by a deficiency of biotin, a B complex vitamin. It is characterized by dermatitis, hyperesthesia, muscle pain, anorexia, slight anemia, and changes in electrocardiographic activity of the heart. The average daily requirement of biotin for an adult is 100 to 200 μg; the average American diet provides 100 to 300 μg of the vitamin. Because biotin is synthesized by intestinal bacteria, naturally occurring deficiency in adults is unknown, although it can be induced by large quantities of raw egg whites in the diet. Symptoms include scaly dermatitis, grayish pallor, extreme lassitude, anorexia, muscle pains, insomnia, some precordial distress, and slight anemia. Some authorities consider seborrheic dermatitis in infants a form of biotin deficiency.

biotope /bī′ətōp/ [Gk, *bios* + *topos*, place], a specific biologic habitat or site.

biotoxin /bī′ətok′in/, any toxin produced by an organism.

biotoxins, poisons produced by and derived from plants and animals. Biotoxins include abrin, from the jequirity bean or rosary pea *(Abrus precatorius);* ricin, from castor beans; and strychnine, from *Strychnos nux vomica.* Biotoxins can be absorbed by ingesting or inhaling the toxin. Inhalation of ricin or abrin causes severe respiratory distress and ingestion of these agents causes nausea and vomiting; multisystem organ failure and death may occur. Strychnine attacks communication between the nerves and muscles and may lead to death from respiratory failure as the respiratory muscles tire. Treatment consists of removal of the toxin from the body and supportive care.

biotransformation /-trans′fôrmā′shən/ [Gk, *bios* + L, *trans,* across, *formare,* to form], the chemical changes a substance undergoes in the body, such as by the action of enzymes. See also **metabolic.**

Biot's respiration /bē·ōz′/ [Camille Biot, French physician, b. 1878], an abnormal respiratory pattern, characterized by short episodes of rapid, uniformly deep inspirations followed by 10 to 30 seconds of apnea. Biot's respiration is symptomatic of meningitis or increased intracranial pressure.

biovular twins. See **dizygotic twins.**

bipalatinoid /bī′palat′inoid, -pal′-/, describing a two-compartment capsule with different medications in each side. It is designed so that the two substances become mixed and activated as the gelatin capsule dissolves.

bipara /bip′ərə/, a woman who has given birth twice in separate pregnancies.

biparental inheritance. See **amphigenous inheritance.**

biparietal /bīpərī′ətəl/ [L, *bis,* twice, *paries,* wall], pertaining to the two parietal bones of the head, such as the biparietal diameter.

biparietal diameter (BPD), the transverse distance between the protuberances of the two parietal bones of the skull.

biparietal suture [L, *bis* + *paries,* wall, *sutura*], the interlocking lines of fusion between two parietal bones of the skull.

biparous /bip′ərəs/ [L, *bis,* twice, *parere,* to produce], pertaining to the birth of two infants in separate pregnancies.

bipartite /bīpär′tīt/, having two parts.

biped /bī′ped/, **1.** having two feet. **2.** any animal with only two feet.

bipedal /bīpē′dəl, -ped′əl/ [L, *bis,* twice, *pes,* foot], capable of locomotion on two feet.

bipenniform /bīpen′ifôrm′/ [L, *bis* + *penna,* feather, *forma,* form], (of body structure) having the bilateral symmetry of a feather, such as the pattern formed by the fasciculi that converge on both sides of a muscle tendon in the rectus femoris. Compare **multipenniform, penniform, radiate.**

biperforate /bī·pər′fə·rāt/ [L, *bis,* twice + *perforatus,* bored through], having two perforations.

biperiden /bīper′idən/, a synthetic anticholinergic agent.

■ INDICATIONS: It may be prescribed in the treatment of Parkinson's disease and drug-induced extrapyramidal disorders. Biperiden hydrochloride is administered orally, and biperiden lactate is administered intramuscularly or intravenously.

■ CONTRAINDICATIONS: Narrow-angle glaucoma, asthma, obstruction of the genitourinary or GI tract, or known hypersensitivity to this drug prohibits its use.

■ ADVERSE EFFECTS: Among the more serious adverse reactions are blurred vision, central nervous system effects, urinary retention, postural hypotension, tachycardia, dry mouth, decreased sweating, and hypersensitivity reactions.

biphasic /bīfā′zik/ [L, *bis* + Gk, *phasis,* appearance], having two phases, parts, aspects, or stages.

bipolar /bīpō′lər/ [L, *bis* + *polus,* pole], **1.** having two poles, such as in certain electrotherapeutic treatments using two poles or in certain types of bacterial staining that affects only the two poles of the microorganism under study. **2.** (of a nerve cell) having an afferent and an efferent process.

bipolar cell, a cell, such as a retinal neuron, with two main processes arising from the cell body.

bipolar disorder, a major mental disorder characterized by episodes of mania, depression, or mixed mood. One or the other phase may be predominant at any given time, one phase may appear alternately with the other, or elements of both phases may be present simultaneously. Characteristics of the manic phase are excessive emotional displays, such as excitement, elation, euphoria, or in some cases irritability accompanied by hyperactivity, boisterousness, impaired ability to concentrate, decreased need for sleep, and seemingly unbounded energy. In extreme mania, a sense of omnipotence and delusions of grandeur may occur. In the depressive phase, marked apathy and underactivity are accompanied by feelings of profound sadness, loneliness, guilt, and lowered self-esteem. Causes of the disorder are multiple and complex, often involving biologic, psychologic, interpersonal, and social and cultural factors. See also **major depressive disorder.**

bipolar electrocautery, an electrocautery in which both active and return electrodes are incorporated into a single handheld instrument, so that the current passes between the tips of the two electrodes and affects only a small amount of tissue.

bipolar lead /lēd/, **1.** an electrocardiographic conductor having two electrodes placed on different body regions, with each electrode contributing to the record. **2.** *informal.* a tracing produced by such a lead on an electrocardiograph.

bipolar version, a method for changing the position of a fetus in which one hand is placed on the abdomen of the mother and two fingers of the other hand are inserted into the uterus.

bipotentiality /bī′pəten′shē·al′itē/ [L, *bis* + *potentia,* power], the characteristic of acting or reacting according to either of two possible states.

bird breeder's lung. See **pigeon breeder's lung.**

bird face retrognathism. See **retrognathism.**

birth [ME, *burth*],   **1.** the event of being born, the entry of a new person out of its mother into the world. Kinds of birth are **breech birth, live birth,** and **stillbirth.** See also **effacement, labor. 2.** the childbearing event, the bringing forth by a mother of a baby. **3.** a medical event, the delivery of a fetus by an obstetric attendant.

birth canal, *informal.* the passage that extends from the inlet of the true pelvis to the vaginal orifice through which an infant passes during vaginal birth. See also **clinical pelvimetry.**

birth center, a health facility with services limited to maternity care for women judged to be at minimum risk for obstetric complications that would require hospitalization.

birth certificate, a legal document recording information about a birth, including, among other details, the date, time, and location of the event; identity of the mother and father; and identity of the attending physician or licensed midwife.

birth control. See **contraception.**

birth defect. See **congenital anomaly.**

birthing, a nursing intervention from the Nursing Interventions Classification (NIC) defined as delivery of a baby. See also **Nursing Interventions Classification.**

birthing chair, a special seat used in labor and delivery to promote the comfort of the mother and facilitate the birthing process. The chair may be specially designed, having many technical features, or it may be a simple three-legged stool with a high, slanted back and a circular seat with a large central hole in it. The newer birthing chairs allow women to sit straight up or to recline. The chair has a lower section that may be removed or folded out of the way. Lights, mirrors, and basins may be attached. The upright position appears to shorten the time in labor, particularly the second or expulsive stage of labor, probably because of gravity and increased participation of the mother. The chair is not suitable for use with anesthesia.

birth injury, trauma suffered by a baby while being born. Some kinds of birth injury are **Bell's palsy, cerebral palsy,** and **Erb's palsy.**

birthmark. See **nevus.**

birth mother, the biologic mother or woman who bears a child. The child may have been conceived in a surrogate mother with sperm of the biologic father.

birth palsy [ME, *burth* + Gk, *paralyein,* to be palsied], a loss of motor or sensory nerve function in some body part caused by a nerve injury during the birth process. Also called **birth paralysis.**

birth paralysis. See **birth palsy.**

birth parent, one of an individual's two biologic parents.

birth rate, the proportion of the number of live births in a specific area during a given period to the total population of that area, usually expressed as the number of births per 1000 of population. Compare **crude birth rate, refined birth rate, true birth rate.**

birth trauma, **1.** any physical injury suffered by an infant during the process of delivery. **2.** the supposed psychic shock, according to some psychiatric theories, that an infant suffers during delivery.

birth weight, the measured heaviness of a baby when born, usually about 3500 g (7.5 pounds). In the United States, 97% of newborns weigh between 2500 g (5.5 pounds) and 4500 g (10 pounds). Babies weighing less than 2500 g at term are considered **small for gestational age.** Babies weighing more than 4500 g are considered **large for gestational age** and are often infants of mothers with diabetes.

bis-, prefix meaning "twice, two": *bisacromial, bisferious.*

bisacodyl /bisak′ōdil/, a cathartic.

■ INDICATIONS: It is prescribed in the treatment of acute or chronic constipation or for emptying of the bowel before or after surgery or before diagnostic radiographic procedures.

■ CONTRAINDICATIONS: Abdominal pain, nausea, vomiting, rectal fissures, ulcerated hemorrhoids, or known hypersensitivity to this drug prohibits its use.

■ ADVERSE EFFECTS: Among the more serious adverse reactions are colic, abdominal pain, and diarrhea.

bisacromial /bīsəkrō′mē·əl/, pertaining to both acromions, the triangular, flat, bony plates at the end of the scapula.

bisalbuminemia /bis′albyōōm′inē′mē·ə/, a condition in which two types of albumin exist in an individual. The two types are expressed by heterozygous alleles of the albumin gene and are detected by differences in the mobility of the types on electrophoretic gels.

bisect /bīsekt′/ [L, *bis* + *secare,* to cut], to divide into two equal lengths or parts.

bisexual /bīsek′shoo·əl/ [L, *bis* + *sexus,* male or female], **1.** hermaphroditic; having gonads of both sexes. **2.** possessing physical or psychologic characteristics of both sexes. **3.** engaging in both heterosexual and homosexual activity. **4.** desiring sexual contact with persons of both sexes.

bisexual libido, (in psychoanalysis) the tendency in a person to seek sexual gratification with people of either sex.

bisferious pulse /bisfer′ē·əs/ [L, *bis* + *ferire,* to beat], an arterial pulse that has two palpable peaks, the second of which is slightly weaker than the first. It may be detected in cases of aortic regurgitation and obstructive cardiomyopathy. Compare **dicrotic pulse.**

bishydroxycoumarin. See **dicumarol.**

bis in die (b.i.d.) /dē′ā/, a Latin phrase, used in prescriptions, meaning "twice a day." It is more commonly used in its abbreviated form.

bismuth (Bi) /biz′məth, bis′-/ [Ger, *wismut,* white mass], a reddish, crystalline, trivalent metallic element. Its atomic number is 83; its atomic mass is 208.98. It is combined with various other elements, such as oxygen, to produce numerous salts used in the manufacture of many pharmaceutic substances.

bismuth gingivitis, a dark bluish line along the gingival margin caused by bismuth administered in the treatment of systemic disease. See also **bismuth stomatitis, gingivitis.**

bismuth stomatitis, an abnormal oral condition caused by the systemic use of bismuth compounds over prolonged periods. It is characterized by a blue-black line on the inner aspect of the gingival sulcus or dark pigmentation of the buccal mucosa, sore tongue, metallic taste, and burning sensation in the mouth. Compare **arsenic stomatitis, Atabrine stomatitis.**

bismuth subsalicylate, a bismuth salt of salicylic acid, administered orally in the treatment of diarrhea and gastric distress, including nausea, indigestion, and heartburn.

bisoprolol /bis′o-pro′lol/, a synthetic beta-adrenergic blocking agent, used as the fumarate salt; administered orally as an antihypertensive agent.

bisphosphonate /bis-fos′fo-nāt/, diphosphonate.

bit /bit/, abbreviation for *bi*nary dig*it*, the smallest unit of information in a computer. Bits are the building blocks for all information processing in digital electronics and computers. Eight bits equals one byte. See also **byte.**

bitart, abbreviation for a *bitartrate carboxylate anion.*

bitartrate /bītär′trāt/, the monoanion of tartaric acid, $C_4H_5O_6^-$.

bitartrate carboxylate anion, an ionotropic agent used in the treatment of cardiovascular patients.

bite [AS, *bitan*], **1.** the act of cutting, tearing, holding, or gripping with the teeth. **2.** the lingual portion of an artificial tooth between its shoulder and its incisal edge. **3.** an occlusal record or relationship between the upper and lower teeth or jaws. Compare **closed bite, open bite.**

bite block. See **occlusion rim.**

bitegauge /bīt′gāj′/ [AS, *bitan* + OFr, *gauge,* measure], a prosthetic dental device that helps attain proper occlusion of the upper and lower teeth.

biteguard [AS, *bitan* + OFr, *garder,* to defend], a resin appliance that covers the occlusal and incisal surfaces of the teeth. It is used to stabilize the teeth, to provide a platform for the excursive glides of the mandible, and to eliminate the effects of nocturnal grinding of the teeth. Also called **biteplane, night guard.** Compare **mouth guard.**

biteguard splint, a device, usually made of resin, for covering the occlusal and incisal surfaces of the teeth and for protecting them from traumatic occlusal forces during immobilization and stabilization processes. See also **Gunning's splint.**

bitelock /bīt′lok′/, a dental device for retaining occlusion rims in the same relation outside and inside the mouth.

bitemporal /bītem′pərəl/ [L, *bis,* twice, *tempora,* temples], pertaining to both temples or both temporal bones.

bitemporal hemianopia [L, *bis,* twice, *tempora,* temples; Gk, *hemi,* half, *opsis,* vision], a loss of the temporal half of the vision in each eye, usually resulting from a lesion in the chiasmal area such as a pituitary tumor.

biteplane /bīt′plān/, **1.** See **occlusal plane. 2.** a metal sheet laid across the biting surfaces of the upper or lower teeth to determine the relationship of the teeth to the occlusal plane. **3.** an orthodontic appliance of acrylic resin worn over the maxillary occlusal surfaces and used to treat pain of the temporomandibular joint and adjacent muscles. Although removable, the device is kept in place by labial wires and wrought wire clasps. **4.** See **biteguard.**

biteplate /bīt′plāt/, a device used in dentistry as a diagnostic or therapeutic aid prosthodontics or for orthodontics. It is made of wire and plastic and worn in the palate. It may also be used in the correction of temporomandibular joint problems or as a splint in restoring the full mouth.

bite reflex, a swift, involuntary biting action that may be triggered by stimulation of the oral cavity. The bite can be difficult to release in some cases, such as when a spoon or tongue depressor is placed in a patient's mouth.

bite wing film [AS, *bitan* + ME, *winge*], a dental x-ray film on which a tab is placed so the teeth can hold the film in position during exposure. Also called **interproximal film.** See also **bite wing radiograph.**

bite wing radiograph, a dental radiograph that reveals the coronal portions of maxillary and mandibular teeth and portions of the interdental septa on the same film. See also **bite wing film.**

Bithynia /bəthin′ē·ə/, a genus of snails, species of which act as intermediate hosts to *Opisthorchis.*

biting in childhood, a natural behavior trait and reflex action in infants, acquired at about 5 to 6 months of age in response to the introduction of solid foods in the diet and the beginning of the teething process. The activity represents a significant modality in the psychosocial development of the child, because it is the first aggressive action the infant learns, and through it the infant learns to control the environment. The behavior also confronts the infant with one of the first inner conflicts, because biting can produce both pleasing and displeasing results. Biting during breastfeeding causes withdrawal of the nipple and anxiety in the mother, yet it also serves as a means of soothing teething discomfort. Infants continue to use biting as a mechanism for exploring

Bite wing radiograph of normal teeth
(Roberson, Heymann, and Swift, 2002)

their surroundings. Toddlers and older children often use biting for expressing aggression toward their parents and other children, especially during play or as a means of gaining attention. Most children normally outgrow the tendency unless they have severe maladaptive or emotional problems. See also **psychosexual development, psychosocial development.**

bitolterol /bi-tol′ter-ol/, a beta-adrenergic receptor agonist used as a bronchodilator; administered by inhalation as the mesylate salt in the treatment of bronchospasm associated with asthma and the treatment and prophylaxis of bronchospasm associated with chronic obstructive airway disease, including bronchitis and pulmonary emphysema.

bitolterol mesylate /bitol′tərol mes′ilāt/, an orally inhaled bronchodilator.

■ INDICATIONS: It is used in the treatment of bronchial asthma and reversible bronchospasm.

■ CONTRAINDICATIONS: This product is contraindicated in patients who are known to be hypersensitive to it.

■ ADVERSE EFFECTS: Among adverse reactions reported are tremor, nervousness, headache, dizziness, palpitations, chest discomfort, tachycardia, coughing, and throat irritation.

Bitot's spots /bitōz′/ [Pierre Bitot, French surgeon, 1822–1888], white or gray triangular deposits on the bulbar conjunctiva adjacent to the lateral margin of the cornea, a clinical sign of vitamin A deficiency. Also called **Bitot's patches.**

Bitot's spots *(McLaren, 1992)*

bitrochanteric lipodystrophy /bī′trōkənter′ik/ [L, *bis* + Gk, *trochanter,* runner; *lipos,* fat, *dys,* bad, *trophe,* nourishment], an abnormal and excessive deposition of fat on the buttocks and the outer aspect of the upper thighs, occurring most commonly in women. See also **lipodystrophy.**

biuret test /bī′yo͞oret/ [L, *bis* + Gk, *ouron*, urine], a method for detecting proteins in serum. In alkaline solution, copper sulfate ions react with the peptide bonds of proteins to produce a pink to purple color, called the biuret reaction. The amount of serum protein in a sample solution is estimated by comparing its color with that of a standard solution whose protein concentration is known.

bivalent /bīvā′lənt/ [L, *bis* + *valere*, to be powerful], **1.** See **divalent.** (in genetics) a pair of synapsed homologous chromosomes that are attached to each other by chiasmata during the early first meiotic prophase of gametogenesis. The structure serves as the basis for the tetrads from which gametes are produced during the two meiotic divisions. **2.** See **valence,** def. 1. —**bivalence,** *n.*

bivalent antibody, an antibody that has two or more binding sites that can cross-link one antigen to another.

bivalent chromosome, a pair of synapsed homologous chromosomes during the early stages of gametogenesis. See also **bivalent.**

bivalirudin /bi-val′īroo-din/, an inhibitor of the clot-promoting activity of thrombin, used in conjunction with aspirin as an anticoagulant in patients with unstable angina pectoris who are undergoing percutaneous transluminal coronary angioplasty; administered intravenously.

bivalved cast [L, *bis* + *valva,* valve], a cast that is cut in half to detect or relieve pressure underneath, especially when a patient has decreased or no sensation in the portion of the body surrounded by the cast. "Windows" are often cut out of the cast over the pressure areas to assess circulation or open wounds under the cast.

bivalve speculum, one with two blades that are adjustable.

biventricular pacing, that in which a lead is used to deliver current directly to the left ventricle, in addition to those used to deliver current to the right atrium and ventricle, so that the ventricles can be induced to pump in synchrony.

bizarre leiomyoma. See **epithelioid leiomyoma.**

Björnstad's syndrome /byôrn′städz/ [R. Björnstad, Swedish dermatologist, 20th century], an autosomal recessive disorder characterized by congenital sensorineural deafness and kinky hair.

Bk, symbol for the element **berkelium.**

BK, abbreviation for **below knee.**

black beauties, *slang,* amphetamines.

black cohosh, a perennial herb that grows throughout the United States and in parts of Canada.

■ USES: This herb is used to treat the symptoms of menopause (hot flashes and nervous conditions associated with menopause) and dysmenorrhea (menstrual cramps, pain, inflammation); generally considered to be effective against mild symptoms but not a substitute for estrogen-containing prescriptions needed to control more severe vasomotor symptoms.

■ CONTRAINDICATIONS: Black cohosh should not be used during pregnancy, since uterine stimulation can occur. It also should not be used during lactation or in children.

Black Creek Canal virus, a virus of the genus *Hantavirus* that causes hantavirus pulmonary syndrome.

black damp. See **damp.**

black death. See **bubonic plague.**

Blackett-Healy method, a positioning procedure for producing x-ray images of the subscapularis area. The patient is placed in a supine position with the affected shoulder joint centered on the midline of the film, the arm abducted, and

the elbow flexed. The opposite shoulder is raised about 15 degrees and supported with a sandbag.

black eye, contusion around the eye with bruising, discoloration, and swelling. It is usually treated for the first 24 hours with ice packs to reduce swelling, then with hot compresses to aid in resorption of blood from the hematoma. Also called **periorbital ecchymosis.**

Blackfan-Diamond anemia. See **Diamond-Blackfan syndrome.**

black fever. See **kala-azar.**

black hairy tongue. See **parasitic glossitis.**

black haw, an herb found in the Eastern United States.

■ USES: This herb is used for dysmenorrhea, menstrual cramps and pain, menopausal metrorrhagia, hysteria, asthma, and heart palpitations. It is also used to lower blood pressure. It is possibly effective at relieving uterine spasms but effectiveness in other instances has not been verified.

■ CONTRAINDICATIONS: Black haw should be used with caution in people with kidney stones since it contains oxalic acid.

blackhead. See **comedo.**

black light. See **Wood's light.**

black lung disease. See **anthracosis.**

black measles [AS, *blac* + OHG, *masala*], hemorrhagic measles characterized by a darkened rash caused by bleeding into the skin and mucous membranes. Also called **hemorrhagic measles.**

blackout, *informal.* a temporary loss of vision or consciousness.

black plague. See **bubonic plague.**

Black's Classification of Caries. See **classification of caries.**

black spots film fault, a defect in a radiograph, seen as dark spots throughout the image area. It is caused by dust particles or developer on the x-ray film before development or by outdated film.

blackwater fever, a serious complication of chronic falciparum malaria, characterized by jaundice, hemoglobinuria, acute renal failure, and passage of bloody dark red or black urine caused by massive intravascular hemolysis. Death occurs in 20% to 30% of all cases; the mortality rate is particularly high among Europeans. See also **falciparum malaria, malaria,** *Plasmodium.*

Blackwell, Elizabeth (1821–1910), a British-born American physician, the first woman to be awarded a medical degree. She established the New York Infirmary, a 40-bed hospital staffed entirely by women, in which she trained nurses in a 4-month course. Her influence helped others establish nursing schools to improve patient care.

black widow spider [AS, *blac* + *widewe;* ME, *spithre*], *Latrodectus mactans,* a species of spider found in the United States, whose bite causes pain and sometimes death.

black widow spider antivenin, a passive immunizing agent.

■ INDICATION: It is prescribed in the treatment of black widow spider bite.

■ CONTRAINDICATIONS: Known hypersensitivity to this drug or to horse serum prohibits its use.

■ ADVERSE EFFECTS: Among the more serious adverse effects are allergic reactions.

black widow spider bite [AS, *blac* + *widewe;* ME, *spithre* + AS, *bitan*], the bite of the spider species *Latrodectus mactans,* a poisonous arachnid found in many parts of the world. Black widow venom contains some enzymatic proteins, including a peptide that affects neuromuscular transmission. The bite is perceived as a sharp pinprick pain, followed by a dull pain in the area of the bite; restlessness; anxiety; sweating; weakness; and drooping eyelids. Muscu-

Black widow spider *(Auerbach, 1995)*

lar rigidity starts at the location of the bite and moves in peripherally to the chest. Small children, elderly adults, or persons with heart disorders are most severely affected and may require hospitalization and the administration of an antivenin. Immediate treatment includes keeping the victim quiet and immobilizing the bite area at the level of the heart.

bladder [AS, *blaedre*], **1.** a membranous sac serving as a receptacle for secretions, such as the gallbladder. **2.** the urinary bladder.

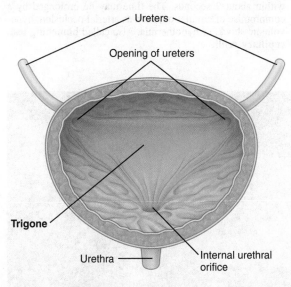

Bladder *(Drake, Vogl, and Mitchell, 2005)*

bladder augmentation, augmentation cystoplasty.

bladder calculus, vesical calculus.

bladder cancer, the most common malignancy of the urinary tract, characterized by multiple growths that tend to recur in a more aggressive form. Bladder cancer occurs 2.3 times more often in men than in women and is more prevalent in urban than in rural areas. The risk of bladder cancer increases with cigarette smoking and exposure to aniline dyes, beta-naphthylamine, mixtures of aromatic hydrocar-

bons, or benzidine and its salts, used in chemical, paint, plastics, rubber, textile, petroleum, and wood industries and in medical laboratories. Other predisposing factors are chronic urinary tract infections, calculous disease, and schistosomiasis. Symptoms of bladder cancer include hematuria, frequent urination, dysuria, and cystitis. Urinalysis, excretory urography, cystoscopy, or transurethral biopsy are performed for diagnosis. The majority of bladder malignancies are transitional cell carcinomas; a small percentage are squamous cell carcinomas or adenocarcinomas. Superficial or multiple lesions may be treated by fulguration or open loop resection. A segmental resection is usually performed if the tumor is at the dome or in a lateral wall of the bladder. Total cystectomy may be performed for an invasive lesion of the trigone. Radiation therapy and/or chemotherapy may be valuable under certain circumstances, such as unresectable tumor growth. Internal irradiation, the introduction of radioisotopes via a balloon of a catheter, or the implantation of radon seeds may be used in treating small localized tumors on the bladder wall. Medications that are often used as palliatives are BCG, 5-fluorouracil, thio-TEPA, and adriamycin. See also **cystectomy.**

Transitional cell carcinoma of bladder cancer
(Fletcher, 2000)

bladder flap, *informal.* the vesicouterine fold of peritoneum incised during low cervical cesarean section so the bladder can be separated from the uterus to expose the lower uterine segment for incision. The flap is reapproximated with sutures during closure to cover the uterine incision. See also **cesarean section.**

bladder hernia, a protrusion of the bladder through an opening in the abdominal wall.

bladder irrigation[1] [AS, *blaedre* + L, *irrigare,* to conduct water], the washing out of the bladder by a continuous or intermittent flow of saline or a medicated solution. The bladder also may be irrigated by an oral intake of fluid.

bladder irrigation[2], a nursing intervention from the Nursing Interventions Classification (NIC) defined as instillation of a solution into the bladder to provide cleansing or medication. See also **Nursing Interventions Classification.**

bladder neck dyssynergia, reduced opening of the bladder neck during urination caused by dyssynergia of the smooth muscle, resulting in partial obstruction of urinary flow; seen primarily in young to middle-aged men. Also called *smooth sphincter d.*

bladder neck incision, surgical incision of the bladder neck, an operation similar to but less serious than bladder neck resection.

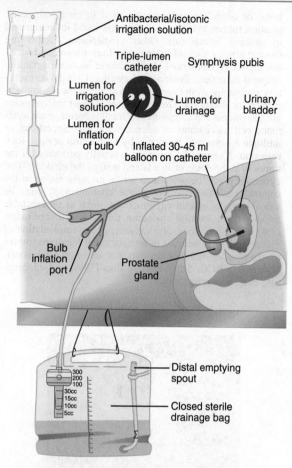

- Antibacterial/isotonic irrigation solution
- Triple-lumen catheter
- Symphysis pubis
- Lumen for irrigation solution
- Lumen for drainage
- Urinary bladder
- Lumen for inflation of bulb
- Inflated 30-45 ml balloon on catheter
- Bulb inflation port
- Prostate gland
- Distal emptying spout
- Closed sterile drainage bag

Bladder irrigation *(Black and Hawks, 2005)*

bladder neck resection, surgical removal of the bladder neck, usually done by the transurethral route to treat obstruction or neurogenic dysfunction.

bladder neck suspension, any of various methods of surgical fixation of the urethrovesical junction area and the bladder neck to restore the neck to a high retropubic position for relief of stress incontinence. The group includes the Marshall-Marchetti-Krantz operation and the Burch, Pereyra, and Stamey procedures. Also called *colposuspension.*

bladder outlet obstruction, any of various blockages in the outflow of urine from the bladder; causes include benign prostatic hyperplasia, bladder neck dyssynergia, prostate cancer or another tumor that presses against the urethra, and a variety of other conditions.

bladder retraining [AS, *blaedre* + L, *trahere,* to draw], a system of therapy for urinary incontinence in which a patient practices withholding urine while maintaining a normal intake of fluid. The interval between urination is increased from about 1 hour to 3–4 hours over a period of 10 days. The patient also learns to recognize and react to the urge to urinate.

bladder sphincter [AS, *blaedre* + Gk, *sphingein,* to bind], a circular muscle surrounding the opening of the urinary bladder into the urethra.

bladder stone. See **vesicle calculus.**

bladder wall, the surrounding structure of the urinary

bladder, consisting of the serous coat, subserous layer, muscular coat, submucous layer, and mucous coat.

Blakemore-Sengstaken tube. See **Sengstaken-Blakemore tube.**

Blalock-Taussig procedure /blā'loktô'sig/ [Alfred Blalock, American surgeon, 1899–1964; Helen B. Taussig, American physician, 1898–1986], surgical construction of a shunt as a temporary measure to overcome congenital heart malformations, such as tetralogy of Fallot, in which there is insufficient pulmonary blood flow. Before surgery, a cardiac catheterization is done to identify the defect or defects, and the arterial blood gases are analyzed. Hypothermia anesthesia and a cardiac bypass machine are used. The subclavian artery is joined end to end with the pulmonary artery, directing blood from the systemic circulation to the lungs. Thrombosis of the shunt is the major postoperative complication. Permanent surgical correction is performed in early childhood. See also **heart surgery.**

blame placing, the process of placing responsibility for one's behavior on others.

blanch /blanch, blänch/ [Fr, *blanchir,* to become white], **1.** to cause to become pale, as a nailbed may be blanched by using digital pressure. **2.** to press blood away and wait for return, such as blanching of fingernails and return of blood. **3.** to become white or pale, as from vasoconstriction accompanying fear or anger.

blanch test [Fr, *blanchir,* to become white; L, *testum,* crucible], a test of blood circulation in the fingers or toes. Pressure is applied to a fingernail or toenail until normal color is lost. The pressure is then removed, and, if the circulation is normal, color should return almost immediately, within about 2 seconds. The time may be prolonged by a compromise of circulation, such as arterial occlusion, hypovolemic shock, or hypothermia. Also called **blanching test, capillary refill.**

Blanch test *(Chapleau, 2004)*

bland [L, *blandus*], mild or having a soothing effect.

bland aerosols, aerosols that consist of water, saline solutions, or similar substances that do not have important pharmacologic action. They are primarily used for humidification and liquefaction of secretions.

bland diet, a diet that is mechanically, chemically, physiologically, and sometimes thermally nonirritating to the GI tract. It is often prescribed in the treatment of peptic ulcer, ulcerative colitis, gallbladder disease, diverticulitis, gastritis, idiopathic spastic constipation, and mucous colitis and after abdominal surgery. Historically, it was first called the "white diet" (or Sippy diet, after Dr. Sippy, who developed it). This allowed the use of only white foods, such as milk, cream, mashed potatoes, and hot cereal (Cream of Wheat). It has progressed to what has been called the "liberal bland diet," which allows all foods except caffeine, alcohol, black pepper, spices, or any other food that could be considered irritating. The clinical value of the traditional bland diet has never been proven.

blank, a solution containing all of the reagents needed for analysis of a substance except the substance tested.

blanket bath [OFr, *blanchet,* a white garment], the procedure of wrapping the patient in a wet pack and then in blankets.

blast, **1.** a primitive cell, such as an embryonic germ cell. **2.** a cell capable of building tissue, such as an osteoblast in growing bone.

-blast, suffix meaning an "embryonic state of development": *megaloblast, osteoblast.*

blast cell [Gk, *blastos,* germ], any immature cell, such as an erythroblast, lymphoblast, or neuroblast.

blastema /blastē'mə/, *pl.* **blastemas, blastemata** [Gk, bud], **1.** any mass of cells capable of growth and differentiation, specifically the primordial, undifferentiated cellular material from which a particular organ or tissue develops. **2.** in certain animals, a group of cells capable of regenerating a lost or damaged part or creating a complete organism in asexual reproduction. **3.** the budding or sprouting area of a plant. See also **anlage. —blastemal, blastematic, blastemic,** *adj.*

-blastema /-blas'təmə/, suffix meaning a "beginning substance or foundation for new growth": *epiblastema, scytoblastema.*

blastemata, blastemal, blastematic, blastemic. See **blastema.**

blastic transformation, a late stage in the progress of chronic granulocytic leukemia; the leukemic cells become more undifferentiated and morphologically and genetically more abnormal, with more aggressive growth patterns. Signs of anemia and blood platelet deficiency are present, and half of the blood cells in the bone marrow are immature forms. Blastic transformation indicates that resistance to therapy has developed in the patient who has entered a terminal stage of leukemia.

blastid /blas'tid/ [Gk, *blastos,* germ], the site in the fertilized ovum where the pronuclei fuse and the nucleus forms. Also called **blastide.**

blastin /blas'tin/ [Gk, *blastanein,* to grow], any substance that provides nourishment for or stimulates the growth or proliferation of cells, such as allantoin.

blasto-, blast-, combining form meaning "an early embryonic or developing stage": *blastocoele, blastema.*

blastocoele /blas'təsēl'/ [Gk, *blastos,* germ, *koilos,* hollow], the fluid-filled cavity of the blastocyst in mammals and the blastula or discoblastula of lower animals. The cavity increases the surface area of the developing embryo to allow better absorption of nutrients and oxygen. Also spelled **blastocoel, blastocele.** Also called **cleavage cavity, segmentation cavity, subgerminal cavity.**

blastocyst /blas'təsist/ [Gk, *blastos + kystis,* bag], the embryonic form that follows the morula in human development. Implantation in the wall of the uterus usually occurs at this stage, on approximately the eighth day after fertilization. The blastocyst consists of an outer layer (trophoblast) which is attached to the inner cell mast.

Blastocyst (Applegate, 2000)

blastocyst cavity, the fluid-filled cavity developing in the morula as it becomes a blastocyst.

blastocyte /blas'təsīt/ [Gk, *blastos + kytos,* cell], an undifferentiated embryonic cell that precedes germ layer formation. **—blastocytic,** *adj.*

blastocytoma. See **blastoma.**

blastoderm /blas'tədurm'/ [Gk, *blastos + derma,* skin], the layer of cells forming the wall of the blastocyst in mammals and the blastula in lower animals during the early stages of embryonic development. It is produced by the cleavage of the fertilized ovum and gives rise to the primary germ layers, the ectoderm, mesoderm, and endoderm, from which the embryo and all of its membranes are derived. Kinds of blastoderm are **bilaminar blastoderm, embryonic blastoderm, extraembryonic blastoderm,** and **trilaminar blastoderm.** Also called **germinal membrane. —blastodermal, blastodermic,** *adj.*

blastodisk /blas'tədisk/, the disklike, yolk-free area of cytoplasm surrounding the animal pole in a yolk-rich ovum, such as that of birds and reptiles. The blastodisk is the site where cleavage occurs after fertilization. As cleavage continues, the blastodisk develops into the embryo. Also spelled **blastodisc.**

blastogenesis /blas'tōjen'əsis/ [Gk, *blastos + genein,* to produce], **1.** asexual reproduction by budding. **2.** the transmission of hereditary characteristics by the germ plasm. Compare **pangenesis. 3.** the early development of an embryo during cleavage and formation of the germ layers. **4.** the process of transforming small lymphocytes in tissue culture into large, blastlike cells by exposure to phytohemagglutinin or other substances, often for the purpose of inducing mitosis. **—blastogenetic,** *adj.*

blastogenic /-jen'ik/, **1.** originating in the germ plasm. **2.** initiating tissue proliferation. **3.** relating to or characterized by blastogenesis.

blastogenic factor, lymphocyte-transforming factor.

blastogeny /blastoj'ənē/, the early stages in ontogeny; the germ plasm history of an organism or species, which traces the history of inherited characteristics.

blastokinin /blas'təkī'nin/ [Gk, *blastos + kinein,* to move], a globulin, secreted by the uterus in many mammals, that may stimulate and regulate the implantation process of the blastocyst in the uterine wall. Also called **uteroglobulin.**

blastolysis /blastol'isis/ [Gk, *blastos + lysis,* loosening], destruction of a germ cell or blastoderm. **—blastolytic,** *adj.*

blastoma /blastō'mə/, *pl.* **blastomas, blastomata** [Gk, *blastos + oma,* tumor], a neoplasm of embryonic tissue that develops from the blastema of an organ or tissue. A blastoma derived from a number of scattered cells is pluricentric; one arising from a single cell or group of cells is unicentric. Also called **blastocytoma. —blastomatous** /blastom′ətəs/, *adj.*

blastomatosis /blast′tōmətō′sis/ [Gk, *blastos* + *oma,* tumor, *osis,* condition], the development of many tumors from embryonic tissue.

blastomatous. See **blastoma.**

blastomere /blas′təmēr/ [Gk, *blastos* + *meros,* part], any of the cells formed from the first mitotic division of a fertilized ovum (zygote). The blastomeres further divide and subdivide to form a multicellular morula in the first several days of pregnancy. Also called **segmentation cell.** See also **blastula. —blastomeric,** *adj.*

blastomere biopsy, a technique for preimplantation genetic diagnosis, in which a blastomere is removed from a 6- or 8-cell embryo and tested for genetic abnormalities.

blastomerotomy /-merot′əmē/ [Gk, *blastos* + *meros,* part, *tome,* cut], destruction of blastomere. Also called **blastotomy.** /blastot′əmē/, **-blastomerotomic,** *adj.*

Blastomyces /blas′tōmī′sēz/ [Gk, *blastos* + *mykes,* fungus], a genus of yeastlike fungi, usually including the species *Blastomyces dermatitidis,* which causes North American blastomycosis, and *Paracoccidioides brasiliensis,* which causes South American blastomycosis.

Blastomyces dermatitidis (Baron, Peterson, and Finegold, 1994)

blastomycosis /blas′tōmīkō′sis/ [Gk, *blastos* + *mykes,* fungus, *osis,* condition], an infectious disease caused by a yeastlike fungus, *Blastomyces dermatitidis.* It usually affects only the skin but may cause acute pneumonitis or disseminated disease and invade the lungs, kidneys, central nervous system, and bones. The disease is most common in river valleys of North America, particularly the southeastern United States, but outbreaks have occurred in Africa and Latin America. Skin infections are almost always a result of hematogenous seeding from a primary infection and often begin as small papules on the hand, face, neck, or other exposed areas where there has been a cut, bruise, or other injury. The infection may spread gradually and irregularly into surrounding areas. When the lungs are involved, mucous membrane lesions resemble squamous cell carcinoma. The person usually has a cough, dyspnea, chest pain, chills, and a fever with heavy sweating. Diagnosis is made by identification of the disease organism in a culture of specimens from lesions. Treatment usually involves the administration of amphotericin B in pulmonary disease or intraconazole or ketoconazole. Recovery usually begins within the first week of treatment. Also called **Gilchrist's disease.** See also **fungus, mycosis.**

Blastomycosis (Callen et al, 2000)

blastopore /blas′təpôr/ [Gk, *blastos* + *poros,* opening], (in embryology) the opening into the archenteron made by invagination of the blastula.

blastoporic canal. See **neurenteric canal.**

blastosphere. See **blastula.**

blastotomy. See **blastomerotomy.**

blastula /blas′tyələ/ [Gk, *blastos,* germ], an early stage of the process through which a zygote develops into an embryo, characterized by a fluid-filled sphere formed by a single layer of cells. The spheric layer of cells is called a blastoderm; the fluid-filled cavity is the blastocoele. The blastula develops from the morula stage and is usually the form in which the embryo becomes implanted in the wall of the uterus. Also called **blastosphere.**

-blastula, suffix meaning an "early embryonic stage in the development of a fertilized egg": *coeloblastula, stero-blastula.*

blastulation, the transformation of the morula into a blastocyst or blastula by the development of a central cavity, the blastocoele.

BLB mask, abbreviation for **Boothby-Lovelace-Bulbulian mask.**

bleaching /blēch′ing/ [ME, *blechen*], the act or process of removing stains or color by chemical means.

bleaching agents, medications and over-the-counter preparations used to depigment the skin. The products may be used by persons whose skin has become hyperpigmented through exposure to sunlight and particularly for melasma associated with pregnancy, the use of oral contraceptives, or hormone replacement therapy. Most agents are sold as creams or lotions and contain hydroquinone.

bleach poisoning, an adverse reaction to ingestion of hypochlorite salts commonly found in household and commercial bleaches. Symptoms include pain and inflammation of the mouth, throat, and esophagus; vomiting; shock; and circulatory collapse.

bleb /bleb/ [ME, blob], an accumulation of fluid under the skin.

bleed [AS, *blod,* blood], **1.** to lose blood from the blood vessels of the body. The blood may flow externally through an orifice or a break in the skin or flow internally into a cavity, into an organ, or between tissues. **2.** to cause blood to flow from a vein or an artery.

bleeder, *informal,* **1.** a person who has hemophilia or any other vascular or hematologic condition associated with a tendency to hemorrhage. **2.** blood vessel that bleeds, especially one cut during a surgical procedure.

bleeding, the release of blood from the vascular system as a result of damage to a blood vessel. See also **blood clotting.**

bleeding diathesis, a predisposition to abnormal blood clotting.

bleeding precautions, a nursing intervention from the Nursing Interventions Classification (NIC) defined as reduction of stimuli that may induce bleeding or hemorrhage in at-risk patients. See also **Nursing Interventions Classification.**

bleeding reduction, a nursing intervention from the Nursing Interventions Classification (NIC) defined as limitation of the loss of blood volume during an episode of bleeding. See also **Nursing Interventions Classification.**

bleeding reduction: antepartum uterus, a nursing intervention from the Nursing Interventions Classification (NIC) defined as limitation of the amount of blood loss from the pregnant uterus during third trimester of pregnancy. See also **Nursing Interventions Classification.**

bleeding reduction: gastrointestinal, a nursing intervention from the Nursing Interventions Classification (NIC) defined as limitation of the amount of blood loss from the upper and lower gastrointestinal tract and related complications. See also **Nursing Interventions Classification.**

bleeding reduction: nasal, a nursing intervention from the Nursing Interventions Classification (NIC) defined as limitation of the amount of blood loss from the nasal cavity. See also **Nursing Interventions Classification.**

bleeding reduction: postpartum uterus, a nursing intervention from the Nursing Interventions Classification (NIC) defined as limitation of the amount of blood loss from the postpartum uterus. See also **Nursing Interventions Classification.**

bleeding reduction: wound, a nursing intervention from the Nursing Interventions Classification (NIC) defined as limitation of the blood loss from a wound that may be a result of trauma, incisions, or placement of a tube or catheter. See also **Nursing Interventions Classification.**

bleeding time, the time required for blood to stop flowing from a tiny wound. A test of bleeding time is the **Ivy method.** See also **hemostasis, simplate bleeding time.**

bleeding time test, a blood test used to evaluate the vascular and platelet factors associated with hemostasis. This test is occasionally performed preoperatively to ensure adequate hemostasis.

blemish [OFr, *bleme,* to deface], a skin stain, alteration, defect, or flaw.

blended family [ME, *blenden,* to mix], a family formed when parents bring together children from previous marriages.

blending inheritance, the apparent fusion in offspring of distinct, dissimilar characteristics of the parents. Blended characteristics are usually of a quantitative nature, such as height, and fail to segregate in successive generations. The phenomenon is the result of multiple pairs of genes that have a cumulative effect. See also **polygene.**

blenno-, blenn-, combining form meaning "mucus": *blennemesis, blennothorax.*

blennorrhea /blen'ərē'ə/ [Gk, *blennos,* mucus, *rhoia,* flow], excessive discharge of mucus. See also pharyngoconjunctival fever. Also called **blennorrhoea, blennorrhagia** /blen'ôrā'jē·ə/.

Blenoxane, trademark for an antineoplastic (bleomycin sulfate).

bleomycin sulfate /blē·əmī'sin/, an antineoplastic antibiotic.

■ INDICATIONS: It is prescribed in the treatment of a variety of neoplasms.

■ CONTRAINDICATION: Hypersensitivity to this drug prohibits its use.

■ ADVERSE EFFECTS: Among the most serious adverse reactions are pneumonitis, pulmonary fibrosis, and a syndrome of hyperpyrexia and circulatory collapse. Rashes and skin reactions commonly occur.

blephar-. See **blepharo-.**

blepharal /blef'ərəl/ [Gk, *blepharon,* eyelid], pertaining to the eyelids.

blepharedema /blef'əridē'mə/, a fluid accumulation in the eyelid, causing a swollen appearance.

-blepharia, suffix meaning "(condition of the) eyelid": *atretoblepharia, macroblepharia.*

blepharitis /blef'ərī'tis/ [Gk, *blepharon + itis*], an inflammatory condition of the lash follicles and meibomian glands of the eyelids, characterized by swelling, redness, and crusts of dried mucus on the lids. **Ulcerative blepharitis** is caused by bacterial infection. **Nonulcerative blepharitis** may be caused by psoriasis, seborrhea, or an allergic response.

■ OBSERVATIONS: Individuals report a foreign-body sensation of the eye.There are red eyelid margins, flaking and scaling around lashes, an itching and burning sensation, and loss of lashes. Light sensitivity, conjunctivitis, and possible corneal inflammation may also occur. In ulcerative blepharitis there are crusts on the eyelids, which bleed when removed. Small pustules develop in lash follicles and eyelids become "glued" together by dried drainage during sleep. Lid margins thicken over time with misdirected growth and/or loss of eyelashes. Corneal pannus, ulcerative keratitis, and lid ectropion can occur in severe cases. Diagnosis is made by clinical examination and lab tests may be run to isolate the causative agent. Individuals with chronic diseases, such as diabetes, gout, anemia, and rosacea; or a history of sties, chalazia, or chronic infections of the mouth and/or throat are at greater risk.

■ INTERVENTION: Blepharitis is stubborn to treat and is often resistant to various therapies. Topical antiinfective ointments and drops are used but the mainstay of treatment is the use of eyelid scrubs.

■ NURSING CONSIDERATIONS: Nurses need to provide individuals with detailed instructions in scrubbing and washing techniques. Eyelid hygiene consists of scrubbing the lid margins and lashes on closed eyelids daily; massaging lid margins to stimulate flow of secretions then cleansing with a cotton swab dipped in a diluted solution of baby shampoo. Careful instructions are needed for the application of antibiotic ointments to lid margins and drops to ocular surfaces. Individuals should also be instructed to use seborrheic dermatitis medicated shampoos and to apply hot compresses for 5 to 10 minutes to closed eyelids to loosen lid debris.

blepharo-, blephar-, combining form meaning "eyelid or eyelash": *blepharochalasis, blepharelosis.*

blepharoadenoma /-ad'inō'mə/, *pl.* **blepharoadenomas, blepharoadenomata,** a glandular epithelial tumor of the eyelid.

blepharoatheroma /-ath'ərō'mə/, *pl.* **blepharoatheromas,** blepharoatheromata, a tumor of the eyelid.

blepharochalasis /blef'ə·rō·kal'ə·sis/ [Gk, *blepharon,* eyelid + chalasis, relaxation], relaxation of the skin of the eyelid because of atrophy of the intercellular tissue.

Blepharitis *(Zitelli and Davis, 1997)*

blepharoclonus /blef′ərok′lōnəs/, a condition characterized by muscle spasms of the eyelid, appearing as increased winking.

blepharoncus /blef′əron′kəs/ [Gk, *blepharon* + *onkos*, swelling], a tumor of the eyelid.

blepharophimosis /blef′ə·rō·fi·mō′sis/ [Gk, *blepharon*, eyelid + *phimōsis*, a muzzling], abnormal narrowness of the palpebral fissure in the horizontal direction, caused by lateral displacement of the medial canthus.

blepharoplasty /blef′əroplas′tē/ [Gk, *blepharon*, eyelid, *plassein*, to mold], the use of plastic surgery to restore or repair the eyelid and eyebrow. Also called **brow lift.**

Removal of excess fat from upper eyelid

Wound closure

Blepharoplasty procedure *(Beare and Myers, 1998)*

blepharoplegia /-plē′jē·ə/ [Gk, *blepharon* + *plege,* stroke], paralysis of muscles of the eyelid.

blepharospasm /blef′ərōspaz′əm/ [Gk, *blepharon*, eyelid, *spasmos*, spasm], the involuntary contraction of eyelid muscles. The condition may be caused by a local lesion of the eye, a neurologic irritation, or psychologic stress.

blessed thistle, an annual herb found in Europe and Asia.

■ USES: This herb is used for loss of appetite, indigestion, and intestinal gas; probably safe when used as recommended but evidence of effectiveness is lacking.

■ CONTRAINDICATIONS: Blessed thistle should not be used during pregnancy, in children, or in those with known hypersensitivity to the herb.

Bleuler, Eugen /bloi′lər/ [Swiss psychiatrist, 1857–1939], a pioneer investigator in the fields of autism and schizophrenia. Bleuler introduced the term *schizophrenia* to replace *dementia praecox* and identified four primary symptoms of schizophrenia, known as Bleuler's "4 A's": ambivalence, associative disturbance, autistic thinking, and affective incongruity.

blighted ovum /blī′tid/, a fertilized ovum that fails to develop. On x-ray or ultrasonic visualization it appears to be a fluid-filled cyst attached to the wall of the uterus. It may be empty, or it may contain amorphous parts. Many first trimester spontaneous abortions represent the expulsion of a blighted ovum. Suction curettage may be necessary if the blighted ovum is retained.

blind [AS, *blind*], the absence of sight. The term may indicate a total loss of vision or may be applied in a modified manner to describe certain visual limitations, as in yellow color blindness (tritanopia) or word blindness (dyslexia). Legal blindness is defined as best corrected visual acuity less than 20/200 in the better eye.

blind fistula [AS, *blind* + L, pipe], an abnormal passage with only one open end; the opening may be on the body surface or on or within an internal organ or structure. Also called **incomplete fistula.**

blindgut. See **cecum.**

blind intubation. See **intubation.**

blind loop [AS, *blind* + ME, *loupe*], a redundant segment of intestine. Bacterial overgrowth occurs and may lead to malabsorption, obstruction, and necrosis. Blind loops may be created inadvertently by surgical procedures, such as side to side ileotransverse colostomy. See also **blind spot.**

blind loop syndrome. See **stasis syndrome.**

blindness. See **blind.**

blind spot, 1. a normal gap in the visual field occurring when an image is focused on the space in the retina occupied by the optic disc. 2. an abnormal gap in the visual field caused by a lesion on the retina or in the optic pathways or resulting from hemorrhage or choroiditis, often perceived as light spots or flashes.

blink reflex [ME, *blenken* + L, *reflectere*, to bend back], the automatic closure of the eyelid when an object is perceived to be rapidly approaching the eye.

blister, a vesicle or bulla.

blister agents/vesicants, chemicals that cause blistering of the skin or mucous membranes on contact. These agents include phosgene oxime, lewisite, distilled mustard, mustard gas, nitrogen mustard, sesqui mustard, and sulfur mustard. Exposure is mainly by inhalation or by contact with the skin or eyes. Inhalation causes shortness of breath, tachypnea, and hemoptysis, and death may result from the accumulation of fluid in the lungs; contact with the skin causes blistering and necrosis; and ocular contact causes swelling of the eyelids and corneal damage and can lead to blindness. Exposure to high doses affects the cardiovascular and nervous systems and may lead to cardiac arrest, convulsions, and coma. If these agents are ingested, nausea, vomiting, hematemesis, and diarrhea result. No antidote exists for most blister agents and treatment consists of removal of clothing, washing of the exposed areas, and supportive care. Lewisite can be neutralized by the application of British anti-Lewisite if it is done soon after exposure.

bloat [ME, *blout*], a swelling or filling with gas, such as distension of the abdomen that results from swallowed air or from intestinal gas. The stomach on percussion will have a tympanic sound.

Blocadren, trademark for a beta-adrenergic receptor blocking agent (timolol maleate).

Bloch-Sulzberger incontinentia pigmenti, Bloch-Sulzberger syndrome. See **incontinentia pigmenti.**

block [OFr, *bloc*], 1. a stoppage or obstruction. The term is commonly used to indicate an obstruction to the passage of a nerve impulse, as an alpha block of an impulse to an alpha-adrenergic receptor or a beta block of an impulse to a beta-adrenergic receptor. 2. an anesthetic injected in a local area, as a spinal block or mandibular block. **3.** a dental device, as a bite block.

blockade /blokād'/, an agent that interferes with or prevents a specific action in an organ or tissue, such as a cholinergic blockade that inhibits transmission of acetylcholine-stimulated nerve impulses along fibers of the autonomic nervous system.

blockage. See **obstruction.**

block anesthesia. See **conduction anesthesia.**

blocked communication, a situation in which communication with a patient is made difficult because of incongruent verbal and nonverbal messages and messages that contain discrepancies and inconsistencies. To clarify blocked communication, therapists may record meetings with patients on videotapes that can be studied for eye contact and other clues to the patient's thinking processes. See also **blocking.**

blocked pleurisy, circumscribed pleurisy, encysted pleurisy.

blocker. See **blocking agent.**

blocking [ME, *blok*], **1.** preventing the transmission of an impulse, such as by an antiadrenergic agent or by the injection of an anesthetic. **2.** interrupting an intracellular biosynthetic process, such as by the injection of actinomycin D or the action of an antivitamin. **3.** an interruption in the spontaneous flow of speech or thought. **4.** repressing an idea or emotion to prevent it from obtruding into the consciousness.

blocking agent, an agent that inhibits a biologic action, such as movement of an ion across the cell membrane, passage of a neural impulse, or interaction with a specific receptor.

blocking antibody, an antibody that fails to cross-link and cause agglutination. When such antibodies are present in high concentration, they interfere with the action of other antibodies by occupying all the antigenic sites. See also **antigen-antibody reaction, hapten.**

blockout /blok'out/ [OFr, *bloc* + AS, *ūt*], in dentistry, elimination in a cast of undesirable undercut areas by filling them in with a suitable material; this includes all areas that would offer interference to placement of the denture framework and those not crossed by a rigid part of the denture.

blood [AS, *blod*], the liquid pumped by the heart through all the arteries, veins, and capillaries. The blood is composed of a clear yellow fluid, called plasma, and the formed elements, and a series of cell types with different functions. The major function of the blood is to transport oxygen and nutrients to the cells and to remove carbon dioxide and other waste products from the cells for detoxification and elimination. Adults normally have a total blood volume of 7% to 8% of body weight, or 70 ml/kg of body weight for men and about 65 ml/kg for women. Blood is pumped through the body at a speed of about 30 cm/second, with a complete circulation time of 20 seconds. Compare **lymph.** See also **blood cell, erythrocyte, leukocyte, plasma, platelet.**

blood agar, a culture medium consisting of blood (usually sheep's blood) and nutrient agar, used in bacteriology to cultivate certain microorganisms, including *Staphylococcus epidermidis, Streptococcus pneumoniae,* and *Clostridium perfringens.*

blood agents, poisons that affect the body by being absorbed into the blood. Blood agents include arsine and cyanide. Exposure to both may occur by inhalation, and cyanide exposure may also occur by ingestion and absorption through the skin and eyes. Arsine causes hemolysis, resulting in generalized weakness, jaundice, delirium, and renal failure; high doses may result in death. There is no antidote and treatment is supportive. Cyanide prevents cells from using oxygen, leading to cell death, and poisoning especially

Blood *(Carr and Rodak, 1999)*

affects the cardiovascular and nervous systems and can lead to heart and brain damage and death from respiratory failure. Treatment consists of the administration of an antidote and supportive care.

blood albumin [AS, *blod* + L, *albus*], the plasma protein circulating in blood serum. Also called **serum albumin.**

blood and urine cortisol, a blood or urine test that assists in the evaluation of adrenal activity. Adrenal hyperfunction may indicate Cushing's disease, adrenal adenoma or carcinoma, ectopic ACTH-producing tumors, or hyperthyroidism, while hypofunction may indicate congenital adrenal hyperplasia, Addison's disease, hypopituitarism, hypothyroidism, or liver disease.

blood and urine uric acid, a blood/urine test that detects levels of uric acid in order to determine the presence of hyperuricemia (elevated uric acid in the blood) and uricosuria (elevated uric acid in the urine). Causes of abnormal uric acid levels may include gout, kidney failure, alcoholism, leukemias, metastatic cancer, multiple myeloma, hyperlipoproteinemia, diabetes mellitus, stress, lead poisoning, and dehydration.

blood bank, an organizational unit responsible for collecting, processing, and storing blood for transfusion and other purposes. The blood bank is usually a subdivision of a laboratory in a hospital and is often charged with the responsibility for serologic testing. See also **bank blood, component therapy, transfusion.**

blood bank technology specialist, an allied health professional who performs both routine and specialized immunohematologic tests in technical areas of the modern blood bank and who performs transfusion services using methodology that conforms to the *Standards for Blood Banks and Transfusion Services* of the American Association of Blood Banks. The individual may be responsible for testing for blood group antigens, compatibility, and antibody identification; investigating abnormalities such as hemolytic diseases of the newborn, hemolytic anemias, and adverse responses to transfusions; supporting physicians and nurses in transfusion therapy, including that for homologous organ transplantation; collecting and processing blood, including selecting donors, drawing and typing blood, and performing pretransfusion tests to ensure patient safety.

blood bilirubin test, a blood test performed in cases of jaundice to help determine whether the jaundice is caused by hepatocellular dysfunction (as in hepatitis) or extrahepatic obstruction of the bile ducts (as with gallstones or tumor blocking the bile ducts). Total serum bilirubin is made up of conjugated (direct) and unconjungated (indirect) bilirubin, with varying ratios of each characterizing different diseases.

blood blister, a blister containing blood; it may be caused by a pinch, a bruise, or persistent friction.

blood-borne pathogens, pathogenic microorganisms that are transmitted via human blood and cause disease in humans. They include, but are not limited to, hepatitis B virus (HBV) and human immunodeficiency virus (HIV). Although a number of pathogens can be transmitted percutaneously HIV-1 remains the most common.

blood-brain barrier (BBB) [AS, *blod* + *bragen* + ME, *barrere*], an anatomic-physiologic feature of the brain thought to consist of walls of capillaries in the central nervous system and surrounding astrocytic glial membranes. The barrier separates the parenchyma of the central nervous system from blood. The blood-brain barrier prevents or slows the passage of some drugs and other chemical compounds, radioactive ions, and disease-causing organisms such as viruses from the blood into the central nervous system.

Blood-brain barrier

blood buffers [AS, *blod* + ME, *buffe,* to cushion], a system of buffers, composed primarily of dissolved carbon dioxide and bicarbonate ions, that functions in maintaining the proper pH of the blood. See also **buffer, arterial pH.**

blood capillaries [AS, *blod* + L, *capillaris,* hairlike], the tiny vessels that convey blood between the arterioles and the venules and allow for internal respiration and nourishment of tissues. The capillary wall generally has a thickness of one cell, permitting easy diffusion of gas molecules; occasional tiny openings permit diapedesis of leukocytes, distribution of nutrients to the tissues supplied by the capillary network, and collection of waste products released by the cells.

blood cell, any of the formed elements of the blood, including red cells (erythrocytes), white cells (leukocytes), and platelets (thrombocytes). Blood cells constitute about 50% of the total volume of the blood. See also **erythrocyte, leukocyte, platelet.**

blood cell casts [AS, *blod* + L, *cella,* storeroom; ONorse, *kasta*], a mass of blood debris released from a diseased body surface or excreted in the urine.

blood chloride test, a blood test performed as part of mul-

tiphasic testing of electrolytes. It is performed along with other electrolyte tests to indicate the patient's acid-base balance and hydrational status.

blood circulation [AS, *blod* + L, *circulare,* to go around], the circuit of blood through the body, from the heart through the arteries, arterioles, capillaries, venules, and veins and back to the heart.

blood clot [AS, *blod* + *clott,* lump], a semisolid, gelatinous mass, the final result of the clotting process in blood. Red cells, white cells, and platelets are enmeshed in an insoluble fibrin network of the blood clot. Compare **embolus, thrombus.** See also **blood clotting, fibrinogen.**

blood clotting, the conversion of blood from a free-flowing liquid to a semisolid gel. Although clotting can occur within an intact blood vessel, the process usually starts with tissue damage. Within seconds of injury to the vessel wall, platelets clump at the site. If normal amounts of calcium, platelets, and tissue factors are present, prothrombin is converted to thrombin. Thrombin acts as a catalyst for the conversion of fibrinogen to a mesh of insoluble fibrin, in which all the formed elements are immobilized. Different pharmacologic agents may interact throughout this process. Also called **blood coagulation.** Compare **hemostasis.** See also **anticoagulant, coagulation.**

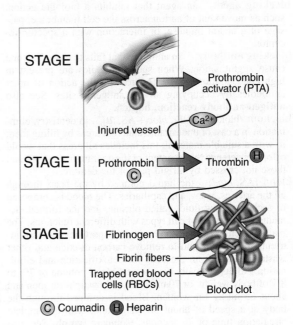

Blood clotting *(Herlihy and Maebius, 2003)*

blood coagulation, a nursing outcome from the Nursing Outcomes Classification (NOC) defined as the extent to which blood clots within a normal period of time.

blood corpuscle [AS, *blod* + L, *corpusculum,* little body], an old term for a blood cell, an erythrocyte, a leukocyte, and sometimes a thrombocyte.

blood count. See **complete blood count.**

blood creatinine test, a blood test that measures the amount of creatinine in the blood, in order to diagnose impaired renal function. Elevated creatinine levels suggest a chronic disease process. This test's results are interpreted in conjunction with those for blood urea nitrogen, as part of a renal function study.

blood crossmatching, the direct matching of donor and recipient blood to prevent the transfusion of incompatible blood types. Crossmatching tests for agglutination of (1) donor red blood cells (RBCs) by recipient serum, and (2) recipient RBCs by donor serum.

blood culture and sensitivity test, a blood culture obtained to detect the presence of bacteria in the blood (bacteremia). Bacteria present are identified and tested for resistance to antibiotics.

blood culture medium, a liquid enrichment medium for the growth of bacteria in the diagnosis of blood infections (bacteremia and septicermia). It contains a suspension of brain tissue in meat broth with dextrose, peptone, and citrate and has a pH of 7.4.

blood donor, anyone who donates blood or blood components. See also **blood bank, transfusion.**

blood doping, the administration of blood, red blood cells, or related blood products to an athlete to enhance performance, often preceded by the withdrawal of blood so that training continues in a blood-depleted state.

blood dyscrasia [AS, *blod* + Gk, *dys,* bad, *krasis,* mingling], a pathologic condition in which any of the constituents of the blood are abnormal in structure, function, or quality, as in leukemia or hemophilia.

blood fluke, a parasitic flatworm of the class Trematoda, genus *Schistosoma,* including the species *S. haematobium, S. japonicum,* and *S. mansoni.* See also *Schistosoma,* **schistosomiasis.**

blood gas, 1. gas dissolved in the liquid part of the blood. Blood gases include oxygen, carbon dioxide, and nitrogen. **2.** a laboratory test to determine the amount of oxygen, carbon dioxide, and nitrogen in blood.

blood gas analysis, the determination of oxygen and carbon dioxide concentrations and pressures with the pH of the blood by laboratory tests; the following measurements may be made: PO_2, partial pressure of oxygen in arterial blood; PCO_2, partial pressure of carbon dioxide in arterial blood; SO_2, percent saturation of hemoglobin with oxygen in arterial blood; the total CO_2 content of (venous) plasma; and the pH.

blood gas determination, an analysis of the pH of the blood and the concentration and pressure of oxygen and carbon dioxide in the blood. It can be performed as an emergency procedure to assess acid-base balance and ventilatory status. Blood gas determination is often important in the evaluation of cardiac failure, hemorrhage, kidney failure, drug overdose, shock, uncontrolled diabetes mellitus, or any other condition of severe stress. The blood for examination is drawn from an artery as ordered in a heparinized syringe, sealed from air, placed in ice, and immediately transported for analysis. Normal adult arterial blood gas values are pH 7.35 to 7.45; PCO_2 35 to 45 mm Hg; HCO^-_3 21 to 28 mEq/L; PO_2 80 to 100 mm Hg; O_2 saturation 95% to 100%. See also **acid-base balance, acidosis, alkalosis, oxygenation, $PaCO_2$, pH, PO_2.**

blood gas tension, the partial pressure of a gas in the blood.

blood glucose. See **blood sugar.**

blood glucose control, a nursing outcome from the Nursing Outcomes Classification (NOC) defined as extent to which plasma glucose levels are maintained in an expected range. See also **Nursing Outcomes Classification.**

blood glucose level [AS, *blod* + OFr, *livel* + Gk, *glykys,* sweet], the amount of glucose found in the bloodstream, usually about 70 to 115 mg/dL after an overnight fast. Concentrations higher or lower than these can be a sign of a variety of diseases, such as diabetes mellitus or pancreatic cancer.

blood glucose test, a blood test used to detect hyperglycemia or hypoglycemia. This test must be performed frequently in patients with newly diagnosed diabetes mellitus, in order to assist in monitoring and adjusting the insulin dose.

Blood glucose meter *(Belchetz and Hammond, 2003)*

blood group, the classification of blood based on the presence or absence of genetically determined antigens on the surface of the red cell. Several different grouping systems have been described. These include ABO, Duffy, high-frequency antigens, I, Kell, Kidd, Lewis, low-frequency antigens, Lutheran, MNS, P, Rh, and Xg. Their relative importance depends on their clinical significance in transfusion therapy, organ transplantation, maternal-fetal compatibility, and genetic studies. See also **ABO blood group.**

blood island, one of the clusters of mesodermal cells that proliferate on the outer surface of the embryonic yolk sac and give it a lumpy appearance.

blood lactate, lactic acid that appears in the blood as a result of anaerobic metabolism when oxygen delivery to the tissues is insufficient to support normal metabolic demands.

blood lavage [AS, *blod* + L, *lavere,* to wash], the removal of toxic elements from the blood by the injection of serum into the veins.

bloodless, **1.** any organ or body part that lacks blood or appears to lack blood. **2.** a surgical field in which the normal local blood supply has been shunted to other areas.

bloodless phlebotomy [AS, *blod* + ME, *les* + Gk, *phleps,* vein, *tomos,* cutting], a technique of trapping blood in a body region by the application of tourniquet pressure that is less than the pressure needed to interrupt arterial blood flow.

bloodletting, the therapeutic opening of an artery or vein to withdraw blood from a particular area. It is sometimes performed to treat polycythemia and congestive heart failure. See also **phlebotomy.**

blood level, the concentration of a drug or other substance in a measured amount of plasma, serum, or whole blood.

blood loss severity, a nursing outcome from the Nursing Outcomes Classification (NOC) defined as the severity of internal or external bleeding/hemorrhage.

blood osmolality [AS, *blod* + Gk, *ōsmos,* impulsion], the osmotic pressure of blood. It measures the amount of solute concentration per unit of total volume of a particular solution. The normal values in serum are 280 to 295 mOsm/L. See also **osmolality.**

blood osmolality test, a blood test that measures the concentration of dissolved particles in the blood. It is useful in evaluating patients with fluid and electrolyte imbalance, seizures, coma, and ascites; and in monitoring and evaluating hydration status, acid-base balance, and suspected antidiuretic hormone (ADH) abnormalities.

blood patch. See **epidural blood patch.**

blood pH, the hydrogen ion concentration of the blood, a measure of blood acidity or alkalinity. The normal pH values for arterial whole blood are 7.35 to 7.454; for venous whole blood, 7.36 to 7.41; for venous serum or plasma, 7.35 to 7.45.

blood plasma [AS, *blod* + Gk, *plassein,* to mold], the liquid portion of the blood, free of its formed elements and particles. Plasma represents approximately 50% of the total volume of blood and contains glucose, proteins, amino acids, and other nutritive materials; urea and other excretory products; and hormones, enzymes, vitamins, and minerals. Compare **serum.** See also **blood, plasma protein, pooled plasma.**

blood platelet. See **platelet, thrombocyte.**

blood poisoning. See **septicemia.**

blood potassium test (K$^+$), a blood test that detects the serum concentration of potassium, the major cation within cells. Potassium levels are followed carefully in patients with uremia, Addison's disease, or vomiting and diarrhea; in those on steroid therapy; in those taking potassium-depleting diuretics; and in those taking digitalis-like drugs.

blood pressure (BP) [AS, *blod* + L, *premere,* to press], the pressure exerted by the circulating volume of blood on the walls of the arteries and veins and on the chambers of the heart. Blood pressure is regulated by the homeostatic mechanisms of the body by the volume of the blood, the lumen of the arteries and arterioles, and the force of cardiac contraction. In the aorta and large arteries of a healthy young adult, blood pressure is approximately 120 mm Hg during systole and 70 mm Hg during diastole. See also **hypertension, hypotension.**

■ METHOD: The indirect blood pressure is most often measured by auscultation, using an aneroid or mercury sphygmomanometer, a stethoscope, and a blood pressure cuff. With the upper arm at the level of the heart, the cuff is placed around the upper arm and inflated to a pressure greater than the systolic pressure, occluding the brachial artery. The diaphragm of the stethoscope is placed over the artery in the antecubital space, and the pressure in the cuff is slowly released. No sound is heard until the cuff pressure falls below the systolic pressure in the artery; at that point a pulse is heard. As the cuff pressure continues to fall slowly, the pulse continues, first becoming louder, then dull and muffled. These sounds, called **sounds of Korotkoff,** are produced by turbulence of the blood flowing through a vessel that is partially occluded as the arterial pressure falls to the low pressure of diastole. When the cuff pressure is less than the diastolic pressure, no pulse is heard. Thus the cuff pressure at which the first sound is heard is the systolic blood pressure, indicative of the pressure in the large arteries during systole; the cuff pressure at which the sounds stop is the diastolic blood pressure, indicative of the pressure in the arteries during diastole. A variation of this method involves the use of palpation in place of auscultation in the antecubital space to determine the systolic pressure (the pressure at which a pulse is first palpated). Another variation uses a transducer in the cuff to translate changes in ultrasound frequency caused by blood movement within the artery to audible sounds. Blood pressure may be monitored directly by means of a strain gauge or mercury manometer after a cannula has been placed in an artery. The flush method is used when blood pressure is difficult to measure by other methods. The cuff is applied, and complete capillary emptying is performed, usually with an elastic bandage. The cuff is inflated, the elastic bandage is removed, and the earliest discernible flush is observed as the cuff is deflated. This method measures mean blood pressure.

■ INTERVENTIONS: The intervals at which the patient's blood pressure is to be taken are specified. The pressure in both arms is taken the first time the procedure is performed; persistent major differences between the two readings is indicative of a vascular occlusion. Alternatively, the blood pressure may be taken using the thigh and the popliteal space when the leg is at the level of the heart. The width of the cuff should be one third to one half the circumference of the limb used. Thus, a larger cuff is required for a large patient or for any patient if the pressure is taken at the thigh.

■ OUTCOME CRITERIA: Any factor that increases peripheral resistance or cardiac output increases the blood pressure. Therefore, it is important to obtain a blood pressure reading when the patient is at rest. Increased peripheral resistance usually increases the diastolic pressure, and increased cardiac output tends to increase the systolic pressure. Blood pressure increases with age, primarily as a result of the decreased distensibility of the veins. As a person grows older, an increase in systolic pressure precedes an increase in diastolic pressure.

blood pressure monitor [AS, *blod* + L, *premere,* to press, *monere,* to warn], a device that automatically measures blood pressure and records the information continuously. Automatic monitoring of blood pressure is often used in surgery or in an intensive care unit where frequent monitoring is required.

blood products administration, a nursing intervention from the Nursing Interventions Classification (NIC) defined as administration of blood or blood products and monitoring of patient's response. See also **Nursing Interventions Classification.**

blood protein [AS, *blod* + Gk, *proteios,* of first rank], any of the large variety of proteins normally found in the blood, such as albumin, globulin, hemoglobin, and proteins bound to hormones or other compounds. See also **plasma protein, serum protein.**

Measurement of blood pressure (Potter and Perry, 1999)

An automated blood pressure monitor
(Courtesy Welch Allyn, Inc.)

Classification of blood pressure for adults

Blood pressure classification	Systolic blood pressure		Diastolic blood pressure
Normal	<120	And	<80
Prehypertension	120-139	Or	80-89
Stage 1 Hypertension	140-159	Or	90-99
Stage 2 Hypertension	≥160	Or	≥100

blood protein test (blood albumin), a blood test that measures levels of albumin, a protein that makes up approximately 60% of the total protein and whose major effect is to maintain colloidal osmotic pressure. Serum protein electro-

phoresis may assist in diagnosing diseases such as myocardial infarction, chronic infection, granulomatous diseases, cirrhosis, rheumatoid-collagen diseases, nephrotic syndrome, advanced cirrhosis, tuberculosis, endocarditis, and myeloma, among others.

blood pump, **1.** a device for regulating the flow of blood into a blood vessel during transfusion. **2.** a component of a heart-lung machine that pumps the blood through the machine for oxygenation and then through the peripheral circulatory system of the body. Also called **mechanical heart-lung.** See also **oxygenation.**

blood relative, a related person who shares some of the same genetic material through a common ancestry.

blood serum. See **serum.**

bloodshot, a redness of the conjunctiva or sclera of the eye caused by dilation of blood vessels in the tissues.

blood smear, a blood test used to provide information concerning drugs and diseases that affect the morphology of red and white blood cells and to help diagnose certain congenital and acquired diseases. A properly performed and analyzed blood smear is the most informative of all hematologic tests, allowing examination of erythrocytes, platelets, and leukocytes.

blood sodium test (Na$^+$), a blood test used to determine the presence of hypo- or hypernatremia by measuring levels of sodium, the major cation in the extracellular space.

bloodstream, the blood that flows freely through the circulatory system.

blood substitute, a substance used for a replacement or volume expansion for circulating blood. Plasma, human serum albumin, packed red cells, platelets, leukocytes, and concentrates of clotting factors are often administered in place of whole blood transfusions in the treatment of various disorders. Substances that are sometimes used to expand blood volume include dextran, hetastarch, albumin solutions, or plasma protein fraction. Perfluorocarbon emulsions, although potentially toxic, have been tested as blood substitutes; they are able to carry oxygen to tissues, have a long shelf life without refrigeration, and do not induce antigen-antibody reactions.

blood sugar, **1.** one of a group of closely related substances, such as glucose, fructose, and galactose, that are normal constituents of the blood and are essential for cellular metabolism. **2.** *nontechnical.* the concentration of glucose in the blood, represented in milligrams of glucose per deciliter of blood. Home monitoring devices make blood glucose measurement both efficient and accurate. Also called **blood glucose.** See also **hyperglycemia, hypoglycemia.**

blood test, any test that yields information about the characteristics or properties of the blood.

blood transfusion [AS, *blod* + L *transfundere,* to pour through], the administration of whole blood or a component, such as packed red cells, to replace blood lost through trauma, surgery, or disease.

■ METHOD: Needed equipment is gathered, physician order is reviewed, transfusion consent completed, and blood component obtained, verified and inspected per institution protocol. It is extremely important that the blood component to be transfused is compatible with the individual receiving the transfusion and that the correct individual is receiving the transfusion. Once verification of product and individual is confirmed, the blood component is hung using the appropriate tubing and setup and infused. A piggybacked 0.9% normal saline solution is set up to follow the infusion or to flush the line in event of a transfusion reaction. Infusion must be completed in under 4 hours to prevent bacterial growth. Individuals must be carefully monitored for a transfusion reaction during infusion. Vital signs should be checked every 5 minutes along with checks for signs and symptoms such as fever, facial flushing, rapid thready pulse, cold clammy skin, itching, swelling at infusion site, dizziness, dyspnea, low back or chest pain. (Stop infusion immediately at any sign of transfusion reaction.) After infusion, IV tubing is cleared with saline solution and the blood bag discarded according to institution policy.

■ OUTCOME CRITERIA: No signs of transfusion reaction. (See **transfusion reaction** for appropriate interventions if reaction occurs.) Laboratory values show positive response to administration of blood component.

blood transfusion reaction control, a nursing outcome from the Nursing Outcomes Classification (NOC) is defined as extent to which complications of blood transfusions are minimized. See also **Nursing Outcomes Classification.**

blood typing, typing of blood, a blood test used to determine the character of the blood of prospective blood donors and of expectant mothers and newborns on the basis of agglutinogens in the erythrocytes. The test detects the presence of ABO antigens as well as the Rh factor. See also **blood group.**

blood urea nitrogen (BUN) [AS, *blod* + Gk, *ouron,* urine, *nitron,* soda, *genein,* to produce], a measure of the amount of urea in the blood. Urea forms in the liver as the end product of protein metabolism, circulates in the blood, and is excreted through the kidney in urine. The BUN, determined by a blood test, is directly related to the metabolic function of the liver and the excretory function of the kidney. Normal findings (in mg/dL) are 10 to 20 for adults, 5 to 18 for children and infants, 3 to 12 for newborns, and 21 to 40 for cord blood. In the elderly, the BUN may be slightly higher than the normal adult range. A critical value of 100 mg/dL indicates serious impairment of renal function. Also called **urea nitrogen, serum urea nitrogen.** See also **azotemia.** Compare **creatinine.**

blood vessel, any one of the network of muscular tubes that carry blood. Kinds of blood vessels are **arteries, arterioles, capillaries, veins,** and **venules.**

blood warming coil, a device constructed of coiled plastic tubing used for the warming of reserve blood before massive transfusions, such as those often required for patients who experience extensive bleeding. Administration of cold blood in such transfusions may cause the patient to go into a state

Setup for blood administration
(Harkreader and Hogan, 2004)

of shock. The blood warming coil is a prepackaged sterile single-use device. Compare **electric blood warmer.**

bloody show. See **vaginal bleeding.**

bloody sputum [AS, *blod* + L, *sputum,* spittle], blood-tinged material expelled from the respiratory passages. The amount and color of blood in sputum expelled by coughing or clearing the throat may indicate the cause and location of the bleeding. Swallowed blood regurgitated from the stomach most often loses its vital coloring, however, thus eliminating the opportunity to judge the origin.

blooming, an increase in x-ray focal spot size due to electrostatic repulsion.

Bloom's syndrome [David Bloom, American physician, b. 1892], a rare genetic disease occurring mainly in Ashkenazi Jews. It is transmitted as an autosomal recessive trait and is characterized by growth retardation, dilated capillaries of the face and arms, sensitivity to sunlight, and an increased risk of malignancy.

blot, 1. a technique transfering electrophoretically separated components from a gel onto a nitrocellulose membrane, chemically treated paper, or filter for analysis. It is frequently used to analyze genetic material. **2.** the substrate containing the transferred material. See also **Northern blot test, Southern blot test, Western blot test.**

blotch, a skin discoloration that may vary in severity from an area of pigmentation to large pustules or blisters.

blow bottles, a device used in respiratory care to provide resistance to expiration. Used to improve airways filling and prevent atelectasis. The bottles are partially filled with water, and the patient is encouraged to blow the water from one bottle to another, a practice that requires deep inspiration and lung expansion to develop increased lung pressure.

blow-out fracture, a break in the floor of the orbit caused by a blow that suddenly increases the intraocular pressure.

blowpipe /blō′pīp/ [AS, *blāwan* + *pīpe*], a tube through which a current of air or other gas is forced on a flame to concentrate and intensify the heat.

BLS, abbreviation for **basic life support.**

blue asphyxia. See **asphyxia livida.**

blue baby [OFr, *blou* + ME, *babe*], an infant born with cyanosis caused by a congenital heart lesion, most commonly tetralogy of Fallot. Other causative lesions include transposition of the great vessels, and incomplete expansion of the lungs (congenital atelectasis). Congenital cyanotic heart lesions are diagnosed by cardiac catheterization, angiography, or echocardiography and are corrected surgically, preferably in early childhood. See also **congenital cardiac anomaly, tetralogy of Fallot, transposition of the great vessels.**

blue cohosh, a perennial herb found in the midwest and eastern regions of the United States.

■ USES: This herb is used to treat menopausal symptoms and uterine and ovarian pain, to improve the flow of menstrual blood, and as an antiinflammatory and antirheumatic. It is also a popular remedy in African American ethnic medicine.

■ CONTRAINDICATIONS: Should not be used for any of these indications since it has caused serious toxicities.

Blue Cross, an independent nonprofit U.S. corporation that functions as a health insurance agency, providing protection for an enrolled patient by covering all or part of the person's hospital expenses. Blue Cross programs vary in different communities because of state laws regulating them.

blue diaper syndrome [OFr, *blou;* ME, *diapre,* patterned fabric], a defect of tryptophan absorption in which, because of intestinal bacterial action on the tryptophan, the urine contains abnormal indoles, giving it a blue color. It is similar to Hartnup's disease.

blue dome cyst, a spherical dilation of a mammary duct in which bleeding has occurred.

Blue dome cyst *(Cotran, Kumar, and Collins, 1999)*

blue dot sign, a tender blue or black spot beneath the skin of the testis or epididymis, a sign of testicular torsion of the appendix testis.

blue fever, *informal,* Rocky Mountain spotted fever, so named for the dark cyanotic discoloration of the skin after the initial rickettsial infection. See also **rickettsiosis, Rocky Mountain spotted fever, typhus.**

blue-green algae, misnomer formerly applied to the group now called the **cyanobacteria.**

blue-green algae poisoning. See **cyanobacteria poisoning.**

blue line, a bluish discoloration sometimes observed on the gingival side of the mouth in cases of gingivitis. It is a sign of chronic lead or bismuth poisoning.

blue nevus [OFr, *blou* + L, *naevus,* mole], a sharply circumscribed, usually benign, steel blue skin nodule with a diameter between 2 and 7 mm. It is found on the face or upper extremities, grows very slowly, and persists throughout life. The dark color is caused by large, densely packed melanocytes deep in the dermis of the nevus. Nodular blue nevi found on the buttocks or in the sacrococcygeal region occasionally become malignant. Any sudden change in the size of such a lesion demands surgical attention and biopsy. Compare **melanoma.**

Blue nevus *(Callen et al, 2000)*

blue phlebitis, a severe form of thrombosis of a deep vein, usually the femoral vein. The condition is acute and fulminating and is usually accompanied by vast edema and cyanosis of the limb distal to the occluding thrombus. Also called **phlegmasia cerulea dolens.**

blue rubber bleb nevus [OFR, *blou,* blue; + ME, *rubben,* to scrape; + ME, *bleb,* blob; + L, *naevus,* mole], a type of congenital nevus, transmitted as an autosomal dominant trait, characterized by blue hemangiomas with soft elevated nipple-like centers, found on the skin surface, in the GI tract, and sometimes on mucous membranes; it may be accompanied by pain, regional hyperhidrosis, or GI bleeding.

blues, *informal,* **1.** a designation for **Blue Cross** (an insurance system that pays the costs of treatment by a hospital or clinic) and **Blue Shield. 2.** *informal.* mild depression.

Blue Shield, an independent nonprofit U.S. corporation that offers patient protection for costs of surgery and other medical services. Although Blue Cross and Blue Shield are

Blue rubber bleb nevus *(Callen et al, 2000)*

technically separate organizations, they generally coordinate their functions in providing benefits covering both hospital costs and physician fees.

blue spot, **1.** also called **macula cerulea** /seroo'lē·ə/, one of a number of small grayish blue spots that may appear near the armpits or around the groins of individuals infested with lice, such as in pediculosis corporis and pediculosis pubis. These spots are usually less than 1 cm in diameter and are caused by a substance in the saliva of lice that converts bilirubin to biliverdin. **2.** one of a number of dark blue round or oval spots that may appear as a congenital condition in the sacral regions of certain children less than 4 or 5 years of age. They usually disappear spontaneously as the affected individual matures. Also called **mongolian spot.**

blunt dissection [ME, *blunt* + L, *dissecare,* to cut apart], a dissection performed by separating tissues along natural lines of cleavage without cutting.

blunt-ended DNA, a segment of DNA in which the ends of both strands are even with each other.

blunthook /blunt'hŏŏk/ [ME, *blunt* + AS, *hoc*], **1.** a sturdy hook-shaped bar used in obstetrics for traction between the abdomen and the thigh in cases of difficult breech deliveries. **2.** a hook-shaped device with a blunt end used in embryotomy.

blunting, a decrease in the intensity of emotional expression from the level one would normally expect as a reaction to a specific situation. It is the opposite of overreaction and may be marked by apathy, minimal response, or indifference.

blurred film fault /blurd'/, a defect in a photograph or radiograph that appears as an indistinct or blurred image. It is caused by film movement during exposure, bending of film during exposure, double exposure, or film emulsion flow during processing in excessively warm solutions.

blush [ME, *blusshen,* to redden], a brief, diffuse erythema of the face and neck, commonly the result of dilation of superficial small blood vessels in response to heat or sudden emotion.

BLV-HTLV retroviruses, a genus similar in morphology and replication to the type C retroviruses; organisms have a long latency and cause B and T cell leukemia and lymphoma and neurological disease. Included in this genus are human T-lymphotropic viruses 1 and 2.

B lymphocyte. See **B cell.**

B/M, abbreviation for *black male,* often used in the initial identifying statement in a patient record.

BMA, abbreviation for **British Medical Association.**

BMD, abbreviation for **Bureau of Medical Devices.**

BMI, abbreviation for **body mass index.**

B-mode, brightness modulation in diagnostic ultrasonography. Bright dots on an oscilloscope screen represent echoes, and the intensity of the brightness indicates the strength of the echo. See also **A-mode, M-mode.**

BMR, abbreviation for **basal metabolic rate.**

BNA, abbreviation for *Basle Nomina Anatomica.*

BOA, abbreviation for **born out of asepsis.**

board. See **custodial care.**

board and care, nonmedical, community-based residential care for individuals who can care for themselves; meals and supervision are provided.

board certification, a process by which physicians are certified in a given medical specialty or subspecialty. Certification is awarded by the 23-member boards of the American Board of Medical Specialties on completion of accredited training and examinations and fulfillment of individual requirements of the board.

board certified, denoting a physician who has completed the certification requirements established by a medical specialty board and has been certified as a specialist in a particular field of medicine.

board eligible, denoting a physician who has completed all of the requirements for admission to a medical specialty board.

boarder baby, **1.** an infant abandoned to a hospital because the mother is unable to care for him or her. Many infants born with human immunodeficiency virus (HIV) or to a mother with HIV infection or infants delivered to mothers who are drug users are boarder babies. **2.** in some hospitals, any infant still in the nursery after the mother's discharge for any reason (even if only very temporarily).

board of health, an administrative body acting on a municipal, county, state, provincial, or national level. The functions, powers, and responsibilities of boards of health vary with the locales. Each board is generally concerned with the recognition of the health needs of the people and the coordination of projects and resources to meet and identify these needs. Among the tasks of most boards of health are disease prevention, health education, and implementation of laws pertaining to health.

bobbing, the act of moving up and down, usually with a jerking motion.

Bodansky unit /bōdăn'skē/ [Aaron Bodansky, American biochemist, 1887–1961], the quantity of alkaline phosphatase that liberates 1 mg of phosphate ion from glycerol 2-phosphate in 1 hour at 37° C and under other standardized conditions.

body [AS, *bodig*], **1.** the whole structure of an individual with all the organs. **2.** a cadaver (corpse). **3.** the largest or the main part of any structure, such as the body of the stomach. Also called **corpus, soma.**

body burden, **1.** the state of activity of a radioactive chemical in the body at a specified time after administration. **2.** chemicals stored in the body that may be detected by analysis.

body cast [AS, *bodig,* body; ONorse, *kasta*], a molded cast that may extend from the chest to the groin to immobilize the spine.

body cavity, any of the spaces in the human body that contain organs. One major cavity, the thoracic cavity, is subdivided into a pericardial and two pleural cavities.

body composition, the relative proportions of protein, fat, water, and mineral components in the body. It varies among individuals as a result of differences in body density and

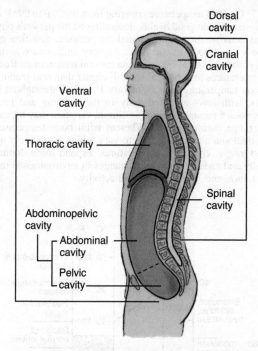

Major body cavities *(Applegate, 2000)*

degree of obesity. Methods for calculating body composition include underwater weighing and injection of radioactive tracers.

body fluid [AS, *bodig* + L, *fluere,* to flow], fluid contained in the three fluid compartments of the body: the plasma of the circulating blood, the interstitial fluid between the cells, and the cell fluid within the cells. See also **blood plasma, interstitial fluid, extracellular fluid (ECF), intracellular fluid.**

body image[1] [AS, *bodig* + L, *imago,* likeness], a person's concept of his or her physical appearance. The mental representation, which may be realistic or unrealistic, is constructed from self-observation, the reactions of others, and a complex interaction of attitudes, emotions, memories, fantasies, and experiences, both conscious and unconscious. A marked inability to conceptualize one's personal body characteristics may be caused by organic brain damage, as in autotopagnosia; by a physical disability, such as the loss of a limb; or by psychologic and emotional disturbances, as in anorexia nervosa.

body image[2], a nursing outcome from the Nursing Outcomes Classification (NOC) defined as positive perception of own appearance and body functions. See also **Nursing Outcomes Classification.**

body image agnosia. See **autotopagnosia.**

body image, disturbed, a nursing diagnosis accepted by the Seventh National Conference on the Classification of Nursing Diagnoses. The condition is defined as a disruption in the way one perceives one's body. The cause of a disturbance in body image may be a biophysical, cognitive, perceptual, psychosocial, cultural, or spiritual factor.

■ DEFINING CHARACTERISTICS: Objective characteristics of the deficit include verbal or nonverbal responses to a real or perceived change in structure or function, a missing body part, trauma to a nonfunctioning part, and a change in the ability to estimate spatial relationship of the body to the

environment. Subjective characteristics include personalization of the missing part by giving it a name, refusal to look at a part of the body, negative feelings about the body, a change in general social involvement or life-style, and a fear of rejection by others.

■ RELATED FACTORS: Related factors include biophysical, cognitive, perceptual, psychosocial, cultural, and spiritual factors. See also **nursing diagnosis.**

body image enhancement, a nursing intervention from the Nursing Interventions Classification (NIC) defined as improving a patient's conscious and unconscious perceptions and attitudes toward his/her body. See also **Nursing Interventions Classification.**

body jacket, an orthopedic cast that encases the trunk of the body but does not extend over the cervical area; it may be equipped with shoulder straps. The cast is used to help position and immobilize the trunk for the healing of spinal injuries and scoliosis and after spinal surgery. Compare **Risser cast.** See also **thoracolumbosacral orthosis.**

body language [AS, *bodig* + L, *lingua,* tongue], a set of nonverbal signals, including body movements, postures, gestures, spatial positions, facial expressions, and body adornment, that give expression to various physical, mental, and emotional states. See also **kinesics.**

body louse. See **lice,** *Pediculus humanus corporis.*

body mass index (BMI), a formula for determining obesity. It is calculated by dividing a person's weight in kilograms by the square of the person's height in meters. A BMI of 27 or greater indicates obesity.

Body mass index calculation

$$BMI = \frac{Weight\ (kg)}{Height\ (m^2)}$$

Body mass index assessment	
19-25	Appropriate weight (19-34 years)
21-27	Appropriate weight (>35 years)
27.5-30	Mild obesity
30-40	Moderate obesity
>40	Morbid obesity

From Thompson JM, Wilson SF: *Health assessment for nursing practice,* St Louis, 1996, Mosby.

body mechanics, the field of physiology that studies muscular actions and the function of muscles in maintaining body posture. Knowledge gained from such studies is especially important in the prevention of injury during the performance of tasks that require the body to lift and move.

body mechanics performance, a nursing outcome from the Nursing Outcomes Classification (NOC) defined as personal actions to maintain proper body alignment and to prevent muscular skeletal strain.

body mechanics promotion, a nursing intervention from the Nursing Interventions Classification (NIC) defined as facilitating the use of posture and movement in daily activities to prevent fatigue and musculoskeletal strain or injury. See also **Nursing Interventions Classification.**

body movement, motion of all or part of the body, especially at a joint or joints. Body movements include **abduction, adduction, extension, flexion, rotation,** and **circumduction.**

body odor, a fetid smell associated with stale perspiration. Freshly secreted perspiration is odorless, but after exposure to the atmosphere and bacterial activity at the surface of the skin, chemical changes occur to produce the odor. Common body odor usually can be eliminated by bathing with soap and water. Body odors can also be the result of discharges from a variety of skin conditions, including cancer, fungus, hemorrhoids, leukemia, and ulcers. See also **bromhidrosis.**

body of Retzius /ret′sē·əs/ [Magnus G. Retzius, Swedish anatomist, 1842–1919], any one of the masses of protoplasm containing pigment granules at the lower end of a hair cell of the organ of Corti in the internal ear.

body plethysmograph [AS, *bodig* + Gk, *plethynein,* to increase, *graphein,* to record], a device for studying alveolar pressures, lung volumes, and airway resistance. The patient sits or reclines in an airtight compartment and breathes normally. The pressure changes in the alveoli are reciprocated in the compartment and are recorded automatically.

body position, attitude or posture of the body. See **anatomic position, decubitus position, Fowler's position, prone, supine,** and **Trendelenburg position.**

body positioning: self-initiated, a nursing outcome from the Nursing Outcomes Classification (NOC) defined as ability to change own body positions. See also **Nursing Outcomes Classification.**

body righting reflex. See **righting reflex.**

body scheme, a piagetian term for a cognitive structure that develops in infants in the sensorimotor period during the first 2 years of life as they learn to differentiate between themselves and the world around them.

body-scheme disorder. See **autotopagnosia.**

body-section radiography, a radiographic technique in which the film and x-ray tube are moved in opposite directions to produce a more distinct image of a selected body plane. The process has the effect of blurring adjacent body structures during exposure. Also called **tomography.**

body stalk, the elongated part of the embryo that is connected to the chorion. See also **allantois.**

body surface area. See **surface area.**

body systems model, (in nursing education) a conceptual framework in which illness is studied in relation to the functional systems of the body, such as the circulatory, nervous, GI, and reproductive. In this model, nursing care is directed to manipulating the patient's environment in such a way that the signs and symptoms of the health problem are alleviated. As the body systems model traditionally focuses on the disease rather than the patient, current educational programs tend to integrate it with other concepts that allow the nurse to approach the patient in a more holistic framework. Also called **medical model.**

body temperature, the level of heat produced and sustained by the body processes. Variations and changes in body temperature are major indicators of disease and other abnormalities. Heat is generated within the body through metabolism of nutrients and lost from the body surface through radiation, convection, and evaporation of perspiration. Heat production and loss are regulated and controlled in the hypothalamus and brainstem. Fever is usually a function of an increase in heat generation; however, some abnormal conditions, such as congestive heart failure, produce slight elevations of body temperature through impairment of the heat loss function. Contributing to the failure to dissipate heat are reduced activity of the heart, lower rate of blood flow to the skin, and the insulating effect of edema. Diseases of the hypothalamus or interference with the other regulatory centers may produce abnormally low body temperatures. Normal adult body temperature, as measured orally, is 98.6° F

(37° C). Oral temperatures ranging from 96.5° F to 99° F are consistent with good health, depending on the person's physical activity, the environmental temperature, and that person's usual body temperature. Axillary temperature is usually from 0.5° to 1° F lower than the oral temperature. Rectal temperatures may be 0.5° to 1° F higher than oral readings. Body temperature appears to vary 1° to 2° F throughout the day, with lows recorded early in the morning and peaks between 6 PM and 10 PM. This diurnal variation may increase in range during a fever. Whereas adult body temperature, normal and abnormal, tends to vary within a relatively narrow range, children's temperatures respond more dramatically and rapidly to disease, changes in environmental temperature, and levels of physical activity.

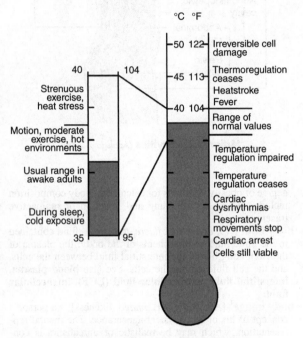

Normal and abnormal body temperatures
(Thibodeau and Patton, 2003)

body temperature, imbalanced, risk for, a nursing diagnosis accepted by the Seventh National Conference on the Classification of Nursing Diagnoses. The condition is a state in which the individual is at risk for failure to maintain body temperature within a normal range.

■ RISK FACTORS: Risk factors are extremes of age; extremes of weight; exposure to cool-to-cold or warm-to-hot environments; dehydration; inactivity or vigorous activity; medications causing vasoconstriction or vasodilation; altered metabolic rate; sedation; clothing inappropriate for environmental temperature; and illness or trauma affecting temperature regulations. See also **nursing diagnosis.**

body type, the general physical appearance of an individual human body. Three commonly used terms for body types are ectomorph, describing a thin, fragile physique; endomorph, denoting a round, soft body; and mesomorph, indicating a muscular, athletic body of average size. See also **asthenic habitus, athletic habitus, ectomorph, endomorph, mesomorph, pyknic.**

body-weight ratio, a relation expressed by dividing the body weight in grams by the height in centimeters.

Boeck's disease, Boeck's sarcoid. See **sarcoidosis.**

Boerhaave's syndrome /bôr′hävz/ [Hermann Boerhaave, Dutch physician, 1668–1738], a condition marked by spontaneous rupture of the esophagus, usually preceded by severe vomiting, leading to mediastinitis and pleural effusion. Clinical manifestations are violent retching or vomiting. Emergency care with surgery and drainage is needed to save the life of the patient.

Bohr effect [Christian Bohr, Danish physiologist, 1855–1911], the effect of CO_2 and H^+ on the affinity of hemoglobin for molecular O_2. Increasing PCO_2 and H^+ decrease oxyhemoglobin saturation, whereas decreasing concentrations have the opposite effect. In humans a decrease of pH from 7.4 to 7.3 at 40 mm Hg PO_2 decreases oxyhemoglobin saturation by 6%. The Bohr effect is particularly significant in the capillaries of working muscles and the myocardium and in maternal and fetal exchange vessels of the placenta.

bohrium (Bh). See **element 107.**

boil [AS, *byle,* sore], a skin abscess. See **furuncle.**

boiling point [ME, *boilen,* to make bubbles; L, *pungere,* to prick], **1.** the temperature at which a substance passes from the liquid to the gaseous state at a particular atmospheric pressure. **2.** the temperature at which the vapor pressure of a liquid equals the external pressure. See also **evaporation.**

-bol, combining form designating an anabolic steroid.

bole /bōl/, any of a variety of soft, friable clays of various colors, although usually red from iron oxide. They consist of hydrous silicate of aluminum, are used as pigments, and were once commonly used as absorbents and astringents.

Bolivian hemorrhagic fever /bəliv′ē·ən/, an infectious disease caused by an arenavirus, generally transmitted by contact with or inhalation of aerosolized rodent urine. After an incubation period of from 1 to 2 weeks, the patient experiences chills, fever, headache, muscle ache, anorexia, nausea, and vomiting. As the disease progresses, hypotension, dehydration, bradycardia, pulmonary edema, and internal hemorrhage may occur. The mortality rate may reach 30%; pulmonary edema is the most common cause of death. There is no specific therapy. Peritoneal dialysis is sometimes performed. Also called **Machupo.** See also **Arenavirus,** Argentine hemorrhagic fever, Lassa fever.

bolus /bō′ləs/ [Gk, *bolos,* lump], **1.** also called **alimentary bolus,** a round mass, specifically a masticated lump of food ready to be swallowed. **2.** a large round preparation of medicinal material for oral ingestion, usually soft and not prepackaged. **3.** a dose of a medication or a contrast material, radioactive isotope, or other pharmaceutic preparation injected all at once intravenously. **4.** (in radiotherapy) material used to fill in irregular body surfaces to improve dose distribution for hyperthermia or to increase the dose to the skin when high-energy photon beams are used. **5.** a clumping in the stomach of ingested foreign material, often the result of habitual behavior.

bolus dose, an amount of IV medication administered rapidly to decrease the response time or to be used as a loading dose prior to an infusion. See also **bolus.**

bombard /bombärd′/, to shower a drug or tissue sample with radioactive particles from a nuclear isotope source.

Bombay phenotype /bombā′/ [Bombay, India, where first reported], a rare genetic trait involving the phenotypic expression of the ABO blood groups. The gene for the H antigen, which in the usual dominant form of HH or Hh is responsible for the precursor necessary for the production of the A and B antigens, is homozygous recessive in individuals with this trait so that the expression of the A, B, and H antigens is suppressed. Cells of such individuals are phenotypically of blood type O, and the serum contains anti-A, anti-B, and anti-H antigens. In such cases the offspring from two phenotypic O blood type parents may be blood type AB. The phenomenon is an example of the intricate interaction of linked genes in which one gene on a chromosome controls the expression or suppression of another gene that is not its allele. See also **ABO blood group.**

bombesin /bom′bə·sin/, a neurohormone and pressor substance found in small amounts in brain and intestinal tissue under normal conditions and in increased amounts in certain pulmonary and thyroid tumors; it is a potent mitogen and its effects on gastrin and other hormones are attributed to increased cell numbers.

bond, a strong coulombic force between atoms in a substance due to attraction of ions of opposite charge for each other or of the nuclei for shared electrons. See also **coulomb, Coulomb's law.**

bonding [ME, *band,* to bind], **1.** (in dentistry) a technique of joining orthodontic brackets or other attachments directly to the enamel surface of a tooth, using orthodontic adhesives. **2.** the reciprocal attachment process that occurs between an infant and the parents, especially the mother. Bonding is significant in the formation of affectionate ties that later influence both the physical and psychologic development of the child. It is usually initiated immediately after birth by placing the nude infant on the mother's abdomen so that both the parents and the child can see and touch one another and begin to interact. The newborn is in an alert, reactive state for about 30 minutes to 1 hour after birth and displays such behaviors as crying, sucking, clinging, grasping, and following with the eyes, which in turn stimulate the expression of parenting instincts. By about the second to third week of the infant's life, a definite, reciprocal pattern of interacting behavior that involves an attention-nonattention cycle occurs during each encounter of parents and child. At the peak of the attention phase, the infant reaches out toward the parent and is very attentive. This peak is followed in a short time by deceleration of excitement in the infant and a turning away from the parent. This nonattentive phase prevents the infant from being overwhelmed by excessive stimuli, and no visual or verbal attempt will regain the infant's attention. Recognizing that the nonattention phase does not represent rejection helps the mother and father develop competence in parenting. Assessment of the attachment process is an important nursing function and requires skillful observation and interviewing. The nurse observes the mother's reactions, especially while feeding, bathing, and comforting her infant, for potential signs of inadequate or delayed mothering. Among the most important actions for bonding are eye contact in the en face position and embracing of the infant close to the body. Many variables determine the development of bonding and parenting, including the parents' fantasies about the child, the conditions surrounding the pregnancy, the arrangements that have been made concerning changes in life-style with the addition of a dependent family member, and the type of parenting the mother and father received as children. Bonding is also seen in adoptive situations and is not limited to the newborn period. Although bonding is considered primarily an emotional response, it is hypothesized that some biochemical and hormonal interaction in the mother may stimulate the response; results of studies testing this hypothesis are inconclusive. Also called **maternal-child attachment.** See also **maternal deprivation syndrome, maternal-infant bonding.**

bond specificity, the nature of enzyme action that causes the disruption of only certain bonds between atoms.

bone [AS, *ban*], **1.** the dense, hard, and somewhat flexible connective tissue constituting the bones of the human skeleton. It is composed of compact osseous tissue surrounding spongy cancellous tissue permeated by many blood vessels and nerves and enclosed in membranous periosteum. **2.** any single element of the skeleton, such as a rib, the sternum, or the femur. Also called *(Latin)* **os.** See also **connective tissue.**

bone age [AS, *ban* + L, *aetas*], the stage of development or decline of the skeleton or its segments, as seen in radio-

Articular cartilage
Epiphysis
Epiphyseal line
Spongy bone
Compact bone
Diaphysis
Medullary cavity
Nutrient foramen
Endosteum
Periosteum
Epiphysis
Articular cartilage

Structure of long bones *(Applegate, 2000)*

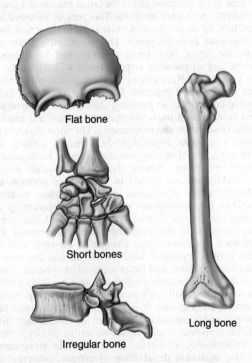

Flat bone

Short bones

Long bone

Irregular bone

Types of bones *(Herlihy and Maebius, 2000)*

graphic examination, when compared with x-ray views of the bone structures of other individuals of the same chronologic age.

bone-anchored hearing aid, a hearing aid that allows direct bone conduction of sound to the cochlea by means of a sound processing device attached to an osseointegrated titanium fixture implanted posterior to the ear.

bone cancer [AS, *ban* + Gk, *karkinos,* crab], a skeletal malignancy occurring as a sarcoma or a myeloma in an area of rapid growth or as metastasis from cancer elsewhere in the body. Primary bone tumors are rare; the incidence peaks during adolescence, decreases, and then rises slowly after 35 years of age. In adults, bone cancer is linked to exposure to ionizing radiation. Paget's disease, hyperparathyroidism, chronic osteomyelitis, old bone infarcts, and fracture callosities increase the risk of many bone tumors. Most osseous malignancies are metastatic lesions found most often in the spine or pelvis and less often in sites away from the trunk. Bone cancers progress rapidly but are often difficult to detect. Alkaline phosphatase levels are elevated in osteoblastic tumors, and serum calcium and urinary calcium levels are increased in highly destructive lesions. X-ray films, radio-isotopic scanning, arteriography, and biopsy are diagnostic. Surgical treatment consists of local resection of slow-growing tumors or amputation, including the joint above the tumor, if the lesion is aggressive. Radiotherapy may be given preoperatively or as the primary form of treatment. See also **chondrosarcoma, Ewing's sarcoma, fibrosarcoma, multiple myeloma, osteosarcoma.**

bone cell [AS, *ban* + L, *cella,* storeroom], an osteocyte osteoblast, or osteoclast, a cell with myriad spidery processes embedded in the matrix of bone. See also **osteoblast.**

bone cutting forceps, a type of forceps that has long handles, single or double joints, and heavy blades for cutting bone.

bone cyst [AS, *ban* + Gk, *kytis,* cyst], **1.** a dilation in the wall of a blood vessel in a bone, usually eccentrically placed. **2.** a sac in bone tissue in the parathyroid disorder osteitis fibrosa.

bone densitometry, any of several methods of determining bone mass by measuring radiation absorption by the skeleton. Common techniques include single-photon absorptiometry (SPA) of the forearm and heel, dual-photon absorptiometry (DPA) and dual-energy x-ray absorptiometry (DXA) of the spine and hip, quantitative computed tomography (QCT) of the spine and forearm, and radiographic absorptiometry (RA) of the hand, and quantitative ultrasound (QU).

Bone densitometry *(Greer et al, 2001)*

bone graft, the transplantation of a piece of bone from one part of the body to another to repair a skeletal defect.

bone healing, a nursing outcome from the Nursing Outcomes Classification (NOC) defined as the extent to which cells and tissues have regenerated following bone injury. See also **Nursing Outcomes Classification.**

bone lamella [AS, *ban,* bone, *lamella,* plate], a thin plate of bone matrix, a basic structural unit of mature bone.

bone marrow [AS, *ban* + ME, *marowe*], the soft, organic, spongelike material in the cavities of bones; also called *medulla ossium.* It is a network of blood vessels and special connective tissue fibers that hold together a composite of fat and blood-producing cells. Its chief function is to manufacture erythrocytes, leukocytes, and platelets. These blood cells normally do not enter the bloodstream until they are fully developed, so that the marrow contains cells in all stages of growth. If the body's demand for leukocytes is increased because of infection, the marrow responds immediately by stepping up production. The same is true if more erythrocytes are necessary, as in hemorrhage or anemia. **Red marrow** is found in many bones of infants and children and in the spongy (cancellous) bone of the proximal epiphyses of the humerus and femur and the sternum, ribs, and vertebral bodies of adults. Fatty **yellow marrow** is found in the medullary cavity of most adult long bones.

Bone marrow (© Ed Reschke/used with permission)

Nuclei   Fat

bone marrow biopsy, a microscopic tissue examination used to help evaluate patients with hematologic diseases. The biopsy may be done to confirm a diagnosis of megaloblastic anemia, to diagnose leukemia or myeloma, to determine the cause of reduced red blood cells in the peripheral bloodstream, to document deficient iron stores, to document bone marrow infiltrative diseases such as neoplasm or fibrosis, to identify tumors, and to diagnose a variety of other conditions.

bone marrow failure, failure of the hematopoietic function of the bone marrow. See also **hematopoietic system.**

bone marrow infusion, a method of injecting a fluid substance through an aspiration needle directly into the marrow cavity of a long bone. The substance is absorbed into the general circulation almost immediately.

bone marrow reserve, a storage pool of mature neutrophils in the bone marrow, which can be released as necessary.

bone marrow suppression, suppression of bone marrow

activity, resulting in reduction in the number of platelets, red cells, and white cells, such as in aplastic anemia. Also called **myelosuppression.**

bone marrow transplantation, the transplantation of bone marrow from a healthy donor to stimulate production of normal blood cells. The marrow may be autologous (from a previously harvested and stored self-donation) or allogeneic (from a living related donor or a living unrelated donor). The bone marrow is removed from the donor by aspiration and infused intravenously into the recipient. Used to treat malignancies, such as leukemia, lymphoma, myeloma, and selected solid tumors; and nonmalignant conditions, such as aplastic anemia, immunologic deficiencies, and inborn errors of metabolism. Transplantation is usually preceded by chemotherapy and total body radiation of the recipient.

bone plate [AS, *ban,* bone; OFr, *plate*], a metal plate used to reconstruct a bone that has been fractured. The plate is designed to hold bone fragments in apposition.

bone recession [AS, *ban* + L, *recedere,* to recede], apical progression of the level of the alveolar crest, resulting in decreased bone support for the teeth. The condition is associated with inflammatory or dystrophic periodontal disease.

bone scan, the injection of a radioactive substance to enable visualization of a bone via the image produced by emission of radioactive particles.

bone tissue [AS, *ban* + OFr, *tissu*], a hard form of connective tissue composed of osteocytes and a calcified collagenous intercellular substance arranged in thin plates. See **connective tissue.** Also called **bony tissue.**

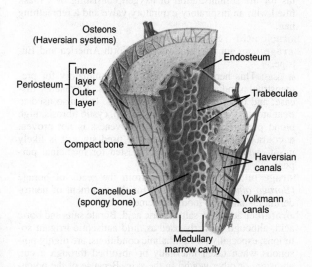

Bone tissue (Thibodeau and Patton, 2003)

Osteons (Haversian systems)
Periosteum — Inner layer / Outer layer
Endosteum
Trabeculae
Compact bone
Haversian canals
Cancellous (spongy bone)
Volkmann canals
Medullary marrow cavity

Bonine, trademark for an antiemetic (meclizine hydrochloride).

Bonnevie-Ullrich syndrome. See **Turner's syndrome.**

Bonnie Pruden myotherapy, a method of applying manual pressure on muscles with the fingers, knuckles, and elbows to defuse trigger points and relax muscle spasm, improve circulation, and alleviate pain.

Bonwill's triangle [William G.A. Bonwill, American dentist, 1833–1899], an equilateral triangle formed by lines from the contact points of the lower central incisors (or the median line of the residual ridge of the mandible) to the mandibular condyle on each side and from one condyle to the other.

bony landmark [AS, *ban* + AS, *land, mearc*], a groove or prominence on a bone that serves as a guide to the location of other body structures. An example is the posterior, superior iliac crest.

bony palate. See **hard palate.**

bony thorax [AS, *ban* + Gk, *thorax,* chest], the skeletal part of the chest, including the thoracic vertebrae, ribs, and sternum.

bony tissue. See **bone tissue.**

book retinoscopy, a type in which the patient focuses on reading a book and is commonly used with children.

booster injection, the administration of an additional dose of antigen within a defined period of time, such as a vaccine or toxoid, usually in a smaller amount than the original immunization. It is given to maintain the immune response at an appropriate level.

booster phenomenon /bōōs'ter/, on a tuberculin test, an initial false-negative result caused by a diminished amnestic response that becomes positive on subsequent testing.

booster response. See **secondary antibody response.**

boot, 1. a shoelike prosthetic device for holding a leg or arm during treatment. **2.** a basketweave bandage that covers the foot and lower leg. **3.** an airtight device in which the arm or leg can be inserted and the air pumped out, creating a partial vacuum to divert blood flow from the surrounding area.

Boothby-Lovelace-Bulbulian (BLB) mask, an apparatus for the administration of oxygen consisting of a mask fitted with an inspiratory-expiratory valve and a rebreathing bag.

boracic acid. See **boric acid.**

borage, an annual herb found in North America and Europe.

■ USES: This herb is used as an antiinflammatory for premenstrual syndrome, rheumatoid arthritis, Raynaud's disease, and other inflammatory conditions. It is also used to treat atopic dermatitis, infant cradle cap, cystic fibrosis, high blood pressure, and diabetes; effectiveness is not proven.

■ CONTRAINDICATIONS: Should not be used since it is likely unsafe when used in amounts ingested for medicinal purpose.

borage oil, the oil extracted from the seeds of borage *(Borago officinalis).* It is used for the treatment of neurodermatitis and as a food supplement.

borate /bôr'āt/, any salt of boric acid. Borate salts and boric acid, although formerly used as mild antiseptic irrigant solutions, especially for ophthalmic conditions, are highly poisonous when taken internally or absorbed through a cut, abrasion, or other wound in the skin. Because of the potential for fatal poisoning, such solutions are rarely used now. See also **boric acid.**

borax bath [Ar, *bauraq* + AS, *baeth*], a medicated bath in which borax and glycerin are added to the water.

borborygmos /bôr'bərig'məs/, *pl.,* **borborygmi** [Gk, *borborygmos,* bowel rumbling], an audible abdominal sound produced by hyperactive intestinal peristalsis. Borborygmi are rumbling, gurgling, and tinkling noises heard in auscultation. The increased intestinal activity noted at times in cases of gastroenteritis and diarrhea result in borborygmi that do not have the intensity or the episodic character of "normal borborygmi." Borborygmi that are high-pitched

and accompanied by vomiting, distension, and intestinal cramps suggest a mechanical obstruction of the small intestine.

border [OFr, *bordure*], an edge or boundary of a body structure.

borderline [OFr, *bordure* + L, *linea*], pertaining to a state of health in which the patient has some of the signs and symptoms of a disease but not enough to justify a definite diagnosis.

borderline personality [OFr, *bordure* + L, *linea* + *personalis*], a personality in which there is a pervasive pattern of instability of self-image, interpersonal relationships, and mood. There is almost always a marked, persistent disturbance of identity, which is frequently manifested by uncertainty about more than one important personal issue. The hallmark of borderline personality is the defense mechanism of "splitting" in which the person views people or situations as being either all good or all bad and acts accordingly.

Bordetella /bôr'ditel'ə/ [Jules J.B.V. Bordet, Belgian bacteriologist, 1870–1961], a genus of gram-negative coccobacilli, some species of which are pathogens of the respiratory tract of humans, including *Bordetella bronchiseptica, B. parapertussis,* and *B. pertussis.* See also **parapertussis, pertussis.**

boric acid /bôr'ik/, a white, odorless powder or crystalline substance used as a buffer and formerly used as a topical antiseptic and eyewash. Also called **boracic acid, orthoboric acid.**

boric acid poisoning, an adverse reaction to the ingestion or absorption through the skin of boric acid, a mild but potentially lethal antiseptic. Symptoms include nausea, vomiting, diarrhea, convulsions, and shock. Absorption of boric acid from diapers is a threat to infants.

Bornholm disease. See **epidemic pleurodynia.**

born out of asepsis (BOA), (in a hospital) denoting a newborn who was not delivered in the usual place in an obstetric unit. Depending on the policy of the institution, a BOA-designated infant may have been born on the way to the hospital or in the hospital, on the way to the delivery suite, or in a labor room.

■ OBSERVATIONS: Initial assessment in the admitting unit includes evaluation of respiration, quality of cry, skin color, apical pulse rate, muscle tone, reflexes, temperature, condition of umbilical cord or cord stump, ability to suck, presence of meconium, congenital defect, skin eruption, or signs of sepsis, including jaundice, anorexia, vomiting, diarrhea, irritability or lethargy, high-pitched cry, and hypothermia or hyperthermia.

■ INTERVENTIONS: The usual steps in caring for a newborn are performed. Head and chest circumferences are measured, weight is taken, and the baby is placed in a warmer until the axillary temperature is 36.5° C. Vitamin K and silver nitrate are usually given, and a bath is given when the body temperature is over 36.5° C and stable. In many hospitals BOA infants are placed in a special nursery and isolated from other infants to prevent contagion if they are infected.

■ NURSING CONSIDERATIONS: Daily care for the BOA infant is the same as that given to other newborns, but, in addition, the BOA baby is closely observed for signs of sepsis. The parents are involved in the care of the infant as soon as possible, and the usual instructions are given at discharge for home care of the baby.

boron (B) /bôr'on/, a nonmetallic element, whose atomic number is 5; its atomic mass is 10.81. Elemental boron occurs in the form of dark crystals and as a greenish yellow amorphous mass. Certain concentrations of this element are toxic to plant and animal life, but plants need traces of boron for normal growth. It is the characteristic element of boric acid, which is used chiefly as a dusting powder and ointment for minor skin disorders. Boric acid in solution was formerly extensively used as an antiinfective and eyewash, but the high incidence of toxic reactions and fatalities associated with these preparations has greatly reduced their use.

Borrelia /bərel′ē·ə/ [Amédée Borrel, French bacteriologist, 1867–1936], a genus of coarse, unevenly coiled helical spirochetes, several species of which cause tickborne and louseborne relapsing fever. The organism is spread to offspring from generation to generation. This does not occur in lice. Many animals serve as reservoirs and hosts for *Borrelia*. The spirochete may be identified by microscopic examination of a smear of blood stained with Wright's stain; it is also easily inoculated onto culture media for bacterial culture and identification.

Borrelia burgdorferi /burg′dôrfer′ī/, the causative agent in Lyme disease. The organism is transmitted to humans by tick vectors, primarily *Ixodes dammini*. In the United States the disease is found primarily in the Northeast, North-Central, and Northwest.

bortezomib, an antineoplastic agent used to treat multiple myeloma when at least two other treatments have failed.

bosentan, a vasodilator used to treat pulmonary arterial hypertension.

boss [ME, *boce*], a swelling, eminence, or protuberance on an organ, such as a tumor or overgrowth on a bone surface. For example, on the forehead it is often a sign of rickets.

Boston exanthem [Boston; Gk, *ex,* out, *anthema,* blossoming], an epidemic disease characterized by scattered, pale red maculopapules on the face, chest, and back, occasionally accompanied by small ulcerations on the tonsils and soft palate. There is little or no adenopathy, and the rash disappears spontaneously in 2 or 3 weeks. It is caused by echovirus 16 and requires no treatment. Compare **herpangina.**

botox, *(informal),* See **botulinum toxin.**

bottle feeding[1], [OFr, *bouteille* + AS, *faeden*], feeding an infant or young child from a bottle with a rubber nipple on the end as a substitute for or supplement to breastfeeding.

■ METHOD: The infant is held on one arm close to the body of the mother or nurse during feeding. The bottle is held at an angle to ensure that the nipple is always filled with liquid so that the infant does not ingest air while feeding. For a newborn, rest periods may be given every several minutes. At least once in the course of the feeding and again at the end the infant is encouraged to burp by being held upright on the mother's or nurse's shoulder or on its stomach on the feeder's lap. Gentle rubbing or patting on the back and pressure on the stomach often help induce burping.

■ INTERVENTIONS: The formula contains protein, fats, carbohydrates, vitamins, and minerals in amounts similar to those in breast milk. The formula may be warmed before feeding by immersing the bottle in warm water for several minutes (although this is not necessary if the formula is kept at room temperature), and the size of the nipple hole is adjusted to the needs of the infant. Smaller infants need larger nipple holes, which require less sucking. Premature or weak infants may be fed by using a long soft nipple through which it is very easy for the infant to feed.

■ OUTCOME CRITERIA: Bottle feeding is used as a substitute for breastfeeding when the mother is unable or unwilling to breastfeed. Bottle feeding can also be substituted for breastfeeding occasionally, once lactation has been established. Bottle feeding is recommended if the mother has active tuberculosis or other active, acute contagious disease; if she has a serious chronic disease, such as cancer or cardiac

disease; or if she has recently undergone extensive surgery. Severe mastitis, narcotic addiction, or concurrent use of medication that is secreted in the breast milk usually requires the mother to bottle feed.

bottle feeding[2], a nursing intervention from the Nursing Interventions Classification (NIC) defined as preparation and administration of fluids to an infant via a bottle. See also **Nursing Interventions Classification.**

bottle mouth caries, early childhood caries.

botulinum toxin /boch′əlī′nəm/ [L, *botulus,* sausage; Gk, *toxikon,* poison], any of a group of potent bacterial toxins produced by different strains of *Clostridium botulinum.* It may be used therapeutically for blepharospasm or cosmetically to relax facial wrinkles. The strains are sometimes identified by letters of the alphabet, such as A, B, or C. Also called **botox, botulinus toxin.**

botulism /boch′əliz′əm/ [L, *botulus,* sausage], an often fatal form of food poisoning caused by an endotoxin produced by the bacillus *Clostridium botulinum.* The toxin is ingested in food contaminated by *C. botulinum,* although it is not necessary for the live bacillus to be present if the toxin has been produced. In rare instances the toxin may be introduced into the human body through a wound contaminated by the organism. Infants may consume spores that produce the toxin, which is associated with eating unpasteurized honey. Botulism differs from most other types of food poisoning in that it develops without gastric distress and occurs from 18 hours up to 1 week after the contaminated food has been ingested. Botulism is characterized by lassitude, fatigue, and visual disturbances, such as double vision, difficulty in focusing the eyes, and loss of ability of the pupil to accommodate to light. Muscles may become weak, and dysphagia often develops. Nausea and vomiting occur in fewer than half the cases. Affected infants are lethargic, feed poorly, are constipated, and have a weak cry and poor muscle tone. Hospitalization is required, and antitoxins are administered. Sedatives are given, mainly to relieve anxiety. Approximately 10% of the cases of botulism are fatal, usually as a result of delayed diagnosis and respiratory complications. Most botulism occurs after eating improperly canned or cooked foods. See also *Clostridium.*

■ OBSERVATIONS: Symptoms usually appear 12 to 36 hours after ingestion of a contaminated food substance. Severity of symptoms is related to the quantity of the botulinum toxin that was ingested and include dry mouth, diplopia, loss of pupillary light reflex; nausea, vomiting, cramps, and diarrhea, which precede dysphagia, dysarthria, and progressive descending muscular paralysis. Botulism is fatal in about 10% of cases, usually because of respiratory paralysis or circulatory failure. Serum may be positive for botulinal toxins and cultures may be taken of stomach contents, feces, or suspected food to confirm the causative organism.

■ INTERVENTIONS: The trivalent botulinal antitoxin is administered as soon as possible after onset and clinical diagnosis. The GI tract is purged using laxatives, gastric lavage, and high colonic enemas to dilute and decrease absorption of the toxin. Tracheostomy and mechanical ventilation may be instituted if necessary. Care is supportive with a long recovery period and the need for rehabilitation to regain muscle tone, strength, and function.

■ NURSING CONSIDERATIONS: Nurses should be alert to signs and symptoms of serum sickness that frequently occur after the administration of the antitoxin, including fever, arthralgia, lymphadenopathy, skin eruption, pain, pruritus, and erythematous swelling at the injection site. Individuals may also report joint and muscle aches, chest pain, and difficulty breathing. Nursing care for acute illness is largely supportive and involves airway management, prevention of aspiration, fluid and electrolyte management, pain management, nutrition management, prevention of skin breakdown and contractures during paralysis, minimization of stimuli, precise communication because of altered vision and loss of speech, and allaying anxiety about paralysis and treatment. Primary prevention targets education of consumers in the safe handling, storage, and preparation of food. Nurses should also be prepared for an effective response should botulinum toxin be used in a bioterrorism event. This includes familiarization of institution policies, procedures and protocols, and maintenance of current knowledge regarding bioterrorism threats.

bouba.   See **yaws.**

Bouchard's node /bo͞oshärz'/ [Charles J. Bouchard, French physician, 1837–1915],   an abnormal cartilaginous or bony enlargement of a proximal interphalangeal joint of a finger, usually occurring in degenerative diseases of the joints, such as rheumatoid arthritis. Compare **Heberden's node.**

Bouchard's nodes *(Phipps et al, 2003)*

Bouchut's tubes /bo͞osho͞oz/ [Jean E.W. Bouchut, French physician, 1818–1891],   a set of short cylindric devices used for intubation of the larynx.

bougie /bo͞o'zhē, bo͞ozhē'/ [Fr, candle],   a thin cylindric instrument made of rubber, waxed silk, or other flexible material for insertion into canals of the body in order to dilate, examine, or measure them.

-boulia.   See **-bulia.**

boulimia.   See **bulimia.**

boundary /boun'dərē/,   (in psychology) an aspect of family health in which the generations are clearly defined and issues dealt with by the appropriate generation. There are also limits between the family "turf" and the larger society. This term can also apply to the roles of patient and therapist in psychotherapy.

boundary lubrication,   a coating of a thin layer of molecules on each weight-bearing surface of a joint to facilitate a sliding action by the opposing bone surfaces.

boundary maintenance mechanisms,   (in psychology) behavior and practices that exclude members of some groups from the customs and values of another group.

bound carbon dioxide,   carbon dioxide that is transported in the bloodstream as part of a sodium bicarbonate molecule, as distinguished from dissolved carbon dioxide or bicarbonate ion.

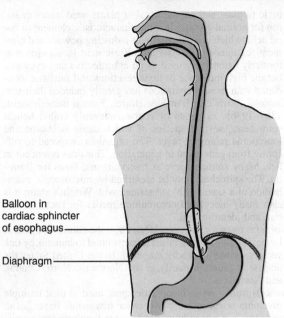

Balloon in cardiac sphincter of esophagus

Diaphragm

Passage of a bougie *(Black and Hawks, 2005)*

bounding pulse [OFr, *bondir,* to leap; L, *pulsare,* to beat],   a pulse that feels full and springlike on palpation as a result of an increased thrust of cardiac contraction or an increased volume of circulating blood within the elastic structures of the vascular system.

bound water,   water in the tissue of the body bound to macromolecules or organelles.

bouquet fever.   See **dengue fever.**

Bourdon regulator,   a commonly used adjustable device with an attached pressure gauge for controlling the flow of oxygen or other gases from cylinders in medical applications.

Bourneville's disease.   See **tuberous sclerosis.**

bouton /bo͞otôN', bo͞o'ton/ [Fr, button],   **1.** a knoblike swelling, such as the expanded end of an axon at a synapse (terminaux) which comes into contact with cell bodies of other neurons. **2.** a lesion associated with cutaneous leishmaniasis. **3.** a small abscess of the intestinal mucosa in amebic dysentery.

boutonneuse fever /bo͞o'təno͞oz'/ [Fr, *bouton,* button; L, *febris*],   an infectious disease caused by *Rickettsia conorii,* transmitted to humans through the bite of a tick. The onset of the disease is characterized by a lesion called a *tache noire* /täshno·är'/, or black spot, at the site of the infection; fever lasting from a few days to 2 weeks; and a papular erythematous rash that spreads over the body to include the skin of the palms and soles. Treatment usually involves administration of antibiotics. There is no prophylactic medication available, and prevention depends primarily on avoiding ticks. See also **rickettsiosis, Rocky Mountain spotted fever.**

boutonnière deformity /bo͞o'tônyer'/ [Fr, buttonhole],   an abnormality of a finger marked by fixed flexion of the proximal interphalangeal joint and hyperextension of the distal interphalangeal joint. The condition occurs in rheumatoid arthritis.

bovine spongiform encephalopathy (BSE),   an infection of cattle characterized by degenerative, clumsy, apprehen-

Boutonnière deformity *(Zitelli and Davis, 1997)*

sive behavior, and death. The BSE brain tissue is perforated and spongy in appearance. The disease was first observed in cattle by veterinarians in 1883. It has been associated with other spongiform encephalopathies such as scrapie in sheep and goats, and Cruetzfeldt-Jakob disease (CJD) in humans. In European "mad cow" disease, it is believed the disease was transmitted to cattle through livestock feed that contained remains of scrapie-infected sheep. The disease was then transmitted to humans who ate BSE-infected beef.

bovine tuberculosis /bō′vīn/ [L, *bos,* ox, *tuber,* swelling; Gk, *osis,* condition], a form of tuberculosis caused by *Mycobacterium tuberculosis* that primarily affects cattle. Mastitis and pulmonary symptoms can occur.

Bowditch's law. See **all-or-none law.**

bowel. See **intestine.**

bowel bypass syndrome, a series of adverse effects that may follow bowel bypass surgery, which include chills, fever, joint pain, and skin inflammation on the arms, legs, and thorax.

bowel continence, a nursing outcome from the Nursing Outcomes Classification (NOC) defined as control of passage of stool from the bowel. See also **Nursing Outcomes Classification.**

bowel elimination, a nursing outcome from the Nursing Outcomes Classification (NOC) defined as ability of the gastrointestinal tract to form and evacuate stool effectively. See also **Nursing Outcomes Classification.**

bowel incontinence. See **incontinence, bowel.**

bowel incontinence care, a nursing intervention from the Nursing Interventions Classification (NIC) defined as promotion of bowel continence and maintenance of perianal skin integrity. See also **Nursing Interventions Classification.**

bowel incontinence care: encopresis, a nursing intervention from the Nursing Interventions Classification (NIC) defined as promotion of bowel continence in children. See also **Nursing Interventions Classification.**

bowel irrigation, a nursing intervention from the Nursing Interventions Classification (NIC) defined as instillation of a substance into the lower gastrointestinal tract. See also **Nursing Interventions Classification.**

bowel management, a nursing intervention from the Nursing Interventions Classification (NIC) defined as establishment and maintenance of a regular pattern of bowel elimination. See also **Nursing Interventions Classification.**

bowel training[1] [OFr, *boel*], a method of establishing regular evacuation by reflex conditioning used in the treatment of fecal incontinence, impaction, chronic diarrhea, and autonomic hyperreflexia. In patients with autonomic hyperreflexia, distension of the rectum and bladder causes paroxysmal hypertension, restlessness, chills, diaphoresis, headache, elevated temperature, and bradycardia.

■ METHOD: The patient's previous bowel habits are assessed, and the necessity of developing a program to induce an evacuation at the same time each day or every other day is explained. Exercises to strengthen abdominal muscles, such as pushing up, bearing down, and contracting the musculature, are demonstrated. The patient is instructed to recognize and respond promptly to signals indicating a full bowel, such as goose pimples, perspiration, and piloerection on arms or legs, and to develop cues to stimulate the urge to defecate, such as drinking coffee, or massaging the abdomen. Fluids to 3000 ml daily are encouraged; exercise is increased as able, and the importance of eating well-balanced meals that include bulk and roughage and of avoiding constipating or gas-producing foods, such as bananas, beans, and cabbage, is discussed. Depending on the patient and the problem, the training program may involve drinking warm fluid, ensuring privacy, and inserting a lubricated glycerin suppository before the set time. The patient is told that no formed stools for 3 days, semiliquid feces, restlessness, and discomfort are signs of impending impaction and that the condition may be treated with a laxative suppository or with a tap water or oil retention enema. The importance of reporting symptoms of autonomic hyperreflexia to the physician is stressed. The possibility that emotional stress or illness may cause accidental incontinence after the program has been established is discussed. Many clients require weeks or months of training to achieve success.

■ INTERVENTIONS: The nurse provides instruction, encourages the patient to establish a program of regular evacuation, and offers positive reinforcement frequently.

■ OUTCOME CRITERIA: Reflex conditioning is often an effective method of developing regular bowel habits for incontinent patients, especially those who are highly motivated and are given good instruction and understanding support. Young persons with spinal cord lesions are able to develop automatic defecation when adequately trained, but some elderly incontinent people may not be able to learn the program.

bowel training[2], a nursing intervention from the Nursing Interventions Classification (NIC) defined as assisting the patient to train the bowel to evacuate at specific intervals. See also **Nursing Interventions Classification.**

bowel urgency, the sudden, almost uncontrollable, need to defecate.

bowenoid papulosis. See **Bowen's disease.**

Bowen's disease [John T. Bowen, American dermatologist, 1857–1941], a form of intraepidermal carcinoma (squamous cell). It is characterized by red-brown scaly or crusted lesions that resemble a patch of psoriasis or dermatitis. Treatment includes curettage and electrodesiccation. A corresponding lesion found on the glans penis is called **erythroplasia of Queyrat.** Also called **Bowen's precancerous dermatosis.** See also **intraepidermal carcinoma.**

Bowen's disease *(Hordinsky, Sawaya, and Scher, 2000)*

Bowen technique, a system of gentle but powerful soft tissue mobilizations using the thumbs and fingers over muscles, tendons, nerves, and fascia to restore the self-healing mechanism of the body. This technique has been used for conditions affecting the musculoskeletal system, including back, neck, hip, and shoulder pain.

bowleg. See **genu varum.**

Bowman's capsule /bō′manz/ [William Bowman, English anatomist, 1816–1892], the cup-shaped end of a renal tubule or nephron enclosing a glomerulus. With the glomerulus, it is the site of filtration in the kidney. Also called **glomerular capsule.**

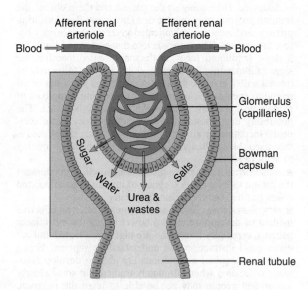

Bowman's capsule (Chabner, 2004)

Bowman's glands [William Bowman; L, *glans,* acorn], branched tubuloalveolar glands in olefactory membrane of the mouth. They keep the mouth surfaces moist.

Bowman's lamina [William Bowman; L, *lamina,* plate], a tough membrane beneath the corneal epithelium. Also called **anterior elastic lamina, Bowman's layer, Bowman's membrane.**

bowtie filter /bō′tī/, a filter shaped like a bow tie that may be used in computed tomography to compensate for the shape of the patient's head or body. It is used with fan-shaped x-ray beams to equalize the amount of radiation reaching the film.

box bath. See **cabinet bath.**

boxer's ear. See **pachyotia.**

boxer's fracture [Dan, *bask,* a blow; L, *fractura,* break], a break in one or more metacarpal bones, usually the fourth or the fifth, caused by punching a hard object. Such a fracture is often distal, angulated, and impacted.

boxing, the forming of vertical walls, most commonly made of wax, to produce the desired shape and size of the base of a dental cast.

boxing wax [L, *buxis,* box; AS, *weax*], (in dentistry) a wax used for boxing.

Boyd's amputation, amputation at the ankle with removal of the talus and fusion of the tibia and calcaneus.

Boyle's law /boilz/ [Robert Boyle, English scientist, 1627–1691], (in physics) the law stating that the product of the volume and pressure of a gas contained at a constant temperature remains constant.

BP, abbreviation for **blood pressure.**

BPD, 1. abbreviation for **biparietal diameter, 2.** abbreviation for **bronchopulmonary dysplasia.**

BPDE-I, abbreviation for **benzopyrene dihydrodiol epoxide.**

BPH, abbreviation for **benign prostatic hypertrophy.**

bpm, abbreviation for *beats per minute.*

Br, symbol for the element **bromine.**

brace [OFr, *bracier,* to embrace], an orthotic device, sometimes jointed, used to support and hold any part of the body in the correct position to allow function and healing, such as a leg brace that permits walking and standing. Compare **splint.**

brachi- /brā′kē-/, prefix meaning "arm": *brachiation, brachiocyllosis.*

-brachia /-brā′kē·ə/, suffix meaning an "anatomic condition involving an arm": *acephalobrachia, monobrachia.*

brachial /brā′kē·əl/ [Gk, *brachion,* arm], pertaining to the arm.

brachial artery, the principal artery of the upper arm that is the continuation of the axillary artery. It has three branches and terminates at the bifurcation of its main trunk into the radial artery and the ulnar artery.

brachialgia /-al′jē·ə/ [L, *brachium,* arm; Gk, *algos,* pain], a severe pain in the arm, often related to a disorder involving the brachial plexus.

brachialis /brā′kē·al′is/ [Gk, *brachion,* arm], a muscle of the upper arm, covering the anterior part of the elbow joint and the distal half of the humerus. It functions to flex the forearm. Compare **biceps brachii, triceps brachii.**

Brachialis

Brachialis

brachial paralysis [L, *brachium,* arm; Gk, *paralyein,* to be palsied], paralysis of an arm or a hand as a result of a lesion of the brachial plexus. See also **Erb palsy.**

brachial plexus [Gk, *brachion* + L, braided], a network of nerves in the neck, passing under the clavicle and into the axilla, originating in the fifth, sixth, seventh, and eighth cervical and first two thoracic spinal nerves. It innervates the muscles and skin of the chest, shoulders, and arms.

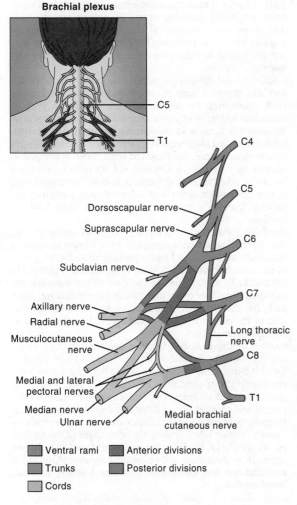

Brachial plexus

Brachial plexus *(Thibodeau and Patton, 2003)*

brachial plexus anesthesia, an anesthetic block of the upper extremity, performed by injecting local anesthetic near the plexis formed by the last four cervical and first two thoracic spinal nerves. The plexus extends from the transverse processes of the spine to the apex of the axilla, where the terminal nerves are formed. Because of the anatomy of this area, many approaches are possible. The axillary approach is most common and has the least risk of producing pneumothorax; supraclavicular and interscalene approaches are also used. Various approaches may result in Horner's syndrome, phrenic nerve block, pneumothorax, recurrent laryngeal paralysis, persistent sensory deficits, venous or arterial puncture, subarachnoid injection, paresthesias, or hematoma. Also called **brachial plexus block.** See also **regional anesthesia.**

brachial plexus block. See **brachial plexus anesthesia.**
brachial plexus paralysis. See **Erb palsy.**
brachial pulse [Gk, *brachion* + L, *pulsare,* to beat], the pulse of the brachial artery, palpated in the antecubital space. See also **pulse.**

Assessment of brachial pulse *(Wilson and Giddens, 2001)*

brachial region, an anatomical term used to refer to the arm (shoulder to elbow), divided into anterior and posterior brachial regions.
brachial vein, a vein in the arm that accompanies the brachial artery and drains into the axillary vein.
brachiocephalic, relating to the arm and head.
brachiocephalic arteritis. See **Takayasu's arteritis.**
brachiocephalic artery, first branch of the aortic arch. See also **innominate artery.**
brachiocephalic trunk. See **innominate artery.**
brachiocephalic vein, the vein feeding the superior vena cava, collecting blood from the subclavian and jugular veins. See also **innominate vein.**
brachiocubital /-kyoo'bitəl/ [Gk, *brachion* + L, *cubitus,* elbow], pertaining to the arm and forearm.
brachioplasty, a surgical procedure to lift and tighten skin of the upper arm.
brachioradialis /-rā'dē·al'is/, the most superficial muscle on the radial side of the forearm. It functions to flex the forearm.
brachioradialis reflex [Gk, *brachion* + L, *radial, reflectare,* to bend backward], a deep tendon reflex elicited by striking the lateral surface of the forearm proximal to the distal head of the radius, characterized by normal slight elbow flexion and forearm supination. It is accentuated by disease of the pyramidal tract above the level of the fifth cervical vertebra. See also **deep tendon reflex.**
-brachium /-brā'kē·əm/, **1.** suffix meaning "the upper arm from shoulder to elbow." **2.** suffix meaning "an arm or armlike growth": *prebrachium, pontibrachium.*
brachy- /brak'ē-/, prefix meaning "short": *brachycheilia, brachyskelous.*
brachybasia /-bā'zhə/, abnormally slow walking, with a short, shuffling gait. The condition is associated with cerebral hemorrhage or pyramidal tract disease, or Parkinson's disease.
brachycardia. See **bradycardia.**
brachycephaly /-sef'əlē/ [Gk, *brachys,* short, *kephale,* head], a congenital malformation of the skull in which premature closure of the coronal suture results in excessive

brachioradialis

Brachioradialis *(Thibodeau and Patton, 2003)*

Brachioradialis reflex testing *(Seidel et al, 2003)*

lateral growth of the head, giving it a short, broad appearance. Also called **brachycephalia** /-səfā'lē·ə/, **brachycephalism** /-sef'əlizəm/. See also **craniostenosis.** —**brachycephalic** /-səfal'ik/, **brachycephalous** /-sef'əl əs/, *adj.*

brachydactyly /-dak'təlē/, a condition in which fingers or toes are abnormally short.

brachygnathia. See **micrognathia.**

brachytherapy [Gk, *brachys,* short, *therapeia,* treatment], the placement of radioactive sources in contact with or implanted into the tumor tissues to be treated for a specific period. The rationale for this treatment is to provide a high absorbed dose of radiation in the tumor tissues and a very limited absorbed low dose in the surrounding normal tissues. Compare **teletherapy.**

bracket /brak'ət/ [Fr, *braguette,* codpiece], a support projecting from the main structure. An **orthodontic bracket** is a small metal attachment soldered or welded to an orthodontic band or cemented directly to the teeth, serving to fasten the arch wire to the band or tooth. Also called **orthodontic attachment.** See also **orthodontic appliance, orthodontic band.**

Bradford frame [Edward H. Bradford, American surgeon, 1848–1926], a rectangular orthopedic frame made of pipes to which heavy movable straps of canvas are attached. The straps run from side to side to support a patient in a prone or supine position. They can be removed to permit the patient to urinate or defecate while remaining immobile.

Bradford solid frame, a rectangular metal orthopedic device that provides support for the entire body and is especially appropriate for patients who are less than 5 years of age, hyperactive, or mentally retarded. The main purpose of the device is to assist in maintaining proper immobilization, positioning, and alignment by controlling movement. To facilitate nursing care, the Bradford solid frame is not placed directly on a bed but is elevated at both ends by plywood blocks or other suitable devices. It is most often used with Bryant traction but never with balanced suspension traction, cervical traction, cervical tongs, or certain other kinds of traction.

Bradford split frame, a rectangular metal orthopedic device covered with two separate pieces of canvas fastened at both ends of the frame. Used especially in pediatrics to aid in the immobilization of children in traction, it is divided in the middle by a large opening designed to accommodate the excretory functions of an incontinent patient in a hip spica cast. The division also allows the upper and lower extremities of the patient to be elevated separately and the cast to be kept clean and dry.

Bradley method [Robert Bradley, twentieth century American physician], a method of psychophysical preparation for childbirth, comprising education about the physiologic characteristics of childbirth, exercise, and nutrition during pregnancy, and techniques of breathing and relaxation for control and comfort during labor and delivery. The father is extensively involved in the classes and acts as the mother's "coach" during labor. Among the advantages of the method are its simplicity, the father's involvement, and the realistic approach to the efforts and discomfort of labor. Also called **husband-coached childbirth.** Compare **Lamaze method, Read method.**

brady- /brad'ē-/, prefix meaning "slow, dull": *bradycardia, bradydiastalsis, bradyphagia.*

bradyarrhythmia /-ərith'mē·ə/ [Gk, *bradys,* slow, *a + rhythmos,* without rhythm], any disturbance of cardiac rhythm in which the heart rate is less than 60 beats/min.

bradycardia /-kär'dē·ə/ [Gk, *bradys,* slow, *kardia,* heart], a condition in which the heart rate is less than 60/min. Bradycardia takes the form of sinus bradycardia, sinus arrhythmia, and second- or third-degree atrioventricular block. Sinus bradycardia may be caused by excessive vagal tone, decreased sympathetic tone, or anatomic changes. It is common in athletes and is relatively benign. It may even be beneficial in acute myocardial infarction (especially inferior). Pathologic bradycardia may be symptomatic of a brain tumor, digitalis toxicity, heart block, or vagotonus. Cardiac output is decreased, causing faintness, dizziness, chest pain, and eventually syncope and circulatory collapse. Treatment may include administration of atropine, implantation of a pacemaker, or change in medical treatment. Also called **brachycardia.**

bradycardia-tachycardia syndrome [Gk, *bradys + kardia, + tachys,* fast, *kardia + syn,* together, *dromos,* course], a disorder characterized by a heart rate that alternates between being abnormally low (less than 60 beats/min) and abnormally high (greater than 100 beats/min). Also called **bradytachycardia, tachycardia-bradycardia syndrome.** See also **sick sinus syndrome, sinus nodal dysfunction.**

bradyesthesia /-esthē′zhə/ [Gk, *bradys,* slow, *aisthesis,* feeling], a slowness in perception.

bradykinesia /-kinē′zhə, -kīnē′zhə/ [Gk, *bradys + kinesis,* motion], an abnormal condition characterized by slowness of all voluntary movement and speech, such as caused by parkinsonism, other extrapyramidal disorders, and certain tranquilizers.

bradykinin /-kī′nin/ [Gk, *bradys + kinein,* to move], a peptide containing nine amino acid residues produced from α_2-globulin by the enzyme kallikrein. Bradykinin is a potent vasodilator.

bradylalia. See **bradyphasia.**

bradyphagia /-fā′jə/, a habit of eating very slowly.

bradyphasia /-fā′zhə/, an abnormally slow manner of speech, often associated with mental illness. Also called **bradylalia.**

bradypnea /-pnē′ə/ [Gk, *bradys + pnein,* to breath], an abnormally low rate of breathing(lower than 12/min). Compare **hypopnea.** See also **respiration rate.**

bradyspermatism /-spur′mətiz′əm/, ejaculation that lacks normal force so that semen trickles slowly from the penis.

bradytachycardia. See **bradycardia-tachycardia syndrome.**

bradyuria /brad′ēyo͞or′ē·ə/, a condition in which urine is passed very slowly.

Bragg curve [William H. Bragg, English physicist, 1862–1942], the path followed by ionizing particles used in a radiation treatment. Because certain particles reach a peak of potential near the end of their path, the Bragg curve can be used to direct the radiation to deep-seated tumors while significantly sparing normal overlying tissues.

Braille /brāl, brä′yə/ [Louis Braille, French teacher of the blind, 1809–1852], a system of printing for the blind consisting of raised dots or points that can be read by touch.

brain [AS, *bragen*], the portion of the central nervous system contained within the cranium. It consists of the cerebrum, cerebellum, pons, medulla, and midbrain. Specialized cells in its mass of convoluted, soft gray or white tissue coordinate and regulate the functions of the central nervous system, integrating the functions of the body as a whole.

brain abscess [AS, *bragen* + L, *abscedere,* to go away], a pocket of infection in a part of the brain. It is usually a result of the spread of an infection from another source, such as the skull, sinuses, or other structures in the head. The infection also may be secondary to a disease in the bones, the nervous system outside the brain, or the heart. Also called **cerebral abscess, intracranial abscess.**

Brain airway. See **laryngeal mask airway.**

brain attack, term signifying that a stroke is in progress and an emergency situation exists. So-called to draw attention to the situation as in heart attack by the American Stroke Association. See also **cerebrovascular accident.**

brain compression. See **cerebral compression.**

brain concussion [AS, *bragen* + L, *concussus,* a shaking], a bruising to cerebral tissues caused by a violent jarring or shaking or other blunt, nonpenetrating injury to the brain resulting in a sudden change in momentum of the head. Characteristically, after a mild concussion there may be a transient loss of consciousness followed, on awakening, by a headache. Severe concussion may cause prolonged uncon-

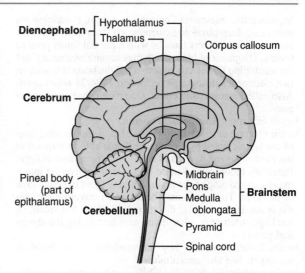

Major structures of the brain
(Phipps et al, 2003)

Brain abscess *(Damjanov and Linder, 2000)*

sciousness and disruption of certain vital functions of the brainstem, such as respiration and vasomotor stability. The treatment for a person recovering from a concussion consists principally of observation for signs of intracranial bleeding and increased intracranial pressure. Also called **concussion.**

brain death [AS, *bragen* + *death*], an irreversible form of unconsciousness characterized by a complete loss of brain function while the heart continues to beat. The legal definition of this condition varies from state to state. The usual clinical criteria for brain death include the absence of reflex activity, movements, and spontaneous respiration requiring mechanical ventilation or life support to continue any cardiac function. The pupils are dilated and fixed. Because hypothermia, anesthesia, poisoning, or drug intoxication may cause deep physiologic depression that resembles brain death these parameters must be within normal limits prior to testing. Diagnosis of brain death may require evaluating and demonstrating that electrical activity of the brain is absent on two electroencephalograms performed 12 to 24 hours apart. Also called **irreversible coma.** Compare **coma, sleep, stupor.**

brain edema. See **cerebral edema.**

brain electric activity map (BEAM), a topographic map of the brain created by a computer that is able to respond to the electric potentials evoked in the brain by a flash of light. Potentials recorded at 4-msec intervals are converted into a many-colored map of the brain, showing them to be positive or negative. The waves may be observed traveling through the brain. If the wave is disordered, blocked, too small, or too large, a tumor or other lesion may be causing the abnormal pattern.

brain fever, *informal,* any inflammation of the brain or meninges. See also **encephalitis.**

brain natriuretic peptide (BNP), a hormone, originally isolated from porcine brain tissue, having biologic effects similar to those of atrial natriuretic peptide and stored mainly in the myocardium of the cardiac ventricles. Blood levels of BNP are elevated in hypervolemic states, such as congestive heart failure and hypertension.

brain scan [AS, *bragen* + L, *scandere,* to climb], a diagnostic procedure using radioisotope imaging to localize and identify intracranial masses, lesions, tumors, or infarcts. Intravenously injected radioisotopes accumulate in abnormal brain tissue and are traced and photographed by a scintillator or scanner. The nature and rate of accumulation of radioisotopes in pathologic tissue are diagnostic of some lesions. Compare **computed tomography.** See also **isotope, radioisotope.**

Brain's reflex [Walter R. Brain, English physician, 1895–1966; L, *reflectere,* to bend back], the reflexive extension of the flexed paralyzed arm of a hemiplegia patient when assuming a quadrupedal posture. Also called **quadrupedal extensor reflex.**

brainstem [AS, *bragen* + *stemm*], the portion of the brain comprising the medulla oblongata, the pons, and the mesencephalon. It performs motor, sensory, and reflex functions and contains the corticospinal and reticulospinal tracts. The 12 pairs of cranial nerves from the brain arise mostly from the brainstem. Compare **medulla oblongata, mesencephalon, pons.**

brainstem auditory evoked response (BAER), the electric activity that may be recorded from the brainstem in the first 10 msec after presentation of an auditory stimulus. In a subject with normal brainstem functioning, seven peaks are observed. A delayed, normally shaped waveform may indicate a hearing loss caused by a middle or inner ear disorder; one or more missing peaks may indicate a neural disorder.

brain swelling. See **cerebral edema.**

brain syndrome, a group of symptoms resulting from impaired function of the brain. It may be acute and reversible, or chronic and irreversible. An organic mental disorder is a specific organic mental syndrome in which the cause is known or presumed. An organic mental syndrome is a temporary or permanent brain dysfunction of any cause.

brain tumor, an invasive neoplasm of the intracranial portion of the central nervous system. Brain tumors cause significant rates of morbidity and mortality but are occasionally treated successfully. In adults 20% to 40% of malignancies in the brain are metastatic lesions from cancers in the breast, lung, GI tract, or kidney or a malignant melanoma. The origin of primary brain tumors is not known, but the risk is increased in individuals exposed to vinyl chloride, in the siblings of cancer patients, and in recipients of renal transplantation being treated with immunosuppressant medication. Symptoms of a brain tumor are often those of increased intracranial pressure, such as headache, nausea, vomiting, papilledema, lethargy, and disorientation. Localizing signs, such as loss of vision on the side of an occipital neoplasm, may occur. Diagnostic measures include visual field and funduscopic examinations, skull x-ray examinations, electroencephalography, cerebral angiography, brain scanning, magnetic resonance imaging, computed tomography, and spinal fluid studies. Gliomas, chiefly astrocytomas, are the most common malignancies. Medulloblastomas occur often in children. Surgery is the initial treatment for most primary tumors of the brain. Radiotherapy is indicated for inoperable lesions, medulloblastomas, and tumors with multiple foci and is used in postoperative treatment of residual tumor tissue. The blood-brain barrier impedes the effect of some antineoplastic agents, but responses are obtained in some cases treated with procarbazine and various nitrosoureas administered alone or with vincristine. Compare **spinal cord tumor.**

Brain tumor
(Mace and Kowalczyk, 2004/courtesy Riverside Methodist Hospitals)

brainwashing, intensive indoctrination, usually of a political or religious nature, applied to individuals to develop in their minds a specific belief and motivation.

brain wave [AS, *bragen* + *wafian*], any of a number of patterns of rhythmic electric impulses produced in different parts of the brain. Most patterns, identified by the Greek letters alpha, beta, delta, gamma, kappa, and theta, are similar for all normal persons and are relatively stable for each individual. Alpha waves are produced when the person is awake but resting, beta waves signal an active phase of cerebral function, delta waves are emitted during deep sleep, and theta waves occur, usually in children but also in adults during emotional stress. Brain waves help in the diagnosis of certain neurologic disorders, such as epilepsy or brain tumors.

bran, a coarse outer covering or coat (seed husk) of cereal grain, such as wheat or rye. It is broken or separated from the meal or flour portion of the grain to provide a source of dietary fiber, B vitamins, iron, magnesium, and zinc.

bran bath [OFr, *bren* + AS, *baeth*], a bath in which bran has been boiled in the water. It is used for the relief of skin irritation.

branch, (in anatomy) an offshoot arising from the main trunk of a nerve or blood vessel.

branched-chain amino acids, leucine, isoleucine, and valine; they are incorporated into proteins or catabolized for energy.

branched chain ketoaciduria. See **maple syrup urine disease.**

branched tubular gland [OFr, *branche*], one of the many multicellular glands with one excretory duct from two or more tube-shaped secretory branches, such as some of the gastric glands.

brancher glycogen storage disease. See **Andersen's disease.**

branchial /brang′kē·əl/ [Gk, *branchia*, gills], pertaining to body structures of the face, neck, and throat area, particularly the muscles.

branchial arches [Gk, *branchia*, gills; L, *arcus*, bow], arched structures in the embryonic pharynx.

branchial cleft [Gk, *branchia*, gills; ME, *clift*], a linear depression in the pharynx of the early embryo opposite a branchial or pharyngeal pouch.

branchial cyst [Gk, *branchia*, gills, *kystis*, bag], a cyst derived from a branchial remnant in the neck.

branchial fistula, a congenital abnormal passage from the pharynx to the external surface of the neck, resulting from the failure of a branchial cleft to close during fetal development. Also called **cervical fistula.**

branching canal. See **collateral pulp canal.**

branchiogenic /brang′kē·ōjen′ik/ [Gk, *branchia*, gills, *genein*, to produce], pertaining to any tissues originating in the branchial cleft or arch. Also **branchiogenous** /-kē·oj′ənes/.

branchio-oto-renal syndrome /brang′kē·ō·ō′tō·rē′nəl/ [Gk, *branchia*, gills + *ous*, ear + L, *ren*, kidney], branchial arch anomalies (preauricular pits, branchial fistulas or pits) associated with congenital deafness resulting from dysgenesis of the organ of Corti, and with renal dysplasia; inherited as an autosomal dominant trait with high penetrance and variable expression.

brand name. See **trademark.**

Brandt-Andrews maneuver [Thure Brandt, Swedish obstetrician, 1819–1895; Henry R. Andrews, English obstetrician, 1871–1942], a method of expressing the placenta from the uterus in the third stage of labor. One hand grasps the umbilical cord while the other is placed on the mother's abdomen with the fingers over the anterior surface of the uterus. While the hand on the abdomen is pressed backward and slightly upward, the other applies gentle traction on the cord.

Braschi valve, a one-way valve put into the inspiratory limb of a ventilator circuit to measure the intrinsic positive end-expiratory pressure.

brass founder's ague. See **metal fume fever.**

brassy cough [AS, *brase*, brassy, *cohhetan*, to cough], a high-pitched cough caused by irritation of the recurrent pharyngeal nerve or by pressure on the trachea.

brassy eye. See **chalkitis.**

Braun's canal. See **neurenteric canal.**

brawny arm, a swollen arm caused by lymphedema, usually after a mastectomy.

Braxton Hicks contractions. See **preterm contractions.**

Braxton Hicks version /brak′stənhiks′/ [John Braxton Hicks, English physician, 1823–1897], one of several types of maneuvers sometimes used to turn the fetus from an undesirable position to one that is more likely to facilitate delivery. See also **version.**

Brazelton assessment. See **Neonatal Behavioral Assessment Scale.**

Brazilian trypanosomiasis. See **Chagas' disease.**

BRCA1, symbol for a breast cancer gene. A healthy BRCA1 gene produces a protein that protects against unwanted cell growth. The protein is packaged by the cell's Golgi apparatus into secretory vesicles, which release their contents on the cell's surface. The protein circulates in the intracellular space, attaching itself to neighboring cell receptors. The receptors signal the cell nuclei to stop growing. When the gene is defective, it produces a faulty protein that is unable to prevent proliferation of abnormal cells as they evolve into potentially deadly breast cancer. BRCA1 may also normally inhibit ovarian cancer.

BRCA2, symbol for a breast cancer gene with activity similar to that of BRCA1.

BRCA3, symbol for a breast cancer gene.

breach of contract, the failure to perform as promised or agreed in a contract. The breach may be complete or partial and may entail repudiation, failure to recognize the contract, or prevention or hindrance of performance.

breach of duty, 1. the failure to perform an act required by law. **2.** the performance of an act in an unlawful way.

breakbone fever. See **dengue fever.**

break test, a test of a person's muscle strength by application of resistance after the person has reached the end of a range of motion. Resistance is applied gradually in a direction opposite to the line of pull of the muscle or muscle group being tested. The resistance is released immediately if there is any sign of pain or discomfort.

breakthrough, (in psychiatry) a sudden new insight into a problem and its solution after a period of little or no progress.

breakthrough analgesia, analgesia administered for the relief of breakthrough pain.

breakthrough bleeding, the escape of uterine blood between menstrual periods, a possible side effect of fibroids or oral contraceptive use.

breakthrough dose, the dose of an analgesic required for the relief of breakthrough pain. Also called *rescue dose.*

breakthrough pain, a transient increase in pain intensity from a baseline pain level of no greater than moderate.

breast [AS, *breast*], **1.** the anterior aspect of the surface of the chest. **2.** a mammary gland.

breast abscess, an abscess of a mammary gland, usually during lactation or weaning.

breast augmentation, popular name for **augmentation mammoplasty.**

breast cancer, a malignant neoplastic disease of breast tissue, a common malignancy in women in the United States. The incidence increases with age from the third to the fifth decade and reaches a second peak at age 65. Risk factors include certain genetic abnormalities, a family history of breast cancer, nulliparity, exposure to ionizing radiation, early menarche, late menopause, obesity, diabetes, hypertension, chronic cystic disease of the breast, and, possibly, postmenopausal estrogen therapy. Women who are above 40 years of age when they bear their first child and individuals

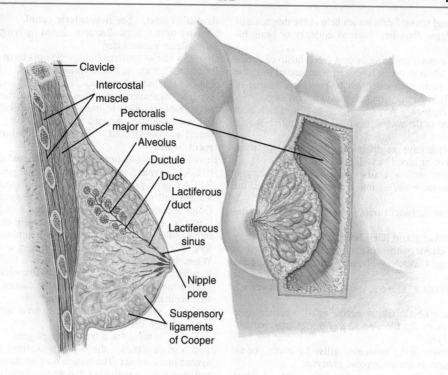

Breast (Seidel et al, 2003)

Breast abscess (Zitelli and Davis, 1997)

who have malignancies in other body sites also have an increased risk of development of breast cancer. Initial symptoms, detected in most cases by self-examination, include a small painless lump, thick or dimpled skin, or nipple retraction. As the lesion progresses, there may be nipple discharge, pain, ulceration, and enlarged axillary glands. The diagnosis may be established by a careful physical examination, mammography, and cytologic examination of tumor cells obtained by biopsy. Infiltrating ductal carcinomas are found in about 75% of cases, and infiltrating lobular, infiltrating medullary, colloid, comedo, or papillary carcinomas in the others. Tumors are more common in the left than in the right breast and in the upper and outer quadrant than in the other quadrants. Metastasis through the lymphatic system to axillary lymph nodes and to bone, lung, brain, and liver is common, but there is evidence that primary carcinomas of the

breast may exist in multiple sites and that tumor cells may enter the bloodstream directly without passing through lymph nodes. Surgical treatment may consist of a mastectomy or a lumpectomy, with dissection of axillary nodes. Postoperative radiotherapy, chemotherapy, or both are often prescribed. Chemotherapeutic agents frequently administered in various combinations are cyclophosphamide, methotrexate, 5-fluorouracil, phenylalanine mustard (L-PAM), thio-TEPA, doxorubicin, vincristine, methotrexate, and prednisone. The presence of estrogen receptors in breast tumors is considered an indication for hormonal manipulation such as the administration of antiestrogens. Implantation of a prosthesis after mastectomy is optional and does not appear to decrease survival probability. Reconstructive surgery is also an option. Fewer than 1% of breast cancers occur in men, but those with Klinefelter's syndrome are at much greater risk than other men. See also **lumpectomy, mastectomy, scirrhous carcinoma.**

■ OBSERVATIONS: Increasing numbers of breast cancers are found on mammogram. The most common presenting sign is a lump in the breast. About 50% of all lumps are found in the upper outer quadrant. Nipple discharge may also be present. A mass detected by breast self-examination, physical examination, or mammogram requires follow-up. Ultrasonography helps distinguish cysts from a solid mass. Definitive diagnosis is made by incisional, excisional, fine needle, or stereotactic core biopsy of the mass. Pain, tenderness, changes in breast shape, dimpling, and nipple retraction rarely occur until the disease reaches an advanced stage. Prognosis dims markedly as the number of involved lymph nodes increases. Pleural effusion, ascites, pathologic fracture, and spinal compression can occur with advanced disease.

■ INTERVENTIONS: The treatment of choice is resection of the lump with removal of varying amounts of surrounding healthy tissue, ranging from a margin of breast tissue to the entire breast, axillary lymph nodes, mammary lymphatic chain, and pectoral muscles. Adjunct systemic multidrug chemotherapy is used primarily for premenopausal node-positive women. Adjunct hormone therapy (estrogens, androgens, and progestins) is used primarily for postmenopausal node-positive or receptor-positive women. Antiestrogen therapy (Tamoxifen and Femara) is used as first line therapy; biological therapy with trastuzumab (Herceptin) is used in select patients for treatment of metastatic disease. Bone marrow/stem cell transplants are under investigation for advanced metastatic disease. Radiation may be used as an adjunct after surgery and for palliation in advanced disease.

■ NURSING CONSIDERATIONS: Nurses have responsibilities for patient care at all levels of the care continuum, from primary care and screening to acute and long-term follow through after diagnosis and medical treatment for breast cancer. Nurses play a large role in early detection and should educate and instruct women age 40 and older and women at increased risk (e.g., family history, genetic tendency, past breast cancer) to get an annual mammogram and clinical breast exam. Women under 40 should be encouraged to get a clinical breast exam every 3 years. All women should perform regular breast self-exams. Nurses work with women who are diagnosed with breast cancer to better understand and cope with treatment options. Acute care management is dictated in part by the treatment intervention. Physical care after surgery includes prevention of infection, incision site care, pain management, and prevention of loss of function or feeling on affected side. Management of radiation side effects, such as erythema, ulceration, edema, and peeling, are necessary. Chemotherapy and radiation protocols and side effects need to be reviewed. Emotional needs, such as fear over a cancer diagnosis, grieving over loss of a breast, and altered body image must be addressed. Counseling may be needed. Referrals can be made for recovery support groups. Referral may also be made for fitting and construction of a breast prostheses or surgical reconstruction of the breast. The need for long-term follow-up of physical and emotional sequelae is stressed.

Breast cancer: invasive ductal carcinoma
(Kumar, Cotran, and Robbins, 2003)

breast cancer genetic screening test (BRCA genetic testing), a blood test used to detect the presence of breast cancer genes, which indicate an increased susceptibility for development of breast cancer. One breast cancer gene also confers an increased susceptibility for ovarian cancer.

Breast cancer *(Swartz, 2002)*

breast examination[1], a process in which the breasts and their accessory structures are observed and palpated in assessing the presence of changes or abnormalities that could indicate malignant disease. See also **self-breast examination.**

■ METHOD: The breasts are observed with the patient sitting with her arms at her sides; sitting with her arms over her head, back straight, then leaning forward; and, finally, sitting upright as she contracts the pectoral muscles by placing hands on hips. The breasts are observed for symmetry of shape and size and for surface characteristics, including moles or nevi, hyperpigmentation, retraction or dimpling, edema, abnormal distribution of hair, focal vascularity, or lesions. With the patient still sitting, the axillary nodes and the supraclavicular and subclavicular areas are palpated. With the patient lying on her back, each breast is shifted medially, and the glandular area in each is palpated with the flat of the fingers of a hand in concentric circles or in a pattern like the spokes of a wheel, from the periphery inward. The areolar areas, the nipples, and the axillary tail of Spence in the upper outer quadrant extending toward the axilla are then palpated. The nipple is squeezed to check for discharge.

■ INTERVENTIONS: The patient should be taught to perform a self-breast examination and encouraged to do it monthly. The American Cancer Society recommends starting at about age 18. Premenopausal women should examine breasts approximately 1 week past the menstrual period, when breasts are less tender and less swollen. Postmenopausal women should choose a specific time each month, such as the first day of the month. Many women find it helpful to check their breasts every time they shower for the first few months after being taught the procedure to practice and to become very familiar with their own breasts.

■ OUTCOME CRITERIA: Early diagnosis greatly improves the rate of cure in cancer of the breast.

breast examination[2], a nursing intervention from the Nursing Interventions Classification (NIC) defined as inspection and palpation of the breasts and related areas. See also **Nursing Interventions Classification.**

breastfeeding [AS, **braest** + ME, *feden*], **1.** suckling or nursing, giving a baby milk from the breast. Breastfeeding encourages postpartum uterine involution and slows the nat-

Palpation of glandular area

Palpation of areolar area

Compression of nipple

Breast examination

ural return of the menses. **2.** taking milk from the breast. See also **breast milk, lactation.**

breastfeeding and human breastfeeding establishment: maternal, a nursing outcome from the Nursing Outcomes Classification (NOC) defined as maternal establishment of proper attachment of an infant to and sucking from the breast for nourishment during the first 2 to 3 weeks. See also **Nursing Outcomes Classification.**

breastfeeding assistance, a nursing intervention from the Nursing Interventions Classification (NIC) defined as preparing a new mother to breastfeed her infant. See also **Nursing Interventions Classification.**

breastfeeding, effective, a nursing diagnosis accepted by the Ninth National Conference on the Classification of Nursing Diagnoses. Effective breastfeeding is a state in which a mother-infant dyad/family exhibits adequate proficiency and satisfaction with the breastfeeding process.

■ DEFINING CHARACTERISTICS: The defining characteristics are the mother's ability to position the infant at the breast to promote a successful latch-on response, regular and sustained suckling/swallowing at the breast, infant content after feeding, appropriate infant weight patterns for age, effective mother-infant communication patterns, signs and/or symptoms of oxytocin release, adequate infant elimination patterns for age, eagerness of the infant to nurse, and maternal verbalization of satisfaction with the breastfeeding process.

■ RELATED FACTORS: Related factors include basic breastfeeding knowledge, normal breast structure, normal infant oral structure, infant gestational age greater than 34 weeks, support sources, and maternal confidence.

breastfeeding establishment: infant, a nursing outcome from the Nursing Outcomes Classification (NOC) defined as proper attachment of an infant to and sucking from the mother's breast for nourishment during the first 2 to 3 weeks. See also **Nursing Outcomes Classification.**

breastfeeding, ineffective, a nursing diagnosis accepted by the Eighth National Conference on the Classification of Nursing Diagnoses. Ineffective breastfeeding is a state in which a mother, infant, and/or family experiences dissatisfaction or difficulty with the breastfeeding process.

■ DEFINING CHARACTERISTICS: The major defining characteristic is the unsatisfactory breastfeeding process. Other characteristics include an actual or perceived inadequate milk supply,

no observable signs of oxytocin release, persistence of sore nipples beyond the infant's first week of life, and maternal reluctance to put the infant to breast as necessary. The infant may be unable to attach to the maternal nipple correctly or may resist latching on, with arching and crying at the breast. Within the first hour after breastfeeding the infant may exhibit fussiness or crying and be unresponsive to other comfort measures. There may also be observable signs of an inadequate infant intake, nonsustained suckling at the breast, suckling at only one breast per feeding, and nursing fewer than seven times in 24 hours.

■ RELATED FACTORS: Related factors in the diagnosis of ineffective breastfeeding are prematurity, infant anomaly, maternal breast anomaly, previous breast surgery, previous history of breastfeeding failure, supplemental feeding of the infant with an artificial nipple, poor infant sucking reflex, nonsupportive partner or family, knowledge deficit, and interruption in breastfeeding. See also **nursing diagnosis.**

breastfeeding, interrupted, a nursing diagnosis accepted by the Tenth National Conference on the Classification of Nursing Diagnoses. Interrupted breastfeeding is a break in the continuity of the breastfeeding process as a result of inability or inadvisability of putting the baby to the breast for feeding.

■ DEFINING CHARACTERISTICS: The major defining characteristic is insufficient nourishment by the infant at the breast for some or all feedings. Minor defining characteristics are a maternal desire to maintain lactation and provide her breast milk for her infant's nutritional needs, separation of mother and infant, and lack of knowledge about expression and storage of breast milk.

■ RELATED FACTORS: Related factors include maternal or infant illness, prematurity, maternal employment, contraindications to breastfeeding (e.g., drugs, true breast milk jaundice), or a need to wean the infant abruptly. See also **nursing diagnosis.**

breastfeeding maintenance, a nursing outcome from the Nursing Outcomes Classification (NOC) defined as continued nourishment of an infant through breastfeeding. See also **Nursing Outcomes Classification.**

breastfeeding: weaning, a nursing outcome from the Nursing Outcomes Classification (NOC) defined as process leading to the eventual discontinuation of breastfeeding. See also **Nursing Outcomes Classification.**

breast implant, the surgical placement of prosthetic material in a breast, either to increase the breast's size or for reconstruction after a mastectomy.

breast milk [AS, *braest + meoluc*], human milk. **nursing considerations:** The nurse should counsel mothers that it is easily digested, clean, and warm and that it confers some immunities (bronchiolitis and gastroenteritis are rare in breastfed babies). Infants fed breast milk are less likely to become obese and to have dental malocclusion. See also **breastfeeding.**

breast milk jaundice, jaundice and hyperbilirubinemia in breastfed infants that occur in the first weeks of life as a result of a metabolite in the mother's milk that inhibits the infant's ability to conjugate bilirubin to glucuronide for excretion. See also **hyperbilirubinemia of the newborn.**

■ OBSERVATIONS: Breast milk jaundice usually occurs after the fifth day of life and peaks toward the end of the second or third week. Serum bilirubin levels usually exceed 5 mg/100 ml but rarely reach dangerous levels of 20 mg/100 ml, at which point kernicterus may develop. The infant seems normal and healthy, but the skin, the whites of the eyes, and the serum are jaundiced (yellow).

■ INTERVENTIONS: If serum bilirubin exceeds acceptable levels, breastfeeding may be interrupted until they decrease to the normal range, usually a period of 1 to 3 days. During this interval the infant is bottle-fed with a supplemental formula and the mother uses a breast pump or manual device to maintain lactation without engorgement. Phototherapy may be used to accelerate excretion of bilirubin through the skin.

■ NURSING CONSIDERATIONS: The primary concerns of the nurse are to observe for signs of increasing jaundice, to monitor serum bilirubin levels, and usually to reassure the mother that her child is well and that the jaundice resolves slowly but completely in time.

breast pump, a mechanical or electronic device for withdrawing milk from the breast.

breast scintigraphy, a nuclear scan used to identify breast cancer in patients whose dense breast tissue precludes accurate evaluation by conventional mammography. The test is also used as a second-line imaging modality in patients with an indeterminate mammogram and in women with lumpy breasts.

breast self-examination. See **self-breast examination.**

breast shadows, artifacts caused by breast tissue that appear on chest radiographs of women. The shadows accentuate the underlying tissue and may cause the appearance of an interstitial disease process. Breast nipples may also appear on the radiograph as "coin lesions," requiring that a second radiograph with special markers attached to the nipples be made so the two films can be compared.

breast sonogram, an ultrasound test that is used primarily to determine if a mammographic abnormality or a palpable lump is a cyst (fluid-filled) or a solid tumor (benign or malignant). It is also used to examine symptomatic women who should not be exposed to mammographic radiation, such as pregnant women and women under the age of 25.

breast transillumination [AS, *braest* + L *trans,* through, *illuminare,* to light up], a method of examining the inner structures of the breast by directing light through the outer wall. See also **diaphanography.**

breath, the air inhaled and exhaled during ventilation of the lungs.

Breathalyzer /breth'əlī'zər/, trademark for a device that analyzes exhaled air. It is commonly used to test for blood alcohol levels; the test is based on the relationship between alcohol in the breath and alcohol in the blood circulating through the lungs. Also spelled **Breathalyser.**

breath-holding /breth-/ [AS, *braeth* + ME, *holden*], a form of voluntary apnea that is usually but not necessarily performed with a closed glottis. Although breath-holding may be prolonged for several minutes, it is invariably terminated either voluntarily or when the person or child loses consciousness.

breathing. See **respiration.**

breathing biofeedback, the monitoring of breathing rate, volume, rhythm, and location by sensors placed on the chest and abdomen, used in the treatment of asthma, hyperventilation, and anxiety. The feedback is displayed to the patient visually and is used by the patient to learn to breathe more slowly, deeply, and rhythmically using the abdominal muscles.

breathing cycle /brē'thing/, a ventilatory cycle consisting of an inspiration followed by the expiration of a volume of gas called the tidal volume. The duration or total cycle time of a breathing cycle is the breathing or ventilatory period. Also called **respiratory cycle.**

breathing frequency (f). See **respiration rate.**

breathing nomogram [AS, *braeth* + Gk, *nomos,* law, *gramma,* a record], a chart that presents scales of data for body weight, breathing frequency, and predicted basal tidal volume arranged so that one can find an unknown value on one scale by drawing a line that connects known values on the other two scales.

breathing pattern, ineffective, a nursing diagnosis accepted by the Fourth National Conference on the Classification of Nursing Diagnoses (revised 1998). An ineffective breathing pattern is a state in which inspiration and/or expiration do not provide adequate ventilation for the individual.

■ DEFINING CHARACTERISTICS: Defining characteristics are dyspnea, shortness of breath; respiratory rate (adults [14 years of age or more], 11 or 24; infants, 25 or 60; ages 1 to 4, 20 or 30; ages 5 to 14, 15 or 25); depth of breathing (adults, VT 500 mL at rest; infants, 6 to 8); timing ratio; nasal flaring (infants); use of accessory muscles; altered chest excursion; assumption of three-point position, pursed lip breathing, prolonged expiratory phases, increased anteroposterior diameter; orthopnea; decreased vital capacity; decreased minute ventilation; and decreased inspiratory/expiratory pressure.

■ RELATED FACTORS: Related factors are neuromuscular dysfunction, pain, musculoskeletal impairment, perception/cognitive impairment, anxiety, hyper/hypoventilation, bone deformity, pain, chest wall deformity, obesity, spinal cord injury, body position, neurological immaturity, respiratory muscle fatigue, and decreased energy/fatigue. See also **nursing diagnosis.**

breathing-related sleep disorder, any of several disorders characterized by sleep disruption caused by some sleep-related breathing problem, resulting in excessive sleepiness or insomnia; included are central sleep apnea, obstructive sleep apnea, and primary alveolar hypoventilation (Ondine's curse).

breathing tube. See **endotracheal tube, nasotracheal tube.**

breathing work, the energy required for breathing movements. It is the cumulative product of the instantaneous pressure developed by the respiratory muscles and the volume of air moved during a breathing cycle.

breathlessness. See **dyspnea.**

breath odor, an odor usually produced by substances or diseases in the lungs or mouth. Certain specific odors are associated with some diseases, such as diabetes, liver failure, uremia, or a lung abscess.

breath sound [AS, *braeth* + L, *sonus*], the sound of air passing in and out of the lungs as heard with a stethoscope. These breath sounds are normal if heard in normal beat ions. Vesicular, bronchovesicular, and bronchial breath sounds are normal. Decreased breath sounds may indicate an obstruction of an airway, collapse of a portion or all of a lung, thickening of the pleurae of the lungs, emphysema, or other chronic obstructive pulmonary disease. Also occur with frail clients who are not physically able to breathe deeply.

breath test, any of various tests in which a person's breath is analyzed for presence of something abnormal. Subgroups called the ^{13}C breath tests and ^{14}C breath tests involve administration of organic compounds labeled with carbon 13 (heavy carbon) or carbon 14 (radioactive carbon) and measuring the subsequent levels of labeled carbon dioxide in the patient's breath; the labeled compound may be found to be metabolized normally, too fast, or too slow in the GI tract.

breath tests, diagnostic tests for intestinal disorders such as bacterial overgrowth, ileal disease, lactase deficiency, and steatorrhea. Lactose malabsorption is treated by giving the patient 12.5 to 25.0 grams of lactose and measuring the amount of hydrogen excreted in the breath. If lactose absorption is impaired in the small intestine, colonic bacteria ferment the lactose, releasing hydrogen, which is excreted in

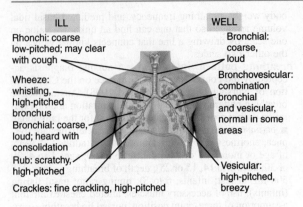

ILL	WELL
Rhonchi: coarse low-pitched; may clear with cough	Bronchial: coarse, loud
Wheeze: whistling, high-pitched bronchus	Bronchovesicular: combination bronchial and vesicular, normal in some areas
Bronchial: coarse, loud; heard with consolidation	
Rub: scratchy, high-pitched	Vesicular: high-pitched, breezy
Crackles: fine crackling, high-pitched	

Breath sounds in the ill and well patient
(Seidel et al, 2003)

Frank breech Full breech Single footling breech

Breech presentation *(McKinney et al, 2000)*

Brenner tumor *(Fletcher, 2000)*

the breath. Bacterial overgrowth is tested with ^{14}C-cholyl-glycine, which is normally absorbed by the ileum and re-cycled via the enterohepatic circulation. In cases of bacterial overgrowth the labeled glycine is removed by conjugation in the small intestine, absorbed, and metabolized, resulting in an increase of $^{14}CO_2$ in the breath.

Breckinridge, Mary (1881–1965), the American nurse who founded the Frontier Nursing Service in Kentucky to improve the obstetric care of women living in remote mountainous areas. The nurses in the service had training in midwifery and reached their patients on horseback and on foot, often encountering personal danger. The service began training midwives and stimulated the establishment of other midwifery schools.

breech birth [ME, *brech* + *burth*], parturition in which the infant emerges feet, knees, or buttocks first. Breech birth is often hazardous. The body may deliver easily, but the aftercoming head may become trapped by an incompletely dilated cervix because infants' heads are usually larger than their bodies. See also **assisted breech, breech presentation, complete breech, footling breech, frank breech, version and extraction.**

breech extraction [ME, *brech* + L, *ex*, out, *trahere*, to pull], an obstetric operation in which an infant being born feet or buttocks first is grasped before any part of the trunk is born and delivered by traction. Compare **assisted breech.**

breech presentation [ME, *brech* + L, *praesentare*, to show], intrauterine position of the fetus in which the buttocks or feet present. It occurs in approximately 3% of labors. Kinds of breech presentation are **complete breech, footling breech,** and **frank breech.** Compare **vertex presentation.** See also **breech birth.**

bregma /breg'mə/ [Gk, the front of the head], the junction of the coronal and sagittal sutures on the top of the skull. —**bregmatic,** *adj.*

bregmacardiac reflex /breg'məkär'dē·ək/ [Gk, *bregma,* front of the head], a phenomenon in which pressure on the anterior fontanel of an infant's skull causes the heart to slow.

bremsstrahlung radiation /brems'shträ'loong/ [Ger, braking radiation], a type of radiation produced by the interaction between electrons and the nuclei of target atoms.

Brenner tumor [Fritz Brenner, German pathologist, b. 1877], an uncommon benign ovarian neoplasm consisting of nests or cords of epithelial cells containing glycogen that are enclosed in fibrous connective tissue. The tumor may be solid or cystic and is sometimes difficult to distinguish from certain granulosa-theca cell neoplasms.

Brethine, trademark for a beta$_2$ receptor agonist agent (terbutaline sulfate).

bretylium tosylate /britil'ē·əm/, an antiarrhythmic agent.
■ INDICATION: It is prescribed in the treatment of selected life-threatening ventricular arrhythmias when other measures have not been effective.
■ CONTRAINDICATION: Known hypersensitivity to this drug prohibits its use.
■ ADVERSE EFFECTS: Among the more serious adverse reactions are hypotension, nausea and vomiting, anginal pain, and nasal stuffiness.

brevi- /brev'ē-/, prefix meaning "short": *brevicollis, breviradiate.*

Brevicon, trademark for a norethindrone-ethinyl estradiol oral contraceptive.

Brevital Sodium, trademark for a barbiturate (methohexital sodium).

brewer's yeast /broo'ərz/ [ME, *brewen,* to boil, *yest,* foam], a preparation containing the dried pulverized cells of a yeast, such as *Saccharomyces cerevisiae,* that is used as a leavening agent and as a dietary supplement. It is one of the best sources of the B complex vitamins and a rich source of many minerals and a high grade of protein.

Bricanyl, trademark for a beta$_2$ receptor agonist agent (terbutaline sulfate).

brick dust urine, a reddish discoloration signaling precipitated urates in acidic urine.

bridge. See **bridgework.**

bridge of Varolius. See **pons.**

bridgework, a fixed partial denture that is cemented permanently to abutment teeth. Also called **bridge.**

bridging [AS, *brycg*], **1.** a nursing technique of positioning a patient so that bony prominences are free of pressure on the mattress by using pads, bolsters of foam rubber, or pillows to distribute body weight over a larger surface. **2.** a nursing technique for supporting a part of the body, such as the testicles in treating orchitis, using a Bellevue bridge made of a towel or other material. **3.** a physical rehabilitation technique that strengthens abdominal and leg muscles. Reclining with knees bent, the patient plants the feet on a firm surface and lifts the buttocks off the surface.

Brief Psychiatric Rating Scale (BPRS), a rating scale for assessing psychopathology on the basis of a small number of items, usually 16 to 24, encompassing psychosis, depression, and anxiety symptoms.

brief psychotherapy, (in psychiatry) treatment directed to the active resolution of personality or behavioral problems rather than to the speculative analysis of the unconscious. It usually concentrates on a specific problem or symptom and is limited to a specified number of sessions with the therapist.

brief psychotic disorder, an episode of psychotic symptoms (incoherence, loosening of associations, delusions, hallucinations, disorganized or catatonic behavior) with sudden onset, lasting less than one month. If it occurs in response to a stressful life event, it may be called **brief reactive psychosis.**

brief reactive psychosis, a short episode, usually less than 2 weeks, of psychotic behavior that occurs in response to a significant psychosocial stressor.

brightness gain /brīt′nes/, the increase in illumination level of a radiograph produced by an image intensifier. It is calculated as the minification gain multiplied by the flux gain. The product is the ratio of the number of photons at the output phosphor to the number at the input phosphor.

Brill-Symmers disease. See **giant follicular lymphoma.**

Brill-Zinsser disease /bril′zin′sər/ [Nathan E. Brill, American physician, 1860–1925; Hans Zinsser, American bacteriologist, 1878–1940], a mild form of epidemic typhus that recurs in a person who appears to have completely recovered from a severe case of the disease years earlier. Some rickettsiae remain in the body after the symptoms of the disease abate, causing the recurrence of symptoms, especially when stress, illness, or malnutrition weakens the person. Treatment with antibiotics may eradicate the organism. See also **epidemic typhus, murine typhus, rickettsiosis, typhus.**

brim, 1. edge or margin. **2.** the edge of the upper border of the true pelvis, or the pelvic inlet. See also **pelvis.**

brim of true pelvic cavity. See **iliopectineal line.**

brimonidine /brĭ-mo′nĭ-dēn/, an alpha-adrenergic receptor agonist used as the tartrate salt in treatment of open-angle glaucoma and ocular hypertension. It is administered topically to the conjunctiva.

Brinnell hardness test [Johann A. Brinnell, Swedish engineer, 1849–1925], a means of determining the surface hardness of a material by measuring the resistance the material offers to the impact of a steel ball. The test result is recorded as the Brinnell hardness number (BHN); harder materials have higher BHNs. The Brinnell hardness test is commonly used to measure abrasion resistance in materials used in dental restorations, such as amalgams, cements, and porcelains. Compare Knoop hardness test.

brinzolamide /brin-zo′lah-mīd/, a carbonic anhydrase inhibitor used in treatment of open-angle glaucoma and ocular hypertension.

Briquet's syndrome. See **somatization disorder.**

Brissaud's dwarf /brisōz′/ [Edouard Brissaud, French physician, 1852–1909], a person affected with infantile myxedema in which short stature is associated with hypothyroidism.

Bristol Cancer Help Center (BCHC) diet, a stringent diet of raw and partly cooked vegetables with proteins from soy. It is claimed to enhance the quality of life and attitude toward illness in cancer patients.

British antilewisite. See **dimercaprol.**

British Medical Association (BMA), a national professional organization of physicians in the United Kingdom.

British Pharmacopoeia (BP), the official British reference work setting forth standards of strength and purity of medications and containing directions for their preparation to ensure that the same prescription written by different doctors and filled by different pharmacists will contain exactly the same ingredients in the same proportions. The first *British Pharmacopoeia* was published in 1864 by the General Medical Council; it superseded the *London Pharmacopoeia,* which had been published since 1618. See also **British Medical Association,** *United States Pharmacopeia* (USP).

British thermal unit (BTU), a unit of heat energy. The amount of thermal energy that must be absorbed by 1 lb of water to raise its temperature by 1° at 39.2° F. It is also equivalent to 1055 joules or 252 calories.

brittle bones. See **osteogenesis imperfecta.**

brittle diabetes, poorly controlled diabetes mellitus in which blood glucose levels are unstable. See also **type 1 diabetes mellitus.**

broach, an elongated, tapering dental instrument used in removing pulpal material.

broad beta disease, a familial type of hyperlipoproteinemia in which a lipoprotein, high in cholesterol and triglycerides, accumulates in the blood. The condition, which affects males in their twenties and females in their thirties and forties, is characterized by yellowish nodules (xanthomas) on the elbows and knees, peripheral vascular disease, and elevated serum cholesterol levels. Persons with this disease are at risk of development of early coronary disease. Therapy includes dietary measures to reduce weight and levels of serum lipids. Also called **dysbetalipoproteinemia, hyperlipidemia type III.** See also **hyperlipidemia, hyperlipoproteinemia.**

broad ligament [ME, *brood* + L, *ligare,* to tie], a folded sheet of peritoneum draped over the uterine tubes, the uterus, and the ovaries. It extends from the sides of the uterus to the sidewalls of the pelvis, dividing the pelvis from side to side and creating the vesicouterine fossa and pouch in front of the uterus and the rectouterine fossa and pouch behind it. Also called **ligamentum latum uteri.** See also **cardinal ligament.**

broad ligament of the liver [ME, *brod* + L, *ligare,* to bind; AS, *lifer*], a crescent-shaped fold of peritoneum attached to the lower surface of the diaphragm, connecting with the liver and the anterior abdominal wall. Also called **falciform ligament of the liver, ligamentum falciforme hepatis.**

broad-spectrum antibiotic, an antibiotic that is effective against a wide range of infectious microorganisms.

Broca's aphasia /brō′kəz/ [Pierre P. Broca, French neurologist, 1824–1880], a type of aphasia consisting of nonfluent speech, with a laconic and hesitant, telegraphic quality caused by a large left frontal lesion extending to the central sulcus. The patient's agrammatic speech is characterized by abundant nouns and verbs but few articles and prepositions, the resulting speech is economical but lacking in syntax.

Broca's area [Pierre P. Broca], an area involved in speech production situated on the inferior frontal gyrus of the brain. See also **aphasia, Broca's aphasia, motor speech areas, speech centers.**

Broca's fissure [Pierre P. Broca], a cleft or groove encircling Broca's area in the left frontal area of the brain.

Broca's plane [Pierre P. Broca], a plane that includes the tip of the interalveolar septum between the upper central incisors and the lowest point of the left and right occipital condyles.

Brödel's bloodless line, a longitudinal light-colored zone on the anterior surface of the kidney near the convex border, considered to be less vascularized than other areas because it is the border between two areas of arterial distribution.

Brodie's abscess [Benjamin Brodie, English surgeon, 1783–1862], a form of osteomyelitis consisting of an indolent staphylococcal infection of bone, usually in the metaphysis of a long bone of a child, characterized by a necrotic cavity surrounded by dense granulation tissue. See also **osteomyelitis.** Also called **circumscribed abscess of bone.**

Brodmann's areas /brod'manz, brŏt'mons/ [Korbinian Brodmann, German anatomist, 1868–1918], the 47 different areas of the cerebral cortex that are associated with specific neurologic functions and distinguished by different cellular components. They control movements of the lips and vocal cords as well as motor speech. Compare **motor area.** See also **cerebral cortex.**

broken cell preparation. See **homogenate.**

brom, abbreviation for a *bromide anion.*

brom-, bromo-, prefix meaning a compound containing bromine or meaning "odor, stench": *bromhidrosis, bromoacetophenon.*

bromazepam /bro-maz'ĕ-pam/, a benzodiazepine used as an antianxiety agent and as a sedative and hypnotic. It is administered orally.

bromelain /brō'məlān/, any of several enzymes that catalyze cleavage of proteins on the carboxyl side of alanine, glycine, lysine, and tyrosine bonds. Differing forms are derived from the fruit (fruit bromelain) and stem (stem bromelain) of the pineapple plant. The enzyme is administered orally as an anti-inflammatory agent (especially to relieve swelling in the nasal and paranasal sinuses) and is also used in immunology to render red cells agglutinable by incomplete antibody.

Bromfed, trademark for a fixed-combination decongestant containing brompheniramine maleate and pseudoephedrine maleate.

bromhidrosis /brō'midrō'sis/ [Gk, *bromos,* stench, *hidros,* sweat], an abnormal condition in which the apocrine sweat has an unpleasant odor. The odor is usually caused by bacterial decomposition of perspiration on the skin. Treatment includes frequent bathing, changing of socks and underclothes, and use of deodorants, antibacterial soaps, and dusting powders. Also called **body odor.**

bromide /brō'mīd/ [Gk, *bromos,* stench], an anion of bromine. Bromide salts, once widely prescribed as sedatives, are now seldom used for that purpose because they may cause serious mental disturbances as side effects.

bromide poisoning, an adverse reaction to ingested bromide. Symptoms include nausea, vomiting, an acnelike rash, slurred speech, ataxia, psychotic behavior, and coma.

bromine (Br) /brō'mēn/, a corrosive, toxic red-brown liquid element of the halogen group. Its atomic number is 35; its atomic mass is 79.904. It exists naturally as a diatomic molecule, Br_2. Bromine is used in industry, in photography, in the manufacture of organic chemicals and fuels, and in medications. Bromine gives off a red vapor that is extremely irritating to the eyes and the respiratory tract. Liquid bromine causes serious skin burns. Compounds of bromine have been used as sedatives, hypnotics, and analgesics and are still used in some nonprescription, over-the-counter preparations. Prolonged use of these products may cause brominism, a toxic condition characterized by acneiform eruptions, headache, loss of libido, drowsiness, and fatigue. See also **bromide.**

bromo-. See **brom-.**

bromocriptine mesylate /brō'mōkrip'tēn/, a dopamine receptor agonist.

■ INDICATIONS: It is prescribed for the treatment of amenorrhea and galactorrhea associated with hyperprolactinemia, female infertility, and Parkinson's disease.

■ CONTRAINDICATIONS: Sensitivity to any ergot alkaloid prohibits its use. The drug was disqualified for use in suppressing postpartum lactation by the FDA in 1994 because of a previously unrecognized increase in intracranial hemorrhages.

■ ADVERSE EFFECTS: Among the more severe adverse reactions are palpitations, hypotension, bradycardia, hallucinations, syncope, nausea, ataxia, dyspnea, dysphagia, and confusion.

bromoderma /brō'mōdur'mə/ [Gk, *bromos,* stench, *derma* skin], an acneiform, bullous, or nodular skin rash, occurring as a hypersensitivity reaction to ingested bromides.

brompheniramine maleate /brom'fənir'əmin/, an antihistamine.

■ INDICATIONS: It is prescribed in the treatment of allergic reactions, including rhinitis, skin reactions, and itching.

■ CONTRAINDICATIONS: Asthma or known hypersensitivity to this drug prohibits its use. It is not given to newborns, lactating mothers, or other people for whom anticholinergic medications are contraindicated.

■ ADVERSE EFFECTS: Drowsiness, skin rash, hypersensitivity reactions, dry mouth, and tachycardia commonly occur.

Brompton's cocktail, an analgesic solution containing alcohol, morphine or heroin, and, in some cases, a phenothiazine. Formulations vary, and recently cocaine has generally been eliminated from the mixture. The cocktail is administered in the control of pain in the terminally ill patient. Given frequently at the lowest effective dose, it may relieve pain for many months. It was developed at the Brompton Hospital in England. Also called **Brompton's mixture.**

bronch-, broncho-, combining form meaning "bronchus": *bronchiectasis, bronchodilation.*

bronch(o)-, prefix meaning relationship to a bronchus. See also **bronchi(o)-.**

bronchi(o)-, prefix meaning relationship to a bronchus. See also **bronch(o)-.**

bronchial /brong'kē-əl/ [Gk, *bronchos,* windpipe], pertaining to the bronchi or bronchioles.

bronchial asthma. See **asthma.**

bronchial atresia, atresia of a lobar or segmental bronchus, usually in the left upper lobe; the affected lung segment is often hyperinflated because of leakage of air through the alveolar pores.

bronchial breath sound [Gk, *bronchos,* windpipe], a normal sound heard with a stethoscope over the main airways of the lungs, especially the trachea. Expiration and inspiration produce noise of equal loudness and duration, sounding like blowing through a hollow tube. The expiratory sound is heard during the greater part of expiration, whereas the inspiratory sound stops abruptly at the height of inspiration, with a pause before the sound of expiration is heard. Also called **tracheal breath sound.**

bronchial cast, a cylindrical solid or semisolid plug that blocks a bronchus and is sometimes expectorated.

bronchial challenge, bronchial challenge test, a challenge test in which a nonspecific agent such as histamine or methacholine is applied to the bronchi and they are assessed for a bronchoconstriction reaction. Also called **bronchial provocation.** See **inhalational challenge.**

bronchial cough, a cough associated with bronchiectasis and heard in early stages as hacking and irritating, becoming looser in later stages.

bronchial drainage. See **postural drainage.**

bronchial fremitus, a vibration that can be palpated or auscultated on the chest wall over a bronchus. It results from congestion by secretions that rattle as air passes during respiration. See also **fremitus.**

bronchial hyperreactivity [Gk, *bronchos* + *hyper,* excess; L, *re,* again, *agere,* to act], an abnormal respiratory condition characterized by reflex bronchospasm in response to histamine or a cholinergic drug, such as methacholine. It is a universal feature of asthma and is used in the differential diagnosis of asthma and heart disease.

bronchial murmur, a murmur heard as a blowing sound, caused by air flowing in and out of the bronchial tubes.

bronchial pneumonia. See **bronchopneumonia.**

bronchial provocation. See **bronchial challenge.**

bronchial secretion, a substance produced in the bronchial tree that consists of mucus secreted by the goblet cells and mucous glands of the bronchi, protein salts released from disintegrating cells, plasma fluid, and proteins, including fibrinogen, that have escaped from pulmonary capillaries.

bronchial spasm. See **bronchospasm.**

bronchial toilet, special care that is given to patients with tracheostomies and respiratory disorders, including stimulation of coughing, deep breathing, and suctioning of the respiratory tract with a tracheobronchial aspiration pump.

bronchial tree, an anatomic complex of the trachea and bronchi. The bronchi branch from the trachea. The right bronchus is wider and shorter than the left bronchus and branches into three secondary bronchi, one passing to each of the three lobes of the right lung. The left bronchus is smaller in diameter and about twice as long as the right bronchus. It branches into the secondary bronchi for the inferior and the superior lobes of the left lung. The bronchus is sometimes described as a **bronchial tube.**

bronchial tube. See **bronchus.**

bronchial washing [Gk, *bronchos,* windpipe; ME, *wasshen,* to wash], irrigation of the bronchi and bronchioles performed during bronchoscopy to cleanse the tubes and to collect specimens for laboratory examination.

bronchiectasis /brong′kē·ek′təsis/ [Gk, *bronchos* + *ektasis,* stretching], an abnormal condition of the bronchial tree characterized by irreversible dilation and destruction of the bronchial walls. The condition is sometimes congenital but is more often a result of bronchial infection or of obstruction by a tumor or an aspirated foreign body. Symptoms include a constant cough producing copious purulent sputum, hemoptysis, chronic sinusitis, clubbing of fingers, and persistent moist, coarse crackles. Some of the complications of bronchiectasis are pneumonia, lung abscess, empyema, brain abscess, and amyloidosis. Treatment includes frequent postural drainage, expectorants, antibiotics, and, rarely, surgical resection of the affected part of the lungs.

■ OBSERVATIONS: The individual is often asymptomatic early in the disease. A chronic cough with sputum production is the most common presenting sign. Hemoptysis, recurrent pneumonia, dyspnea, wheezing, and fatigue are also frequently seen. Fever, night sweats, weight loss, fetid breath, and hemoptysis may also be present. Moist crackles in lung bases may be heard on auscultation. Sputum appears purulent and foamy with sediment and has a large number of WBCs. Sputum cultures and gram stain are used to identify microorganisms. Chest x-rays reveal increased markings, honeycombing, and tram tracking. Pulmonary function studies show a decrease in vital capacity and expiratory flow. CT scans are used to detect cystic lesions and rule out neoplastic obstruction. Bronchography may be used when surgery is contemplated to visualize bronchiectatic areas. Clubbed fingers, pulmonary hypertension, right ventricular failure, and cor pulmonale are complications associated with long-standing disease.

■ INTERVENTIONS: Acute treatment includes medications, such as mucolytics to clear secretions; antibiotics to treat bacterial infection; and bronchodilators to reduce dyspnea. Chest physiotherapy, with postural drainage, is used to clear secretions. Adequate hydration and a vaporizer help liquefy secretions. Supplemental oxygen is administered for hypoxemia. Bronchial resection is used to treat confined disease, which is unresponsive to conservative therapy.

■ NURSING CONSIDERATIONS: The focus of nursing care during acute episodes is to promote airway clearance and effective breathing patterns through respiratory monitoring, cough enhancement, anxiety reduction, and rest. Preventive and chronic care focuses on avoidance of air pollution and contact with individuals with respiratory infections; prompt identification and treatment of respiratory infection; maintenance of adequate nutrition and hydration; smoking cessation as applicable; and use of flu and pneumonia vaccines for prophylaxis.

Bronchiectasis *(Wilson and Giddens, 2001)*

bronchioalveolar adenocarcinoma, bronchioalveolar carcinoma. See **bronchioloalveolar carcinoma.**

bronchiolar. See **bronchiole.**

bronchiolar adenocarcinoma. See **bronchioloalveolar carcinoma.**

bronchiolar carcinoma. See **alveolar cell carcinoma.**

bronchiolar collapse /brong′kyələr/ [L, *bronchiolus,* little windpipe, *conlabi,* to fall], a condition in which bronchioles, which are pliable and lack cartilaginous support, become compressed by surrounding structures in the absence of inflowing air needed to keep them inflated. The condition occurs in disorders such as emphysema, cystic fibrosis, and bronchiectasis.

bronchiole /brong′kē·ōl/ [L, *bronchiolus,* little windpipe], a small airway of the respiratory system extending from the bronchi into the lobes of the lung. There are two divisions of bronchioles: The terminal bronchioles passively conduct inspired air from the bronchi to the respiratory bronchioles and expired air from the respiratory bronchioles to the bronchi. The respiratory bronchioles function similarly, allowing the exchange of air and waste gases between the alveolar ducts and the terminal bronchioles. —**bronchiolar** /brongkē′ələr/, *adj.*

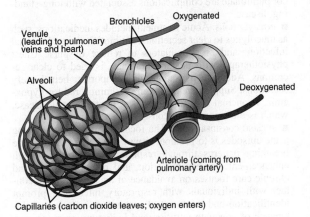

Bronchioles *(Chabner, 2004)*

bronchiolitis /brong′kē·ōlī′tis/ [L, *bronchiolus,* little windpipe; Gk, *itis,* inflammation], an acute viral infection of the lower respiratory tract that occurs primarily in infants less than 18 months of age. It is characterized by expiratory wheezing, respiratory distress, inflammation, and obstruction at the level of the bronchioles. The most common causative agents are the respiratory syncytial viruses (RSVs) and the parainfluenza viruses. *Mycoplasma pneumoniae,* rhinoviruses, enteroviruses, and measles virus are less common causative agents. Transmission occurs by infection with airborne particles or by contact with infected secretions. The diagnosis consists of evidence of hyperinflation of the lungs through percussion or chest x-ray.

■ OBSERVATIONS: The condition typically begins as an upper respiratory tract infection with serous nasal discharge and often with low-grade fever. Increasing respiratory distress follows, characterized by tachypnea, tachycardia, intercostal and subcostal retractions, a paroxysmal cough, an expiratory wheeze, and often an elevated temperature. The chest may appear barrel-shaped; x-ray films show hyperinflated lungs and a depressed diaphragm. Respiration becomes more shallow, causing increased alveolar oxygen tension and leading to respiratory acidosis. Complete obstruction and absorption of trapped air may lead to atelectasis and respiratory failure. Blood gas determinations indicate the degree of carbon dioxide retention.

■ INTERVENTIONS: Routine treatment includes administering humidity and oxygen via a mist tent, vaporizer, or Croupette, generally combined with oxygen; ensuring an adequate fluid intake, usually given intravenously because of tachypnea, weakness, and fatigue; suctioning the airways to remove secretions; and promoting rest. Endotracheal intubation is indicated when carbon dioxide retention occurs, when bronchial secretions do not loosen and clear, or when oxygen therapy does not alleviate hypoxia. Such medications as an-

tibiotics, bronchodilators, corticosteroids, cough suppressants, and expectorants are not routinely used. Ribovarin may be used when RSV is the causative agent. Sedatives are contraindicated because of their suppressant effect on the respiratory tract. The infection typically runs its course in 7 to 10 days, with good prognosis. A major complication is bacterial infection, most commonly after prolonged use of a mist tent. The disorder is often confused with asthma. A family history of allergy, the presence of other allergic manifestations, and improvement with epinephrine injection are usually indicative of asthma, not bronchiolitis. Cystic fibrosis, pertussis, the bronchopneumonias, and foreign body obstruction of the trachea are other disorders that may be confused with bronchiolitis.

■ NURSING CONSIDERATIONS: The focus of nursing care is to promote rest and to conserve the child's energy by reducing anxiety and apprehension; to increase the ease of breathing with humidity and oxygen as needed; to aid in changing position for comfort; and to induce drainage of secretions or to suction when necessary. Fever is usually controlled by the cool atmosphere of the mist tent and by administration of antipyretics as needed. Frequent changing of clothing and bed linen is often necessary in a mist environment to reduce chilling. Vital signs and chest and breath sounds are continuously monitored to detect early signs of respiratory distress.

bronchiolitis obliterans, a form of bronchiolitis in which the exudate is not expectorated but becomes organized and obliterates the bronchial tubes, causing collapse of the affected part of the lungs.

bronchioloalveolar carcinoma /brong′kē·ō′lō·al·vē′ə·lər/, a less common variant of adenocarcinoma of the lung, with columnar to cuboidal epithelial cells lining the alveolar septa and projecting into alveolar spaces in branching papillary formations. Also called **alveolar adenocarcinoma, alveolar carcinoma, alveolar cell carcinoma, bronchioalveolar adenocarcinoma, bronchiolar adenocarcinoma, bronchiolar carcinoma, bronchoalveolar adenocarcinoma, bronchoalveolar carcinoma.**

bronchiospasm. See **bronchospasm.**

bronchitis /brongkī′tis/ [Gk, *bronchos,* windpipe, *itis,* inflammation], acute or chronic inflammation of the mucous membranes of the tracheobronchial tree. **Acute bronchitis** is characterized by a productive cough, fever, hypertrophy of mucus-secreting structures, and back pain. Caused by the spread of upper respiratory viral or sometimes bacterial infections to the bronchi, it is often observed with or after childhood infections, such as measles, whooping cough, diphtheria, and typhoid fever. Treatment includes bed rest, antipyretics, expectorants, and appropriate antibiotic therapy. See also **chronic bronchitis, chronic obstructive pulmonary disease, respiratory syncytial virus.**

bronchoalveolar /-alvē′ələr/ [Gk, *bronchos,* windpipe; L, *alveolus,* little hollow], pertaining to the terminal air sacs at the ends of the bronchioles.

bronchoalveolar adenocarcinoma. See **bronchioloalveolar carcinoma.**

bronchoalveolar carcinoma (BAC), a peripheral well-differentiated neoplasm that spreads locally through the air spaces of the alveoli. A variant of adenocarcinoma, BAC constitutes about 5% of all lung cancers.

bronchoalveolar lavage (BAL), a diagnostic procedure in which small amounts of physiologic solution are injected through a fiberoptic bronchoscope into a specific area of the lung, while the rest of the lung is sequestered by an inflated balloon. The fluid is then aspirated and inspected for pathogens, malignant cells, and mineral bodies.

Chronic bronchitis (Thibodeau and Patton, 2003)

Bronchogenic carcinoma (Kumar, Cotran, and Robbins, 2003)

bronchoaortic constriction, thoracic constriction of esophagus.

bronchoconstriction [Gk, *bronchos,* windpipe; L, *constringere,* to draw tight], a narrowing of the lumen of the bronchi, restricting airflow to and from the lungs.

bronchodilation /-dil′ətā′shən/ [Gk, *bronchos,* windpipe; L, *dilatare,* to widen], a widening of the lumen of the bronchi, allowing increased airflow to and from the lungs.

bronchodilator /-dilā′tər/, a substance, especially a drug, that relaxes contractions of the smooth muscle of the bronchioles to improve ventilation to the lungs. Pharmacologic bronchodilators are prescribed to improve aeration in asthma, bronchiectasis, bronchitis, and emphysema. Commonly used bronchodilators include albuterol, terbutaline, and various derivatives and combinations of these drugs. The adverse effects vary, depending on the particular class of the bronchodilating drug. Bronchodilators are given with caution to people with impaired cardiac function. Nervousness, irritability, gastritis, or heart palpitations may occur.

bronchofibroscopy, the visual examination of the tracheobronchial tree through a fiberoptic bronchoscope. It is also used for diagnosing/treating hemoptysis. See also **fiberoptic bronchoscopy.**

bronchogenic /-jen′ik/ [Gk, *bronchos* + *genein,* to produce], originating in the bronchi.

bronchogenic adenocarcinoma, the more common type of adenocarcinoma of the lung, as distinguished from the type called **bronchioloalveolar carcinoma.**

bronchogenic carcinoma, one of the more than 90% of malignant lung tumors that originate in bronchi. Lesions, usually resulting from cigarette smoking, may cause coughing and wheezing, fatigue, chest tightness, and aching joints. In the late stages, bloody sputum, clubbing of the fingers, weight loss, and pleural effusion may be present. Diagnosis is made by bronchoscopy, sputum cytologic examination, lymph node biopsy, radioisotope scanning procedures, or exploratory surgery. Surgery is the most effective treatment, but well over 50% of cases are unresectable when first detected. Palliative treatment includes radiotherapy and chemotherapy.

bronchogenic cyst, a cyst that develops in the lungs or mediastinum. It may be asymptomatic or cause cough, stri-

dor, wheezing, or dyspnea. It may also become infected or malignant, requiring surgical removal.

bronchogram /brong′kō·gram/ [Gk, *bronchos,* windpipe + *gramma,* something drawn or written], the radiogram obtained by bronchography.

bronchography /brongkog′rəfē/, an x-ray examination of the bronchi after they have been coated with a radiopaque substance.

broncholithiasis /-lithī′əsis/, inflammation of the bronchi caused by an accumulation of hard concretions or stones on their lining.

bronchomotor tone, the state of contraction or relaxation of the smooth muscle in the bronchial walls that regulates the caliber of the airways.

bronchophony /brongkof′ənē/ [Gk, *bronchos* + *phone,* voice], an increase in the intensity and clarity of **vocal resonance** that may result from an increase in lung tissue density, such as in the consolidation of pneumonia. Assessed by having patient repeat a phrase such as 99 during auscultation.

bronchopleural fistula /-ploor′əl/, an abnormal passageway between a bronchus and the pleural cavity.

bronchopneumonia [Gk, *bronchos* + *pneumon,* lung], an acute inflammation of the lungs and bronchioles, characterized by chills, fever, high pulse and respiratory rates, bronchial breathing, cough with purulent bloody sputum, severe chest pain, and abdominal distension. The disease is usually a result of the spread of infection from the upper to the lower respiratory tract, most common caused by the bacterium *Mycoplasma pneumoniae, Staphylococcus pyogenes,* or *Streptococcus pneumoniae.* Atypical forms of bronchopneumonia may occur in viral and rickettsial infections. The most common cause in infancy is the respiratory syncytial virus. Bronchopneumonia may lead to pleural effusion, empyema, lung abscess, peripheral thrombophlebitis, respiratory failure, congestive heart failure, and jaundice. Treatment includes administration of an antibiotic, oxygen therapy, supportive measures to keep the bronchi clear of secretions, and relief of pleural pain. Also called **bronchial pneumonia, catarrhal pneumonia.** Compare **aspiration pneumonia, eosinophilic pneumonia, interstitial pneumonia.** See also **lobar pneumonia, respiratory syncytial virus.**

bronchoprovocation inhalation test, a pulmonary function test performed on patients with a history of asthma who have normal pulmonary function at rest. In a specific test, the patient inhales a particular antigen while the forced expira-

Bronchopneumonia (Kumar, Abbas, and Fausto, 2005)

Fiberoptic bronchoscope (Courtesy Olympus America)

tory volume (FEV) is measured. In a nonspecific test, the patient inhales a substance such as histamine periodically at increasing concentrations while the FEV is measured.

bronchopulmonary /-pul′mōner′ē/ [Gk, *bronchos* + L, *pulmonis*, lung],   pertaining to the bronchi and the lungs.

bronchopulmonary dysplasia (BPD) /-pōōl′məner′ē/,   a chronic respiratory disorder characterized by scarring of lung tissue, thickened pulmonary arterial walls, and mismatch between lung ventilation and perfusion. It often occurs in infants who have been dependent on long-term artificial ventilation.

bronchopulmonary hygiene,   the care and cleanliness of the respiratory tract and of ventilatory/respiratory therapy. Hygienic care may include providing assistance with postural drainage and controlled coughing techniques, percussion, vibration, and rib shaking. Respiratory care equipment is a potential source and reservoir of infectious organisms and must be cleaned and sterilized periodically.

bronchopulmonary lavage [Gk, *bronchos,* windpipe; L, *pulmonis,* lung; Fr, *lavage,* washing out],   the irrigation or washing out of the bronchi and bronchioles to remove pulmonary secretions.

bronchoscope /brong′kəskōp′/,   a curved, flexible tube for visual examination of the bronchi. It contains fibers that carry light down the tube and project an enlarged image up the tube to the viewer. The bronchoscope is used to examine the bronchi, to secure a specimen for biopsy or culture, or to aspirate secretions or a foreign body from the respiratory tract. See also **fiberoptic bronchoscopy. —bronchoscopic,** *adj.*

bronchoscopy /brongkos′kəpē/,   the visual examination of the tracheobronchial tree, using the standard rigid, tubular metal bronchoscope or the narrower, flexible fiberoptic bronchoscope. The procedure also may be used for suctioning, for obtaining a biopsy specimen and fluid or sputum for examination, for removing foreign bodies, and for diagnosing such conditions as localized atelectasis, bronchial obstruction, lung abscess, and tracheal extubation. See also **bronchoscope.**

bronchospasm /-spaz′əm/,   an excessive and prolonged

Broncoscopy (Elkin, Perry, and Potter, 2004)

contraction of the smooth muscle of the bronchi and bronchioles, resulting in an acute narrowing and obstruction of the respiratory airway. The contractions may be localized or general and may be caused by irritation or injury to the respiratory mucosa, infections, or allergies. A cough with generalized wheezing usually indicates the condition. Bronchospasm is a chief characteristic of asthma and bronchitis. Treatment includes the use of active bronchodilators, catecholamines, corticosteroids, or methylxanthines and preventive drugs such as cromolyn sodium. Also called **bronchial spasm, bronchiospasm.** See also **asthma, bronchitis.**

bronchospirometry /-spīrom′ətrē/, a technique for the study of the ventilation and gas exchange of each lung separately by the introduction of a catheter into either the left or the right mainstem bronchus. A double-lumen tube permits simultaneous but separate sampling of the gas from both lungs.

bronchotomogram /-tom′əgram/, an image of the respiratory system from the trachea to the lower bronchi produced by tomography. The procedure is used to detect tumors or other causes of obstruction of the respiratory tract.

bronchotracheal. See **tracheobronchial.**

bronchovesicular /-vesik′yələr/, pertaining to the bronchi, bronchioles, and alveoli.

bronchovesicular sounds [Gk, *bronchos,* windpipe; L, *vesicula,* small bladder, *sonus,* sound], one of three normal breath sounds that occur between the sounds of the bronchial tubes and those of the alveoli, or a combination of the two sounds.

bronchus /brong′kəs/, *pl.* **bronchi** /-kī/ [L; Gk, *bronchos,* windpipe], any one of several large air passages in the lungs through which pass inhaled air and exhaled air. Each bronchus has a wall consisting of three layers. The outermost is made of dense fibrous tissue, reinforced with cartilage. The middle layer is a network of smooth muscle. The innermost layer consists of ciliated mucous membrane. Kinds of bronchi are **lobar bronchus (secondary bronchus), primary bronchus,** and **segmental bronchus (tertiary bronchus).** Also called **bronchial tube.** See also **bronchiole.** —**bronchial,** *adj.*

Bronkodyl, trademark for a smooth muscle relaxant (theophylline).

Bronkosol, trademark for a bronchodilator (isoetharine hydrochloride).

Brönsted acid [Johannes N. Bronsted, Danish physical chemist, 1879–1947], a molecule or an ion that acts as a hydrogen ion donor.

Brönsted base [Johannes N. Bronsted], a molecule or an ion that acts as a hydrogen ion acceptor.

brontophobia. See **tonitrophobia.**

bronze diabetes. See **exogenous hemochromatosis.**

broth, **1.** a fluid culture medium, such as a solution of lactose or thioglycollate, used to support the growth of bacteria for laboratory analysis. **2.** a beverage or other clear fluid made with meat extract and water, such as chicken bouillon.

brow, the forehead, particularly the eyebrow or ridge above the eye.

brow lift, forehead lift. It is the removal or alteration of muscles and tissues of forehead to raise the eyebrows and minimize frown lines. See also **blepharoplasty.**

brown fat [ME, *broun* + AS, *faett,* filled], a type of fat present in newborns and rarely found in adults. Brown fat is a unique source of heat energy for the infant because it has greater thermogenic activity than ordinary fat. Brown fat deposits occur around the kidneys, neck, and upper chest.

brownian motion /brou′nyən/ [Robert Brown, Scottish botanist, 1773–1858], a random movement of microscopic particles suspended in a liquid or gas, such as the continuing erratic behavior of dust particles in still water. The movement is produced by the natural kinetic activity of molecules of the fluid that strike the foreign particles. Also called brownian movement.

brownian movement. See **brownian motion.**

brown recluse spider, a small poisonous arachnid, *Loxosceles reclusa,* also known as the brown or violin spider, found in both North and South America. The bite of the brown or violin spider, *Loxosceles reclusa,* produces a characteristic necrotic lesion. The venom from its bite usually creates a blister surrounded by concentric white and red circles. This so-called bull's-eye appearance is helpful in distinguishing it from other spider bites. There is little or no initial pain, but localized pain develops in about an hour. The patient may experience systemic symptoms; nausea, fever, and chills are common, but the reaction is usually self-limited. Immediate treatment includes keeping the victim quiet and immobilizing the bite area at the level of the heart. A bleb forms, sometimes in a target or bull's-eye pattern. The blood-filled bleb increases in size and eventually ruptures, leaving a black scar. Antivenin is not available in the United States.

Brown recluse spider
(Auerbach, 2001/courtesy Indiana University Medical Center)

Brown recluse spider bite after 48 hours
(Auerbach, 2001)

Brown-Séquard's syndrome /broun′sākärz′/ [Charles E. Brown-Séquard, French physiologist, 1817–1894], a traumatic neurologic disorder resulting from compression or transaction of one side of the spinal cord, above the tenth thoracic vertebrae, characterized by spastic paralysis and loss of postural sense (proprioception) on the body's injured side, and loss of the senses of pain and heat on the other side of the body.

Brown-Séquard's treatment. See **organotherapy.**

brown spider. See **brown recluse spider.**

brow presentation, an obstetric situation in which the brow, or forehead, of the fetus is the first part of the body to enter the birth canal. Because the diameter of the fetal head at this angle may be greater than that of the mother's pelvic outlet, a cesarean section may be recommended. However, the fetus usually converts to a face presentation.

Brucella abortus. See **abortus fever.**

brucellosis /broo'səlō'sis/ [David Bruce, English pathologist, 1855–1931], a disease caused by any of several species of the gram-negative coccobacillus *Brucella*. Brucellosis is most prevalent in rural areas among farmers, veterinarians, meat packers, slaughterhouse workers, and livestock producers. Laboratory workers are also at risk. It is primarily a disease of animals (including cattle, pigs, sheep, camels, goats, and dogs); humans usually acquire it by ingestion of contaminated milk or milk products or raw meat or marrow, through a break in the skin, contact with an infected animal or through inhalation of dust from contaminated soil. It is characterized by fever, chills, sweating, malaise, and weakness. The fever often occurs in waves, rising in the evening and subsiding during the day, at intervals separated by periods of remission. Other signs and symptoms may include anorexia and weight loss, headache, muscle and joint pain, and an enlarged spleen, and orchiepididymitis in young men. In some victims the disease is acute; more often it is chronic, recurring over a period of months or years. Although brucellosis itself is rarely fatal, treatment is important because serious complications such as pneumonia, endocarditis, meningitis, and encephalitis can develop. Tetracycline plus streptomycin is the treatment of choice; bed rest is also important. A vaccine is available outside the United States. This organism is considered a potential agent of bioterrorism due to its low infectious dose (10-100 organisms) and method of infection by way of aerosol, allowing distribution over a large area. Also called **Cyprus fever, dust fever, Gibraltar fever, Malta fever, Mediterranean fever, rock fever, undulant fever.** See also **abortus fever.**

Bruch's disease. See **Marseilles fever.**

Brudzinski's sign /broodzin'skēz/ [Josef Brudzinski, Polish physician, 1874–1917], an involuntary flexion of the arm, hip, and knee when the neck is passively flexed. It occurs in patients with meningitis.

Elicitation of Brudzinski's sign
(Barkauskas, Baumann, and Darling-Fisher, 2002)

Brueghel's syndrome. See **Meige's syndrome** (def. 1).

Brugia /bruj'ə/ [S.L. Brug, Dutch parasitologist in Indonesia, 1879–1946], a genus of nematodes of the superfamily Filarioidea that parasitize humans and other mammals. See also **filariasis.**

bruise. See **contusion, ecchymosis.**

bruit /broo'ē/ [Fr, noise], an abnormal blowing or swishing sound or murmur heard while auscultating a carotid artery,

organ, or gland, such as the liver or thyroid, and resulting from blood flowing through a narrow or partially occluded artery. The specific character of the bruit, its location, and the time of its occurrence in a cycle of other sounds are all of diagnostic importance.

Brunnstrom hemiplegia classification, an evaluation procedure that assesses muscle tone and voluntary control of movement patterns in a stroke patient. Results indicate the patient's progress through stages of recovery.

brush biopsy, the use of a catheter with bristles that is inserted into the body to collect cells from tissues.

brush border, microvilli on the free surfaces of certain epithelial cells, particularly the absorptive surfaces of the intestine and the proximal convoluted tubules of the kidney.

Brushfield's spots [Thomas Brushfield, English physician, 1858–1937; ME, *spotte,* stain], pinpoint white or light yellow spots on the iris of a child with Down syndrome. Occasionally, they are seen in normal infants.

Bruton's agammaglobulinemia [Ogden C. Bruton, American physician, b. 1908], a sex-linked, inherited condition characterized by the absence of gamma globulin in the blood. Those (usually children) affected by the syndrome are deficient in antibodies and susceptible to repeated infections. Compare **agammaglobulinemia.**

bruxism /bruk'sizəm/ [Gk, *brychein,* to gnash the teeth], the compulsive, unconscious grinding or clenching of the teeth, especially during sleep or as a mechanism for releasing tension during periods of extreme stress in the waking hours. Also called **bruxomania.**

bruxomania. See **bruxism.**

bry-, prefix meaning "tree moss": *bryocyte, bryocytole.*

Bryant's traction [Thomas Bryant, English physician, 1828–1914; L, *trahere,* to pull], an orthopedic mechanism used to immobilize both lower extremities in the treatment of a fractured femur or in the correction of a congenital hip dislocation. The mechanism consists of a traction frame supporting weights, which are connected by ropes that run through pulleys to traction foot plates. The traction pull elevates the lower extremities to a vertical position with the patient supine, the trunk and the lower extremities forming a right angle. The weight applied to the traction mechanism is usually less than 35 pounds. Compare **Buck's traction.**

Bryant's traction *(Lewis, Heitkemper, and Dirksen, 2000)*

BSA, 1. abbreviation for **body surface area.** See **surface area.** 2. abbreviation for *bovine serum albumin.*

BSE, 1. abbreviation for **breast self-examination.** See **self-breast examination.** 2. Abbreviation for **bovine spongiform encephalopathy.**

BSN, abbreviation for **Bachelor of Science in Nursing.**

BSP, abbreviation for **Bromsulphalein.**

BT, abbreviation for **bleeding time.**

BTPD, abbreviation for *body temperature, ambient pressure, dry.*

BTPS, abbreviation for *body temperature, ambient pressure, saturated* (with water vapor). See also **volume BTPS.**

BTU, abbreviation for **British thermal unit.**

buba. See **yaws.**

bubble-diffusion humidifier, a device that provides humidified oxygen or other therapeutic gases by allowing the gas to bubble through a reservoir of water.

Bubble diffusion humidifiers *(Courtesy Allied Health Care)*

bubble goniometer, a device used for measuring joint angles, consisting of a spirit level and a pendulum.

bubble oxygenator, a heart-lung device that oxygenates the blood while it is diverted outside the patient's body.

bubo /byoo´bo/, *pl.* **buboes** [Gk, *boubon,* groin], a greatly enlarged, tender, inflamed lymph node usually in the groin that is associated with diseases such as chancroid, lymphogranuloma venereum, and syphilis. Treatment includes specific antibiotic therapy, application of moist heat, and sometimes incision and drainage.

bubonic plague /byoobon´ik/ [Gk, *boubon,* groin; L, *plaga,* stroke], the most common form of plague. It is characterized by painful buboes in the axilla, groin, or neck; fever often rising to 106° F (41.11° C); prostration with a rapid, thready pulse; hypotension; delirium; and bleeding into the skin from the superficial blood vessels. The symptoms are caused by an endotoxin released by a bacillus, *Yersinia pestis,* usually introduced into the body by the bite of a rat flea that has bitten an infected rat. Inoculation with plague vaccine confers partial immunity; infection provides lifetime immunity. Treatment includes antibiotics, supportive nursing care, surgical drainage of buboes, isolation, and stringent precautions against spread of the disease. Conditions favor a plague epidemic when a large infected rodent population lives with a large nonimmune human population in a damp, warm climate. Improved sanitary conditions and eradication of rats and other rodent reservoirs of *Y. pestis* may prevent outbreaks of the disease. Killing the infected rodents, which may include ground squirrels and rabbits, and not the fleas

allows a continued threat of human infection. Also called *(informal)* **black death, black plague.** Compare **pneumonic plague, septicemic plague.** See also **bubo, plague,** *Yersinia pestis.*

bucardia /bookär´de-ə/, extreme enlargement of the heart.

bucca-. See **bucco-.**

buccal /buk´əl/, *pl.* **bucca** [L, *bucca,* cheek], pertaining to the inside of the cheek, the surface of a tooth, or the gum beside the cheek.

buccal administration of medication, oral administration of a drug, usually in the form of a tablet, by placing it between the cheek and the teeth or gum until it dissolves.

buccal bar, a portion of an orthodontic appliance consisting of a rigid metal wire that extends anteriorly from the buccal side of a molar band. See also **arch bar, labial bar, lingual bar.**

buccal cavity, the vestibule of the mouth, specifically the area lying between the teeth and cheeks.

buccal contour [L, *bucca + cum,* together with, *tornare,* to turn], the shape of the buccal side of a posterior tooth. It is usually characterized by a slight occlusocervical convexity that has its largest prominence at the gingival third of the clinical buccal surface.

buccal fat pad, a fat pad in the cheek under the subcutaneous layer of the skin, over the buccinator. It is particularly prominent in infants and is often called a sucking pad.

buccal flange [L, *bucca + OFr, flanche,* flank], the portion of a denture base that occupies the cheek side of the mouth and extends distally from the buccal notch. Compare **labial flange, lingual flange.** See also **flange.**

buccal frenum, a fold of mucous membrane connecting the alveolar ridge to the cheek and separating the labial vestibule from the buccal vestibule.

buccal glands [L, *bucca,* cheek, *glans,* acorn], small salivary glands located between the buccinator muscle and the mucous membrane in the vestibule of the mouth.

buccal mucosa, the mucous membrane lining the inside of the mouth.

buccal notch, a depression in a denture flange that accommodates the buccal frenum. See also **labial notch.**

buccal smear, a sample of cells removed from the buccal mucosa for purposes of obtaining a karyotype to determine the genetic sex of an individual.

buccal splint, material, usually plaster, that is placed on the buccal surfaces of fixed partial denture units to hold the units in position for assembly.

buccal vestibule, that portion of the vestibule of the mouth that lies between the cheeks and the teeth and gingivae or residual alveolar ridges.

bucci-. See **bucco-.**

buccinator /buk´sinā´tər/ [L, *buccina,* trumpet], the main muscle of the cheek, one of the 12 muscles of the mouth. It is pierced by the duct of the parotid gland opposite the second molar tooth. The buccinator, innervated by buccal branches of the facial nerve, compresses the cheek, acting as an important accessory muscle of mastication by holding food under the teeth.

bucco-, bucc-, bucca-, bucci-, combining form meaning "cheek": *buccodistal, buccal, buccinator.*

buccoclusion /buk´ə-kloo´zhən/ [L, *bucca,* cheek + *occludere,* to close up], malocclusion in which the dental arch or a quadrant or group of teeth is buccal to the normal.

buccogingival /buk´ōjinji´vəl/, pertaining to the internal mouth structures, particularly the cheeks and gums.

buccolinguomasticatory triad /buk´ōling´wōmas´təkə -tôr´e/ [L, *bucca,* cheek, *lingua,* tongue, *masticare,* to gnash

Parotid
duct (cut)

Buccinator muscle

Pterygomandibular raphe

Superior pharyngeal
constrictor muscle

Buccinator *(Drake, Vogl, and Mitchell, 2005)*

the teeth], a complex of involuntary lip, tongue, jaw, and head movements seen in tardive dyskinesia.

buccopharyngeal /buk′ōfərin′jē·əl/, pertaining to the cheek and the pharynx or to the mouth and the pharynx.

buccopharyngeal membrane. See **pharyngeal membrane.**

buccula /buk′yələ/ [L, *bucca,* cheek], a fold of fatty tissue, literally a "little cheek" beneath the chin. Also called **double chin.**

bucket handle fracture [OFr, *buket,* tub; ME, *handel,* part grasped; L, *fractura,* break], a fracture that produces a tear in a semilunar cartilage along the medial side of the knee joint.

bucking, *informal,* **1.** gagging on an endotracheal tube. **2.** involuntarily resisting positive pressure ventilation. Treatment for either is to sedate or extubate as appropriate.

buck knife, a periodontal surgical knife with a spear-shaped cutting point, used to make an interdental incision associated with a gingivectomy.

Buck's fascia [Gurdon Buck, American surgeon, 1807–1877], the deep fascia encasing the erectile tissue of the penis.

Buck's skin traction [Gurdon Buck], an orthopedic procedure that applies traction to the lower extremity with the

hips and the knees extended. It is used in the treatment of hip and knee contractures, in postoperative positioning and immobilization, and in disease processes of the hip and the knee. This type of traction may be unilateral, involving one leg, or bilateral, involving both legs.

Buck's traction [Gurdon Buck; L, *trahere,* to pull], one of the most common orthopedic mechanisms by which pull is exerted on the lower extremity with a system of ropes, weights, and pulleys. Buck's traction, which may be unilateral or bilateral, is used to immobilize, position, and align the lower extremity in the treatment of contractures and diseases of the hip and knee. The mechanism commonly consists of a metal bar extending from a frame at the foot of the patient's bed, supporting traction weights connected by a rope passing through a pulley to a cast or a splint around the affected body structure. Compare **Bryant's traction.**

Buck's traction *(Lewis, Heitkemper, and Dirksen, 2004)*

buckwheat allergy, an allergic reaction to buckwheat *Fagopyrum esculentum,* characterized primarily by photosensitivity. It is seen in susceptible humans who eat the grain and ruminants that eat excessive numbers of buckwheat plants. Also called *fagopyrism.*

Bucky diaphragm [Gustav P. Bucky, American radiologist, 1880–1963; Gk, *diaphragma,* partition], a moving grid that limits the amount of scattered radiation reaching a radiographic film, thereby increasing the film contrast. Also called **Bucky grid.**

buclizine hydrochloride /boo′kləzēn/, an antiemetic/antivertigo drug derived from piperazine that has anticholinergic and antihistaminic properties. It is used to treat nausea, vomiting, and dizziness of motion sickness.

bud [ME, *budde*], any small outgrowth that is the beginning stage of a living structure, as a limb bud from which an arm or leg develops.

Budd-Chiari syndrome /bud′kē·är′ē/ [George Budd, English physician, 1808–1882; Hans Chiari, Czech-French pathologist, 1851–1916], a disorder of hepatic circulation, marked by venous obstruction, that leads to liver enlargement, ascites, extensive development of collateral vessels, and severe portal hypertension. Also called **Chiari's syndrome, Rokitansky's disease.**

budding [ME, *budde*], a type of asexual reproduction in which an organism produces a budlike projection containing chromatin that eventually detaches and develops into an independent organism. It is common in simple organisms, such as sponges, yeasts, and molds.

buddy splint, a splinting technique commonly used after a finger or toe injury requiring immobilization. The injured and an adjacent digit are typically taped together to limit the

Budd-Chiari syndrome *(Kumar, Cotran, and Robbins, 2003)*

Buffalo hump *(Zitelli and Davis, 1997)*

Budding *(Baron, Peterson, and Finegold, 1994)*

range of motion of the affected digit. Also called **buddy tape.**

buddy tape.   See **buddy splint.**

budesonide,   a nasal corticosteroid antiinflammatory agent. It is available under the brand name Pulmicort as a turboinhaler (used in the mouth) and for use in nebulizers.

■ INDICATIONS: It is prescribed in the management of symptoms of seasonal or perennial allergic rhinitis or perennial nonallergic rhinitis. Neublizer solutions are used for the treatment of asthma in children.

■ CONTRAINDICATIONS: The drug should not be given to patients who have an allergic reaction to the drug or to any of its components or to patients with an untreated infection of the mucous membranes.

■ ADVERSE EFFECTS: The side effects most often reported include nasal or throat irritation, stinging, burning, or dryness in the respiratory system, nosebleeds, sneezing, and congestion.

Buerger's disease.   See **thromboangiitis obliterans.**

Buerger's postural exercises [Leo Buerger, American physician, 1879–1943; L, *ponere,* to place, *exercere,* to continue working],   exercises designed to maintain circulation in a limb.

buffalo hump,   an accumulation of fat on the back of the neck associated with the prolonged use of large doses of glucocorticoids or the hypersecretion of cortisol caused by Cushing's syndrome.

buffer [ME, *buffe,* to cushion],   a substance or group of substances that tends to control the hydrogen ion concentration in a solution by reacting with hydrogen ions of an acid added to the system and releasing hydrogen ions to a base added to the system. Buffers minimize significant changes of

pH in a chemical system. Among the functions carried out by buffer systems in the body is maintenance of the acid-base balance of the blood and of the proper pH in kidney tubules. See also **blood buffers, pH.**

buffer anions,   the negatively charged bicarbonate, protein, and phosphate ions that comprise the buffer systems of the body.

buffer cations,   the positively charged ions associated with the buffering anions of the body's electrolytes, including sodium, potassium, and magnesium.

buffered insulin human,   human insulin buffered with phosphate. It is used particularly in continuous infusion pumps, but also administered subcutaneously, intramuscularly, or intravenously.

buffer solution [ME, *buffet* + L, *solutus,* dissolved],   a solution that will minimize changes in pH value despite dilution or addition of a small amount of base or acid.

buffy coat [ME, *buffet* + Fr, *cote*],   a grayish white layer of white blood cells and platelets, mixed with some red blood cells, that accumulates on the surface of sedimented erythrocytes when blood plasma is allowed to stand.

buffy coat transfusion,   light stratum of a blood clot seen when the blood is centrifuged or allowed to stand in a test tube. See also **granulocyte transfusion.**

bug,   an error in a computer program (software bug) or a design flaw in computer hardware (hardware bug), usually resulting in an inability to process data correctly.

bulb [L, *bulbus,* swollen root],   any rounded structure, such as the eyeball, hair roots, and certain sensory nerve endings.

bulbar /bul'bər/ [L, *bulbus*],   **1.** pertaining to a bulb. **2.** pertaining to the medulla oblongata of the brain and the cranial nerves.

bulbar ataxia [L, *bulbus,* swollen root; Gk, *ataxia,* without order],   a loss of motor coordination caused by a lesion in the medulla oblongata or pons.

bulbar conjunctiva.   See **conjunctiva.**

bulbar myelitis [L, *bulbus,* swollen root; Gk, *myelos,* marrow, *itis,* inflammation],   an inflammation of the central nervous system involving the medulla oblongata.

bulbar palsy [L, *bulbus,* swollen root; Gk, *paralyein,* to be palsied],   a form of paralysis resulting from a defect in the motor centers of the medulla oblongata. See also **bulbar poliomyelitis.**

bulbar paralysis, a degenerative neurologic condition characterized by progressive paralysis of cranial nerves and involving the lips, tongue, mouth, pharynx, and larynx. The condition occurs most commonly in people above 50 years of age, in multiple sclerosis, and in amyotrophic lateral sclerosis.

bulbar poliomyelitis [L, *bulbus,* swollen root; Gk, *polios,* gray, *myelos,* marrow, *itis,* inflammation], a form of poliomyelitis that involves the medulla oblongata and gradually progresses to bulbar paralysis, with respiratory and circulatory failure.

bulbiform /bul′bifôrm/, shaped like a bulb.

bulbocavernosus /bul′bōkav′ərnō′səs/ [L, *bulbus,* swollen root, *cavernosum,* full of hollows], a muscle that covers the bulb of the penis in the male and the bulbus vestibuli in the female. Also called **accelerator urinae, ejaculator urinae,** (*in females*) sphincter vaginae.

bulbocavernosus reflex, bulbospongiosus reflex, the contraction of the bulbospongiosus muscle when the dorsum of the penis is tapped or the glans penis is compressed. Also called *penile reflex.*

bulbourethral gland /-yōōrē′thrəl/, one of two small glands located on each side of the prostate, draining to the wall of the urethra. Bulbourethral glands secrete a fluid component of the seminal fluid. Also called **Cowper's gland.**

bulbous [L, *bulbus,* swollen root], pertaining to a structure that resembles a bulb or that originates in a bulb.

bulb syringe, a device with a flexible bulb that replaces the plunger for instillation or aspiration. Bulb syringes can be used to irrigate an external orifice, such as the auditory canal. See also **syringe.**

bulbus oculi. See **eye.**

-bulia, -boulia, suffix meaning "(condition of the) will": *abulia, hyperbulia.*

bulimia /bōōlim′ē·ə/ [Gk, *bous,* ox, *limos,* hunger], a disorder characterized by an insatiable craving for food, often resulting in episodes of continuous eating and often followed by purging, depression, and self-deprivation. Also spelled **boulimia.** Also called **binge eating.** See also **anorexia nervosa.**

bulimic /bōōlim′ik/, pertaining to bulimia.

bulk. See **dietary fiber.**

bulk cathartic [ME, *bulke,* heap; Gk, *kathartikos,* evacuation of bowels], a cathartic (laxative) that acts by softening and increasing the mass of fecal material in the bowel. Bulk cathartics contain a hydrophilic agent such as methylcellulose or psyllium seed.

bulla /bōōl′ə, bul′ə/, *pl.* **bullae** [L, bubble], a thin-walled blister of the skin or mucous membranes greater than 1 cm in diameter containing clear, serous fluid. Compare **vesicle.** **—bullous,** *adj.*

bulldog forceps, short spring forceps for clamping an artery or vein for hemostasis. The jaws may be padded to prevent injury to vascular tissue.

bullet forceps, a kind of forceps that has thin, curved, serrated blades that are designed for extracting a foreign object, such as a bullet, from the base of a puncture wound.

bullous. See **bulla.**

bullous disease /bōōl′əs/, any disease marked by eruptions of blisters, or bullae, filled with fluid, on the skin or mucous membranes. An example is pemphigus.

bullous emphysema, single or multiple large cystic alveolar dilations of lung tissue. Also called **cystic emphysema.**

Bulla *(du Vivier, 1993)*

Bulldog forceps *(Brooks-Tighe, 1989)*

bullous impetigo, a form of impetigo in which the skin lesions are bullae instead of vesicles. The crusts are thin and greenish yellow. Infection is treated with oral anti-staphylococcal antibiotics.

bullous myringitis [L, *bulla* + *myringa,* eardrum], an inflammatory condition of the ear, characterized by fluid-filled vesicles on the tympanic membrane and the sudden onset of severe pain in the ear. The condition often occurs with bacterial otitis media. Treatment includes administration of antibiotics and analgesics and surgical draining of the vesicles. See also **otitis media.**

bullous pemphigoid [L, *bulla,* bubble; Gk, *pemphix,* bubble, *eidos,* form], a rare, relatively benign subepidermal autoimmune blistering disease of the elderly. It is of unknown origin.

bullseye rash. See **erythema migrans.**

bumetanide /bōōmet′ənīd/, a loop (high ceiling) diuretic related to furosemide.

■ INDICATIONS: It is prescribed for edema caused by cardiac, hepatic, or renal disease.

■ CONTRAINDICATIONS: Anuria, electrolyte depletion, or known sensitivity to this drug prohibits its use.

■ ADVERSE EFFECTS: Among the most serious adverse reactions are hypokalemia, hyperuricemia, and azotemia.

Bumex, trademark for a diuretic (bumetanide).

Buminate, trademark for a blood volume expander (human albumin).

Bullous myringitis (Swartz, 2002)

Bullous pemphigoid (Callen et al, 2000)

BUN, abbreviation for **blood urea nitrogen.**

-bund, suffix meaning "prone to" something specified: *moribund.*

bundle, a group of nerve fibers or other threadlike structures running in the same direction. See also **fasciculus.**

bundle branch [Dan, *bondel* + Fr, *branche*], a segment of the network of specialized conducting fibers that transmit electrical impulses within the ventricles of the heart. Bundle branches are a continuation of the atrioventricular (AV) bundle, which extends from the upper part of the intraventricular septum. The AV bundle divides into a left and a right branch, each going to its respective ventricle by passing down the septum and beneath the endocardium. Within the ventricles the bundle branches subdivide and terminate in the Purkinje fibers.

bundle branch block (BBB), an inability of cardiac impulses to be conducted down the bundle branches, causing a broaded and abnormally shaped QRS complex. BBB is commonly seen in high-risk, acute, anterior wall myocardial infarction. It may be caused by ischemia or necrosis of the bundle branches, trauma (as in surgical manipulation), or mechanical compression of the branches by a tumor. A pacemaker may be inserted if further deterioration of conduction is anticipated. See also **left bundle branch block, right bundle branch block.**

bundle of His. See **atrioventricular (AV) bundle.**

bunion /bun′yən/ [Gk, *bounion,* turnip], an abnormal, medial enlargement of the joint at the base of the great toe. It is caused by inflammation of the bursa, usually as a result of heredity, degenerative joint disease, or chronic irritation and pressure from poorly fitted shoes. It is characterized by soreness, swelling, thickening of the skin, and lateral displacement of the great toe.

Bunion (du Vivier, 1993)

bunionectomy /bun′yənek′təmē/, excision of a bunion.

bunionette /bun′yənet′/, an abnormal enlargement and inflammation of the joint at the base of the small toe. Also called **tailor's bunion.**

Bunnell block, trademark for a small wooden block used in exercise of the fingers after surgery. The exercises with the block allow each joint to be exercised individually with full tendon excursion while the other joints are held extended.

Bunsen burner /bŏŏn′sən, bun′sən/ [Robert E.W. Bunsen, German chemist, 1811–1899], a standard laboratory gas burner designed to produce nearly complete combustion in a smokeless flame.

Bunyamwera virus infection /bun′yəmwir′ə/ [Bunyamwera, town in Uganda where the type species was isolated], one of a group of arthropod-borne viruses that infect humans and are carried by mosquitoes from rodent hosts. Related viruses cause California encephalitis, Rift Valley fever, and other diseases characterized by headache, weakness, low-grade fever, myalgia, and a rash. Convalescence is prolonged. Outbreaks have occurred in North America, South America, Africa, and Europe.

buoyant density, the thickness or compactness of a substance that allows it to float in a standard fluid.

buphthalmos. See **congenital glaucoma.**

bupivacaine hydrochloride /byŏŏpiv′əkān/, a local anesthetic.

■ INDICATIONS: It is prescribed for caudal, epidural, peripheral, or sympathetic anesthetic block.

■ CONTRAINDICATIONS: Known hypersensitivity to this drug or to any of the amide class of local anesthetics prohibits its use.

■ ADVERSE EFFECTS: Among the more serious adverse reactions are central nervous system disturbances, cardiovascular depression, respiratory arrest, cardiac arrest, and hypersensitivity reactions.

Buprenex, trademark for a parenteral analgesic (buprenorphine hydrochloride).

buprenorphine /bu′prĕ-nor′fēn/, a synthetic opioid agonist-antagonist derived from thebaine, used in the form of the hydrochloride salt as an analgesic for moderate to severe pain and as an anesthesia adjunct. Administered sublingually or by intramuscular or IV injection.

■ INDICATIONS: It is administered parenterally for the relief of moderate to severe pain and is used in tablet form to treat opiod dependence.

■ CONTRAINDICATIONS: This Schedule V controlled substance is contraindicated for patients who may be opioid dependent.

■ ADVERSE EFFECTS: Among the reported adverse effects are respiratory depression, sedation, nausea, dizziness, vertigo, headache, vomiting, miosis, diaphoresis, and hypotension.

buPROPion /bo͞oprō′pē-on/, a heterocyclic mood-elevating drug used to treat some types of depression (trademark: Wellbutrin) and also to promote smoking cessation (trademark: Zyban).

bur. see **burr.**

Burch procedure /berch/, a type of bladder neck suspension for stress incontinence, consisting of fixation of the lateral vaginal fornices to the iliopectineal ligaments.

burden, 1. load. **2.** a heavy, oppressive load, as a disabling clinical load.

burdock root, a perennial herb found in the United States, China, and Europe.

■ USES: This herb is used for skin diseases, inflammation, rashes, colds and fever, cancer, gout, and arthritis; insufficient data to know if it is effective.

■ CONTRAINDICATIONS: Burdock is probably safe except in those who are hypersensitive to this plant. Burdock also should be used cautiously in people with diabetes or cardiac disorders.

Bureau of Medical Devices (BMD), an agency of the U.S. Food and Drug Administration organized in 1976 with the responsibility of providing standards for and regulation of the manufacture and uses of medical devices.

buret /byo͞oret′/ [Fr, small jug], a laboratory utensil used to deliver a wide range of volumes accurately. Also spelled **burette.**

burette /bu-ret′/, buret.

buried penis, concealed penis.

buried suture [L, *sutura*], a suture that is inserted to draw together soft tissues between the viscus and the skin.

Burkholderia /bərk′holdĕr′ēə/, a genus of gram-negative, rod-shaped bacteria that includes several species formerly classified in the genus *Pseudomonas,* including the agents of glanders and melioidosis.

Burkholderia cepacia, formerly *Pseudomonas cepacia.* A group of bacteria that are often resistant to common antibiotics. Immunocompromised persons or those with chronic lung disease, especially cystic fibrosis, are susceptible to infection. In patients without cystic fibrosis, *B. cepacia* infections are almost all nosocomial or related to intravenous drug abuse. Outbreaks have been related to intra aortic balloon pumps, contaminated water sources, respiratory therapy equipment such as reusable electronic ventilator probes or contaminated disinfectants. A variety of approaches including strict segregation of cystic fibrosis patients based on the presence of this organism have been tried in order to reduce nosocomial transmission. Even a single significant nosocomial infection with *B. cepacia* may warrant investigation.

Burkholderia mallei, a nonmotile species that causes glanders. It is pathogenic chiefly for horses, but may also infect humans and other animals. Potential agent for bioterrorism.

Burkholderia pickettii, formerly *Pseudomonas pickettii. B. pickettii* has been responsible for epidemics of blood-stream infections associated with contaminated distilled or sterile water.

Burkholderia pseudomallei, a species that inhabits water and soil and causes melioidosis. Infection is spread via contact with a contaminated source and is a predominant disease of tropical climates. Also called Whitemore's disease.

Burkitt's lymphoma /bur′kits/ [Denis P. Burkitt, English surgeon in Africa, b. 1911], a malignant neoplasm composed of undifferentiated lymphoreticular cells that form a large osteolytic lesion in the jaw or, in children, an abdominal mass. The tumor, which is seen chiefly in Central Africa, is characteristically a gray-white mass sometimes containing areas of hemorrhage and necrosis. Central nervous system involvement often occurs, and other organs may be affected. The Epstein-Barr virus (EBV), a herpesvirus, is associated with this lymphoma. Chemotherapy can often cure the disease. Also called **African lymphoma, Burkitt's tumor.**

Burkitt's lymphoma *(Kumar, Abbas, and Fausto, 2005)*

burn [AS, *baernan*], any injury to tissues of the body caused by hot objects or flames, electricity, chemicals, radiation, or gases in which the extent of the injury is determined by the nature of the agent, length of time exposed, body part involved, and depth of burn. The treatment of burns includes pain relief, careful asepsis, prevention of infection, regulation of body temperature, maintenance of the balance in the body of fluids and electrolytes, and good nutrition. First priority with burns of the airway is airway control. Severe burns of any origin may cause shock, which is treated before the wound. Burns are sometimes classified as first, second, third, and fourth degree. First-degree burns involve only a superficial layer of epidermal cells. Second-degree burns may be divided into superficial partial-thickness and deep partial-thickness wounds. Damage in second-degree burns extends through the epidermis to the dermis, but is usually not sufficient to prevent skin regeneration. In third-degree burns the entire thickness of the epidermis and dermis is destroyed. Fourth-degree burns are full-thickness injuries that penetrate the subcutaneous tissue, muscle, and periosteum or bone. See also **chemical burn, electrocution, thermal burn.**

burn center, a health care facility that is designed to care for patients who have been severely burned. A number of burn centers has been established throughout the United States and Canada to provide sophisticated advanced techniques of care for burn victims.

burner syndrome, a condition of burning pain, especially in the upper extremities, and sometimes accompanied by shoulder girdle weakness. It may be experienced during con-

First-degree burn *(Sanders et al, 2000)*

Superficial partial-thickness second-degree burn

First-degree burn: damaged epidermis and edema

Deep partial-thickness second-degree burn
(Sanders et al, 2000/courtesy St. John's Mercy Medical Center)

Superficial partial-thickness second-degree burn
(Sanders et al, 2000/courtesy St. John's Mercy Medical Center)

Deep partial-thickness second-degree burn

Third-degree burn
(Sanders et al, 2000/courtesy St. John's Mercy Medical Center)

Third-degree burn

tact sports, such as football, as a result of a blow to the head or shoulder. It is attributed to an upper trunk neuropathy of the brachial plexus.

Burnett's syndrome. See **milk-alkali syndrome.**

burning drops sign, a sensation of hot liquid dripping into the abdominal cavity caused by a perforated stomach ulcer.

burning feet syndrome, a neurologic disorder characterized by symptoms of a burning sensation in the sole of the foot. The burning tends to be more intense at night and may also involve the hands. Possible causes include causalgia from injury to the sciatic nerve, degeneration of the spinal cord, and acute polyneuropathy. The condition is also associated with diabetes mellitus, kidney disease, and a B vitamin deficiency. Also known as **Gopalan's syndrome.**

burning mouth syndrome, a burning sensation in the mouth that is often associated with menopause.

burning pain [AS, *baernan,* to burn; L, *poena,* penalty], the pain experienced as a result of a thermal burn. The term is also used sometimes to describe heartburn or myocardial pain.

burnisher /bur'nishər/ [ME, *burnischen,* to make brown], a dental instrument with one end shaped as a beveled nib, used to smooth rough edges of restorations.

burnishing /bur'nish·ing/ [ME, *burnischen,* to make brown], **1.** (in dentistry) condensation and polishing under the sliding pressure of a smooth hard instrument, as in finishing the surface of a gold filling. **2.** (in dentistry) smoothing out the margins of a thin, annealed sheet metal to form a band about a tooth root or fit a matrix for porcelain.

burnout, a popular term for a mental or physical energy depletion after a period of chronic, unrelieved job-related stress characterized sometimes by physical illness. The person suffering from burnout may lose concern or respect for other people and often has cynical, dehumanized perceptions of people, labeling them in a derogatory manner. Causes of burnout peculiar to the nursing profession often include stressful, even dangerous, work environments; lack of support; lack of respectful relationships within the health care team; low pay scales compared with physicians' salaries; shift changes and long work hours; understaffing of hospitals; pressure from the responsibility of providing continuous high levels of care over long periods; and frustration and disillusionment resulting from the difference between job realities and job expectations.

burn therapy, the management of a patient burned by flames, hot liquids, explosives, chemicals, or electric current. Partial thickness burns may be first degree, involving only the epidermis, or second degree, involving the epidermis and dermis, whereas full thickness or third-degree burns involve all skin layers. Second-degree burns covering more than 30% of the body and third-degree burns on the face and extremities, or more than 10% of the body surface, are critical. In the first 48 hours of a severe burn, vascular fluid, sodium chloride, and protein rapidly pass into the affected area, causing local edema, blister formation, hypovolemia, hypoproteinemia, hyponatremia, hyperkalemia, hypotension, and oliguria. The initial hypovolemic stage is followed by a shift of fluid in the opposite direction, resulting in diuresis, increased blood volume, and decreased serum electrolyte level. Potential complications in serious burns include circulatory collapse, renal damage, gastric atony, paralytic ileus, infections, septic shock, pneumonia, and stress ulcer (Curling's ulcer), characterized by hematemesis and peritonitis.

■ METHOD: The extent of the burn, its cause, its time of occurrence, and the patient's age, weight, allergies, and any preexisting illness are recorded. If respiratory distress is present, endotracheal intubation or tracheostomy may be performed. Specimens are obtained for urinalysis, blood type, blood urea nitrogen level, hematocrit, prothrombin time, electrolyte levels, blood gases, and cultures of nasal, throat, wound, and stool organisms. Parenteral fluids and electrolytes, antibiotics, tetanus prophylaxis, and pain medication are administered as ordered; large doses of analgesics and sedatives are avoided when possible to prevent depression of respiration and masking of symptoms. An indwelling urinary catheter is inserted, and a nasogastric tube and catheter for monitoring central venous pressure may be indicated. Local treatment of the burn may use the closed method or the more frequently used open method, in which the injured area is cleaned and exposed to air and the patient is kept warm by a blanket or linen over a bed cradle or by a heater or lamp. In the closed method, a germicidal or bacteriostatic cream, ointment, or solution is applied to the burn, and the wound is covered with a dressing. A porcine heterograft may be used to cover the wound temporarily; this technique prevents fluid loss and reduces the risk of infection, but the graft dries in 1 or 2 days and may pull and cause pain. Newly developed artificial skin holds great promise for treating severe burns.

During the acute stage of a burn, the patient's blood pressure, pulse, respiration, and cerebrovascular pressure are checked every 30 to 60 minutes, and the rectal temperature every 2 to 4 hours. Oral hygiene and assistance in turning, coughing, and deep breathing are provided every 2 hours, and the patient's sensorium is evaluated hourly. If oral fluids are ordered, juices and carbonated drinks are offered, but plain water and ice chips are avoided. Fluid intake and output are measured hourly; if a child excretes less than 1 mL/kg of urine or an adult less than 0.5 mL/kg, a diuretic or an increase in IV infusion of fluid may be necessary. Blood transfusions, steroid therapy, and antipyretics may be ordered; aspirin is contraindicated. Excessive chilling and exposure to upper respiratory and wound infections are carefully prevented. Burned extremities are elevated, and contractures are prevented by using firm supports to keep affected areas properly aligned. The patient is weighed daily at the same time on the same scale, and, after the initial acute period, an adequate intake of a high-calorie, high-protein diet is encouraged; to stimulate appetite, the patient is offered frequent small meals of preferred foods and beverages that are high in potassium. Vitamins may be required. Tranquilizers may be given before wound care, but narcotics for pain usually are not needed after the acute phase. The patient is encouraged to stand for a few minutes every hour or every second hour and is generally able to walk in 7 to 10 days, but convalescence may be prolonged. Burn patients often are frightened, withdrawn, and disoriented initially, but after a few days they may become angry, depressed, or rebellious and need emotional support to help them cooperate with their treatment and rehabilitation. Extensive plastic surgery and repeated skin grafts may be required to restore function and the physical appearance of burn patients.
■ INTERVENTIONS: The burn patient requires intensive, prolonged care to prevent complications and disfiguring contractures. The nurse administers parenteral fluids and medication, implements wound care, closely monitors the patient's condition, limits physical discomfort, provides emotional support and diversion, and encourages the family to visit regularly and become involved in the patient's care.
■ OUTCOME CRITERIA: The outcome for the severely burned patient depends greatly on the detailed, near-constant care required during the acute phase of treatment. Scarring may cause residual dysfunction and discouragement. Encouragement to participate fully in physical therapy and to continue treatments may be helpful. Although protection from infection is essential, the nurse does not isolate the patient unless necessary.

Burow's solution /byŏŏr′ōz/ [Karl A. Burow, German physician, 1809–1874], a liquid preparation containing aluminum sulfate, acetic acid, precipitated calcium carbonate, and water, used as a topical astringent, antiseptic, and antipyretic for a wide variety of skin disorders. Also called **aluminum acetate solution.**

burp, *informal,* **1.** to belch, or eructate; to expel gas from the stomach through the mouth. **2.** a belch, or eructation.

burr, a rotary instrument fitted into a handpiece and used to cut teeth or bone. Also spelled **bur.**

burr cell [ME, *burre* + L, *cella,* storeroom], a form of mature erythrocyte in which the cells or cell fragments have spicules, or tiny projections, on the surface.

burr holes, holes drilled in the skull to drain and irrigate an abscess.

burrowing flea. See **chigoe.**

bursa /bur′sə/, *pl.* **bursae** [Gk, *byrsa,* wineskin], **1.** a fibrous sac between certain tendons and the bones beneath

Burr cell *(Carr and Rodak, 1999)*

Burr hole used to drain subdural hematoma
(Beare and Myers, 1998)

them. Lined with a synovial membrane that secretes synovial fluid, the bursa acts as a small cushion that allows the tendon to move over the bone as it contracts and relaxes. See also **adventitious bursa, bursa of Achilles, olecranon bursa, prepatellar bursa. 2.** a sac or closed cavity. See also **omental bursa, pharyngeal bursa.**

bursa-equivalent tissue, bursal equivalent tissue, a hypothesized lymphoid tissue in nonavian vertebrates, including human beings, equivalent to the bursa of Fabricius in birds: the site of B lymphocyte maturation. It now appears that B lymphocyte maturation occurs primarily in the bone marrow.

bursal abscess /bur′səl/, a collection of pus in the cavity of a bursa.

bursa of Achilles, bursa separating the tendon of Achilles and the calcaneus.

bursectomy /bərsek′təmē/ [Gk, *byrsa,* wineskin, *ektomē,* cutting out], the excision of a bursa.

bursitis /bərsī′tis/, inflammation of the bursa, the connective tissue structure surrounding a joint. Bursitis may be precipitated by arthritis, infection, injury, or excessive or traumatic exercise or effort. The chief symptom is severe pain of the affected joint, particularly on movement. Treatment goals include the control of pain and the maintenance of joint motion. Acute pain is often treated with an intrabursal injection of an adrenocorticosteroid. Other common treatments are analgesics, antiinflammatory agents, cold, and immobilization of the inflamed site. After the inflammation has subsided, heat may be helpful. In chronic cases surgery may be required to remove calcium deposits. Kinds of bursitis include **housemaid's knee, miner's elbow,** and **weaver's bottom.** See also **rheumatism.**

Bursitis
(Mace and Kowalczyk, 2004/
courtesy Ohio State University Medical Center)

burst, to break suddenly while under tension or expansion.
burst fracture [ME, *bersten* + L, *fractura*, break], any fracture that disperses multiple bone fragments, usually at or near the end of a bone. It frequently occurs in a vertebra.
Burton's line [Henry Burton, English physician, 1799–1849], a dark blue stippled line along the gingival margin, which is a sign of lead poisoning. See also **blue line.**
Buruli ulcer /bōo′rə·le/ [Buruli, district in Uganda], a cutaneous infection caused by a species of *Mycobacterium*, manifested by a small, firm, painless, movable subcutaneous nodule that enlarges and ulcerates. It occurs principally in Central Africa, but has also been seen in other tropical areas.
bus, a set of parallel wires in a computer to which the central processing unit and all input-output units are connected. Each separate wire carries the electric current representing 1 bit. Buses interconnect the parts of the computer that communicate with each other, such as a video card or modem.
Buschke's disease. See **cryptococcosis.**
bushy chorion, the region of the chorion that bears villi.
BuSpar, trademark for an oral antianxiety drug (buspirone hydrochloride).
busPIRone hydrochloride /bōospir′ōn/, an antianxiety agent not related chemically to others. Administered orally as the hydrochloride salt. Unlike benzodiazepines, does cause sedation, has low abuse potential, takes several days to weeks to exert its effect, and does not intensify the effects of other CNS depressants.

■ INDICATIONS: It is prescribed for generalized anxiety disorders.
■ CONTRAINDICATIONS: This drug is contraindicated in patients with severe hepatic or renal impairment. Patients taking a benzodiazepine drug should be gradually withdrawn from that medication before starting therapy with buspirone.
■ ADVERSE EFFECTS: Among adverse reactions reported are dizziness, headache, lightheadedness, excitement, and nausea.
busulfan /bōosul′fən/, an alkylating agent.
■ INDICATION: It is prescribed in the treatment of chronic myelocytic leukemia.
■ CONTRAINDICATIONS: Radiation therapy, depressed neutrophil or platelet counts, concurrent administration of neoplastic medication, or known hypersensitivity to this drug prohibits its use.
■ ADVERSE REACTIONS: Among the more serious adverse reactions are alveolar hyperplasia (busulfan lung), depression of the bone marrow, and severe nausea and diarrhea. Amenorrhea commonly occurs.
butabarbital sodium /byōo′təbär′bitôl/, a sedative; intermediate-acting barbiturate.
■ INDICATIONS: It is prescribed for the relief of anxiety, nervous tension, and insomnia.
■ CONTRAINDICATIONS: Porphyria, seizure disorders, or known hypersensitivity to this drug prohibits its use.
■ ADVERSE EFFECTS: Among the more serious adverse reactions are jaundice, skin rash, and paradoxical excitement.
butamben picrate /byōotam′bən pik′rāt/, a topical local anesthetic for the temporary relief of pain from minor burns.
butanamide. See **acebutolol.**
butane (C_4H_{10}), a colorless petroleum-based gas. It is the fourth member of the paraffin series of hydrocarbons.
butanoic acid. See **butyric acid.**
butanol. See **butyl alcohol.**
Butazolidin, trademark for an antirheumatic (phenylbutazone).
butenafine /bu-ten′ah-fēn/, a topical antifungal agent used as the hydrochloride salt in the treatment of athlete's foot, jock itch, and ringworm.
Butisol Sodium, trademark for a sedative (butabarbital sodium).
Butler-Albright syndrome, a type of distal renal tubular acidosis occurring later than infancy and having autosomal-dominant inheritance.
butoconazole nitrate /byōo′təkō′nəzōl/, an intravaginal antifungal cream.
■ INDICATIONS: It is prescribed for the treatment of vulvovaginal fungal infections caused by *Candida* species.
■ CONTRAINDICATIONS: Its use is contraindicated during the first trimester of a pregnancy.
■ ADVERSE EFFECTS: Adverse reactions include vulvar and vaginal burning and itching.
butorphanol tartrate /byōotôr′fənôl/, an agonist/antagonist opioid of the phenanthrene family.
■ INDICATIONS: It is administered parentally for surgical premedication, as an analgesic component of balanced anesthesia, and for prompt relief of moderate to severe pain associated with surgical procedures, and as a nasal spray for the relief of migraine pain.
■ CONTRAINDICATIONS: Butorphanol tartrate is not given to patients known to be sensitive to phenanthrenes or to persons dependent on opioids because it may provoke withdrawal symptoms.
■ ADVERSE EFFECTS: Toxicity may result from the use of butorphanol with other opioids.

butt, 1. to place two surfaces together to form a joint. **2.** (in dentistry) to place directly against the tissues covering the residual alveolar ridge.

butter, a soft, solid substance, such as the oily mass produced by churning cream.

butterfly bandage [AS, *buttorfleoge*], a narrow adhesive strip with broader winglike ends used to approximate the edges of a superficial wound and to hold the edges together as they heal. It is used in place of a suture in certain cases. Also called **butterfly.**

butterfly fracture, a bone break in which the center fragment contained by two cracks forms a triangle.

butterfly needle, a short needle attached to plastic stabilizers at 90 degrees. It is used for IV access of small veins of adults and children. Usual gauge is 25 to 22 length.

Butterfly needle (Courtesy Medline Industries)

butterfly rash, an erythematous eruption of both cheeks joined by a narrow band of rash across the nose. It may be seen in lupus erythematosus, rosacea, and seborrheic dermatitis.

Butterfly rash (Habif, 2004)

buttermilk [Gk, *boutyron,* butter; AS, *meoluc*], **1.** the slightly sour tasting liquid remaining after the solids in cream have been churned into butter. It is nearly fat free and is nutritionally comparable to whole milk. **2.** cultured milk made by the addition of certain organisms to fat-free milk.

butter stools, a fatty fecal discharge from the bowels, as may occur in steatorrhea.

buttock, the fleshy hillocks at the lower posterior part of the torso comprising fat and the gluteal muscles. Also called **nates.**

buttock augmentation, a reconstructive procedure in cosmetic surgery for reshaping the buttocks.

button /but'ən/ [OFr, *boton*], **1.** a knoblike elevation or structure. **2.** a small appliance shaped like a spool or disk, used in surgery for construction of an intestinal anastomosis.

buttonhole [OFr, *boton* + AS, *hol*], a small slitlike hole in the wall of a structure or a cavity of the body.

buttonhole fracture, a fracture caused by a straight perforation of a bone, such as by a bullet.

buttonhole stenosis, an extreme narrowing of a vessel. The term usually refers to the mitral valve, in which the valve cusps are contracted to form an opening shaped like a buttonhole.

buttonhook, an adaptive device designed to help patients with limited finger range of motion, dexterity, or weakness fastening buttons on clothing.

button suture, a technique in suturing in which the ends of the suture material are passed through buttons on the surface of the skin and tied. It is used to prevent the suture from cutting through the skin.

buttressing, a phenomenon of osteoarthritis in which osteophytes at the hip joint extend across the femoral neck inferior to the femoral head and combine, with a proliferation along the medial aspect of the femoral neck.

buttress plate, a thin, flat metal plate used to provide support in the surgical repair of a fracture.

butyl /byoo'til/ [Gk, *boutyron,* butter, *hyle,* matter], a hydrocarbon radical (C_4H_9), most compounds of which are obtained from petroleum. Butyl compounds, some of which are toxic and irritating, are used in a variety of industrial and medical applications, including anesthesia.

butyl alcohol (C_4H_9OH), a clear, toxic liquid used as an organic solvent. It exists as four isomers, *n*-butyl, isobutyl, secondary butyl, and tertiary butyl alcohol. Also called **butanol.**

butyr-, combining form meaning "butter": *butyric, butyrinase.*

butyric acid (C_4H_7OOH) /byootir'ik/, a clear, colorless liquid with an odor of rancid butter or vomit that is miscible with water, alcohol, glycerin, and ether. Butyric acid is obtained commercially from 1-butanol by oxidation, and can be obtained from carbohydrates by butyric fermentation. It is used in the production of artificial flavors. Also called **butanoic acid** /byoo'tənō'ik/, **propylformic acid.**

butyric fermentation, the conversion of carbohydrates to butyric acid.

butyrophenone /byoo'tərōfē'nōn/, one of a small group of major tranquilizers. They are used in treating psychosis, to decrease the choreic symptoms of Huntington's disease and the tics and coprolalia of Gilles de la Tourette's syndrome, and are used as an adjunct in neuroleptanesthesia. Principal butyrophenones are haloperidol and droperidol. Butyrophenones are pharmacologically and clinically similar to phenothiazines.

Buzzard's maneuver [Thomas Buzzard, English neurologist, 1831–1919], a modified patellar reflex in which the patient's toes are firmly pressed on the floor while the quadriceps muscle is tapped.

BWS, abbreviation for **battered woman syndrome.**

Byler's disease, progressive familial intrahepatic cholestasis.

bypass [AS, *bi,* alongside; Fr, *passer*], **1.** any one of various surgical procedures to divert or shunt the flow of blood or other natural fluids from normal anatomic courses. A bypass may be temporary or permanent. Bypass surgery is commonly performed in the treatment of cardiac and GI disorders. **2.** a term used by some hospitals to signal that its emergency department lacks the personnel and equipment to handle additional patients, thereby advising that ambulances transporting new patients be diverted to other hospitals.

by-product material, the radioactive waste of nuclear reactors.

byssinosis /bis'inō'sis/ [Gk, *byssos,* flax, *osis,* condition], an occupational respiratory disease characterized by shortness of breath, cough, and wheezing. The condition is an allergic reaction to dust or fungi in cotton, flax, and hemp fibers. The symptoms are typically more pronounced on Mondays when workers return after a weekend break. They are reversible in the early stages, but prolonged exposure results in chronic airway obstruction, bronchitis, and emphysema with fibrosis, leading to respiratory failure, pulmonary hypertension, and cor pulmonale. Treatment is symptomatic for the irreversible changes of emphysema and chronic bronchitis. Compare **pneumoconiosis.** See also **organic dust.**

byte /bīt/, the amount of memory required to encode one character of information (letter, number, or symbol) in a computer system; it is normally 8 bits. See also **bit.**

Byzantine arch palate /biz'əntēn/, a congenital anomaly of the roof of the mouth marked by incomplete fusion of the palatal process and the nasal spine.